SYMPTOMS

The Complete Home Medical Encyclopedia

SYMPTOMS

The Complete Home Medical Encyclopedia

edited by

Sigmund Stephen Miller

M

First published 1979 simultaneously by
Macmillan London Limited
London and Basingstoke
(Associated companies in Delhi, Dublin,
Hong Kong, Johannesburg, Lagos, Melbourne,
New York, Singapore and Tokyo)
and Pan Books Limited

Filmset in Great Britain by
Northumberland Press Ltd, Gateshead, Tyne and Wear
Printed and bound in Great Britain by
William Clowes (Beccles) Limited, Beccles and London

ISBN 0 333 27104 1

Contents

Introduction

The uniqueness of *Symptoms: the complete home medical encyclopedia* is that it combines and interrelates a book of symptoms (*Part 1*) with an up-to-the-minute medical reference book of disease (*Part 2*).

The average person knows little about disease, but he does have a keen and intimate knowledge of symptoms. Outside of a few common disorders, he has no idea what he is suffering from. In *Symptoms: the complete home medical encyclopedia*, he will quickly know whether his symptoms are unimportant, potentially serious, or serious. In other medical encyclopedias he is obliged to look up his ailment first and then try to find his symptoms – a difficult and frustrating search.

In this book he has some of the best medical minds to help him; he can identify his symptoms, resolve them into a specific ailment, understand the nature of his disease, and decide the best form of procedure.

The saying that a little bit of knowledge can do more harm than good is in itself a statement that does more harm than good. More light is surely better than less light. Our present understanding of the human body is certainly small compared to the ultimate total revelation of how the human body works, yet even with that little bit of knowledge countless numbers of lives have been saved. This book makes expert knowledge easily available to the reader.

We all know that a show of blood in the urine is a dangerous sign, which may be indicative of cancer and/or nephritis. But access to this book and a quick glance under the symptom heading *Blood in the urine* will show that besides several forms of cancer and nephritis, blood in the urine is also a common symptom in such disorders as stones in the kidney or bladder, benign tumours in the kidney or bladder, prostate disorders, and vitamin K deficiency – not minor ailments true, but neither are they life-threatening. Such information is readily available in this book.

Another major objective of this book is to enlighten the reader about his own vast potential in fighting disease and maintaining ebullient good health. The aid of the physician, empowered by a great armamentarium of knowledge and constant new discoveries, is often lifesaving, but the patient's own efforts, armed with an equally great armamentarium of will, a thrust for life, and other profound inner resources, can often mean the difference between succumbing and survival.

Part 2 is a comprehensive reference book defining some five hundred ailments that afflict man. Most of these disorders are described in terms of cause (if known), incidence, type of contagion (if any), the dangers, symptoms (usually in greater detail than found in *Part 1*), treatment, prevention (when possible), and outlook.

Part 3 contains chapters on *Early warning signals*, *Tablets, tests, and guides*, and *A briefing for good health and long life*. A *Glossary of medical terms* follows, as well as an *Index of symptoms* and an *Index of diseases*.

Early warning signals discusses a considerable number of diseases that fortunately warn the patient very early, long before the full-blown disease arrives. Knowing these signals beforehand can often forestall the disease or minimize its consequence.

Tables, tests, and guides presents a variety of information to help the reader know the condition of his own body and how to correct some deficiencies.

A briefing for good health and long life describes the age in which we live, an age that is under great pressure and has lost most of its social and physical values. While most of the world is close to starvation, we are being overfed with sugar, baby food (milk), saturated fatty foods, salt, adulterants, and additives. We are recklessly over-medicated and shockingly under-exercised to the point of degenerative physical indolence. In addition, we are being overwhelmed with every kind of pollution.

How to survive and live out a full life in such a world needs vigilance and a willingness to pay the price.

In the twenty-one rules to achieve good health and long life, a guide through this dangerous planet, the emphasis is on prevention rather than cure, on the avoidance of poor health rather than the restoration of good health.

The *Glossary* contains words and phrases often used in the medical world. Although usually explained where originally used, they are also defined here.

Special note: this book is not male oriented, although all references are made to 'he' rather than 'she'. Diseases in general are impartial, striking males as well as females. All doctors and patients are indicated as 'he', since there is no precise pronoun in the English language that means a human being of either sex. In almost all cases where 'he' is used it also means 'she'. Where the diseases are specifically female, 'she' is used.

The book has been compiled and written by a distinguished panel of doctors and represents not only their expert thinking but also the latest available research and medical knowledge at the time of publication. Periodically this book will be updated.

Acknowledgements

The editorial board

8

How to use this book

The more than 600 symptoms included in this book cover practically the entire spectrum of disease in man. In *Part 1: Symptoms*, the various indications of illness are grouped according to the part of the body affected and alphabetized within each group. (The section *Symptoms affecting the whole body* lists those symptoms that cannot be associated with any specific part of the body, such as weakness or weight loss.) The diseases indicated by a particular symptom are listed below each symptoms category.

Each disease is identified by a reference number; to know more about a particular ailment, refer to *Part 2: Diseases*, and locate the disease by its reference number; the reference numbers are consecutive.

Every disease is reviewed, emphasizing all the pertinent facts. Such questions are answered as, Is it serious? Can this disorder be regarded with intelligent neglect or should a doctor be seen at once? Every vital question about the disease is revealed and keynoted. The advice given represents the best thinking of some of the best medical minds.

Preface

The purpose of this book is to describe signs and symptoms of the diseases of the body. It is not meant to act as a substitute for the services of a doctor, nor is it meant to encourage diagnosis and treatment of diseases by the layman. Proper diagnosis and treatment can only be performed by a qualified doctor.

However, preventive medicine and the early diagnosis and treatment of disease are two of the most important areas of modern medicine; they are moreover the areas in which the layman must work with his doctor for better health. By acquainting the reader of *Symptoms: the complete home medical encyclopedia* with both the early and later manifestations of disorders and disease, it is hoped that he will be better able to determine when to seek appropriate medical advice.

Abner J. Delman

Part 1
Symptoms of disease

TABLE OF SYMPTOMS

Symptoms

Symptoms

Muscle
Muscular atrophy 194
Cramps in the muscles 195
  Cramps, ache or spasm in the muscles and headache 196
Loss of muscle control 195
Pain in the muscles (see *Cramps in the muscles*)
Pulled or strained muscle 196
Soreness, spasm (see *Cramps in the muscles*)
Swollen muscle 196
Twitching, tremors of a muscle (see *Symptoms affecting the whole body*)
Weakness of a muscle 196

Shoulder
Dislocation of the shoulder 197
Frozen shoulder 197
Pain in the shoulder 197

Round shoulders 197
Weak shoulders 197

Spine
Disorders of the spine 197
Inability to straighten up 197

The toes
Bump on the toe joint 197
Pain in the toe 197

Walking
Abnormal fatigue or pain in walking 198
Abnormal walking speed (see *Symptoms affecting the whole body*)
Waddling gait 199

The wrist
Lump on the wrist 199
Pain in the wrist 199
Swollen wrist (see *Pain in the wrist*)

Symptoms affecting the whole body

Abnormal walking speed

Parkinson's disease 1: A running gait to avoid losing balance. The arms do not swing, hands trembling, face immobile, eyes unblinking, drooling.

Anaemia

Anaemia means lack of sufficient blood or a shortage of red blood cells, a deficiency due to faulty body function, disease, or the intake of certain drugs. Anaemia is a disease entity in itself, but is also symptomatic of a considerable number of ailments. The symptoms of anaemia include first of all pallor of the skin. (Some people are naturally pale so look for unusual paleness in the mucous membrane and in the fingernail beds.) Weakness and great fatigability are other symptoms. Quite often there is dizziness, breathlessness, palpitation, and drowsiness.

Anaemia, Anaemia with jaundice, Anaemia with skin disorders, Anaemia with weight loss, Anaemia with weight loss and swollen lymph nodes

Anaemia

Rheumatic heart disease and rheumatic fever 127: Including rapid heartbeat, inflammation of the joints, sweating, malaise, weight loss or failure to gain weight in the case of a growing child.

Atrial fibrillation 132: Anaemia plus irregular fluttering of the heart.

Hiatus hernia 149: Pain radiating out behind the breastbone simulating a heart attack. Insidious bleeding into the stools, causing anaemia, pallor. Also heartburn.

Chronic nephritis 198: Blood in urine, puffiness of the face, swelling of the ankles, breathlessness on slight exertion, late night urination, impaired vision from bleeding into the retina. (Rise in blood pressure.)

Nephrosis 199: Swelling of face, ankles, abdomen.

Dietary deficiencies in pregnancy 236: Particular symptoms are fatigue and breathlessness.

Anaemia 322: Considerable weakness, palpitation, tongue is flabby, pale, or sore, hair is lustreless. In some cases, jaundice, numbness of limbs, thirst, poor memory, spoon-shaped (concave) fingernails, and finally, shock.

Pernicious anaemia 323: All the anaemic symptoms, including palpitations, pins-and-needles sensation in hands and feet, general pain, sore, beefy, red tongue, weight loss, jaundice, difficulty walking, impotence and frigidity.

Haemolytic anaemia 324: All the anaemic symptoms (pallor, breathlessness, fatigue), jaundice, dizziness, fainting, weak, rapid pulse, rapid breathing, chills, fever, and aches in the extremities and in the abdomen.

All-vegetarian diet deficiency 355: Anaemic symptoms. Also palpitations, inflammation of the tongue, twitching, occasional numbness.

Hookworm 387: Extreme fatigue, very marked pallor, shortness of breath, weakness, great hunger, black stools, malnutrition, blister or pimple on sole of foot.

Anaemia with jaundice

Anaemia 322: Considerable weakness, palpitations, tongue is flabby, pale or sore, hair lustreless. In several cases jaundice, numbness of limbs, thirst, poor memory, spoon-shaped fingernails, and finally, shock.

Pernicious anaemia 323: All anaemic symptoms including palpitations, pins-and-needles sensation in hands and feet, general pain, red, sore tongue, weight loss, jaundice, difficulty walking, impotence and frigidity.

Haemolytic anaemia 324: Anaemic symptoms, jaundice, faintness, dizziness, rapid, weak pulse, chills and fever, aches in extremities and abdomen.

Sickle cell anaemia 325: Acute anaemic symptoms, jaundice, severe arthritic pain, poor development resulting in long arms and legs, short trunk; in infants, swollen hands and feet.

Aplastic anaemia 326: Severe anaemia, brown pigmentation on pale, waxy skin, bleeding from the nose and mouth, black-and-blue marks on the skin.

Cancer of the liver 433: Anaemic symptoms, nausea, vomiting, pressure in abdomen, constipation, dull ache in liver area, jaundice, weight loss.

Anaemia with skin disorders

Endocarditis 135: Worsening anaemia symptoms, especially fatigue, unexplained intermittent fever, pain in joints, red and purplish spots all over body, bleeding from nose. Blood is also found in urine.

Allergic drug reactions 289: From Chloramphenicol, an antibiotic; from arsenical medications. Analgesics can also give rise to anaemia and various skin reactions.

Pemphigus 297: Besides anaemia and itching, large water blisters all over the body.

Lupus erythematosus 320: Red butterfly-like patches on cheeks or bridge of nose and elsewhere. As old one heals, new ones form. The patches itch and are scaly. In the systemic lupus variation, patient can be feverish, anaemic, and emaciated. Complications besides joint pains are lung, heart, and kidney disorders.

Aplastic anaemia 326: Severe anaemia, brown spots on skin, black-and-blue marks on body, bleeding from nose and mouth.

Bilharziasis 383: Abdominal pains, skin rash, swelling of face, limbs, genitalia, chronic fatigue, great malaise, anaemia.

Hodgkin's disease and other lymphomas 416: Painless enlarged lymph nodes on neck (often the size of an orange). If enlargements are only on one side, the disease is Hodgkin's; if on both, it is another lymphoma. Other symptoms are itchy skin, weakness, weight loss, swelling of legs, difficulty breathing, persistent recurrent fever.

Anaemia with weight loss

Rheumatic heart disease and rheumatic fever 127: Symptoms include rapid heartbeat, inflammation of the joints, sweating, malaise, weight loss or failure to gain weight in a growing child.

Postgastrectomy syndrome 161: Explosive diarrhoea, palpitations, periods of dizziness ranging in intensity from light-headedness to fainting, sweating, weakness, and pain in the upper abdomen.

Regional enteritis 168: Growing anaemia with malnutrition, migratory arthritis, weight loss, mid-abdominal cramps.

Sprue 180: Diarrhoea, fatty, frothy, light-coloured, foul-smelling stools, distended stomach, emaciation, brown pigment on the skin, pallor, anaemia, apathy, pinpoint bleeding under the skin, very sore, red tongue. Children: retarded growth, deformities of bone and muscle, spontaneous fractures.

Pernicious anaemia 323: All anaemic symptoms including palpitations, pins-and-needles sensation in hands and feet, general pains, sore, red tongue, weight loss, jaundice, difficulty walking, impotence and frigidity.

Multiple myeloma 419: Neuralgic arthritic bone pain which can be extreme and which worsens with exercise, swelling on ribs and skull, spontaneous fractures, severe anaemia. Bones most often affected are the thigh, pelvis, upper arm.

Cancer of the kidney 427: Blood in urine, palpable mass in kidney region, pain in ribs and spine, anaemia is frequent.

Wilms' tumour 428: Children: first sign is large abdominal mass on one side of the abdomen, frequent appearance of blood in urine, loss of appetite. Later, pain, anaemia and weight loss.

Cancer of the oesophagus 429: Difficulty swallowing, some pressure or pain under the breastbone, rapid weight loss, emaciation, dehydration, thirst, cough, heavy salivation, flatulence. Later anaemia, loss of voice, fever, foul breath.

Cancer of the stomach 430: Prolonged periods of indigestion, upper abdominal distress after meals, rapid satiation at meals, inexplicable distaste for some foods like meat, especially red meat. Great fatigue, progressive weight loss, vomiting of blood, black, tarry stools. Occasionally the first sign is sudden pain in the abdomen.

Cancer of the liver 433: Nausea, vomiting, pressure in abdomen, constipation, dull ache in liver area, jaundice, and weight loss.

Cancer of the colon and rectum 434: Discomfort in rectum not relieved by bowel movement, change in bowel habits, narrowing of stools, constipation followed by diarrhoea and vice versa, pain on defecation. Later, persistent bleeding into stools, excessive gas, cramping pain, loss of weight.

Anaemia with weight loss and swollen lymph nodes

Malignant tumours of the nervous system 413: Infants, children: rapid weight loss, distension of the abdomen, loss of strength, discoloration around the eyes, swelling of the lymph nodes, pain in the bones.

Leukaemia 415: Bleeding all over body from gums, skin (in tiny red spots), nose, etc. Always anaemia with great pallor, fatigue, malaise, pain in the joints. Children: (acute form) sore throat, rapid pulse, bruised body appearance. Adults: (chronic form) enlarged lumph nodes, night sweats, weight loss.

Hodgkin's disease and other lymphomas 416: Painless enlarged lymph nodes on the neck (often the size of an orange). If on one side only, the disease is Hodgkin's; if on both, lymphoma. Other symptoms are itchy skin, weakness, weight loss, swelling of the legs, difficulty breathing, persistent, recurrent fever.

Bleeding, general

Endocarditis 135: Bleeding from nose, mucous membranes, in the urine. Pain in the joints, deep fatigue, red and purple spots all over the body (bleeding into the skin), clubbing of fingers, unexplained fever.

Cirrhosis of the liver 191: Loss of weight, flatulence, foetid breath, abdominal distension. Later, severe jaundice, emaciation, spider angiomas (red spots with red lines radiating out), puffiness in feet and legs, enlarged vein on the abdomen, general bleeding and blood in the faeces. In men, atrophy of the testicles and enlarged breasts.

Acute yellow atrophy 193: High fever, severe headache, jaundice, severe abdominal pain, vomiting of black material, apathy, confusion, bleeding under the skin and from the mouth, dilated pupils, foul breath, scanty, bloody urine and rapid, feeble pulse.

Aplastic anaemia 326: Pallor, shortness of breath, fatigue, palpitations, brown pigmentation on pale, waxy skin, bleeding from nose and gums, black-and-blue marks.

Purpura 328: Small reddish-blue spots on skin (pinpoint bleeding), bleeding from the mucous membranes and gums on slight injury, pain in abdomen and joints, slow clotting of blood from cuts and wounds, black-and-blue marks.

Haemophilia 329: Spontaneous bleeding, uncontrolled bleeding, deformity of the joints.

Vitamin C deficiency (scurvy) 352: Weakness, bleeding into the skin (pinpoint bleeding) causing small reddish-purple spots, bleeding from the gums and mucous membranes, loose teeth, skin rash. Infants: loss of appetite and weight, irritability, very painful, swollen legs.

Vitamin K deficiency 354: General bleeding from nose, gums, vagina, bleeding into urine and stools.

Leukaemia 415: Prolonged general bleeding from nose, gums, mucous membranes, skin (small reddish-purple spots). Other symptoms are acute anaemia, fatigue, malaise, marked pallor. Children: (acute form) sore throat, rapid pulse, bruised body appearance. Adults: (chronic form) enlarged lymph nodes, night sweats, weight loss.

Bruised body appearance

Cushing's disease 343: Weight gain on trunk, back, and face (moon face), excessive hair growth, easy bruising, loss of menstrual periods, muscle weakness, easily broken bones.

Leukaemia 415: Children only: (acute form) general bleeding from gums, mucous membrane, nose, skin (in the form of small red-purple spots); fatigue, pain in the joints, malaise, anaemia, sore throat, rapid pulse and bruised body appearance.

Chills and fever

also see **Fever**

Fevers resulting from viral or blood diseases rarely cause chills.
Chills and fever, Chills and fever with headache, Severe chills and high fever

Chills and fever

Tonsillitis 70: Chills, fever, pain in tonsillar region and in back of the jaw or in the neck. Painful swallowing. Tonsils are enlarged with white-amberish streaks.

Empyaema 119: Sweating, sharp pain in affected side, short, dry cough, emaciation, clubbing of fingers, strong malaise.

Diverticulitis 173: Pain in lower left quadrant of abdomen, distension of the abdomen, nausea and vomiting. In the severe form, chills and fever; in the chronic form, constipation alternating with diarrhoea.

Childbed fever 247: Chills and high fever, fast pulse, abdominal pain, vomiting.

Prostatitis 249: Males: flu-like chills and fever, severe pain between the scrotum and anus, difficult, painful urination without being able to empty bladder completely. Occasionally blood in urine. Frequent incidence of impotency.

Orchitis (mumps orchitis) 253: Males: pain and swelling of the testicles and scrotum, hiccups, occasional vomiting, swelling of the salivary glands.

Epididymitis 254: Males: swelling and pain in scrotum and testicles.

Haemolytic anaemia 324: Anaemia symptoms, jaundice, faintness, dizziness, weak, rapid pulse, aches in abdomen and extremities.

Gout 334: Sharp agonizing pain in the large toe or other joints which become red and swollen, rapid pulse, lumps (painless tumours) around the ears and around various joints. Urine may be dark and scanty.

The plague 365: Chills and high fever, buboes (egg-size lymph nodes in the groin, which fester and burst), rapid heartbeat, black spots on the skin, stupor, coma.

Chills and fever with headache

Sinusitis 66: Heavy, yellow nasal discharge, frontal headache, swelling around eye sockets.

Acute kidney infection 200: Pain in the kidney can range from dull to acute, radiating to the lower abdomen and groin. Urination is frequent, urgent, urine is scanty, burning and cloudy with a decaying odour. In numerous cases there may be total arrest of the urine, high pulse rate, nausea and vomiting.

Erysipelas 300: Raised rash from dull red to scarlet with advancing margins, chills and high fever, intense headache, swollen face and lymph nodes.

Sunburn 314: Skin red to angry red, painful and itching. In severe cases blisters, chills and fever, headache. Later, peeling of skin.

Lymphangitis 330: Chills and high fever, red streaks or lines on arms or legs going upwards, swelling of lymph nodes, headaches, body aches.

Relapsing fever 369: Chills and high fever, severe headache, recurrent attacks of fever, fast heartbeat, muscle and joint pain, profuse sweating.

Chicken pox 372: Itching body rash becoming pimply then blistering and finally crusting. In adults, headache, body aches, and chills.

Flu 376: Mild cold symptoms, flushed face, severe headache, extreme fatigue, prostration from weakness, sweating.

Dengue fever 380: Chills and high fever, pain in back of the eyeball, headache, pain in the muscles and joints severe enough to cause prostration, measles-like rash over the body.

Toxoplasmosis 385: Chills, high fever, swollen lymph nodes, severe headache.

Severe chills and high fever

Pneumonia 109: Very severe shaking chills, high fever, pain in chest, painful cough with rusty phlegm, rapid breathing, rapid pulse.

Lung abscess 115: Repeated attacks of severe chills, high fever, drenching sweats, great malaise, painful cough with bloodstained, foul, purulent phlegm, shortness of breath on exertion, weakness and weight loss.

Cholangitis 196: Severe chills, high fever, jaundice, clay-coloured stools.

Blood poisoning 360: Shaking chills, irregular high fever, severe headache, periods of profuse sweating, severe diarrhoea, rash, small purplish bleeding spots on the skin, collapse.

Malaria 381: Teeth-chattering chills and high fever, drenching sweats, severe headache, vomiting, diarrhoea, rapid pulse, rapid breathing.

Common cold symptoms

Common cold symptoms, Common cold symptoms with fever

Common cold symptoms

Common cold 63: Obstructed running nose, sneezing, tearing, irritated throat.

Chronic rhinitis 64: Postnasal drip, conjunctivitis, loss of taste and smell, frequent running nose, often accompanied by irritation in the throat.

Acute bronchitis 103: Cold symptoms which turn into a prolonged racking cough, unproductive at first, then producing purulent, heavy, yellowish phlegm. There may be shortness of breath. Fever is slight.

Whooping cough 357: Whooping cough, loss of appetite, heavy phlegm, vomiting.

German measles 371: Begins with a slight cold, then the appearance of swollen lymph nodes in neck, finally a rosy-coloured rash on face and neck, later over the entire body. Slight fever.

Common cold symptoms with fever

Meningitis 7: Cold symptoms worsen rapidly to very high fever with the characteristic stiff neck and overwhelming headache. In children, twitching, convulsions, vomiting and delirium.

Pharyngitis (streptococcal throat) 73: Starts with cold symptoms which develop into acute sore throat, high fever, difficulty swallowing, plus rapid and irregular pulse.

Laryngotracheobronchitis (croup) 107: At first gasping unproductive cough, later with sticky, tenacious phlegm, breathing is gasping and strident, high fever. In severe cases, cyanosis. Patient is anxious, frightened.

Pneumonia 109: Starts like a cold, then develops into severe shaking chills, high fever, pain in chest, painful cough with rusty phlegm, rapid breathing, rapid heartbeat.

Diphtheria 358: From the initial cold symptoms it moves rapidly to unusually deep fatigue, very sore, swollen throat with difficult swallowing and greyish false membrane in throat and nose.

Typhoid fever 363: Develops into flu-like symptoms, severe temple or frontal headaches, very high, sustained fever, nosebleeds, distended stomach, stupor, slow, double pulse beat, diarrhoea, rosy spots mostly on abdomen.

Measles 370: Can simulate a cold except for the telltale sign: body rash.

Flu 376: Begins like a common cold but soon the malaise and fever become quite severe, with strong aches in back and legs plus extreme fatigue, weakness.

*

Craving for salt

Adrenal insufficiency (Addison's disease) 344: Easily fatigued, nervous and mental disorders, vomiting, abdominal pain, dizziness, fainting, dehydration, craving for salt, intolerance for cold, black freckles, bronzing and/or piebald skin, loss of pubic hair.

Crying infant

There's nothing more common or normal than a crying baby but when the cry is feeble, prolonged, or different in tone, it is then a symptom of disorder.

Low birth weight 396: Infants: feeble cry, weakness, irregular breathing, large head, prominent eyes, protruding abdomen, small genitals, slowness in gaining weight.

Colic 401: Infants: excessive, prolonged crying, screaming, fretfulness diarrhoea, vomiting, passing of gas, distended stomach.

Cerebral palsy 406: In infancy, high-pitched crying, vomiting, jaundice, lack of alertness, twitching limbs, irritability, lack of muscular control, convulsions, difficulty in movement, tremors, difficulty swallowing.

Cyanosis

Cyanosis is caused by an insufficiency of oxygen, and is a serious sign.
Cyanosis, Cyanosis with shock

Cyanosis

Foreign body in the bronchi 106: Severe shortness of breath, heavy cough with bloodstained, foul phlegm, gagging and high fever.

Asthma 108: Laboured, gasping breathing, wheezing. Appearance is either pale or flushed, with some cyanosis. Later, coughing with profuse, heavy phlegm.

Emphysema 113: Hard, tiring cough bringing up small amounts of thick, heavy phlegm. Shortness of breath on slight exercise. Barrel chest. Loss of vital capacity.

Oedema of the lung 116: Breathing is difficult, laboured, and rapid. Asthmatic and wheezing cough occasionally producing bloody phlegm. Cold extremities, cyanosis, anxiety, oppression in the chest.

High altitude lung oedema 116a: Shortness of breath, cough becoming bloody, noisy breathing.

Heart failure 126: Shortness of breath on slight exertion, palpitations, sweating.

Congenital heart disorders 128: Cyanosis plus easy fatigue, shortness of breath. Child fails to grow properly.

Acute gastritis (erosive) 155: Severe pain in stomach, collapse, very fast pulse, difficulty swallowing, excessive thirst, clammy skin. Possibly vomiting with blood.

Diphtheria 358: Major sympton is grey false membrane in the throat, high fever, foul breath, vomiting. In extreme cases prostration, closing of the throat, cyanosis, difficulty breathing, paralysis of palate and larynx.

Cholera 364: Onset sudden, extreme, continuous diarrhoea, great dehydration, voluminous rice-water stools, stomach and leg cramps, violent vomiting, intense thirst, cyanosis, cold, clammy, wrinkled skin, and finally, total collapse.

Coccidioidomycosis 394: Pain in lungs, deep malaise. In progressive form, weakness, shortness of breath, cyanosis, weight loss, and occasionally spitting up of blood.

Cyanosis with shock

Atelectasis 114: Severe shortness of breath, pain on the affected side, rapid heartbeat, cyanosis, weakness, and shock.

Shock 133: Great pallor, cold, clammy skin, cyanosis of the lips, nailbeds, or fingertips, shortness of breath, dilated pupils, anxiety state; can become comatose.

Pulmonary embolism 140: Initially pain in the leg. Later, acute shortness of breath, pain in the lungs, bloody phlegm, profound shock.

Acute pancreatitis 166: Writhing pain high in the abdomen, severe vomiting, feeble, rapid pulse, skin bluish and cold or clammy, accompanied by shock.

Dehydration

Dehydration is a gross loss of water from the body or tissues. It is a complex of symptoms such as pinched face (often with sharp, outstanding nose), sunken eyeballs, livid skin, muscle cramps, dry mucous membrane, scanty urine. If unattended, it may result in shock.
Dehydration, Dehydration with thirst

Dehydration

Obstruction in peptic ulcer 158: Major symptom is vomiting. Additionally there is dehydration, distension of the stomach, and foul belching.

Infected food gastroenteritis 163: Dehydration in severe forms only, accompanied by kidney failure and shock. In milder forms, nausea, vomiting, cramps, diarrhoea without dehydration. Symptoms appear twelve or more hours after eating.

Hypertrophic pylonic stenosis 169: Infants: projectile vomiting, constipation, loss of weight, lump in abdomen.

Diabetes (ketoacidosis, diabetic coma) 332: Severe dehydration, shortness of breath, nausea and vomiting, dizziness, abdominal pain. Eventually shock, stupor, coma.

Adrenal insufficiency (Addison's disease) 344: Easily fatigued, weakness, nausea and vomiting, abdominal pain, mental and nervous disorders, intolerance for cold, fainting, dizziness, black freckles, piebald skin, bronzing of skin, loss of pubic hair, weight loss, craving for salt.

Cancer of the oesophagus 429: Difficulty swallowing, vague pressure beneath breastbone, rapid weight loss, dehydration, cough, salivation, flatulence, loss of voice, anaemia, fever, foul-smelling breath.

Dehydration with thirst

Intestinal obstruction 170: Intermittent pain around navel, heavy vomiting, thirst, constipation, abdominal distension. Later (serious stage), dehydration, sunken features, anxiety, total suppression of urine, shock.

Peritonitis 179: Persistent vomiting, extreme pain in abdomen, which is rigid and distended, considerable thirst, hiccups, patient is anxious and very ill.

Diabetes insipidus 338: Massive excretion of urine (up to several gallons daily), nocturia (night awakening to urinate), severe dehydration, extreme thirst.

Cholera 364: Constant voluminous, watery diarrhoea, massive dehydration, severe cramps in stomach, legs, intense thirst, sunken eyes, clammy, wrinkled skin.

Bacillary dysentry 366: Constant diarrhoea, blood, pus, and mucus in stools, pain, thirst, urgency to defecate without ability, nausea and vomiting.

Cancer of the oesophagus 429: Difficulty swallowing, some pressure or pain under the breastbone, rapid weight loss, emaciation, dehydration, thirst, cough, heavy salivation, flatulence. Later, anaemia, loss of the voice, fever, foul breath.

Failure to gain weight or grow

Although growth rate in a child is continuous, one should bear in mind that the rate is rarely constant, even when the child is healthy. In the absence of other symptoms, slow growth rate or temporary failure to gain weight is generally not significant.

Failure to gain weight or grow, Failure to gain weight or growth with body malformations

Failure to gain weight or grow

Tonsillitis (chronic) 70: Low fever, frequent colds and sore throats, low energy level.

Rheumatic heart disease and rheumatic fever 127: Inflammation of joints, rapid heartbeat, easily fatigued, sweating, St Vitus's dance, nosebleeds, rashes, red and purple spots over the body. Occasionally difficulty swallowing.

Congenital heart disorders 128: Breathlessness, cyanosis, easy fatigue.

Hypertrophic pyloric stenosis 169: Infants: projectile vomiting, lump in abdomen, dehydration, constipation, loss of weight.

Megacolon 175: Constipation, slight anaemia, poor nutrition.

Vitamin A deficiency 348a: Night blindness, horny skin, ulceration of cornea.

Vitamin A toxicity 348b: Pain in joints, irritability, severe pressure headaches, falling hair, loss of appetite.

Threadworm 389: Visible white worms in the stools, painful anal scratching, restless sleep, poor appetite.

Failure to gain weight or growth with body malformations

Sprue 180: Children: retarded growth, deformities of bone and muscle, spontaneous fractures, diarrhoea three or four times daily with faeces that are fatty, frothy, foul, and light-coloured, red, sore tongue, distended stomach, emaciated body, and small bleedings under the skin.

Coeliac disease 181: Children: a recurrent childhood disease, beginning with an attack of diarrhoea that is usually touched off by an upper respiratory infection. Faeces are loose, fatty, and foul. Other symptoms include weakness, low appetite, irritability, protuberant stomach with thin body and growth significantly retarded.

Sickle cell anaemia 325: Severe anaemic symptoms, severe general pain, arthritic pains, jaundice, poor physical development, long arms and legs, short trunk. In infants, painful, swollen hands and feet.

Hypothyroidism 339: Children: goitre, mental and physical retardation, 'good', undemanding child, apathy, coarsening of the face, puffy hands and feet, dry skin becoming wrinkled, flat nose, pot-belly, subnormal temperature (36°C, 96°F).

Vitamin D toxicity 353b: Infants: physical retardation, loss of appetite, weakness, excessive urination, weight loss.

Low birth weight 396: Infants: irregular breathing, protruding stomach, slow to gain weight, weakness, large head, prominent eyes, small genitals.

Cystic fibrosis 407: Infants, children: slow development, extreme thinness, ravenous appetite, bulky, greasy, foul-smelling stools, chronic cough, rapid breathing, runny nose, protruding stomach, very salty sweat.

Fatigue
also see **Lethargy, Weakness**

Without other significant symptoms,

fatigue by itself is most often of a psychogenic nature.
Fatigue, Fatigue with anaemic symptoms, Fatigue with fever, Fatigue with headache

Fatigue

Congenital heart disorders 128: Easily fatigued, frequent cyanosis, shortness of breath, child fails to grow properly.

Botulism 165: Symptoms appear 18–36 hours after eating. Double or blurred vision, extreme fatigue, fixed, dilated pupils, difficulty breathing or talking, nausea and vomiting, diarrhoea, cramps, eventual paralysis of respiratory tract.

Adrenal insufficiency (Addison's disease) 344: Easily fatigued, weakness, black freckles, piebald and bronzing skin, nausea, vomiting, abdominal pain, craving for salt, nervous and mental disorders, loss of pubic hair, dehydration, dizziness, fainting, weight loss.

Primary aldosteronism 345: Fatigue, muscle weakness, numbness, tingling, excessive urination, thirst. (Hypertension.)

Vitamin B₁ (thiamine) deficiency 349: Fatigue, appetite and weight loss. Prickly numbness of the hands and feet, emotional instability, cramps in the legs, difficulty walking, rapid heartbeat, difficulty breathing, swelling and fluid in the tissues.

Vitamin C deficiency (scurvy) 352: Weakness, lethargy, bleeding of the gums, under the skin, and from the mucous membranes, loose teeth, fragile bones. Infants: loss of appetite, failure to gain weight, irritability, swollen gums, bone pain.

Roundworm 388: Vague cramping pains in abdomen, malnutrition, weight loss.

Histoplasmosis 393: Ulcerations on nose, ear, pharynx, vomiting, diarrhoea, black stools, enlarged lymph nodes, emaciation. In severe cases, simulates tuberculosis with cough, bloody phlegm, loss of weight, extreme fatigue and drenching sweats.

Fatigue with anaemic symptoms

Bronchiectasis 105: Easily fatigued, anaemia, periodic cough bringing up foul-smelling phlegm, shortness of breath.

Endocarditis 135: Deep fatigue, anaemia, unexplained fever, pain in the joints, spots on the body, clubbing of fingers, bleeding from the nose and into urine.

Dietary deficiencies in pregnancy 236: Anaemia, breathlessness, fatigue.

Anaemia 322: Anaemic symptoms, palpitations, tongue flabby or red and sore, noises in the ear, vertigo, fingernails longitudinally ridged and spoon-shaped, lustreless hair. In severe cases, jaundice, numbness of limbs, excessive thirst, poor memory, and finally shock.

Sickle cell anaemia 325: Severe anaemic symptoms, acute general body pain, jaundice, poor physical development (long arms and legs, short trunk). Infants: painful, swollen hands and feet.

Aplastic anaemia 326: Severe anaemia, brown pigmentation on pale, waxy skin, bleeding from the nose and mouth, black-and-blue marks.

All-vegetarian diet deficiency 355: Anaemia, inflammation of the tongue, nervous disorders. In iodine deficiency: fatigue, puffy hands and face, enlarged tongue, mental apathy.

Bilharziasis 383: Chronic fatigue, abdominal pains, skin rash, swelling of face, limbs and genitalia, anaemia, general ill health.

Leukaemia 415: Bleeding of the gums, nose, skin (in tiny red spots), fatigue, pain in the joints, anaemia with great pallor. Children: (acute form) sore throat, bruised body appearance, rapid pulse. Adults: (chronic form) swollen lymph nodes, night sweats, weight loss.

Stomach cancer 430: Heartburn, abdominal distension, rapid satiation at meals, sudden distaste for certain foods (particularly meat), gradual weight loss, anaemia. Often the first sign is sudden pain, vomiting blood, and black, tarry stools.

Fatigue with fever

Atypical pneumonia (virus) 110: Paroxysmal, incessant cough, phlegm scant but rarely bloodstained, moderate fever, prolonged fatigue in long convalescence.
Pulmonary tuberculosis 112: Deep fatigue, slight to severe cough with bloody phlegm, drenching sweats at night, loss of appetite, loss of weight, pain in the chest, possible fever.

Lung abscess 115: Severe malaise, repeated chills and high fever, painful cough with bloodstained, foul phlegm, shortness of breath on exertion.
Rheumatic heart disease and rheumatic fever 127: Inflammation of the joints, rapid heartbeat, sweating, St Vitus's dance, rash over the body, nosebleeds.
Flu 376: Cold symptoms, chills and fever, flushed face, severe headache, aches in the muscles and joints, sweating, prostration, extreme fatigue.
Infectious mononucleosis 377: Fever, often headache, sore throat, painful swelling of the lymph nodes under the jaw, on the neck, in the armpits and groin, weakness and occasional jaundice.

Fatigue with headache

High blood pressure 138: Pulsating headache in the back of the head appears late in the disease; most common in the morning upon awakening, it then wears off. Later symptoms may include dizziness and nosebleeds.
Acute infectious hepatitis 187 and **Serum hepatitis 188:** Jaundice, deep fatigue, dark urine, light-coloured stools, red, itching wheals, sweet, foul breath, tenderness in the liver area. Nausea, vomiting, severe headache.
Menopause 221: In some women no symptoms at all, but for most hot flushes, chills, sweating, headache, fatigue, frequent urination, giddiness, palpitation, insomnia, appetite loss, dyspepsia, nausea, nervous irritability, emotional instability, crying bouts, periods of depression and anxiety.
Polycythaemia 327: Bluish-red, itching

skin, often with blueness of lips and fingernail beds, dizziness, constant dull headache, ringing in the ears, breathlessness, bleeding in the gastro-intestinal tract causing bloody or tarry stools.
Infectious mononucleosis 377: Daily recurrent headaches, fatigue, sore throat. Painful swelling of lymph nodes under the jaw, in the armpits and groin.

Fever
also see **Chills and fever**

Fever, Erratic fever, High fever, High fever and headache, High fever and shortness of breath, Sustained high fever

A thermometer should be shaken down to below 35°C, 95°F, and kept in place for several minutes, especially if it is taken orally. Oral readings are unreliable in children and those who breathe primarily through the mouth. Strong exertion or heavy exercise will cause a considerable rise in temperature. The peak of fever is almost always late afternoon or early evening. Ordinarily a rise of one degree will also show up as a rise of ten heartbeats per minute – except in cases of tuberculosis or rheumatic fever where the pulse rate goes much higher, or in viral and blood diseases, where the pulse rate is considerably slowed. A serious infection can exist in the absence of fever, especially among the elderly.

Fever

Herpetic stomatitis 80: Inflamed gums, white plaques and ulcers appear on the mucous membrane of the mouth producing a foul taste. In a child, pain may be so severe as to prevent him from taking food.
Atypical pneumonia (virus) 110: Moderate although incessant paroxysmal coughing, phlegm copious but rarely bloodstained. Fever remains for about ten days. Recovery is prolonged.
Rheumatic heart disease and rheumatic fever 127: Inflammation of the large and small joints, rapid heartbeat, St Vitus's dance, malaise, pallor, sweat-

ing, failure to gain weight, skin rash, and loss of appetite. In severe cases, shortness of breath, coughing, and pain in the chest.

Pericarditis 136: Moderate fever, pain in the chest, fluids in the abdomen and chest, veins in the neck are prominent.

Phlebitis 141: Low-grade fever with painful, sensitive, white legs, upon which surface veins are prominent.

Acute infectious hepatitis 187: Fever up to 38·7°C, 102°F, severe headache, jaundice, deep fatigue, dark urine, light-coloured stools, red, itching wheals, tenderness in liver area, nausea and vomiting.

Cholecystitis 195: Agonizing abdominal pain radiating to the back, right shoulder, and pelvis, profuse sweating, jaundice, nausea, vomiting, and rapid heartbeat.

Tuberculosis of the joints and bones 264: Swelling of the joints without pain. If in the leg, weakness, stiffness, and limp; if in the back, rigid spine, postural change, fever and night sweats.

Heat exhaustion 313b: Headache, dizziness, profuse sweating. Skin is cool and moist. Temperature only slightly above normal. Nausea, faintness.

Infectious mononucleosis 377: Painful swelling of the lymph nodes, mostly in the neck but also under the arms and groin. Sore throat, weakness, fatigue, jaundice, occasional headache.

Erratic fever

Meningitis 7: High, erratic fever, overwhelming headache radiating to the neck, vomiting, photophobia, convulsions, confusion, spots on the skin.

Pulmonary tuberculosis 112: Deep fatigue, moderate, erratic fever, slight to severe cough with bloody phlegm, drenching night sweats, weight loss, low appetite, pain in the chest.

Endocarditis 135: Irregular fever, nosebleed, blood in urine, pain in the joints, patient is very sick with great fatigue. Late, crop of small red-purplish spots all over body accompanied by clubbing of the fingers identifies the disease.

Relapsing fever 369: (See *Chills and fever*)

Malaria 381: (See *Severe chills and fever*)

High fever

High fever is considered above 39·4°C, 103°F orally, 40°C, 104°F rectally.

Acute otitis media 58a: Severe earache which may radiate to the side of the head, sensation of fullness in the ear, tinnitus, and tenderness over the mastoid bone. Loss of hearing.

Mastoiditis 59: Begins as a sore throat with a moderate earache which soon becomes severe. The area behind the ear becomes red and tender. There may be a discharge from the ear canal.

Tonsillitis (acute) 70: High fever, extreme pain in tonsillar region and in back of the jaw. Tonsils are clearly enlarged, very red and spotted with amber streaks. Difficulty in swallowing.

Juvenile rheumatoid arthritis 260: Unexplained high fever, iritis; later, painful inflammation and swelling of the joints.

Osteomyelitis 265: Deep pain in the affected bones and joints, very high fever, sweating, overlying muscles are painful, swollen and festering.

Scarlet fever 359: Frequent vomiting, high fever, sore throat, white, coated, furry tongue, possible yellow-grey false membrane in the mouth, body rash, blanching in squeezed spots. Later, rash on skin peels and flakes, face is flushed except around the mouth.

Measles 370: Cold symptoms, hacking cough, white spots inside mouth, brownish-pink body rash, photophobia.

Roseola 399: High fever accompanied by a profuse rash on chest and abdomen, which lessens on face and extremities when fever drops.

High fever and headache
also see **Fever and severe headache** p32

Acute yellow atrophy 193: Jaundice, weakness, severe abdominal pain, black vomit, apathy, confusion, bleeding under the skin and from the mouth, dilated pupils, foul breath, scanty, bloody urine and rapid feeble pulse.

Erysipelas 300: Raised rash ranging in colour from full red to scarlet with advancing margins on the face, chills, high intermittent fever, swollen face and lymph nodes.

Sunstroke 313a: Headache, dizziness, no sweating. Skin is flushed, hot, and dry, very high temperature, very fast pulse, very rapid respiration.

Chicken pox 372: In adult form, headache, backache, chills and high fever. Rash developing to pimples, then to blisters and finally, to crusts.

Smallpox 373: High fever, violent frontal headache, severe muscle pains, crops of small reddish spots over the body which become pimply, turn into purulent blisters and finally, into foul-smelling scabs. Convulsions in children.

Polio 374: High fever, severe headache, major sign is stiff neck, sore throat. In severe cases, prostration, pain in muscles, great weakness, twitching muscles, paralysis in various parts of the body, difficulty swallowing.

Yellow fever 379: High fever, flushed face, prostration, severe headache, pain in the limbs and back, scanty urine. In second attack, jaundice, vomiting with black blood, bleeding from mucous membranes.

Trichinosis 386: High fever, swelling of face around the eyes and forehead, pain in and swelling of the muscles, profuse sweating, diarrhoea. Shortness of breath in severe cases.

High fever and shortness of breath

Foreign body in bronchi 106: High fever, heavy cough with bloodstained, foul phlegm, severe shortness of breath accompanied by cyanosis.

Laryngotracheobronchitis (croup) 107: Children: high fever, breathing is gasping, strident, cough is at first nonproductive, later, phlegm is sticky, tenacious. Cyanosis, hoarseness. Patient appears anxious and frightened.

Pulmonary embolism 140: Major symptom is acute shortness of breath with accompanying cyanosis. Rapid, erratic heartbeat and chest pains.

Sunstroke 313a: Headache, dizziness, no sweating. Skin is flushed, hot, and dry. Temperature very high, pulse very fast, breathing very rapid.

Diphtheria 358: Sore throat, false membrane in throat, high fever, foul mouth odour, difficulty swallowing. In severe cases, prostration, difficulty breathing, paralysis of the palate.

Sustained high fever

Encephalitis 8: High fever abates about the tenth day, severe pounding headache, lack of alertness ranging from drowsiness to stupor, stiff neck. In severe cases, delirium, convulsions, vomiting. Infants: sudden high fever, convulsions, bulging fontanelles.

Pneumonia 109: (See *Severe chills and high fever*)

Typhoid fever 363: Severe, persistent temporal or frontal headaches, sustained high fever, distended stomach, rosy spots on abdomen which disappear in a few days, slow, feeble, double pulse, diarrhoea, nosebleed, slight cough.

Typhus 392: High fever lasting ten days accompanied by severe headache, prostration, mottled rash with small red spots which turn purple, contracted pupils, dark, scanty urine, furry white tongue, twitching of muscles, stupor, delirium, coma. Profuse sweating when fever breaks.

Hodgkin's disease and other lymphomas 416: Painless enlarged lymph nodes in neck (often the size of an orange). If only one side of neck, evidence of Hodgkin's, if both sides, other lymphoma. Later, all lymph nodes of the body are affected. Other symptoms are itchy skin, anaemia, weakness, recurrent fever, weight loss.

*

Hiccups

Almost all cases of hiccups are trivial and transient, occurring without known cause. Occasionally, however, it is symptomatic of serious disorders.

Encephalitis 8: High fever, pounding headache, drowsiness to stupor. In severe cases, convulsions and delirium, persistent hiccups, stiff neck, vomiting, and coma.

Hiccups 12: Most attacks last less than a half hour. Babies' hiccuping is natural and should not be restrained.

Hiatus hernia 149: Pain behind breastbone radiating to left shoulder and accompanied by belching and hiccups. Heartburn, vomiting of blood, insidious bleeding into stools causing symptoms of anaemia.

Peritonitis 179: Pain in abdomen so severe as to be prostrating, abdominal distension and rigidity, persistent vomiting and frequent hiccups, dehydration, rapid heartbeat, thirst. Patient is gravely ill and anxious.

Orchitis (mumps orchitis) 253: Males: swelling and pain in the scrotum and testes, chills and fever, vomiting, in some cases swelling of the salivary glands, hiccups.

Hunger

In the absence of other symptoms unusual hunger can be a manifestation of psychogenic problems.

Diabetes 332: Excessive thirst, urination, and hunger, blurred vision, weakness, sweet, fruity breath, red, sore, dry tongue, pins-and-needles sensation, weight loss. In hypoglycaemic shock (insulin shock) there is weakness, trembling, sweating, excessive hunger and in severe cases, fainting and coma.

Cystic fibrosis 407: Infants, children: slow development, failure to gain weight, ravenous appetite, bulky, greasy, foul-smelling stools, chronic cough, rapid breathing, protruding stomach, emaciation, very salty sweat.

Loss of appetite

Besides disease, the appetite can be depressed by great stress, anxiety, fear, and emotional conflicts.

Loss of appetite, Loss of appetite and weakness, Loss of appetite and weight loss, Loss of appetite, weight loss, and pain in the chest

Loss of appetite

Acute gastritis (simple) 155: Pain and pressure at pit of stomach, nausea, vomiting, coated tongue.

Acute gastritis (infectious toxic) 155: Vomiting, sensation of fullness of stomach. Loss of appetite is a very characteristic symptom.

Chronic gastritis 156: Pain in the stomach ranging from mild to acute, mild nausea, constipation, distension of the stomach, foul taste in the mouth and foul breath, furred or red-tipped tongue.

Acute nephritis 197: Sudden loss of appetite, bloody but scanty urine, severe headache, nausea and vomiting, furred tongue, puffiness of the face, swelling of the ankles. (Rise in blood pressure.)

Menopause 221: In some women, no symptoms at all, but for most, hot flushes, chills, sweating, headache, fatigue, frequent urination, giddiness, palpitation, insomnia, loss of appetite, dyspepsia, nausea, nervous irritability, emotional instability, crying bouts and periods of depression and anxiety.

Vitamin A toxicity 348b: Pain in the joints, irritability, severe pressure headaches, retarded growth in children, falling hair.

Vitamin B$_1$ (thiamine) deficiency 349: Numbness in hands and feet, and legs, emotional instability, palpitations, difficulty breathing, general swelling and fluid in tissues.

Whooping cough 357: Cold symptoms, whooping type of cough, heavy, gagging phlegm, vomiting.

Loss of appetite and weakness

Sprue 180: Diarrhoea, fatty, frothy, light-coloured and foul-smelling stools, distended stomach, emaciation, brown pigment on the skin, pallor, anaemia, apathy, pinpoint bleeding under the skin, very sore, red tongue. Children: retarded growth, deformities of bone and muscle, spontaneous fractures.

Acute infectious hepatitis 187: Nausea at the sight of food, dark urine, jaundice, red, itching wheals, weakness, tenderness in liver area, headache, vomiting, nausea.

Vitamin B complex (niacin) deficiency 351: Weakness, gastric disturbances, red spots turning brown and scaly all over the body, mucous membrane and margins of the tongue becoming scarlet, inflamed gums, excessive salivation, diarrhoea later becoming bloody.

Vitamin D toxicity 353b: Nausea, weakness, excessive urination, yellow deposits under the skin, kidney failure.

Infectious mononucleosis 377: Feeling unwell for weeks or months, low daily fever, daily recurrent headaches, sore throat. Major symptom is painful swelling under the jaw, under the arms, and in the groin.

Tapeworm 390: Abdominal cramps, diarrhoea, exhaustion. Segments of worm visible in stools.

Cancer of the gallbladder 432: Sharp pain in upper right abdomen, jaundice, inability to digest certain foods, progressively increasing weakness, possible vomiting.

Loss of appetite and weight loss

Obstruction in peptic ulcer 158: Vomiting, sometimes with blood, distension of the stomach, loss of appetite and weight, foul belching, and dehydration.

Sprue 180: Diarrhoea, fatty, frothy, light-coloured and foul-smelling stools, distended stomach, emaciation, brown pigment on the skin, pallor, anaemia, apathy, pinpoint bleeding under the skin, very sore, red tongue. Children: retarded growth, deformities of bones and muscles, and spontaneous fractures.

Coeliac disease 181: Children: recurrent disease touched off by upper respiratory infection, persistent diarrhoea, loose

stools that are bulky, fatty, and foul-smelling. Protuberant abdomen, thin body, fretfulness, weakness, and retarded growth.

Pernicious anaemia 323: Anaemic symptoms, palpitations, pins-and-needles sensation in hands, feet, and elsewhere, sore, beefy, red tongue, jaundice, difficulty walking, impotence and frigidity, weight loss.

Hypopituitarism 337: Children: stunted growth, dwarfism. Adults: fatigue, diminished libido, poor appetite, weight loss, apathy, loss of pubic and axillary hair, slow, feeble pulse, pale, sallow skin, loss of menstrual periods.

Adrenal insufficiency (Addison's disease) 344: Easily fatigued, appetite and weight loss, dark pigmentation, nausea, .vomiting, abdominal pain, craving for salt, loss of hair, dehydration, fainting, dizziness, and mental disorders.

Vitamin B₁ (thiamine) deficiency 349: Loss of appetite and weight, prickling numbness of the hands, legs, and feet, heavy palpitation, difficulty breathing, swelling and fluid in the tissues, emotional instability.

Vitamin C deficiency 352: Infants: irritability, loss of appetite and weight, swollen painful legs. Adults: weakness, bleeding from gums and mucous membrane, bleeding into the skin, loose teeth, skin rash, easily broken bones.

Vitamin D toxicity 353b: Excess vitamin D can cause loss of weight and appetite, nausea, weakness, excessive urination and kidney failure.

Threadworm 389: Painful anal scratching, restless sleep, failure to gain weight, visible white worms in stools.

Loss of appetite, weight loss, and pain in the chest

Pulmonary tuberculosis 112: Deep fatigue, drenching sweats, pain in the chest, cough with bloody phlegm, fever, appetite and weight loss.

Empyaema 119: Pain in the chest, short, dry cough, chills, fever, sweating, cheeks flushed with the rest of the face and body quite pale, foul breath, clubbing of the fingers, loss of appetite and weight.

Rheumatic heart disease and rheumatic fever 127: Pain in the joints, rapid heartbeat, rash over the body, loss of appetite and weight, St Vitus's dance, loss of energy. Pain around the heart is a not infrequent complaint.

Endocarditis 135: Small red-purplish spots over the body, chills, fever, pain in the chest and joints, fatigue, clubbing of the fingers, nosebleeds, blood in the urine, loss of appetite and weight. (Enlarged spleen.)

Ulcer of the oesophagus 147: Pain radiating from under the breastbone, vomiting (frequently with blood), diarrhoea, heartburn, loss of appetite and weight.

Oesophagitis 148: Pain behind the breastbone, difficulty swallowing accompanied by heartburn, loss of appetite and weight.

*

Low birth weight

Low birth weight is usually considered to be less than 2·5kg, 5½lb.

Low birth weight 396: Infants: weakness, irregular breathing, large head, prominent eyes, slow to gain weight, small genitals, protruding stomach.

Sudden infant death 398: Infants: there are no symptoms except that a third of all S.I.D.s are infants with low birth weight.

Mental retardation 403: Infants: low birth weight is common, abnormal size of head, jaundice. In infancy development is slow and the subject lethargic.

Pains in the body

Late syphilis (tabes dorsalis) 210: Loss of sense of balance and space when eyes are closed, 'lightning pains' and spasms in various parts of the body, and pain in the throat and stomach.

Pernicious anaemia 323: Anaemic symptoms, palpitations, beefy, red, sore tongue, weight loss, jaundice, pins-and-needles sensation in hands, feet, and else-

where, difficulty walking, impotence, frigidity, nausea.

Haemolytic anaemia 324: Anaemic symptoms, aches in extremities and the abdomen, jaundice, fainting, dizziness, weak, rapid pulse, chills, fever.

Sickle cell anaemia 325: Severe anaemic symptoms, brown body spots, bleeding from nose and mouth, black-and-blue marks, jaundice. Infants: painful, swollen hands and feet, general arthritic pains, poor physical development (long arms and legs, short trunk), severe general pain.

Lymphangitis 330: Red streaks or lines going upwards on arms or legs, swelling of lymph nodes, chills, high fever, headache, aches all over the body.

Pallor

also see **Anaemia**

Pallor can be deceptive; some people look white normally. In such cases the inner part of the lower eyelid, the lips, the inside of the mouth, and the nailbeds will show up pale if the patient has pallor.
Pallor, Extreme pallor

Pallor

Angina pectoris 124: Intense pain or distress lasting a few minutes which radiates from the heart to either shoulder or arm, or to the jaw. There may be shortness of breath, cold sweats, palpitations, and dizziness.

Rheumatic heart disease and rheumatic fever 127: Rapid heartbeat, inflammation of the joints, sweating, malaise, failure to gain weight in a growing child.

Rapid heartbeat 130a: Nausea, weakness, and in extreme cases, shock.

Atrial fibrillation 132: Pallor plus irregular, fluttering heartbeat, and an eerie feeling in the chest.

Endocarditis 135: Worsening anaemia particularly characterized by fatigue, recurrent fever, pain in the joints, purplish spots over the body, blood in the urine, and nosebleeds.

Hiatus hernia 149: Pain behind breastbone radiating outward (may simulate heart attack). Insidious bleeding into stools will cause anaemia, pallor. Heartburn is a frequent symptom.

Anaemia 322: Pallor, shortness of breath, palpitations, vertigo, noises in the ear, tongue flabby or red, sore, and burning. In some cases, jaundice, numbness of the limbs, thirst, poor memory, fingernails longitudinally ridged and spoon-shaped.

Pernicious anaemia 323: Anaemic symptoms (pallor, weakness, and shortness of breath), numbness, palpitations, sore, red tongue, jaundice, difficulty walking, impotence, frigidity, loss of appetite and weight loss.

Phaeochromocytoma 346: Recurrent pounding headaches, profuse sweating, pallor, and tremors. (High blood pressure.)

Extreme pallor

Motion sickness 61: Nausea, vomiting, cold sweat, greenish pallor, difficulty breathing.

Coronary thrombosis 125: Crushing pain in the chest, cold sweat, extreme anxiety, severe pallor.

Ventricular fibrillation 132a: This is a *Medical Emergency*. Total collapse, no pulse, extreme pallor. Get an ambulance.

Shock 133: Great pallor, cold clammy skin, cyanosis of the lips and fingertips, fast, weak pulse, shortness of breath, anxious state, dilated pupils. Patient can become comatose.

Perforation in peptic ulcer 160: Sudden agonizing pain in the stomach, rigidity of the abdomen, rise in pulse and temperature, pain in shoulder tip. Patient is breathless and ashen grey.

*

Posture, rigid and stooped

Parkinson's disease 1: Usually one arm is still, held at side and bent, slow, shuffling step, tremor of hands, eyes wide and staring, drooling.

Tuberculosis of the joints and bones 264: Swelling of the joints (no pain), rigid

spine, postural change, rise in temperature, night sweats.

Premature ageing

Hypopituitarism (dwarfism) 337: The body is properly proportioned but remains small. Diminished libido, apathy, fatigue, slow pulse, loss of weight, loss of hair, skin is wrinkled and pale. These changes give the appearance of premature ageing.

Prostration (collapse)

Prostration, Prostration with pain in the abdomen, Prostration with shock or coma

Prostration

Lung abscess 115: Painful cough with bloody phlegm, repeated severe chills, high fever, great malaise, breathlessness on exertion, weight loss.

Toxic hepatisis 189: Jaundice, itchy skin rash, vomiting, diarrhoea.

Diphtheria 358: False membrane in the throat, sore throat, fever, foul breath, difficulty swallowing. In severe cases, prostration, paralysis of the palate.

Polio 374: High fever, severe headache, sore throat. Stiff neck can be a distinctive symptom. Muscle pain. In severe cases, prostration, extreme weakness, twitching muscles, paralysis of the arms or legs. Difficulty swallowing and nasal speech indicates brain stem involvement.

Flu 376: Chills, high fever, severe headaches and back and muscle pains. Great weakness and prostration. Excessive fatigue, sweating, dry or hacking cough, cold symptoms, flushed face. In intestinal flu, diarrhoea and vomiting.

Yellow fever 379: Flushed face, high fever, quick prostration, severe headache, pain in the back and limbs, scanty urine. After a period of remission of the disease, it returns with jaundice, black vomiting, and bleeding from the mucous membranes.

Dengue fever 380: Sudden onset of chills, high fever, severe headache. Distinctive symptom is pain at the back of the eye. Also pain in the muscles and joints to the prostration point. There is an intermission of the disease; then the fever returns with a rash.

Prostration with pain in the abdomen

Acute gastritis (erosive) 155: Severe pain in the pit of the stomach, fast heartbeat, cyanosis, excessive thirst, vomiting of blood, blood in stools, stomach rigid and tender.

Massive haemorrhage in peptic ulcer 159: Profuse blood in vomit, blood in stools, heavy sweating, symptoms of shock.

Postgastrectomy syndrome 161: Explosive diarrhoea, palpitations, dizziness, ranging from lightheadedness to fainting, sweating, weight loss, anaemia and weakness.

Acute gastroenteritis 162: Distension and cramps of the stomach, nausea, vomiting, diarrhoea, rapid pulse and weakness.

Staphylococcus gastroenteritis 164: Stomach cramps begin two to four hours after eating contaminated food, and are followed by vomiting, nausea, diarrhoea and sweating. In severe cases, prostration, blood and mucus in the stools.

Inguinal hernia (groin) 255: (Strangulated form of hernia only.) Sudden bulge in groin, severe abdominal pain, fainting, vomiting.

Cholera 364: Onset is sudden and violent, constant diarrhoea, great dehydration, voluminous rice-water stools, violent vomiting, intense thirst, cyanosis, cramps in the stomach and legs and finally, total collapse.

Amoebic dysentry 382: Run-down body, extreme diarrhoea, pussy, bloody stools, pain on the right side of the abdomen, weight loss, prostration.

Tapeworm 390: Abdominal cramps, diarrhoea, exhaustion, loss of appetite.

Prostration with shock or coma

Ventricular fibrillation 132a: This is a *Medical Emergency*. Total collapse, coma, no pulse. Fatal if not immediately treated.

Intestinal obstruction 170: In persistent cases, besides abdominal pain there is distension of the abdomen, constipation, increased vomiting becoming brown, thirst, high fever, total suppression of the urine, anxious, sunken features, rectal bleeding, dehydration, collapse and shock.

Blood poisoning 360: Shaking chills, irregular fever, severe headaches, periods of profuse sweating, diarrhoea, small purplish, haemorrhaging pinpoints in the skin, rash, collapse into shock or coma.

Gas gangrene 362: Bubbles emanating from material oozing from a wound, plus crackling sounds of gas in the tissues when pressed. Skin around wound is discoloured then dusky and finally black. Eventually coma.

The plague 365: Onset is sudden. Chills, very high fever, rapid heartbeat, staggering gait while still ambulant, stupor, prostration. Important sign is development of buboes in the groin and axilla (inflamed lymph nodes varying in size from a crab apple to an apple). These may suppurate and drain. Minute bleeding spots on the skin which turn black. Final stages are shock and coma.

Rabies 378: The healed bite remains reddened. Depression, irritability, then excitability and wildness. Swallowing becomes impossible. Drooling, collapse, and coma.

Typhus 392: Ten day high fever, body ache, severe headache, prostration, mottled rash with minute bleeding points turning purple, highly coloured, scanty urine, twitching muscles, furry, white tongue, contracted pupils, stupor, delirium, coma. Profuse sweating when the fever breaks.

*

Recurrent fever attacks

Typhoid fever 363: Severe, sustained high fever, frontal and temporal headaches, distended stomach, rosy spots on abdomen which disappear in a few days, slow feeble double pulse beat, diarrhoea, nosebleeds, slight cough.

Bacillary dysentry 366: Constant diarrhoea, blood, pus, and mucus in the stools, dehydration, abdominal pain, thirst, vomiting. Relapses and reinfection are frequent.

Relapsing fever 369: Chills, very high fever, severe headache, fast heartbeat, pain in muscles and joints, profuse sweating. Recurrent attacks of the disease with repeated incidence of high fever.

Yellow fever 379: High fever, quick prostration, severe headache, pain in the back and limbs, scanty urine. A period of remission is followed by another attack with jaundice, vomiting of black blood, bleeding from mucous membranes.

Dengue fever 380: Chills, high fever, pain in back of eyeball, headache, pain in muscles and joints causing prostration, measle-like rash over the body.

Malaria 381: Teeth-chattering chills, high fever, drenching sweats, intense headaches, vomiting, diarrhoea, rapid pulse, rapid breathing.

Sensitivity to cold

Chilblains 313: The affected extremity (fingers, toes, nose, ears, feet) develops an itching, burning sensation. Later red and swollen. Blisters may form and break. If not treated can turn to frostbite.

Hypothyroidism 339: Children: goitre, mental and physical retardation, apathetic, undemanding child, puffy hands and feet, coarsening of the face, dry skin becoming wrinkled, flat nose, pot-belly, sensitivity to cold weather, scanty hair, subnormal temperature of 35·5°C, 96°F or less. Adults: apathy, slower thinking process, slow heartbeat, obesity, drowsiness, puffy hands and face especially around the eyes, dry, cool, sandpapery skin, dull, falling hair, gravel voice, heavy menstrual bleeding, sensitivity to cold, subnormal temperature of 35·5°C, 96°F or less. (Enlarged heart.)

Adrenal insufficiency (Addison's disease) 344: Mental and nervous disorders, weakness, fainting, dizziness, vomiting, craving for salt, abdominal pain, weight loss, black freckles, bronzing and/or piebald skin, dehydration, loss of pubic hair, intolerance for cold.

Slow clotting of blood

Purpura 328: Crops on the body of tiny red spots first turning purple, later becoming black-and-blue marks. Bleeding of the mouth and mucous membranes at the slightest injury. Pain in abdomen and joints. Slow clotting of the blood.

Haemophilia 329: Hard to control or uncontrollable bleeding from a small cut or wound. Deformity and painful swelling of the joints.

Spastic gait

A stiff movement with toes dragging and seeming to catch together.

Multiple sclerosis 6: Tremor of hands, tingling of extremities, problems with bladder control, poor attention span and judgement, impaired vision, difficulty in speech, spastic gait.

Spasticity

Muscular dystrophy 405: Infants: difficulty walking or standing, waddling gait, frequent falling, loss of muscular control of the face which becomes mask-like. Later, loss of control strikes the pelvis and the legs.

Cerebral palsy 406: Infants: twitching limbs and muscles, loss of muscle control, spasticity, loss of normal balance, lack of alertness, partial paralysis of the face, difficulty swallowing, high-pitched crying, susceptibility to infection, vomiting, jaundice, slow development.

Subnormal temperature

Low temperature, often as low as 35°C, 95°F, can persist for several days following recovery from a serious infection such as pneumonia. However, a marked drop in temperature in a very sick person is a very grave indication. A low temperature is also a characteristic sign of several poisons which affect heat regulation of the body such as barbiturates, morphine, opium, alcohol, chlorpromazine (a tranquillizer), and some anaesthetics. Subnormal temperature is also significant as a sign of shock after severe injury and after major surgery, and is often noted in persons having acute pancreatitis or a gastric ulcer.

Hypothyroidism 339: Children: occasional goitre, mental and physical retardation, apathy, puffy feet and hands, coarsening of the face, short stocky body, flat nose, pot-belly, temperature 35·5°C, 96°F or less. Adults: mental apathy, slower thinking process, slow pulse, obesity, puffy hands and face (especially around eyes), gravel voice, heavy menstrual bleeding. Temperature 35·5°C, 96°F or less. (Enlarged heart.)

Sweating

Sweating is a normal function when due to excessive heat or strenuous exercise. It can also be a manifestation of anxiety, fear, or great emotion and is then often confined to the palms, soles, and armpits. Foul-smelling sweat is caused by bacteria. *Sweating, Sweating and headache, Profuse sweating, Profuse sweating and fever, Drenching night sweats*

Sweating

Motion sickness 61: Nausea, vomiting, and greenish pallor.

Asthma 108: Gaspy, wheezing breathing, face pale or flushed and often cyanotic. Later, coughing with profuse, tenacious phlegm.

Coronary thrombosis (heart attack) 125: Severe, crushing pain or pressure in the chest, shortness of breath, pallor, fear of impending death, cold sweats.

Rheumatic heart disease and rheumatic fever 127: Sweating is a characteristic symptom. Also inflamed joints, rapid heartbeat, St Vitus's dance (in age levels of ten to thirteen years), failure to gain weight, malaise, easily fatigued, red or purple spots over the body.

Postgastrectomy syndrome 161: Symptoms appear fifteen minutes after meals. Sweating, palpitation, dizziness, ranging from light-headedness to fainting, explosive diarrhoea.

Staphylococcus gastroenteritis 164: Stomach cramps within 2–4 hours after eating contaminated food. Nausea, vomiting, diarrhoea, excessive salivation. In severe cases, blood and mucus in the stools, prostration and shock.

Kidney stones 202: Excruciating intermittent kidney pain which may radiate to the groin, blood in the urine, chills, vomiting, sweating and shock.

Painful menstruation 220: Malaise, sweating, mild to severe lower abdominal cramps, low backache.

Osteomyelitis 265: Intense pain in the affected bone or joint, very high fever, sweating, overlying muscle is swollen, rigid, painful, and festering.

Cystic fibrosis 407: Infants, children: ravenous appetite, emaciation, bulky, greasy, foul-smelling stools, protruding stomach, cough, rapid breathing.

Sweating and headache

Cluster headache 13c: Throbbing headache pain radiating to either eye, to the nose, mouth, or neck. Pallor. Prominence of blood vessels on affected side.

Menopause 221: Hot flushes, chills, sweating, frequent urination, headache, dizzy spells, anxiety, depression, dyspepsia.

Acromegaly and gigantism 336: In growing children gigantism produces enlarged skeletons and abnormal tallness. In adults acromegaly will cause an overgrowth of various parts of the body including the internal organs, coarse face, large, stubby hands and feet, low, husky voice, severe headaches, excessive sweating, and joint pains.

Flu 376: Flushed face, chills, high fever, severe headaches, aches in muscles and joints, prostration from weakness and extreme fatigue.

Profuse sweating

Oedema of the lungs 116: Breathing is

difficult, laboured and rapid. Asthmatic wheezing, bloody cough, cyanosis, anxiety, oppression in the chest.

Massive haemorhhage in peptic ulcer 159: Vomiting with considerable blood, blood persistently present in the stools, collapse, profuse sweating, shock symptoms.

Heat exhaustion 313b: Headache, dizziness, heavy sweating but temperature only slightly raised, nausea, faintness, vertigo, but skin cool and moist.

Diabetes (insulin shock) 332: Weakness, trembling, profuse sweating, hunger. If severe, fainting and coma.

Hypoglycaemia 333: Weakness, dizziness, palpitations, shaking, profuse sweating, blurring of vision, headache, poor concentration, irrational or psychotic behaviour, blackouts, coma.

Hyperthyroidism 340: Profuse sweating, hot, moist skin, great weakness, irritability, and nervousness, increase of appetite but loss of weight. Bulging or staring eyes, overactive, overheated body, palpitation, scanty menstruation, enlarged thyroid gland. (High basal metabolism.)

Phaeochromocytoma 346: Severe pounding headache, pallor, profuse sweating, palpitation, flushing, tingling in the extremities.

Profuse sweating and fever

Pneumonia 109: Severe, shaking chills, high fever, pain in the chest, painful cough, rusty phlegm, rapid breathing and rapid pulse.

Lung abscess 115: Painful cough with phlegm, repeated severe chills, high fever, great malaise, breathlessness on exertion, and weight loss.

Empyaema 119: Pain in the chest, short, dry cough, chills, cheeks flushed but rest of face and body quite pale, foul breath, emaciation and clubbing of the fingers.

Blood poisoning 360: Shaking chills, irregular fever, severe headache, periods of profuse sweating, rash, purple haemorrhagic spots under the skin, extreme diarrhoea, collapse.

Relapsing fever 369: Chills, very high fever, intense headache. Recurrent attacks of the disease, rapid heartbeat, muscle and joint pain, profuse sweating.

Malaria 381: Teeth-chattering chills, high fever, soaking sweats, severe headache, vomiting, diarrhoea, rapid pulse, rapid breathing.

Trichinosis 386: High fever, profuse sweating, swelling around the eyes and forehead, pain and swelling in the muscles, diarrhoea. In severe cases, breathlessness.

Typhus 392: Ten day high fever (profuse sweating when fever breaks), severe headache, mottled rash with small haemorrhagic purple spots, contracted pupils, highly coloured, scanty urine, twitching muscles, stupor, delirium, coma.

Drenching night sweats

Pulmonary tuberculosis 112: Drenching sweats at night. Cough producing a bloody phlegm can wax and wane, deep fatigue, loss of weight and appetite. Pain in chest, loss of vital capacity, fever mostly in the morning.

Lung abscess 115: Drenching sweats at night, repeated attacks of severe chills, high fever, painful cough with blood-stained, foul, and purulent phlegm, great malaise, shortness of breath on exertion, weakness and weight loss.

Tuberculosis of the joints and bones 264: Swelling of the joints (no pain). If in the leg, weakness, stiffness, limping; if in the back, rigid spine, postural change, fever, and night sweats.

Histoplasmosis 393: Ulceration on ear, nose, or pharynx, diarrhoea, black stools, enlarged lymph nodes, emaciation. The disease can simulate tuberculosis with cough, bloody phlegm, loss of weight, drenching sweats, extreme fatigue.

Lung cancer 411: May start with a mild cough, wheezing, shortness of breath becoming worse, pain in the chest behind the breastbone may be stabbing or dull. Later, cough becomes persistent and hacking. Loss of weight, hoarseness and night sweats. Coughing up blood is usually a late sign but in some cases, can show up as a first sign.

Leukaemia 415: Prolonged general bleeding from gums, nose, skin (small red-purplish spots). Great fatigue and pallor, anaemia, pain in the joints. Children: (acute) sore throat, rapid pulse, bruised body appearance. Adults (chronic) characteristic enlarged lymph nodes, night sweats, nervousness, weight loss.

Swelling (oedema)

General swelling over the body is usually a sign of kidney trouble, whether directly or indirectly, from some other ailment affecting the kidneys. If no other symptoms are observable, the kidneys should be suspect.

Swelling, general body, Swelling, specific parts of the body

Swelling, general body

Premenstrual tension 219: Irritability, nervousness, variable headache, pain in the breast, puffiness, especially around the abdomen.

Contraception (the 'pill') 233: Varying general puffiness over the body, sore breasts, vaginal bleeding, dizziness, nausea, and vomiting.

Toxaemia of pregnancy (preeclampsia) 246: Large gain in weight (about 700gm, 1½lb per week), severe, persistent headaches, visual disturbances, dizziness, vomiting, jaundice, drowsiness, amnesia.

Anaphylactic shock 292: Giant rash and swelling all over the body, obstructed breathing, rapid pulse, shock.

Vitamin B$_1$ (thiamine) deficiency 349: Loss of appetite and weight, prickling and numbness in hands, legs, and feet, alarming palpitations, difficulty breathing, swelling and fluid in the tissues, emotional instability.

Swelling, specific parts of the body

Heart failure 126: Growing shortness of breath upon exertion, paroxysm of rapid and slow breathing, wheezing, dry cough, swelling around legs and ankles, very rapid heartbeat on slight exertion, prominent jugular vein.

Cirrhosis of the liver 191: Nausea, vomiting, flatulence, loss of weight. Later, severe jaundice, emaciation, abdominal distension (ascites), red spots on body with red lines radiating out (spider angiomas), puffiness in the feet and legs, general bleeding, bleeding into the faeces. In men, enlarged breasts, atrophy of the testicles, loss of pubic hair, and impotence.

Acute nephritis 197: Low output of urine with blood (and albumin), swelling of face, ankles, headache, sharp loss of appetite, vomiting, furred tongue. (Rise in blood pressure.)

Chronic nephritis 198: Excessive late night urination, blood in urine, puffiness of face and ankles, great distension of abdomen, poor vision from bleeding into retina, anaemia, shortness of breath on slight exertion. (Rise in blood pressure.)

Nephrosis 199: Mostly in children: swelling all over the body called dropsy, resulting from fluids collecting in the tissues. Extreme puffiness of face, abdomen distended to twice normal size, swelling of ankles and feet, anaemia, great pallor, great weakness.

Sickle cell anaemia 325: Severe anaemic symptoms, severe general pain, arthritic pains, jaundice, poor physical development – long arms and legs, short trunk. Infants: painful swelling of the hands and feet.

Bilharziasis 383: Abdominal pains, skin rash, swelling of face, limbs, and genitalia, anaemia, chronic fatigue.

Bone cancer 418: Pain in the affected bone, often with swelling around it.

Swelling of the lymph nodes (glands)

Lymph nodes are located in the neck, under the arms (axilla), and in the groin,

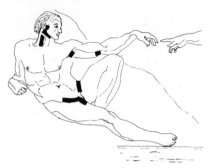

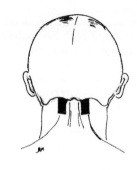

Lymph nodes: major areas. (*Julian A. Miller*)

where they act as filter traps for bacteria to arrest infection.
Swelling of the lymph nodes, Painful swelling of the lymph nodes

Swelling of the lymph nodes

Early syphilis 209: Secondary stage: from one to six months after the infection a widespread varying rash appears. Mouth ulcers, arthritic pains, sore throat, and severe headache. The lymph nodes become enlarged all over the body.

Serum sickness 288: Swelling of lymph nodes, particularly those near injection site. Itching wheals, inflamed joints. Fever occurs in some cases, and may range from mild to high.

Lice infestation 310: Severe itching, tiny red bite marks, occasionally lymph nodes become swollen, small wheals. Lice can be seen; nits are attached to hair or clothing.

African sleeping sickness 384: Weight loss, lethargy, coma, skin eruptions, muscle tremors, weakness, swelling of all lymph nodes.

Toxoplasmosis 385: Chills, high fever, all lymph nodes are swollen, severe headache.

Histoplasmosis 393: Ulcerations on ear, nose, pharynx, vomiting, diarrhoea, black stools, emaciation. In chronic form will simulate tuberculosis with cough, bloody phlegm, loss of weight, drenching sweats, extreme fatigue.

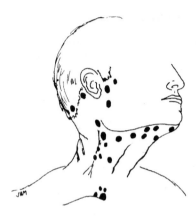

Lymph nodes: head and neck. (*Julian A. Miller*)

Malignant tumours of the nervous system 413: Infants, children: rapid weight loss, distension of abdomen, loss of strength, anaemia, discoloration around eyes, bone pain. Lymph node enlargement may be the first symptom.

Leukaemia 415: General bleeding all over the body from the gums, skin (pinpoint red spots), nose, and elsewhere. Anaemia, great pallor, fatigue, malaise, feverish periods, pain in the joints. Children: (acute form) sore throat, rapid pulse, bruised body appearance. Adults: (chronic form) characteristic enlarged lymph nodes, night sweats and weight loss.

Hodgkin's disease and other lymphomas 416: Swollen but painless lymph nodes, starting in the neck (often as large as an orange). If only on one side of the neck, Hodgkin's; if on both sides, other lymphoma. Later, all body lymph nodes are affected. Also itching, weight loss, anaemia, weakness, leg swelling, difficulty breathing, recurrent fever.

Painful swelling of the lymph nodes

Erysipelas 300: Raised rash on the body ranging in colour from dull red to scarlet with advancing margins, chills, high fever, intense headache, swollen face, painful swollen lymph nodes.

Lymphangitis 330: Red streaks or lines going upwards on arms or legs, swelling of the lymph nodes, chills, high fever, pain all over body, headache.

Lymphadenitis 331: Enlarged, painful lymph nodes, tender red skin over infected node which may abscess.

Infectious mononucleosis 377: Fever, sore throat, headache, painful swelling of all the lymph nodes, weakness, fatigue, occasional jaundice.

Thirst

Excessive thirst, Excessive thirst with excessive urination

Excessive thirst

Acute gastritis (erosive) 155: Severe stomach pains, collapse, vomiting of blood, blood in stools, stomach rigid and tender, excessive thirst.

Intestinal obstruction 170: Pain around the navel, constipation, vomiting, abdominal distension. In persistent, severe cases, dehydration, total suppression of the urine, thirst, anxiety, shock.

Peritonitis 179: Extreme abdominal pain, rigidity and distension, hiccups, dehydration, persistent vomiting. Patient is very ill and anxious.

Anaemia 322: Anaemic symptoms, excessive thirst, jaundice, burning, red tongue, numbness of limbs, poor memory, palpitation, vertigo, fingernails longitudinally ridged and spoon-shaped, shock.

Cholera 364: Constant diarrhoea, voluminous, watery stools, massive dehydration, severe cramps in stomach and legs, intense thirst, violent vomiting, sunken eyes.

Bacillary dysentery 366: Constant diarrhoea, blood and mucus in stools, severe cramps in stomach, dehydration, urgency but difficulty defecating, nausea, vomiting.

Cancer of the oesophagus 429: Difficulty swallowing, distress in chest, heavy salivation, cough, foul breath, loss of voice, flatulence, thirst, emaciation.

Excessive thirst with excessive urination

Diabetes 332: Excessive urination, thirst and hunger. Weight loss, weakness, sweet, fruity breath, blurred vision, pins-and-needles sensation and cramps in the legs, skin and vaginal infections, impotence. In ketoacidosis complication (diabetic shock), breathing is deep and rapid, severe dehydration, dizziness, poor skin tone, nausea and vomiting, abdominal pain, sunken eyeballs, great thirst, stupor, shock and coma.

Diabetes insipidus 338: Cardinal symptom is massive urination, up to several gallons daily causing nocturia (night awakening), severe dehydration, and thirst.

Primary aldosteronism 345: Excessive urination, thirst, fatigue, muscle weakness, numbness and tingling in different parts of the body. (High blood pressure.)

*

Tremors
also see **Twitching**

A tremor is an involuntary trembling or quivering of a limb or other part of the body. Transient tremors are of no medical significance occurring in healthy persons as a result of anxiety, cold, extreme fatigue, old age, physical exertion that is prolonged or violent, excitement, and of course, fear.

Alcoholism is a familiar cause characterized by rapid coarse movements involving the head, fingers, arms, hands, or tongue. Tremors may be even more manifest on the morning after a drinking spree.

Anxiety and hysteria can produce a fine, rapid tremor plus other signs of emotional or mental stress such as rapid heartbeat or palpitations, and sweating.

Drugs such as morphine and cocaine will induce rapid tremor of face and fingers most especially on withdrawal. Other drugs such as barbiturates (taken over a long period of time) and bromides (consistent users), mercury poisoning and tetraethyl lead (an additive of petrol) will cause some condition of tremors.

Parkinson's disease 1: Coarse tremors present during rest, diminishing upon movement. Mask-like face, spastic gait.

Multiple sclerosis 6: Intention tremor, general tremor worsening into weakness and paralysis, tremors of the hand, spastic walk. Disturbances of vision, paralysis or palsy of the eyeball, speech impairment, monotone voice.

Diabetes (insulin shock) 332: Weakness, confusion, nervousness, trembling, sweating, hunger. When severe, fainting and coma.

Hypoglycaemia 333: Weakness, dizziness, palpitation, sweating, blurring of vision, headaches, poor concentration, irrational or psychotic behaviour, blackouts, convulsions, coma.

Hyperthyroidism 340: Bulging eyeballs, goitre, tremor of the fingers, rapid heartbeat, profuse sweating, vomiting, diarrhoea, skin eruptions, emaciation, nervous irritability, anaemia. (Increased metabolism.)

Pheochromocytoma 346: Recurrent pounding headache, profuse sweating, pallor, tremors. (High blood pressure.)

Twitching

also see **Tremors** *and* **Convulsions**, p51 and p58

Twitching is a sudden involuntary contraction of a muscle. Compare with tremor, which is a movement of a limb or part of the body

Neuralgia (tic douloureux) 4: Pains running from forehead to the lips, nose, tongue, or gums.

Tics 11: Jerking of thigh, shrugging of shoulders, grimacing, eye blinking, pulling corners of the mouth, swallowing, clearing of the throat, head shaking.

Rheumatic heart disease and rheumatic fever 127: Inflammation of the joints, especially around the ankles, wrists, and knees, rapid heartbeat. St Vitus's dance, malaise, pallor, sweating, failure of growing child to gain weight, skin rash, and loss of appetite. In severe cases, shortness of breath, cough, and chest pains.

Uraemia 207: Severe headache, contracted pupils may herald coma, urinous odour on breath, urea frost, drowsiness, double vision, nausea, vomiting, diarrhoea, swelling, puffiness of the face.

All-vegetarian diet deficiency 355: Anaemia, palpitation, twitching, inflammation of the tongue, various nerve disorders.

Salt deficiency 356: Stomach cramps, loss of skin elasticity, sharp drop in urinary output, twitching, very faint, rapid pulse; finally, convulsions.

Polio 374: High fever, severe headache, sore throat, stiff neck. In serious cases, prostration, painful, twitching muscles, extreme weakness, difficulty swallowing, paralysis in different parts of the body.

Typhus 392: Ten day high fever, severe headache, prostration, mottled rash over the body with small red spots which turn purple, contracted pupils, furry, white tongue, flushed face, profuse sweating when fever breaks. Stupor and coma.

Cerebral palsy 406: Infants: twitching of limbs and muscles, loss of muscle control, loss of sense of balance, lack of alertness, partial paralysis of face, difficulty swallowing, high-pitched crying, vomiting, susceptibility to infections, general spasticity, jaundice, slow development.

Urea frost

White flaky deposits of urea seen on the skin.

Uraemia 207: Severe headache, contracted pupils may herald coma, urinous odour on breath, drowsiness, double vision, nausea, vomiting, diarrhoea, swelling of different parts of the body and especially puffiness of the face.

Weakness

Weakness, Severe weakness, Severe weakness and shortness of breath

Weakness

Rapid heartbeat 130a: Nausea, pallor. In extreme cases, fainting and shock.

High blood pressure 138: Weakness is a late symptom, as are dizziness, headache, shortness of breath.

Acute yellow atrophy 193: High fever, severe headache, jaundice, weakness, severe abdominal pains, black vomiting, apathy, confusion, bleeding under the skin and from the mouth, dilated pupils, scanty, bloody urine, foul breath, rapid, feeble pulse.

Diabetes 332: Excessive thirst, urination, hunger. Weight loss, sweet, fruity breath, blurred vision, skin and/or vaginal infections, pins-and-needles sensation and cramps in the legs, impotency.

Vitamin B$_2$ (riboflavin) deficiency 350: Cracks at the corners of the mouth, impaired vision, burning sensation in the conjunctiva, photophobia, cloudy or ulcerated cornea.

Vitamin B complex (niacin) deficiency (pellagra) 351: Loss of appetite and weight, red spots on the body turning brown and scaly, tongue margins scarlet, mucous membrane and gums inflamed and scarlet, excessive salivation, diarrhoea later becoming bloody, poor memory and emotional instability.

Vitamin C deficiency (scurvy) 352: Bleeding gums and mucous membrane, bleeding under the skin, loose teeth, easily broken bones, skin rash. In infants, loss of appetite and weight, irritability, severe pains in the legs and swollen gums.

Vitamin D deficiency 353a: Infants: restlessness, softening and thinning of head bones, bow legs, cannot walk or stand at usual age, badly formed teeth. Older infants, children: scoliosis, lordosis. Adults: progressive weakness, rheumatic pains in the spine, limbs, pelvis.

Vitamin D toxicity 353b: Loss of appetite and weight, nausea, excess urination, yellow deposits under the skin, kidney failure.

Infectious mononucleosis 377: Feeling unwell for weeks or months, low daily fever, daily, recurrent headaches, sore throat. Major symptom: painful swelling of the lymph nodes under the jaw; also swelling of the lymph nodes under the arm (axilla) and in the groin.

Severe weakness

Diabetes (insulin shock) 332: Besides weakness, trembling, hunger, and sweating. In severe cases, fainting, convulsions, and coma.

Hypoglycaemia 333: Severe weakness, palpitation, dizziness, trembling, blurring of vision, headache, inability to concentrate, blackouts and coma.

Hyperthyroidism 340: Goitre, heavy heartbeat, profuse sweating, hot, moist skin, extreme weakness, increased appetite but loss of weight, irritability and nervousness, bulging eyes, overactivity, overheated body.

Polio 374: High fever, severe headache, sore throat and very stiff neck. In serious cases, severe weakness, prostration, twitching, painful muscles, paralysis in different parts of the body, difficulty swallowing.

Flu 376: Chills, high fever, severe head pains, back and muscle aches. Great weakness and prostration. Excessive fatigue and sweating, dry or hacking cough, cold symptoms, flushed face. Intestinal flu has in addition diarrhoea and vomiting.

Amoebic dysentery 382: Run-down body, severe diarrhoea, bloody, purulent stools, abdominal pain on the right side, weight loss, prostration.

Malignant tumours of the nervous system 413: Infants, children: rapid weight loss, distension of the abdomen, anaemia, great loss of strength, discoloration around the eyes, swelling of the lymph nodes, bone pain.

Cancer of the gallbladder 432: Pain in the upper right abdomen near the centre, jaundice, weight loss; possibly vomiting, increasing weakness.

Severe weakness and shortness of breath

Atelectasis 114: Severe weakness and considerable shortness of breath, cyanosis, pain on one side of the chest, rapid heartbeat, shock.

Coccidioidomycosis 394: Pain in lungs, cough (often with blood). In progressive form great weakness, loss of weight, cyanosis, shortness of breath.

*

Weight gain

Toxaemia of pregnancy (preeclampsia) 246: Puffiness of the body, severe headache, visual disturbances, drowsiness, dizziness, vomiting, pain in the abdomen.

Hypothyroidism 339: In the adult version: goitre, mental apathy, slower thinking process, slow heartbeat, obesity, drowsiness, puffiness of hands and face (especially around the eyes), dry, cool, sandpapery skin, gravel voice, sensitivity to cold, heavy menstrual periods, dull, falling hair. (Low basal metabolism and enlarged heart.)

Cushing's disease 343: Weight gain especially on trunk, back, and face (moon face), excessive hair growth, acne, easy bruising, loss of menstrual periods, muscle weakness, bones fracture easily.

Obesity 347: (Weight gain of over twenty per cent of normal.) In severe cases, aching back and feet, shortness of breath.

Weight loss

Loss of weight is always a serious symptom; it is one of the chief indications of cancer and other grave disorders. Unexplained loss of weight requires the immediate attention of a doctor.

Although not listed below, cancer of the cervix, ovary, and uterus, as well as metastatic cancer, are all characterized by weight loss.

Weight loss, Weight loss and anaemia (see Anaemia with weight loss, *p30, and* Anaemia with weight loss and swollen lymph nodes, *p31), Weight loss and loss of appetite (see* Loss of appetite and weight loss, *p42, and* Loss of appetite, weight loss, and pain in the chest, *p42), Weight loss and jaundice, Weight loss and weakness or fatigue, Rapid weight loss*

Weight loss

Zenker's diverticulum of the oesophagus 145: Chief complaint is difficulty in swallowing which cuts down intake of food with consequent weight loss. Regurgitation and night cough.

Ulcer of the oesophagus 147: Radiating pain under the breastbone, heartburn, belching, diarrhoea.

Hypertrophic pyloric stenosis 169: Infants: projectile vomiting, constipation, dehydration, lump in abdomen.

Cystic fibrosis 407: Infants, children: slow development, failure to gain weight, emaciation, ravenous appetite, protruding stomach, bulky, greasy, foul-smelling stools, chronic cough, rapid breathing, very salty sweat.

Lung cancer 411: Early major symptoms are chronic bloody cough, wheezing breath, hoarseness, persistent fever, pain in the chest, night sweats, and shortness of breath.

Cancer of the thyroid 417: Nodule (growth) in the thyroid gland. Later, hoarseness, difficulty breathing and swallowing, sensation of fullness in the neck, vocal paralysis, weight loss.

Cancer of the cervix 421: Irregular menstruation, bloody discharge from vagina, bleeding after intercourse or after exertion. Later, yellowish discharge, pain in lower back, urinary aberrations, vomiting, constipation, weight loss.

Weight loss and jaundice

Chronic relapsing pancreatitis 167: Considerable weight loss after a while, mild to raging pain high in the abdomen, nausea and vomiting, occasional jaundice, fatty, frothy, foul stools, fast pulse.

Cirrhosis of the liver 191: Jaundice, abdominal distention, enlarged veins on the abdomen, red dots on skin with red lines radiating out, foetid breath, emaciation, haemorrhoids. In men, enlarged breasts, atrophy of testes, loss of pubic hair, impotence.

Pernicious anaemia 323: Anaemic symptoms, palpitations, general pain, pins-and-needles sensation in hands, feet, and elsewhere, sore, red tongue, jaundice, difficulty in walking, impotence, frigidity.

Cancer of the pancreas 431: Boring pain in the upper abdomen extending to the back, jaundice, brown urine, clay-coloured stools, weight loss, indigestion.

Cancer of the gallbladder 432: Pain in the upper right abdomen towards centre, jaundice, occasional vomiting, progressive weakness.

Cancer of the liver 433: Nausea, vomiting, pressure in the abdomen, dull ache in liver area, anaemia, jaundice, constipation.

Weight loss and weakness or fatigue

Lung abscess 115: Repeated severe chills, high fever, painful cough, drenching sweats, great malaise, phlegm blood-stained and particularly foul, shortness of breath on exertion, weakness.

Regional enteritis 168: Anaemia, malnutrition, migratory arthritis, abscesses around anus, mid-abdominal cramps.

Diabetes 332: Excessive urination, thirst, hunger. Weight loss, weakness, sweet, fruity breath, blurred vision, red, sore, dry tongue, impotence, tingling sensation in extremities.

Hyperthyroidism 340: Goitre, heavy heartbeat, profuse sweating, great weakness, hot moist skin, increased appetite but loss of weight, bulging eyes, over-activity, overheated body, nervousness and irritability.

Amoebic dysentery 382: Run-down body, severe diarrhoea, bloody purulent stools, abdominal pain on the right side, prostration.

Roundworm 388: Vague colicky pain in the abdomen, malnutrition, fatigue.

Histoplasmosis 393: Ulceration on ear, nose, pharynx; black stools, diarrhoea, vomiting, emaciation, swollen lymph nodes. In severe cases it mimics tuberculosis with bloody phlegm, loss of weight, cough, extreme fatigue, drenching sweats.

Coccidioidomycosis 394: Pain in the lungs, cough (often with blood). In the progressive form, great weakness, weight loss, cyanosis, shortness of breath.

Hodgkin's disease and other lymphomas 416: Painless enlarged lymph nodes growing to any size, anaemia, backache, swollen legs, difficulty breathing and swallowing. Later, severe general itching, weakness, weight loss and recurrent fever.

Stomach cancer 430: Heartburn, abdominal distension, rapid satiation at meals, quick fatigue, sudden distaste for certain foods (particularly meat), gradual weight loss and anaemia. Often the first sign is sudden pain, vomiting of blood and black, tarry stools.

Rapid weight loss

Morning sickness (pregnancy) 243: Nausea, vomiting. In extreme cases, severe loss of weight, jaundice, rapid heartbeat.

Malignant tumours of the nervous system 413: Infants, children: rapid loss of weight, distension of the stomach, anaemia, discoloration around the eyes, swelling of the lymph nodes, bone pain.

Cancer of the oesophagus 429: Difficulty swallowing, distress or pain in the chest, heavy salivation, cough, loss of voice, rapid weight loss, emaciation, flatulence, thirst, foul breath.

Symptoms of the brain and nervous system

Anxiety

Anxiety, Anxiety and pallor or cyanosis

Anxiety

Anxiety is most often an expression of tension ranging in intensity from uneasiness to panic. It is abnormal when it does not relate to a real situation. It is by far the most common of all emotional reactions in response to pressure. In a small percentage of cases, anxiety is a symptom of disease, as indicated below.

Hyperventilation 121: Oppression in the heart area causing anxiety, palpitation, fainting, numbness or coldness in the extremities.

Cardiac neurosis 144: Vague or stabbing pains in the chest, shortness of breath, great anxiety and fatigue.

Intestinal obstruction 170: Pain around the navel, vomiting, constipation, abdominal distension. In severe, persistent cases, dehydration, thirst, high fever, total suppression of urine. The patient presents an anxious face and sunken features.

Menopause 221: Depression and anxiety, hot flushes, sweating, frequent urination, headaches, dizzy spells, dyspepsia, irregular periods.

Impotence 257: Anxiety is the major cause and symptom. Possibly prostatitis and inflammation of the testes.

Tetanus 361: Stiffness of the jaw and neck, restlessness and apprehension, difficulty swallowing. Later jaw and neck are fixed and immovable, perpetual grin, body racked by agonizing muscle spasms.

Anxiety and pallor or cyanosis

Laryngotracheobronchitis 107: Children: begins with cold symptoms followed by gasping breath, croupy cough with tenacious phlegm, hoarseness, high fever, cyanosis, fear and anxiety.

Lung abscess 115: Patient is anxious, pale, sweating with a sense of oppression; breathing is laboured, rapid, asthmatic. Also cyanosis, cough with bloodstained phlegm and cold extremities.

Coronary thrombosis 125: Crushing pain in the chest, cold sweat, extreme anxiety.

Shock 133: Great pallor, cold clammy skin, cyanosis (lips, nails, fingertips), shortness of breath, sunken eyes, fast, weak pulse, anxiety state, coma.

*

Attention span, limited

Minimal brain dysfunction 404: Visual perception errors, learning disabilities, disorders of attention span, lack of concentration, hyperactivity, restlessness, emotional instability, poor coordination and occasional loss of sense of balance.

Coma

also see **Fainting**

Coma is a state of unconsciousness from which the patient cannot be roused.
Coma, Coma preceded by stupor or convulsions

Coma

Epilepsy (grand mal) 2a: Nausea, ringing in the ears, flashing lights before the eyes, loss of consciousness, contracted muscles, clenched fists, eyeballs rolled upwards, twitching of muscles and limbs, foaming at the mouth and deep coma.

Brain tumours 9: Coma is a late development. Earlier there are headaches and vomiting.

Shock 133: Great pallor, cold, clammy skin, cyanosis of the lips, nails, and fingertips, fast, weak pulse, shortness of breath, sunken eyes, dilated pupils, anxiety state, finally coma.

Stroke 139: Paralysis, coma, with stertorous breathing, loss of speech, equilibrium, sense, and memory, confusion, impairment of mental abilities. In grave cases, recurrent coma, continuous high fever, fast pulse and rapid breathing.

Acute yellow atrophy 193: Jaundice, black vomiting, severe headache, emotional instability, confusion, bleeding under the skin, severe abdominal pain, scanty, bloody urine, coma.

The plague 365: Onset is sudden. Chills, very high fever, rapid heartbeat, stupor, prostration. Important sign is buboes (inflamed lymph nodes varying in size from a crab apple to an apple) in the groin and under the arms. These may suppurate and drain. Minute bleeding points under the skin which turn black. Final stages: shock and coma.

Rabies 378: Healed bite remains reddened. Depression, irritability changing to excitability, wildness. Swallowing becomes impossible. There is drooling, collapse and finally coma.

Coma preceded by stupor or convulsions

Brain injury (concussion) 10: Bleeding from the mouth, nose, and ears. Dilated pupils, pale, clammy skin, drowsiness, dizziness, headache. If severe, vomiting, pupils of unequal size and coma.

Uraemia 207: Scanty urine, severe headache, impaired vision, contracted pupils, urinous breath odour, urea frost over body, swelling face, ankles, abdomen, vomiting, convulsions, diarrhoea.

Toxaemia of pregnancy (eclampsia) 246: Twitching, violent convulsions, coma.

Diabetes (ketoacidosis, diabetic coma) 332: Rapid, hungry breathing, nausea and vomiting, severe dehydration, abdominal pain, poor skin tone, sunken eyes. Eventually stupor, shock, coma. In insulin shock: weakness, trembling, sweating, hunger. If severe, fainting and coma.

Hypoglycaemia 333: Weakness, dizziness, palpitation, shaking, sweating, blurring, headache, poor concentration, irrational or psychotic behaviour, blackouts, convulsions, coma.

Typhus 392: High fever, severe headaches, prostration, mottled rash with small red spots turning purple, contracted pupils, scanty urine, tremors, stupor, delirium, coma. When fever breaks, profuse sweating.

*

Concentration lack

Minimal brain dysfunction 404: Visual perception errors, learning disabilities, attention span disorders, hyperactivity, restlessness, emotional instability, poor coordination and occasional loss of sense of balance.

Confusion

Stroke 139: Paralysis, coma, stertorous breathing, loss of speech, memory, and equilibrium, impairment of mental abilities. In grave cases recurrent coma, continuous high fever, fast pulse, and rapid breathing.

Acute yellow atrophy 193: Jaundice, black vomiting, severe headache, emotional instability, bleeding under the skin, severe abdominal pain, scanty, bloody urine and coma.

Pernicious anaemia 323: Anaemic symptoms (pallor, weakness, shortness of breath), palpitations, nosebleeds, numbness, sore, red tongue, appetite loss, weight loss, yellow-lemony skin colour. In severe cases, cardiac failure, difficulty walking, and impotence or frigidity.

Diabetes (insulin shock) 332: Weakness, trembling, sweating, hunger. In severe cases, fainting and coma.

Convulsions

Convulsions, Convulsions and headache

Convulsions

Epilepsy (grand mal) 2a: When in convulsions, hands are clenched, arms and legs jerking, muscles twitching, face darkened, incontinence, then deep coma. In non-epileptic seizure, patient does not fall but staggers, making purposeless movements, unintelligible sounds, displaying confusion.

Rheumatic heart disease and rheumatic fever 127: Most common in children aged 10–13 years. Attacks of chorea last six to eight weeks and can recur often (nervous muscular twitching, jerking of limbs, grimacing). Other symptoms are inflammation of the joints, rapid pulse, sweating.

Acute kidney failure 208: Convulsions without warning, very scanty urine, breathing difficulties, lethargy or drowsiness, dry skin, dry mucous membrane, odour of urine in the breath, twitching, nausea, vomiting, diarrhoea.

Toxaemia of pregnancy (eclampsia) 246: Convulsions is a late and ominous symptom, twitching and coma, cyanosis.

Salt deficiency 356: Loss of skin elasticity, stomach cramps, drop in urinary output, twitching muscles, faint, rapid pulse, finally, convulsions.

Tetanus 361: Stiffness of the jaw and neck, apprehension, restlessness, yawning, difficulty swallowing. Later, fixed jaw and neck, perpetual grinning appearance, agonizing muscle spasms in the neck and elsewhere.

Mental retardation 403: Abnormalities occurring during labour and delivery, abnormal size of head, jaundice, low birth weight. In infancy, lethargy, lack of alertness or responsiveness to the environment. Slow development in feeding skills and other normal development.

Cerebral palsy 406: Infants: high-pitched crying, jaundice, lack of alertness, difficulty in movement, lack of muscular control, tremors and twitching.

Convulsions and headache

Meningitis 7: Convulsions in children, overwhelming headache radiating to the neck, stiff, painful neck, intolerance for light or sound, delirium, maybe small irregular red or purple spots all over the body, vomiting.

Brain tumours 9: Severe headaches, vomiting, dizziness, convulsions. Later, mental deterioration.

Uraemia 207: Convulsions without warning, very scanty urine, severe headaches, impaired vision, contracted pupils, odour of urine on the breath, urea frosts on the body, swelling of face, ankles, and abdomen, nausea and vomiting, diarrhoea, coma.

Hypoglycaemia 333: Weakness, palpitation, shaking, dizziness, sweating, blurring of vision, headache, inability to concentrate, irrational or psychotic behaviour, blackouts, convulsions, and finally, coma.

Smallpox 373: Begins with high fever, violent frontal headaches, intense muscular pain, large crop of small reddish spots over the body, becoming pimply, turning to blisters then foul-smelling crusts. Convulsions occur in children.

*

Delirium

Delirium is always serious. All infections with sustained high fever, all infections of the nervous system (some of which are listed below), and all cerebral disorders (from brain tumour to senile dementia) can cause this symptom.

Withdrawal from a drug habit and the following drugs can induce disordered mental function: arsenic, lead, belladonna, quinine, camphor, bromides, as well as overdosing with insulin, mushroom poisoning, and a bite from some insect, spider, or snake.

Alcoholism is the most common malady that will incite delirium. The 'DTs' (delirium tremens) of the alcoholic is well known. Other symptoms of delirium tremens are great confusion, the 'shakes' (tremors) and terrifying visual hallucinations – all of which can last for several hours or days.

Meningitis 7: Overwhelming radiating headache, stiff, painful neck, red or purple spots all over the body, photophobia, high fever, and often delirium.

Encephalitis 8: High temperatures up to 42°C, 108°F, severe pounding, unremitting headache, stiff neck, vomiting. Delirium is common.

Hypoxia 122: Headache, palpitations, blueness of the lips, shortness of breath. Concentration and judgement are impaired. Delirium is a frequent occurrence.

Sunstroke 313a: Headache, dizziness, collapse, pulse as high as 160 per minute, respiration very rapid, skin flushed, hot, and dry, extremely high temperature, convulsions, delirium, coma.

Typhoid fever 363: Frontal and bitemporal headaches for a week, fever mounting to 40·5°C, 105°F, semi-consciousness, delirium, nosebleeds, rosy spots on the trunk and abdomen, distension of the abdomen, slow pulse, white-coated tongue with reddened edges, and constipation giving way to bloody diarrhoea.

Typhus 392: Ten day high fever, severe headache, prostration, mottled rash over body with small red spots turning purple, contracted pupils, highly coloured, scanty urine, tremor, flushed face, stupor, delirium, coma. Profuse sweating when fever breaks.

Depression

Depression is normal when it is a response to failure or a result of genuine grief in reaction to a real situation. However, when the depression is out of proportion to the reality, or when there is no cause at all, it is a destructive emotion.

Depression afflicts a large number of middle-aged people and does them considerable mischief: it impairs mental acuity, lowers sexual libido, causes indigestion, fatigue, and headaches. In women, it can even inhibit menstruation. But worst of all, it lowers resistance, making the subject susceptible to every kind of disease.

There are many diseases which by their chronicity or by their continuous distress will produce a persistent depression, especially gastrointestinal disorders such as *Chronic gastritis* **156**.

Motion sickness 61: This transient disorder is always marked by severe depression in no way commensurate with the degree of seriousness of the disease.

Dizziness (vertigo)

Vertigo is not only a distressing sign of disorder but also a serious one. For the high-strung personality this symptom can be quite catastrophic.

Almost all cases of vertigo are due to some disturbance or disorder of the balancing mechanism situated in the inner ear. Thus, dizziness can be produced by any ear disorder, such as *Wax in the ear* **51**, *Perforation of the eardrum* **56**, *Blockage of the ear canal or eustachian tube* **57**, all forms of *Otitis media* **58**, and *Ménière's syndrome* **60**.

Eyestrain and glaucoma will occasionally cause dizziness.

Poisoning from overdose, or from sensitivity to the following drugs will occasion loss of equilibrium: alcohol, salicylates, quinine, medication designed to lower high blood pressure, opium, and nicotine. Infectious diseases such as flu, diphtheria, typhoid, encephalitis, syphilis, even measles and mumps, may have vertigo as a symptom.

High or low blood pressure, heart failure, stroke, and senility are frequent causes of dizziness. Both forms of epilepsy can often induce severe vertigo. *Dizziness, Dizziness on changing position, Dizziness and headache, Dizziness and severe headache, Dizziness and vomiting*

Dizziness

Angina pectoris 124: Major symptom is intense pain or distress radiating from the heart towards the shoulder, arm or jaw and lasting a few minutes, accompanied by pallor, palpitation and dizziness. There may be shortness of breath and sweating.

Stroke 139: Loss of equilibrium is common in strokes along with severe vertigo, confusion, paralysis, impairment of vision.

Late syphilis (tabes dorsalis) 210: Loss of balance when eyes are closed, episodic 'lightning pains' and spasms in various parts of the body, throat and stomach pains.

Anaemia 322: Symptoms of anaemia, palpitations, flabby or red and burning tongue, noises in the head. In severe cases, jaundice, dizzy spells, numbness of the limbs, excessive thirst, fingernails longitudinally ridged, poor memory and shock.

Haemolytic anaemia 324: All the anaemic symptoms (pallor, fatigue, breathlessness), jaundice, dizziness, fainting, weak, rapid pulse, rapid breathing, chills, fever, ache in the extremities and in the abdomen.

Hypoglycaemia 333: Weakness, dizziness, palpitations, shaking, sweating, blurring of vision, headache, inability to concentrate, irrational or psychotic behaviour, blackouts, convulsions, finally, coma.

Minimal brain dysfunction 404: Children: lowered mental ability, impaired judgement, stuttering, hyperactive, restlessness, emotional instability, occasional loss of balance.

Muscular dystrophy 405: Infants: difficulty standing or walking, weakness in legs, waddling gait, loss of muscle control in face causing expressionless face, then loss in pelvis and legs.

Dizziness on changing position

Some people experience a drop in blood pressure when changing from a recumbent position to an erect one causing a transient giddiness or dizziness. Dizziness can also occur in old age with a sudden head movement, particularly when looking upwards.

In the absence of other significant signs or diseases, this condition is generally benign.

Heart block 134: Getting out of bed, jumping up from a seat, or any sudden change of position can cause a syndrome of dizziness and fainting. Other symptoms of heart block are palpitation, an occasional missed beat, and a fluttering in the chest.

Dizziness and headache

Brain injury 10: Dilated pupils, headache, bleeding from mouth, nose, and ears, pale clammy skin. In more serious cases, vomiting, loss of balance, drowsiness, unequal pupils.

Hypoxia 122: Difficulty concentrating, poor judgement, shortness of breath on exertion, headache, lassitude, dizzy spells, cyanosis of the lips, palpitation, nausea, euphoria.

High blood pressure 138: No symptoms early in the disease; later, throbbing headache, increasing fatigue, dizziness. Some random symptoms are nosebleeds, bloodshot eyes, rapid pulse.

Menopause 221: Hot flushes, sweating, frequent urination, headaches, dizzy spells, depression, anxiety, dyspepsia, irregular periods.

Sunstroke 313a: Headache, dizziness, very high temperature but no sweating, skin flushed, dry, and very hot, very rapid pulse, rapid breathing.

Heat exhaustion 313b: Headache, dizziness, profuse sweating, skin cool, moist, temperature normal or slightly raised, nausea, faintness.

Polycythaemia 327: Bluish-red skin, often with cyanosis of lips and fingernail beds, dizziness, constant dull headaches, fatigue, ringing in the ears (tinnitus), breathlessness, itching, bleeding in gastrointestinal tract causing bloody or tarry stools.

Hypoglycaemia 333: Palpitation, blurring, sweating, inability to concentrate, irrational or psychotic behaviour and blackout. In severe cases, convulsions and coma.

Brain cancer 412: Headache, vomiting, disturbances of vision, loss of balance. Any symptom possible such as weakness of muscle, hallucination, lethargy, obtuseness, psychotic episodes, etc.

Dizziness with severe headache

Brain tumours 9: Slow progressive disturbance of balance, sight, and smell, unexplained weakness in the muscles of the extremities. Later, constant, severe headache, vomiting, convulsions, impairment of mental function.

Migraine headache 13b: Deep, intense headache, pain radiating to and from the eye, nausea, vomiting, photophobia, intolerance for loud sounds, disturbances of vision, dizzy spells.

Toxaemia of pregnancy (preeclampsia) 246: Puffiness of the body, large gain in weight, severe, persistent headaches, visual disturbances, vomiting, amnesia, drowsiness, pain in the abdomen, jaundice.

Dizziness and vomiting

Ménière's syndrome 60: Loss of balance and severe vertigo, noises in ear, increasing deafness, nausea, vomiting, inability to place a finger on an indicated part of the body.

Motion sickness 61: Vomiting, greenish pallor, dizziness.

Botulism 165: Symptoms appear from 18 to 36 hours after eating contaminated food. Fatigue, blurred sight, double vision, dry mouth, speaking and swallowing become difficult, weakening of the muscles (especially of the trunk) causing difficulty breathing. There may be nausea, cramps, diarrhoea and dilated, fixed pupils.

Contraception (the 'pill') 233: Nausea, vomiting, sore breasts, vaginal bleeding, dizzy spells, varying general puffiness over the body.

Diabetes (diabetic coma, ketoacidosis) 332: Breathing is rapid, deep, hungry. Severe dehydration, dizziness, poor skin tone, nausea and vomiting, abdominal pain, sunken eyeballs, stupor, shock, finally, coma.

Adrenal insufficiency (Addison's disease) 344: Bronzing skin, dizziness, freckles, piebald spots, intolerance for cold, dehydration, easily fatigued, weight loss, vomiting, craving for salt, abdominal pains, fainting, nervous and mental disorders, loss of hair.

Cerebral palsy 406: Infants, children: twitching muscles, tremor of limbs, loss of equilibrium, spasticity, lack of muscle control, lack of alertness, partial paralysis of the face, difficulty swallowing, vomiting, jaundice, convulsions, and susceptibility to infections.

*

Drowsiness

also see **Stupor**

Drowsiness is actually a milder form of stupor when it is due to illness. Often these two terms are used interchangeably.

Uraemia 207: Very scanty urine, severe headache, impaired vision, contraction of pupils, odour of urine on breath, urea frost on body, swelling of face, ankles, and abdomen, vomiting, diarrhoea, convulsions, drowsiness deepening into coma.

Acute kidney failure 208: Scanty urine, breathing difficulties, lethargy, odour of urine on breath, dry skin, twitching, vomiting, diarrhoea, drowsiness, convulsions.

Detection of pregnancy 234: Missed period, larger, fuller breasts, larger, darker, more sensitive nipples, frequent urination, drowsiness in the first few months.

Toxaemia of pregnancy (preeclampsia) 246: Puffiness of the body, large gain in weight, severe, persistent headache, visual disturbances, amnesia, drowsiness to stupor, vomiting, abdominal pain, frequently jaundice.

Anaemia 322: Anaemic symptoms, palpitation, vertigo, noises in the ear, flabby or sore, burning tongue. In severe cases, jaundice, numbness of the limbs, thirst, poor memory, nails longitudinally ridged and spoon-shaped, drowsiness, shock.

Hypothyroidism 339: Adults: apathy, slowed mentality, skin dry and rough, puffy eyelids, weak muscles, slow pulse, slow reflexes, dull, brittle hair, low, husky voice, subnormal temperature (35·5°C, 96°F or less). Patient is usually obese.

Brain cancer 412: Headache, vomiting, muscle weakness, failing vision, loss of sense of balance and coordination, changes in personality, drowsiness, lethargy, and disorderly conduct.

Emotional instability

Menopause 221: In some women no symptoms at all, but for most, hot flushes, chills, sweating, headache, fatigue, frequent urination, giddiness, palpitation, insomnia, loss of appetite, dyspepsia, nausea, nervousness, emotional instability, crying bouts, and periods of depression and anxiety.

Hypoglycaemia 333: Weakness, palpitation, dizziness, shaking, sweating, blurring of vision, headache, inability to concentrate, irrational or psychotic behaviour, blackouts, convulsions, finally, coma.

Vitamin B₁ (thiamine) deficiency (beriberi) 349: Loss of appetite, weight, prickling numbness in hands, legs, and feet. Palpitations, rapid heartbeat, difficulty breathing, swelling in the tissues due to presence of excess fluid.

Vitamin B complex (niacin) deficiency (pellagra) 351: Loss of appetite and weight, weakness, red spots on body which turn brown, large, and scaly. The tongue margins, gums, and mucous membranes become inflamed and scarlet. Excessive salivation, diarrhoea later becoming bloody. Poor memory and emotional instability.

Rabies 378: Healed bite remains reddened, depression, irritability, changing to excitability and wildness, swallowing becomes impossible, collapse, coma.

Minimal brain dysfunction 404: Children: lowered mental ability, stuttering, restlessness, hyperactivity, poor coordination.

Brain cancer 412: Headache, vomiting, failing vision. Any symptom is possible: one-sided muscular weakness, loss of balance, clouding of consciousness, lethargy, obtuseness, disordered personality, psychotic episodes.

Euphoria

Euphoria can be induced by alcohol and various drugs, but most of the time this state of exaggerated and unwarranted elation and well-being is due to mental disorders or disturbance of the brain, as in boxers who are punch-drunk.

Multiple sclerosis 6: Mood often ranging from apathy to euphoria, spastic gait, tremor of the hands, impairment of vision, speech difficulties, poor bladder control.

Hypoxia 122: Headache, blueness of the lips, shortness of breath, rapid heartbeat, restlessness, impairment of concentration and judgement, euphoria or delirium.

Fainting

Fainting is a transient form of unconsciousness from which the patient can be roused, as opposed to coma. Fainting is fairly common, particularly in susceptible people; women, for example, tend to faint more readily than men. Often this symptom may be due to minor conditions such as prolonged standing, high, humid temperature, long hours of work, lack of sleep, overheated, poorly ventilated rooms, abrupt changes in altitude (rapid descent or ascent), and fatiguing exertion.

Pain can induce fainting, as can early pregnancy, blood loss, or a sharp blow in the testicles, solar plexus, or knee cap. Many drugs can cause fainting: most blood-pressure-lowering medications, an overdosage of insulin, phenacetin (used in headache preparations), diuretics, and procaine.
Fainting, Fainting preceded by dizziness

Fainting

Hyperventilation 121: A fainting attack is usually preceded by a feeling of oppression in the heart, a fast heartbeat, rapid, deep breathing, and numbness or coldness in the extremities.
Slow heartbeat 130: If very slow can cause fainting.
Rapid heartbeat 130a: Fainting in extreme cases only. Other signs are palpitation, nausea, pallor, weakness.
Inguinal hernia (groin) 255: (Strangulated form of hernia only.) Sudden bulge in the groin, severe abdominal pain, collapse, fainting.
Physical allergy 290: Frequently there is strong reaction to cold water when swimming, causing large hives, rapid pulse, loss of consciousness.

Fainting preceded by dizziness

Heart block 134: A sudden change of position such as jumping out of bed or bending down suddenly can cause dizziness and fainting.
Stroke 139: Paralysis of limbs or eyeball on one side of the body, loss of equilibrium, confusion, severe headache, impairment of vision, fainting.
Haemolytic anaemia 324: All the anaemic symptoms (pallor, breathlessness, fatigue), jaundice, dizziness, faint-ing, weak, rapid pulse, rapid breathing, chills, fever, ache in the extremities and abdomen.
Hypoglycaemia 333: Weakness, dizziness, palpitations, shaking, sweating, headaches, blurring, poor concentration, irrational or psychotic behaviour, blackouts, convulsions, coma.
Adrenal insufficiency (Addison's disease) 344: Weakness, bronzing or piebald skin, black freckles, abdominal pain, vomiting, craving for salt, intolerance for cold, dehydration, dizziness, fainting, mental and nervous disorders, weight loss, loss of pubic hair.
*

Hyperactivity

Hyperthyroidism 340: Goitre, rapid heartbeat, profuse sweating, hot, moist skin, weakness, nervousness, irritability, increased appetite but loss of weight, bulging eyes, overactivity, overheated body.
Minimal brain dysfunction 404: Children: lowered mental ability, stuttering, restlessness, poor coordination, emotional instability, overactiveness.

Insomnia

The failure to obtain a normal amount of sleep is due to a multitude of causes. Normal hours of sleep vary, ranging from nine to six hours or even less. The average is eight. A teenager needs nine hours; a child of twelve, ten; a child of four, twelve; a year old infant, fifteen; at age six months, eighteen, and at one month, twenty-one hours.

Most people underestimate the amount of sleep they have had, often saying they didn't sleep a wink when in fact they have slept for hours with intervals of wakefulness.

A primary cause of insomnia is discomfort and pain from disease such as shortness of breath, gastrointestinal disorders, diseases of the heart and kidneys, the anaemias and more commonly from high blood pressure.

Anxiety is probably the most common

basis for sleeplessness. Excitement and depression will also produce insomnia.

Some comparatively minor faulty habits will induce insomnia such as sleeping in a stuffy, airless, noisy room, overheating the bedroom, insufficient or too many bedclothes, going to bed after a very heavy meal, drinking coffee or tea before bedtime, and fatigue, especially extreme fatigue.

Certain medications, particularly ephedrine and amphetamines, will prevent a full night's sleep.

In infants: the causes are indigestion, discomfort, hunger, and teething.

In children: the same as in infants. Some diseases (encephalitis for example) will often cause reversal of rhythm; insomnia at night and somnolence during the day.

Irritability

Irritability when induced by fatigue or by frustration and failure is within the environs of normal behaviour; almost any form of mental disorder can produce irritability as one of its symptoms. Also, almost any distressing disease will incur irritability. However, in the following disorders irritability is a characteristic of the disease rather than a result of it.

Premenstrual tension 219: Nervousness, variable headache, pain in the breasts and puffiness, especially around the abdomen.

Menopause 221: For most women, hot flushes, chills, headache, fatigue, frequent urination, giddiness, palpitation, insomnia, loss of appetite, dyspepsia, irritability, cyring bouts and periods of depression and anxiety.

Anaemia 322: Irritability is a specific sign in infants besides pallor, breathlessness, and fatigue.

Vitamin A toxicity 348b: Loss of appetite, falling hair, pain in the joints, severe pressure headaches, retarded growth in children, irritability.

Vitamin C deficiency (scurvy) 352: Weakness, bleeding from gums, mucous membranes and under the skin, loose teeth, easily broken bones, skin rash.

Infants: loss of appetite, irritability, swollen and very painful joints.

Tetanus 361: First real sign is stiffness of the jaw, difficulty opening the mouth and swallowing. Restlessness, apprehension, muscle stiffness and spasms, persistent fixed grin and yawning.

Rabies 378: There is first depression, irritability, then excitability and wildness. Swallowing becomes impossible, drooling, collapse, coma.

Colic 401: Infants: excessive, prolonged crying, fretfulness, vomiting and diarrhoea, passage of gas, distended stomach.

Learning disability

Minimal brain dysfunction 404: Visual perception errors, attention span disorders, hyperactivity, restlessness, emotional instability, poor coordination and occasional loss of balance.

Cystic fibrosis 407: Failure to grow normally, ravenous appetite, greasy, foul-smelling stools, chronic cough, rapid respiration, wheezing, running nose, irritability, and thin, protuberant abdomen.

Lethargy

Lethargy, Lethargy and mental impairment

Lethargy

Lethargy is often the beginning of stupor, as is noted in *Brain tumours 9*, in *Brain injury* **10**, and in *Brain cancer* **412**; but often it is a sign of chronic fatigue or state of weakness after a prolonged illness.

Encephalitis 8: High fever (up to 42°C, 108°F), stiff neck, severe headache, vomiting, lethargy, delirium.

Shock 133: Great pallor, cold, clammy skin, cyanosis of the lips, fingernails and fingertips, sunken eyeballs, fast, weak pulse, anxiety and coma.

Vitamin C deficiency 352: (Extreme form is scurvy.) Weakness, easily fatigued, lethargy, bleeding of the gums, under the skin, and from the mucous membranes,

Symptoms of the brain and nervous system

loose teeth and fragile bones. Infants: loss of appetite, failure to gain weight, swollen gums, painful, swollen feet, and pain in the bones.

German measles 371: Slight sore throat, light, rosy-coloured rash over the body, swollen lymph nodes under the jaw, in neck. Adults: lassitude, stiffness of joints.

Infectious mononucleosis 377: Feeling unwell for weeks or months, low daily fever, daily recurrent headaches, sore throat. Major symptom is painful swelling of the lymph nodes under the jaw, and in the axilla and groin.

Cerebral palsy 406: Infants: general spasticity, twitching of muscles, loss of muscle control, loss of balance, lack of alertness, partial paralysis of the face, difficulty swallowing, vomiting, susceptibility to infections, jaundice.

Lethargy and mental impairment

Multiple sclerosis 6: Apathy or euphoria, tremor of the hands, spastic gait, impairment of vision and judgement, speech difficulties.

Hypothyroidism 339: Children: possible goitre, physical and mental retardation, apathy, 'good', undemanding behaviour, puffy hands and feet, coarsened face, dry, wrinkled skin, flat nose, pot-belly, scanty hair, subnormal temperature.

Mental retardation 403: Infants: abnormal size of head at birth, jaundice, low birth weight. The infant is lethargic and develops slowly.

Brain cancer 412: Headache, vomiting, muscle weakness, failing vision, loss of balance and coordination, personality changes, drowsiness, lethargy, and disorderly conduct.

Memory impairment

The causes of memory loss are multifold, ranging from inattention to brain degeneration. Inattention can be due to anxiety, lack of interest, hearing difficulties, or a psychotic condition. Head injuries can engender a mild to extensive amnesia, often not dependent on the severity of the injury. Serious infections (most especially meningitis and encephalitis), including pneumonia, typhoid, malaria, and blood poisoning, can ravage the retentive faculty.

Mental fatigue, drugs (habitual use of barbiturates, cocaine, bromides, as well as intoxication with quinine, scopolamine and overdosage with vitamins A and D), cerebral arteriosclerosis, and any mental disorder can also cause considerable impairment of the memory.

Brain tumours 9: Prolonged severe headaches, persistent nausea, vomiting, dizziness, convulsions, hallucinations, deterioration of mental faculties, memory loss, disorders of personality.

Heart failure 126: A late development is impairment of mental faculties, judgement and memory. Other symptoms include severe shortness of breath, prominent neck veins, swollen ankles.

Stroke 139: Confusion, memory loss, paralysis, severe headache, impaired vision.

Late syphilis (paresis) 210: Severe headache, first memory degeneration then degeneration of all mental faculties, growing slovenliness, tremors of lips and tongue, premature senility.

Toxaemia of pregnancy (preeclampsia) 246: Body puffiness, weight gain, severe headache, dizziness, vomiting, pain in abdomen, amnesia, drowsiness, jaundice.

Anaemia 322: Anaemic symptoms, palpitations. In severe cases numbness of the limbs, jaundice, excessive thirst, vertigo, memory loss, red, sore tongue, shock.

Vitamin B complex (niacin) deficiency (pellagra) 351: Loss of appetite and weight, weakness, red spots on the body which become large, brown, and scaly. The tongue margins, gums, and mucous membranes become inflamed and scarlet. Excessive salivation, diarrhoea later turning bloody. Poor memory and emotional instability.

65

Mental ability impairment

Most mental impairment is genetic or congenital but a few instances are brought on by disease. In the case of a child, suspicion is usually aroused when his rate of development is below average – his learning to talk or walk lags far behind that of other children. Mental impairment is usually attended by an unstable disposition.

Mental ability impairment, Mental ability impairment and headache

Mental ability impairment

Multiple sclerosis 6: Poor attention span, speech difficulties, impaired judgement, impaired vision, tremor of the hands, tingling in the extremities, spastic gait.

Adenoiditis 71: Breathing through the mouth, nasal speech, decreased mental ability.

Heart failure 126: A late development is impairment of judgement, mental faculties, and memory. Other symptoms include severe shortness of breath, prominent neck veins, swelling of the ankles.

Stroke 139: Paralysis, impairment of vision, clouding of the mind, loss of equilibrium, and deterioration of personal habits.

Late syphilis (paresis) 210: Severe headache, growing slovenliness, failing memory, severe degeneration of the mind, tremors of lip and tongue, early senility.

Hypothyroidism 339: Children: physical and mental retardation (cretin), short, stocky body, coarse face, broad, flat nose, pot-belly, skin rough and dry. 'Good', undemanding child, occasional goitre. Low temperature. Adults: mental apathy, skin dry and rough, puffy eyelids, weak muscles, slow pulse, slow reflexes, occasional goitre. Weight gain.

Mental retardation 403: Infants: lethargy, slow development, abnormal head size at birth, low birth weight.

Minimal brain dysfunction 404: Stuttering, hyperactivity, emotional instability, poor coordination, lowered mental ability.

Mental ability impairment and headache

Brain tumours 9: Severe headaches, vomiting, nausea, dizziness, convulsions, lethargy. Diminished mental acuity is a late development.

Hypoxia 122: Impairment of concentration and judgement, shortness of breath on exertion, headache, giddiness, cyanosis of the lips, palpitations, nausea.

Hypoglycaemia 333: Weakness, dizziness, palpitation, shaking, sweating, headache, blurring of vision, inability to concentrate, bizarre behaviour, blackouts, coma.

Acromegaly and gigantism 336: In growing children gigantism produces enlarged skeleton and abnormal tallness. In adults acromegaly will cause an enlargement of hands and feet, overgrowth of internal organs, low, husky voice, joint pains, enlarged coarsened face, protruding jaw, severe headache, excessive sweating, and mental deterioration.

*

Nervousness

In disorders such as *Brain tumours* **9** and *Stroke* **139**, nervousness is a symptom of fear and uneasiness.

Multiple sclerosis 6: Poor attention span, speech difficulties, impaired vision, tremor of the hands, tingling of extremities, spastic gait, general nervousness.

High blood pressure 138: Nervousness is a later development as is headache, dizziness, and fatigue. There are rarely any early signs.

Stroke 139: Paralysis of limb and eyeball, confusion, severe headache, agitation.

Premenstrual tension 219: Nervousness, mild to severe headaches, puffiness, especially of the abdomen, pain in the breasts.

Menopause 221: Hot flushes, anxiety, nervousness, sweating, frequent urination, headaches, dizzy spells, dyspepsia, irregular periods.

Diabetes (insulin shock) 332: Weakness, trembling, profuse sweating, agitation, confusion, hunger. If severe, fainting and coma.

Hyperthyroidism 340: Goitre, rapid heartbeat, profuse sweating, hot, moist skin, increased appetite but loss of weight, bulging eyes, severe weakness, overactivity, and overheated body.

Adrenal insufficiency (Addison's disease) 344: Easy fatigue, bronzing and/or piebald skin, black freckles, vomiting, abdominal pain, craving for salt, nervous and mental disorders, intolerance for cold, dehydration, fainting, dizziness, loss of pubic hair.

Paralysis

Stroke 139: Often one whole side of the body, but more often affects only the leg or the arm. Confusion, loss of speech and memory, disturbances of vision, vomiting, severe headaches, dizziness.

Botulism 165: Paralysis is a symptom in the final stages of the disease.

Allergic drug reactions 289: Some muscle relaxing drugs can occasion prolonged paralysis and inhibition of breathing.

Diphtheria 358: Grey false membrane in the throat, high fever, foul breath, vomiting. In extreme cases, closure of the throat, paralysis of the palate and larynx.

Polio 374: In serious cases, stiff neck, prostration from extreme weakness, painful, twitching muscles, high fever, paralysis in different parts of the body.

Personality changes

Multiple sclerosis 6: Poor attention span, speech difficulties, impaired vision, tremor of the hands, spastic gait.

Brain tumours 9: Mental deterioration is a late symptom, as are severe headache, nausea, vomiting, dizziness, convulsions, lethargy and drowsiness.

Late syphilis (paresis) 210: Development of slovenly habits, failing memory, degeneration of mental acuity, tremor of lips and tongue, premature senility.

Brain cancer 412: Headache, vomiting, muscle weakness, failing vision, loss of balance and coordination, personality changes, drowsiness, lethargy, and disorderly conduct.

Restlessness

Hypoxia 122: Shortness of breath on exertion, night blindness, cyanosis of the lips, giddiness, palpitation, headache, difficulty in concentration, poor judgement, restlessness and nausea.

Coronary thrombosis 125: Crushing pain in the chest, pallor, cold sweat, great anxiety, extreme restlessness.

Anaemia 322: Considerable weakness, palpitations, flabby, red, or sore tongue. In severe cases, jaundice, numbness of limbs, extreme pallor, thirst, poor memory, longitudinally ridged fingernails, restlessness.

Vitamin D deficiency 353a: Infants: restlessness, softening and thinning of the head bones, bow-legs, badly formed teeth, infant cannot sit, stand, nor walk at the proper age. Children: scoliosis and lordosis. Adults: rheumatic pain in the pelvis, limbs, spine, progressive weakness.

Tetanus 361: Stiffness in jaw and neck, apprehension, yawning, restlessness, difficulty swallowing, fixed and frozen jaw, perpetual grin, agonizing muscular spasms.

Pinworm 389: Worms in the stools are visible to the naked eye. Also, restlessness, disturbed sleep, painful anal scratching, poor appetite, failure to gain weight.

Minimal brain dysfunction 404: Children: lowered mental ability, stuttering, hyperactiveness, emotional instability, poor coordination, restlessness.

Shock

Shock is a syndrome of symptoms which may result from a massive haemorrhage, severe trauma, surgery, dehydration, heart attack, serious infections, poisoning, and reaction to various drugs. *Shock* is described in **133** as characterized by great pallor, very dry mouth, cold, clammy skin, cyanosis of the lips, nails, fingertips, and earlobes. The pulse is rapid and weak, and there is shortness of breath. Anxiety which may turn to expressionless apathy is usual. Pupils may be dilated. Thirst may be extreme. If not promptly treated the patient will become comatose and may die.

Shock, Shock and severe shortness of breath, Shock and vomiting

Shock

Rapid heartbeat (tachycardia) 130a: In extreme cases, nausea, weakness, pallor and shock.

Stroke 139: Paralysis, loss of equilibrium, headache, disturbances of mind and vision, shock and coma.

Anaemia 322: Anaemia symptoms. In severe cases, shock, jaundice, numbness of the limbs, excessive thirst, palpitations, and burning, red tongue.

The plague 365: Sudden onset. Chills, high fever, rapid pulse, stupor, prostration. Important sign is development of buboes in the groin and axilla (inflamed lymph nodes ranging from crab apple to apple size). These may suppurate and drain. Minute bleeding spots under the skin which turn black. Final stages are shock and coma.

Shock and severe shortness of breath

Atelectasis 114: Severe shortness of breath, weakness, cyanosis, pain on one side of the chest. Shock is frequent.

Pneumothorax (spontaneous) 120: Sharp pleuritic pain on the affected side, severe shortness of breath, cyanosis, prostration and shock.

Pulmonary embolism 140: Acute shortness of breath, pain in lung, cyanosis, bloody phlegm and shock.

Rupture and/or foreign body in the oesophagus 153: Severe chest pains, breathlessness, and shock.

Anaphylactic shock 292: Giant hives all over the body, body swelling, obstructed breathing, rapid pulse and shock.

Diabetes (ketoacidosis, diabetic coma) 332: Severe dehydration, shortness of breath, nausea, vomiting, dizziness, and abdominal pain. Eventually shock, stupor, and coma.

Shock and vomiting

Massive haemorrhage in peptic ulcer 159: Profuse blood in vomit as well as in the stools, collapse, heavy sweating, shock symptoms.

Infected food gastroenteritis 163: In milder form nausea, vomiting, cramps and diarrhoea; in severe form additionally kidney failure, dehydration, and shock.

Staphylococcus gastroenteritis 164: Reaction occurs two or four hours after eating. Severe cases produce prostration and shock with blood and mucus in stools. Vomiting, cramps, diarrhoea, and excessive salivation.

Acute pancreatitis 166: Writhing pain high in the abdomen, vomiting, feeble, rapid pulse, cyanosis, shock.

Intestinal obstruction 170: Persistent obstruction will cause pain around navel, vomiting, constipation, abdominal distention, dehydration, and thirst. Anxiety, sunken features, and total suppression of urine, finally, shock.

Peritonitis 179: Pain severe enough to cause shock, distended abdomen, acute nausea, rigid abdominal wall, persistent vomiting, fever, sunken eyes, hollow cheeks, and anxiety.

Kidney stones 202: Excruciating spasmodic pain in the kidneys, radiating to the groin. Nausea, vomiting, sweating, chills, occasionally blood in the urine.

*

Stupor
also see **Drowsiness**

Encephalitis 8: Stiff neck, severe headache, vomiting, very high fever, delirium, persistent hiccups.

Brain injury 10: Bleeding from mouth,

nose, and ears, dilated pupils, skin pale and clammy, giddiness, headache. In severe cases, vomiting, pupils of unequal size, stupor, coma.

Toxic hepatitis 189: Nausea, vomiting, collapse, diarrhoea. Always jaundice. In more severe cases, apathy, stupor, and coma.

Diabetes (ketoacidosis, diabetic coma) 332: Breathing is rapid, deep, and hungry. Severe dehydration, dizziness, poor skin tone, nausea, vomiting, abdominal pain, sunken eyeballs, stupor, shock, and finally, coma.

Typhoid fever 363: Severe sustained frontal and temporal headache, sustained and very high fever, distended stomach, rosy spots on abdomen disappearing in few days, diarrhoea, nosebleeds, slow double heartbeat.

The plague 365: Chills and very high fever, rapid pulse, buboes (large egg-sized lymph nodes in the groin which may suppurate and burst), black skin spots; finally, coma.

African sleeping sickness 384: Enlarged lymph nodes, weight loss, skin eruptions, tremors, weakness, stupor and coma.

Typhus 392: High fever, severe headache, prostration, bloodshot eyes, flushed face, body rash with pinpoint bleeding in the centre of spots, which turn purple. Rapid, weak pulse, stupor which may change to coma, muscular twitching, and highly coloured, scanty urine.

Brain cancer 412: Headache, vomiting, faulty vision, one-sided weakness, loss of balance, visual hallucinations, cloudy consciousness, obtuse, and disordered conduct.

Visual perception, lacking

Minimal brain dysfunction 404: Visual perception errors, learning disabilities, attention span disorders, lack of concentration, hyperactivity, restlessness, emotional instability, poor coordination and occasional loss of balance.

Cerebral palsy 406: Infants: twitching of the limbs and muscles, loss of muscle control, spasticity, loss of sense of balance, lack of alertness, partial paralysis of the face, difficulty swallowing, susceptibility to infections. In the ataxic form, lack of depth perception.

Symptoms of the face and head

THE FACE

Adenoidal face (adenoidal facies) (dull, lethargic, open-mouthed)

Adenoiditis 71: Breathing through mouth, nasal speech, nasal obstruction, lowered mental ability, snoring, dull, lethargic appearance.

Blisters or ulcerations on the face

Congenital syphilis 211: Infants: blisters on face and buttocks, also on soles and palms, nose sniffles, curved shinbone, symptoms of meningitis. Later, saddle-backed nose and deformed teeth.

Histoplasmosis 393: Ulcers on the ear, nose, legs, pharynx, larynx, and extremities. Irregular fever, emaciation, anaemia, swollen lymph nodes. Nausea, vomiting, diarrhoea with black stools, debilitation.

Coarsening of the face

Acromegaly and gigantism 336: In growing children gigantism produces abnormal tallness; in adults acromegaly will cause increased size of face, hands, and feet, overgrowth of internal organs, sweating, severe headache, joint pains, protruding jaw, loss of libido, mental deterioration.

Hypothyroidism 339: Children: goitre, mental and physical retardation, apathy, puffy hands and face, grossness of features, dry, wrinkled skin, flat nose, pot-belly, cold intolerance and low body temperature, scanty hair.

Elfin features of the face

Vitamin D toxicity 353b: Infants: physical and mental retardation as well as possible elfin features.

Flushing

Empyaema 119: Pain in the chest, short, dry cough, chills, fever, sweating, cheeks flushed but rest of face and body pale or grey. Foul breath, emaciation, clubbing of the fingers.

Menopause 221: Hot flushes, sweating, frequent urination, headaches, dizzy spells, depression, anxiety, dyspepsia and irregular, fading menstrual periods.

Diabetes (ketoacidosis, diabetic coma) 332: This is a complication of diabetes. Breathing is deep, rapid, and hungry, excessive thirst and urination, severe dehydration, nausea, vomiting, poor skin tone, stupor, shock and finally, coma.

Pheochromocytoma 346: Palpitation, pounding headache, sweating, trembling, nausea and vomiting. (High blood pressure.)

Scarlet fever 359: Flushing except for telltale paleness around mouth, vomiting, high fever, sore throat, white furry tongue turning raspberry, greyish-yellow false membrane forming in mouth, throat. Body rash. Blanching in squeezed spots. Later, skin peels, flakes. Dark red lines appear on skin folds.

Flu 376: Cold symptoms, chills, fever, severe headache, aches in muscles and joints, prostration from weakness, extreme fatigue, sweating.

Yellow fever 379: Fever, prostration, severe headaches, pain in the back and limbs, scanty urine. After the characteristic intermission period, jaundice, vomiting with black blood, bleeding from mucous membranes.

Typhus 392: Ten day high fever, severe headache, prostration, flushed or dusky face, mottled rash on body with small red spots turning purple, contracted pupils, highly coloured, scanty urine, tremors, stupor, delirium, and finally, coma. Profuse sweating when fever breaks.

Grinning (from disease)

Tetanus 361: Stiffness of jaw and neck, restlessness, apprehension, yawning, difficulty swallowing. Later, jaw and neck become fixed, perpetual grin appears, general agonizing muscular spasms.

Immobile face

Parkinson's disease 1: Wide-eyed, unblinking, staring appearance, drooling, slowness, posture is rigid, stooped, slow, shuffling steps, tremor of hands.

Scleroderma 321: The skin swells, becoming mottled, red, and shiny, then hard, rigid, leathery in a process beginning at hands and feet and spreading over the rest of the body. Hands are claw-like, face is mask-like.

Muscular dystrophy 405: Infants: difficulty standing or walking, waddling gait, frequent falls, loss of muscular control.

Hard nodules on the face

Leprosy 368: Red and brown patches with whitish centres appear on the skin. Loss of feeling in these patches as well as elsewhere on the body. Masses of hard nodules particularly on the face but also over the body, atrophy of muscles, open sores, hoarseness, loss of toes and fingers.

Pain in the face

Neuritis (Bell's palsy) 3: Begins with mild ache near the ear which develops into facial paralysis and distortion of the face on the affected side. Eyes cannot close, smiling and speech impeded.

Neuralgia (tic douloureux, trigeminal neuralgia) 4: Lightning-like pain along course of the nerve from any region of the head to lips, nose, tongue or gums which can be triggered off in these areas by a touch, a breath of air, washing or eating.

Cancer of the pharynx (throat) 438: Pain and/or difficulty in eating or swallowing. Pain may radiate to entire side of face, difficulty opening mouth or coughing, lymph nodes in neck may swell. Possibly a visible mass in throat or on back of tongue.

Paralysis of the face

Neuritis (Bell's palsy) 3: Temporary paralysis of face, torturous facial pain, distortion on affected side, eyes cannot close, smiling and speech impeded.

Cerebral palsy 406: Infants: partial paralysis of the face, twitching muscles in the legs, spasticity, loss of muscle control, loss of sense of balance, loss of alertness, difficulty swallowing, jaundice, high-pitched crying and susceptibility to infections.

Puffiness of the face
also see **Swelling**, p49

Any tooth infection such as *Dental caries* **89**, *Pulpitis* **90**, *Tooth abscess* **91** will cause a swelling at the site involved.

Gangrenous stomatitis 81: Grey or black tissues appear on mucous lining of the mouth, cheeks become swollen, red, then black, pain, fever. Always a *Medical Emergency.*

Acute nephritis 197: Puffiness of face and ankles, scanty but bloody urine, severe headache, sudden loss of appetite, nausea, vomiting, furred tongue. (Rise in blood pressure.)

Chronic nephritis 198: Puffiness of face and ankles, distended abdomen, excessive late night urination, bloody urine, breathlessness on slight exertion, impaired vision from bleeding into the retina, anaemia. (Rise in blood pressure.)

Nephrosis 199: Puffiness of face, swelling of ankles and abdomen, anaemia.

Uraemia 207: Puffiness of face, swelling of ankles and abdomen, very scanty urine, severe headaches, convulsions, impaired vision, urinous breath odour, urea frost on body, nausea, vomiting, diarrhoea, and finally, coma.

Erysipelas 300: Swollen face, raised rash with advancing margins, ranging in colour from dull red to scarlet, swollen lymph nodes, chills, high fever, intense headaches.

Hypothyroidism 339: Adults: goitre, mental apathy, thinking process is slowed, slow heart rate, obesity, puffiness of hands and face especially around the eyes, dry, sandpapery skin, gravelly voice, heavy menstrual periods, dull, falling hair, cold intolerance, low body temperature.

Trichinosis 386: Swelling around eyes and forehead, high fever, pain and swelling in the muscles, joint pains, profuse sweating, and diarrhoea. In severe cases, shortness of breath.

Staring appearance

Parkinson's disease 1: The face is immobile, wide-eyed, unblinking, often staring. Mouth is partially open with drooling of saliva, posture rigid and stooped, shuffling walk with body pitched forward, running gait and tremor.

THE HEAD
Bulges in the head

Encephalitis 8: Infants: bulging fontanelles, convulsions, temperature ranging between 41°C, 106°F and 41·5°C, 107°F.

Paget's disease 267: Grotesque enlargement of the head, intermittent, shifting bone pain, spontaneous fractures, impaired hearing.

Headache

The headache is without doubt the most common symptom of man. Almost any body disorder can initiate an attack. A vast number of people express their mental or emotional distress by some form of headache.

Headache symptoms vary widely from moderate and mild to agonizing and unbearable. They can be general or regional, concentrated in the frontal, temporal (one-sided or both), or occipital areas; they can be intermittent, recurrent, penetrating, throbbing, radiating, pressured, and bursting. A disease with a characteristic dull form of headache may develop a severe form and some disorders with known severity of headache may develop only a mild version.

Acute temporary headaches are often due to diseases of the eye, ear, nose, or throat, to acute infections or to injury. Usually other symptoms will dominate the disorder in such cases.

Chronic headaches may be induced by emotional and mental distress, neurotic factors, metabolic diseases, and endocrine ailments. Any form of toxicity will cause headaches such as stale air from inadequate ventilation, fumes of any kind, alcohol, ammonia, barbiturates, benzene, ephedrine, gasoline, kerosene, morphine, nitrous oxide, opium, privine, scopolamine, the sulfa drugs, high doses of vitamin A or D, tetracycline, chlorpromazine (used in tranquillizers), oral contraceptives, and excessive dosage of steroids. (There are 150 other chemicals and medications that can cause headaches.)

Anaemia (due to iron or B$_{12}$ deficiency) as well as hunger and fatigue will produce a headache; the latter can be readily alleviated by food or resting.

The severity of the headache usually does not indicate the severity of the diseases. For example, nothing can be more intense and agonizing than the dismal but not lethal migraine or cluster headache, as opposed to the grave brain tumour headache which, although often severe, can just as often be deceptively mild.

Most headaches are of minor significance; nevertheless, some types of headache are significant of an underlying major disorder. Examples include:
• A severe headache that appears suddenly and without reason, especially in a subject who rarely suffers from this discomfort.
• A headache accompanied by convulsions, confusion, or a drop in mental acuity.
• A headache with pain in a bloodshot eye, or an eye which seems stone-hard, or a headache that is accompanied by seeing coloured halos around lights.
• A headache which awakens one from sleep.
• A headache which worsens every day.
• A throbbing headache in the back of the head which appears on arising and wears off by midday.
• A headache worsened by coughing, bending down or straining.
• A headache accompanied by a fever attributable to no known infection.
• Any of the above symptoms requires consultation with a doctor without delay. They can be indicative of a serious condition.
Chills and fever with headache (see p32), Convulsions and headache (see p58), Dizziness and headache (see p60), Dizziness and severe headache (see p61), Fatigue with headache (see p38), Fever with severe headache, High fever and headache (see p39), Headache in infants and children, Moderate or dull headache, Muscular cramps (aches or spasms) and headache (see p196), Radiating headache, Severe and intermittent headache, Sweating and headache (see p47), Throbbing headache, Variable headache,
Vomiting and headache (see p148), Vomiting and severe headache

Fever and severe headache

Blood poisoning 360: Shaking chills, intense headache, irregular fever. Periods of profuse sweating, severe diarrhoea, small purplish haemorrhagic spots on the skin, collapse.

Typhoid fever 363: Extreme frontal or temporal headache, slow rise to very high fever, slow double pulse rate, nosebleeds, diarrhoea, rosy spots on abdomen.

Relapsing fever 369: Chills, very high fever, constant headache, recurrent attacks of the disease, rapid heartbeat, profuse sweating, muscle and joint pain.

Smallpox 373: High fever, violent frontal headache, intense muscle pain; convulsions may appear in children. Large crop of small reddish spots all over the body becoming pimply then pussy blisters and finally, foul-smelling crusts.

Polio 374: High fever, constant severe headache, stiff neck, sore throat. In serious form, prostration, extreme weakness, acute muscle pain, twitching muscles, paralysis of legs, arms, or other parts of the body.

Flu 376: Flushed face, chills and fever, severe pain in head and back, prostration, excessive fatigue, sweating.

Yellow fever 379: Flushed face, fever, prostration, pain in back and in limbs, scanty urine. Jaundice appears after temporary remission of the disease. Then, vomiting of black blood and bleeding from mucous membranes.

Typhus 392: Very severe headache, ten day high fever, mottled rash with red spots turning purple, contracted pupils, highly coloured, scanty urine, tremors, furry, white tongue, stupor, delirium, coma. Profuse sweating when fever breaks.

Headache in infants and children

Infants express their headaches in a number of ways: by rolling their heads, rubbing hands over the head or over the ear. They are fussy and irritable. If an infant shows any of these particular signs, he is most surely suffering from some headache. Other additional symptoms will help identify the disorder.

The most common headache in children is migraine which is of a paroxysmal nature that does not follow the classic pattern of adults. Second most common headache is tension headache which occasionally occurs in the late afternoon particularly among hard working students. It is of a less intense nature than migraine and is felt at the back of the head or as a tight band about the head. Lying down and massage will relieve it.

Headache is often the only symptom of an underlying disease.

Moderate or dull headache

Brain injury 10: Mild headache, some giddiness, occasionally there is some unconsciousness. (Determination between mild and grave can only be made by a doctor.)

Tension headache 13a: A steady pressing ache, generalized over the top of the head, often throbbing, often feels like a tight hat. Muscles of the jaw and neck, the area in the back of the head and the temples may become tense and tender.

Menstrual headache 13d: General, over the entire head. Pelvic discomfort and general malaise.

Premenstrual headache 13e: General, over the entire head. Appears seven to ten days before the menstrual flow with irritability, volatile emotions, and inability to concentrate. Can hang on until the first day of menstruation.

Postcoital headache 13g: A minor throbbing headache, usually fleeting but can last an hour.

Sinusitis 66: Location of the headache is suggested by the sinus infected (usually frontal). This headache is often worse in the morning and in damp weather. Usually a pressure form of headache with a nasal or postnasal drip. Heavy air

pollution or a smoke-filled room can bring it on. Chills, fever are common.

Menopause 221: Often no symptoms at all but in most women there may be many or all of the following: hot flushes, sweating, fatigue, frequent urination, giddiness, slight puffiness, palpitation, insomnia, nausea, irritability, headaches, crying bouts and periods of depression and anxiety.

Polycythaemia 327: Bluish-red skin often with cyanosis of the lips and fingernail beds, breathlessness, constant dull headache, ringing in the ears (tinnitus), general itching, dizziness, fatigue, bleeding in digestive tract causing bloody or tarry stools.

Radiating headache

Neuralgia (tic douloureux) 4: Extremely intense, jabbing pain radiating from the nose, lips, mouth to the temples or forehead. Although of short duration occurs frequently. Can be triggered by chewing, a touch, or a breath of wind.

Meningitis 7: Headache is intense, usually over the entire head but often occipital, aggravated by the slightest head movement. The headache may radiate to the neck. Stiffness of the neck a cardinal sign, vomiting, high, erratic fever, skin breaks out in small red or purplish spots, intolerance for light and sound, confusion, convulsions, delirium and coma.

Encephalitis 8: (See *Throbbing headache*)

Migraine headache 13b: The patient knows it's coming. Deep intense pain radiating to or from an eye. Disturbances of vision, intolerance for bright lights, intolerance for sounds, nausea, vomiting.

Cluster headache 13c: (See *Severe and throbbing headache*)

Farsightedness 15: Due to eyestrain, the pain is steady but rarely severe, radiating from the eyes to the temples or back of the head. Fatigue will worsen the pain. Mostly farsighted people are affected.

Glaucoma 23a and **23b:** Headache over the forehead radiating to and from the eye. Pain in the eye is very acute. Eyeball is hard. Vomiting. Patient sees coloured halos around lights.

Temporal arteritis 33: Boring, constant headache radiating to an eye; pain in the temple of the affected eye. Arteries and veins of the affected temple become knobbed, knotted, and painful. The headache worsens at night.

Severe and intermittent headache

Brain tumours 9: A rare disorder. Headache is severe but can be occasionally moderate. Begins at area of tumour but soon becomes general. Headache can last several hours every day. A sudden change of position will bring it on. Often the patient will awaken from sleep with intense headache. Persistent nausea, vomiting, convulsions, hallucinations. Later, deterioration of personality and mental faculties.

Erysipelas 300: Intense, mostly intermittent headache, raised rashes ranging in colour from dull red to scarlet with advancing margins, chills, high fever, swollen face, enlarged lymph nodes.

Vitamin A toxicity 348b: Rare, due mostly to overenthusiasm by faddists (overindulgence in vitamin A). Loss of appetite, falling hair, pain in joints. Can mimic brain tumour by severe internal pressure headaches. In children, growth can be retarded.

Brain cancer 412: Vomiting, faulty vision, loss of balance, any type of headache mostly severe and intermittent, lethargy, obtuseness, psychotic episodes, clouding of consciousness.

Throbbing headache

Almost all fevers from infectious diseases will bring on a pounding headache either frontal or occipital. But headache is rarely the important symptom.

Most toxic poisoning will produce a severe throbbing headache. Acute alcoholism (not to be confused with a hangover) from overconsumption will cause a constant, severe, pounding headache in addition to muscular incoordination, drunken gait, double vision, loss of consciousness and feeling. Carbon monoxide poisoning produces a severe constant throbbing in the temples. Cherry-red patches appear on the face or body. Dizziness, dilated pupils, dusky skin, and muscular rigidity of the jaw are other signs. Lead poisoning can cause intense, constant throbbing headache. There may be abdominal distress or pain, bluish lines on the gums, and great weakness. Morphine poisoning (including all its derivatives: codeine, heroin and others) can cause a constant throbbing headache. Pupils are pinpoint or dilated. Patient is usually emaciated from undernourishment. There may be cyanosis.

Encephalitis 8: Extreme throbbing pain which frequently appears suddenly, accompanied by high fever. Headache may radiate to the neck. Stiff neck, stupor, convulsions, vomiting, persistent hiccups.

Migraine headache 13b: The patient knows the headache is coming by tingling in the limbs, depression, noises in the ear, scintillating lights before the eyes. Throbbing pain most often in the same location, frequently radiating to or from an eye, nausea, vomiting, intolerance for light or sound.

Cluster headache 13c: This headache is excruciating, unremitting, pounding; it can also radiate to the nose, mouth, or neck. Usually one-sided. The eye on the affected side may be bloodshot, and the arteries and veins prominent.

High blood pressure 138: Headaches do not appear in this disease until quite late. The headache is a rhythmic pulsation in the back of the head brought on or worsened by straining or bending over. Most common in the morning upon awakening but wears off as the day progresses. Other symptoms that appear late are dizziness, fatigue, nosebleeds.

Uraemia 207: An acute throbbing headache with nausea and vomiting. The identifying symptom is the urine odour on the breath or perspiration.

Whiplash 272: Stiffness and pain in the neck which can be mild or agonizing and can radiate to the hands causing tingling and numbness. Disturbed vision and pounding headache.

Phaeochromocytoma 346: The headache is recurrent and pounding, episodes of profuse sweating, pallor and tremor. (High blood pressure.)

Variable headache

As the name indicates, headaches in this category can be of any type and of any intensity.

Contraceptive pill headache 13f: This headache may appear suddenly. Usually it is the pressure type, feeling like a tight band around the head; it may also be throbbing. There may be depression, irritability, and insomnia. Breasts may be heavier or lumps may appear on the breasts. Additionally there may be skin discolorations, visual disturbances, and unusual vaginal bleeding. A doctor should be seen.

Postcoital headache 13g: This headache is usually throbbing but can take on any form. Most often it is a dull ache, usually fleeting but can last an hour.

Hay fever and allergic rhinitis 65: Headache can range from moderate to severe. Usually it is one-sided. Swollen sockets will appear below the eyes, running nose and tearing.

Acute nephritis 197: Varying headache, sharp loss of appetite, scanty but often bloody urine, puffiness of face, swelling of ankles, furred tongue, nausea, vomiting. (Rise in blood pressure.)

Uraemia 207: From moderate to severe headache, convulsions, contraction of pupils, impaired vision, urine odour on the breath, swelling over the body, urea frost on the body, nausea, vomiting, diarrhoea, coma.

Early syphilis 209: Second stage (only after the disappearance of the ulcer on genitalia): varying headache is usually severe, widespread body rash, enlarged lymph nodes, mouth ulcers, arthritic pain, sore throat, possible eye disorders.

Late syphilis (paresis) 210: Headache, quite often severe, development of slovenly habits, tremors of lip and tongue, failing memory, premature senility, mental loss.

Premenstrual tension 219: Irritability, nervousness, mild to severe headache, pain in the breasts, puffiness especially around abdomen.

Menopause 221 (see also *Menopausal headache* **13h**): Any form of intensity; may also be constant or intermittent. Other symptoms such as hot flushes, depression are more definitive.

Minor disorders of pregnancy 235: Constipation, dyspepsia, possible haemorrhoids, backache, slight shortness of breath, toothache and excessive salivation.

Heat exhaustion 313b: Headache, dizziness, cool, moist skin, profuse sweating. Temperature is either normal or slightly raised. Nausea, faintness, muscle cramps.

Vomiting and severe headache

Brain injury 10: Serious: constant intense headache accompanied by vomiting, lethargy, confusion, dilated pupils of unequal size (a serious sign). Bleeding from nose, mouth, or ears. Skin pale and clammy. Prolonged unconsciousness.

Stroke 139: Overwhelming headache comes on suddenly, can be temporal but usually at the base of the skull. Followed by vomiting, dizziness, visual failures, stupor, paralysis, and coma.

Acute infectious hepatitis 187 and **Serum hepatitis 188:** Severe headache, jaundice, dark urine, light-coloured stools, weakness, red itching wheals, tenderness in liver area, nausea and vomiting.

Acute yellow atrophy 193: Severe headache, jaundice, extreme abdominal distension, black vomiting, emotional instability, coma.

Toxaemia of pregnancy (preeclampsia) 246: Intense headache, body puffiness, large gain in weight, dizziness, considerable vomiting, visual disturbances, amnesia, jaundice.

Yellow fever 379: Flushed face, fever, prostration, pain in the back and in the limbs, scanty urine. Jaundice appears after temporary remission of the disease. Then vomiting of black blood and bleeding from the mucous membranes.

Malaria 381: Teeth-chattering chills, very high fever, drenching sweats, vomiting, diarrhoea, rapid pulse, rapid breathing. Headache is a prominent symptom.

*

Large head (abnormal)

Paget's disease 267: Intermittent shifting bone pain, spontaneous bone fracture, grotesque enlargement of the head, height loss, impaired hearing.

Low birth weight 396: Infant: irregular breathing, abnormally enlarged head, prominent eyes, protruding abdomen, slow to gain weight.

Mental retardation 403: Infants: abnormally large head at birth, low birth weight, may be jaundice, lethargy, slow development, slow learning to feed.

Prominent blood vessels in the head

Cluster headache 13c: Veins and arteries in the affected temple stand out. Headache radiates to the eyes, nose, mouth, or neck, sweating, pallor.

Temporal arteritis 33: Pain in the temporal artery which becomes prominent and often nodular. Pulsation can be felt. Radiating pain to and from the eye.

Softening of bones in the head

Vitamin D deficiency 353a: Infants: restlessness, thinning of head bones, bow legs, badly formed teeth. Infant cannot walk, stand, sit at proper age. Lordosis and scoliosis are other signs.

Twisting head to the side

Stiff neck 271: Painful stiff neck. Abnormal twisting of head to a side. Inability to move head.

Symptoms of the eye

AROUND THE EYE (PERIORBITAL)
Discoloration around the eye

A blow on the eye will often produce discoloration periorbitally (around the eye). A black eye is a classic example. Discoloration may also occur in blood abnormalities.

Pain around the eye

Neuralgia is a common cause of pain around the eye.

Glaucoma 23a and **23b:** Severe eye pain as well as pain around the eye, rainbow seen around lights, loss of vision, hard eyeball, brow ache.

Redness and swelling below the eye

Dacryocystitis 24: Also pain around the eye, profuse tearing and conjunctivitis.

Yellow nodules around the eyelids

Xanthelasma 38: Painless yellow nodules around the eyes.
Hyperlipidaemia 335: Painless yellow

lumps around the eyelids, palms, knees, elbows, buttocks and in the tendons of the hands and legs.

THE CORNEA
Cloudy cornea

Glaucoma 23a and **23b:** Seeing rainbows around lights, blurring vision, stony-hard eyeball, severe pain (in acute form only), brow ache, dilated pupils, vomiting.
Keratitis 31: Blurred vision, heavy tearing, pain in the eye, redness, photophobia.
Vitamin A deficiency 348a: Dryness of the eyes, lowered vision in dim light. In children, retarded growth. Kidney inflammation, horny skin.

White ring around the cornea

Arcus senilis 42: An opaque, thin ring around the iris.

THE EYEBALL
Bloodshot eye

A blow, injury or foreign object can make an eye bloodshot.

Contact lens intolerance 19: Irritation and redness of the eye is common.

Conjunctivitis 21: Red eyes, tearing, itching, burning plus inflamed, swollen eyelids.

Trachoma 22: Tearing, swollen and granular eyelids which can become permanently scarred. Red eyes, ulcerated cornea, obstructed vision.

Iritis 26: Pain in the eye, redness, blurred vision, swollen, muddy iris, tearing, photophobia, contracted pupils.

Measles 370: Begins like a cold, then high fever, harsh, hacking cough, bloodshot burning eyes, intolerance for light, red spots with white centres in the inside of the cheeks, brownish-pink rash over the body consisting of slightly elevated spots which run into each other. Rash disappears in a few days.

Typhus 392: Sustained high fever, severe headache, prostration, bloodshot eyes, flushed face, body rash with pinpoint centres of bleeding turning purple, rapid weak pulse, stupor may change to coma, muscular twitching, high coloured, scanty urine.

Blood spot on eyeball

A blood spot must not be confused with a bloodshot eye. The former is usually benign and is only serious if coupled with a loss of vision, in which case it should be immediately looked at by a doctor.

Burning, smarting feeling in the eye

Many allergies will induce this symptom.

Conjunctivitis 21: Also inflamed eyelids and bloodshot eyes.

Blepharitis 36: Inflammation of the eyelids as well, tearing, falling out of lashes.

Sty 37: Inflammation of eyelids as well, small, red boil at base of eyelash.

Vitamin B$_2$ (riboflavin) deficiency 350: Weakness, tongue is swollen at the tip and edges, inflamed, chapped lips, cracks around the corners of the mouth, dry, red, scaly skin around nose, ear, scrotum. Cloudy ulcerated cornea, impairment of vision, photophobia, burning sensation in the eyes.

Measles 370: Begins like a cold, then high fever, harsh, hacking cough, bloodshot, burning eyes, photophobia, red spots with white centres in the inside of the cheeks, brownish-pink rash consisting of slightly elevated spots which run into each other. Rash disappears in a few days.

Enlarged eyeball

Hypothyroidism 339: Protruding eyes, retarded physical and mental development, apathy, rough skin. Children: coarse face, thick lips, flat nose.

Hyperthyroidism 340: Bulging eyes, visual disturbances, nervousness, intolerance for heat, sweating, fatigue, loss of weight, rapid pulse, pounding heart.

Cancer of the retina 414: Whitish pupil and squinting are the first signs, followed by loss of vision, enlarged eyeball.

Feeling something in the eye

A foreign object in the eye is the most frequent cause of this symptom. A speck of dust or some other substance will irritate the eyelid or eyeball. If not embedded, object may be washed out by tear flow; if irritation persists, a doctor should be seen.

Conjunctivitis 21: Burning feeling in the eye, bloodshot eye, tearing.

Keratitis 31: Pain in the eye, cloudy cornea, blurred vision, photophobia.

Blepharitis 36: Burning feeling in the eye, inflammation, tearing, falling out of lashes, tenacious crusts, itching of the eyelid.

Sty 37: Boil on the eyelid, swelling, itching of the eyelid.

Opaque or coloured spot on the eyeball

Brown spots on the white part of the eye

may lead to malignancy. A doctor should be consulted.

Keratitis 31: Blurring, cloudy cornea, feeling something in the eye, heavy tearing, pain in eyeball, redness, photophobia.
Diabetic retinopathy 45: Blood spots, opaque spots from ruptured vessels. Impaired vision which may terminate in blindness.
Pterygium 43: Triangular white growth over the cornea and pupil.

Palsied eyeball (nystagmus) and paralysed eye muscles

Palsied eyeball is a constant, rather quick motion of the eyeball.

Multiple sclerosis 6: In early stages, fleeting palsied eyeball, later partial blindness, inability to control eyeball, speech difficulties, hand tremors, spastic gait.
Eye disorders resulting from tobacco and alcohol 34: Chronic alcoholism can cause eye muscle palsy.
Stroke 139: Paralysis of the eye muscles, legs, arms, or whole side of the body. Loss of speech, memory. Confusion and severe headaches.

Protruding eyeball

Exophthalmos 41: Absence of blinking and large amounts of the white of the eye showing.
Hyperthyroidism 340: Bulging or staring eyes, enlarged goitre, very heavy heartbeat, profuse sweating, severe weakness, increased appetite but loss of weight, overheated body, nervousness.

Sunken eyeball

Shock 133: Great pallor, cold, clammy skin, cyanosis (lips, nails, fingertips), fast, weak pulse, shortness of breath, dilated pupils, anxiety state, coma.
Diabetes (ketoacidosis, diabetic coma) 332: Rapid, deep, hungry breath-

ing, severe dehydration, excessive thirst and urination, nausea, vomiting, abdominal pain, poor skin tone. Eventually stupor, shock, and coma.
Cholera 364: Constant voluminous watery diarrhoea, massive dehydration, severe stomach cramps, violent vomiting, intense thirst, clammy, wrinkled skin.

Ulceration on eyeball

Pterygium 43: Triangular white growth over the cornea and pupil.
Vitamin B$_2$ (riboflavin) deficiency 350: Ulceration or cloudiness of the cornea, impaired vision, developing cataracts, fissured tongue, cracks in the corners of the mouth, burning feeling in the eye.

THE EYELIDS
Drooping eyelids (ptosis) or lid lag

Drooping of the eyelids is characteristic of myasthenia gravis, a neuromuscular disease. It is also seen in palsy of the nerves of the eye.
  Sagging of the lower lid is not infrequent in older people when the eyelid loses its tonicity. This is particularly apt to occur in rough weather when the eyes will tear.

Exophthalmos 41: Protrusion of the eyeball with frequent pain in the eyeball. In exophthalmic goitre there is also lid lag and absence of blinking.

Granular eyelid

Trachoma 22: Upper eyelid becomes scarred and swollen. Vision is disturbed and ulcers appear on the cornea.

Inflamed eyelid (redness)

This is a major symptom in *Conjunctivitis* 21, *Trachoma* 22, and *Blepharitis* 36.

Dacryocystitis 24: Profuse tears, pain, redness and swelling around the eye.

Blepharitis 36: Margins of the eyelid become thickened, lashes fall out, tenacious crusts on the eyelids, tearing.

Sty 37: Small boil on the eyelid which is also swollen and painful.

Early syphilis (secondary) 209: Iritis, conjunctivitis, pain in the eye, body rash, headache, arthritic pains, enlarged lymph nodes.

Itching eyelid

This is a characteristic symptom of *Conjunctivitis* **21**, *Blepharitis* **36** and *Trachoma* **22**.

Pain in the eyelid

Trachoma 22: Upper lids become swollen, granular, scarred. Vision is obstructed, ulcers appear on the cornea.

Sty 37: The eyelid is inflamed and swollen, with a small boil on the margin.

Small boil on the eyelid

Sty 37: Pain, redness and swelling of the eyelid.

Swollen eyelids

This is a constant symptom of *Conjunctivitis* **21**, *Trachoma* **22**, and *Sty* **37**

Dacryocystitis 24: Profuse tears, pain, redness and swelling below the eye.

Iritis 26: Pain in the eye, redness of the eyelids, swollen, muddy iris, blurred vision, tearing, photophobia.

Blepharitis 36: Inflamed, thickened, itching eyelid margins, falling out of lashes, tenacious crusts on the eyelids.

Trichinosis 386: Swelling of the face particularly around the eyes and forehead, high fever, pain and swelling in the muscles, profuse sweating, gastric distress, nausea, and occasionally diarrhoea. In some cases shortness of breath.

Twitching eyelid

Tics 11: A common symptom of fatigue or chronic eye irritation. This tic is frequently seen in children.

IMPAIRED VISION
Blindness

A large number of eye disorders as well as systemic diseases can end up in blindness if left untreated. Only a very small number of these disorders cannot be helped. Over ninety per cent of all blindness is tragically unnecessary. Alert awareness will almost always save the eyesight.

The following diseases can result in total blindness: *Trachoma* **22**, *Glaucoma* **23a** and **23b**, *Retinitis pigmentosa* **29**, *Optic neuritis* **32**, *Temporal arteritis* **33**, *Eye disorders resulting from tobacco and alcohol* **34**, *Diabetic retinopathy* **45**, *Arterio-atherosclerosis* **47** and **123**, *Stroke* **139**, *Late syphilis* **210**, *Cancer of the retina* **414**.

Blind spots (scotomas)

Migraine headache 13b: Double vision, headache radiating to the eye, photophobia, nausea, vomiting, dizziness. Blind spots are usually temporary.

Glaucoma 23a and **23b:** Seeing rainbows around lights, blurred vision, brow ache, hard eyeballs, dilated pupils.

Eye disorders resulting from tobacco and alcohol 34: Methyl (wood) alcohol can cause blindness; the lucky victims will just develop blind spots.

Diabetic retinopathy and eye disorders 45 and **332:** Vision becomes impaired, usually after a long history of diabetes.

Arterio-atherosclerosis 47 and **123:** Blind spots can develop, usually after a long history of the disease.

Stroke 139: Blind spots or blindness is a frequent symptom.

Cancer of the retina 414: Children before age of four: progressive blindness, chronic squint. Later sign is enlarged eyeballs.

Blurring

Blurring, Blurring of distant vision, Blurring and double vision, Blurring of near vision, Blurring and pain in the eye

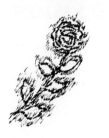
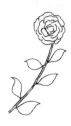

Blurring vision. (*Julian A. Miller*)

Blurring

Choroiditis 27: Blank or grey areas in the visual field, considerable blurring, occasional flashes of light.

Retinitis 28: Blurring, contraction of the visual field, distortion of objects.

Eye disorders resulting from side effects of commonly used drugs 35: Sensitivity to or overuse of belladonna, atropine, prolonged use of cortisone and most tranquillizers.

Diabetic retinopathy 45 and **332:** Impaired vision from prolonged diabetes. Blurring. (See *Diabetes* **332**)

Chronic nephritis 198: Blurring from bleeding into the retina. Swelling of face, abdomen, ankles. Bloody urine, breathlessness on slight exertion, anaemia.

Heat exhaustion 313b: Profuse sweating, clammy, cold skin, faintness, weakness and blurring of vision, no real rise in temperature.

Hypoglycaemia 333: Weakness, dizziness, palpitations, shaking, sweating, headaches, poor concentration, irrational or psychotic behaviour, blackouts, convulsions, coma.

Vitamin A deficiency 348a: Dryness of the eyes, blurring, night blindness, cloudy cornea, rough dry skin. Children: retarded growth.

Vitamin B_2 (riboflavin) deficiency 350: Weakness, tongue is swollen with the tip and edges inflamed, chapped lips, cracked corners of the mouth, dry, red, scaly skin around the nose, ear, scrotum, and cloudy, ulcerated cornea.

Blurring of distant vision

Nearsightedness 14: Distant vision is blurred; near objects are seen clearly.

Blurring and double vision

Multiple sclerosis 6: Early sign is fleeting palsy of eyeball; later, blurring to partial blindness. Occasionally double vision, inability to control eyeball, tremors of the hand, spastic gait, numbness, speech difficulties.

Botulism 165: Besides blurring there may be double vision. Pupils are fixed and dilated. Difficulty in breathing, talking. Cramps, diarrhoea, nausea and vomiting. Paralysis of the respiratory tract. Symptoms appear 18–36 hours after eating contaminated food.

Uraemia 207: Severe headache, drowsiness, contracted pupils may herald coma, muscular twitching, urine odour on breath, urea frost, nausea, vomiting, diarrhoea. In children, swelling and puffiness of the face.

Toxaemia of pregnancy (preeclampsis) 246: Spots before the eyes, blurring and double vision, puffiness of the body, large gain in weight, severe headache, dizziness, vomiting, pain in the abdomen, anaemia.

Blurring of near vision

Farsightedness 15: Near vision is blurred; distant objects are seen clearly.

Blurring and pain in the eye

Acute glaucoma 23b: Rainbow around lights, severe pain (acute form only), stony eyeballs, brow ache, vomiting.

Iritis 26: Pain in the eye, redness, swollen, muddy iris, swelling of eyelids, tearing, photophobia.

Early syphilis (secondary) 209: Swollen eyelids, eye pain radiating to the temple, splotchy body rash, enlarged lymph nodes, arthritic pains, severe headache.

*

Distortion of colour

This is usually due to some form of poisoning. Very heavy indulgence in alcohol can also produce this symptom, as can usage of LSD and mescaline, both hallucinatory drugs.

Distortion in size and shape

Choroiditis 27: Blank or grey areas in the visual field, blurring, occasional flashes of light.
Retinitis 28: Besides distortion of size and shape, there is blurring and reduction of the visual field.

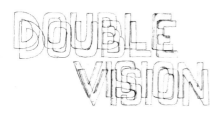

Double vision. (*Julian A. Miller*)

Double vision (diplopia)

Many commonly used drugs such as barbiturates, digitalis (heart medication), insulin, scopolamine, ergot, Dilantin, antipyrine, and caffeine can cause double vision.
Multiple sclerosis 6: Blurring, partial vision, eyeball palsy and double vision. Also tremor of the hands, spastic gait, numbness, speech difficulties.
Migraine headache 13b: Partial temporary blindness, often with double vision, radiating headache to an eye, nausea, vomiting, intense headache, strong photophobia.
Temporal arteritis 33: Double vision may occur at the beginning. Pain in the eye radiating to the temple, pain in temporal artery which becomes prominent and pulsates. This disorder can cause frequent loss of vision.
Eye disorders resulting from tobac-
co and alcohol 34: Methyl (wood) alcohol poisoning begins with double vision and ends in loss of sight.
Eye disorders resulting from side effects of commonly used drugs 35: Such drugs as cocaine, morphine, and the birth control pill (for some women) can induce this symptom.
Botulism 165: Blurring, double vision, pupils fixed and dilated, difficulty breathing and talking, cramps, diarrhoea, nausea and vomiting. Paralysis of the repiratory tract. Symptoms occur 18–36 hours after eating contaminated food.
Brain cancer 412: Double vision is a distinctive symptom. Also headache, vomiting, muscle weakness, generally failing vision, loss of balance and coordination, personality changes, lethargy, and disorderly conduct.
Uraemia 207: Breath has an odour of urine. Double vision, contraction of pupils, swelling of face and ankles, nausea, vomiting, diarrhoea, severe headaches, scanty urine, urea frost, convulsions and eventually coma.
Toxaemia of pregnancy (preeclampsia) 246: Besides double vision, there are spots before the eyes and dimness of sight. Puffiness of the body, large gain in weight, severe, persistent headache, dizziness, vomiting, nausea.

Narrowing of the visual field

Glaucoma 23a and **23b:** Progressive narrowing of visual field. In acute form, severe eye pain, rainbow around lights, brow ache, blurring.
Retinitis 28: Distortion of size and shape of objects seen, blurring.
Retinitis pigmentosa 29: Tunnel vision (gradual narrowing of the visual field).
Optic neuritis 32: Painful movement of the eye, sudden loss of vision.
Temporal arteritis 33: Often begins with double vision, pain radiating to temple from affected eye, pain in temporal artery which pulsates and is prominent, sudden loss of vision.

Hypoxia 122 (mountain sickness) 122a: Above 5000m, 17,000ft loss of peripheral vision, dimness, and muscular incoordination.

Night blindness

Choroiditis 27: Blurring, spots on the eyeball, black areas in the visual field, occasional flashes of light.

Vitamin A deficiency 348a: Dryness of the eyes, ulceration of the cornea. In children, retarded growth, inflammation of the kidneys, horny skin.

Rapid loss of vision

Many victims of stroke suffer rapid loss of vision.

Optic neuritis 32: Pain in socket when eyeball is moved. Usually sudden loss of vision.

Temporal arteritis 33: Pain radiating to the temple, pain in the temporal artery which becomes prominent and pulsating. Sudden loss of vision may occur. Double vision at the beginning.

Eye disorders resulting from tobacco and alcohol 34: Poisoning from methyl alcohol causes a rapid loss of vision.

Late syphilis 210: Severe headache, loss of memory, loss of balance, rapid loss of vision, severe pains and spasms all over the body.

Slow loss of vision

Glaucoma 23a and **23b:** In chronic form, the loss may be slow, insidious, and painless. In acute form, severe eye pain, rainbow around lights, brow ache, hard eyeball, dilated pupils, blurring.

Cataract 25: Loss of vision is gradual, painless. Growing opacity of the lens may be noticeable.

Congenital syphilis 211: Cloudy cornea, heavy tearing, pain in the eyeball, slow loss of sight. Also saddle-backed nose.

Brain cancer 412: Headache, vomiting, muscle weakness, failing vision, double

vision, loss of balance and coordination, personality changes, drowsiness, lethargy, and disorderly conduct.

Cancer of the retina 414: Children: whitish pupil and squinting are the first signs. Loss of vision, enlarged eyeball.

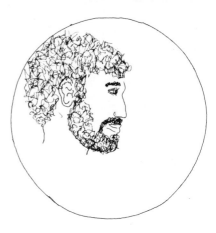

Normal and tunnel vision. (*Julian A. Miller*)

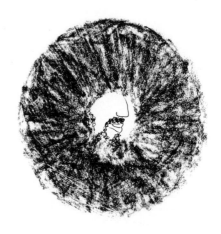

Tunnel vision

Diminishing visual field as if peering through two narrow tubes.

Retinitis pigmentosa 29: Gradual narrowing of the area of sight.

THE IRIS
Muddy or clouded iris

Iritis 26: Iris is swollen. Pain in the eye, redness, narrowed pupils, blurred vision.
Juvenile rheumatoid arthritis 260: High fever, pain in the eye radiating to the temple, loss of vision, contracted pupils. Burning and swelling in the joints, morning joint stiffness.

THE LENS
Clouding the lens

Cataract 25: Gradual painless loss of vision. Noticeable growing opacity in the lens.

PAIN IN THE EYE
Pain in the eyeball

Pain in the eye is not a characteristic symptom of any eye disease but it is a frequent complaint.

High fevers, notably those due to the flu, measles, typhoid, and others will also painfully affect the eyes. Painful eye symptoms are common in secondary syphilis; they are also frequent in sinusitis.

Acute glaucoma 23b: Severe pain, rainbow around lights, blurring, severe headache, and vomiting.
Retinitis 28: Eye discomfort, blurring, distortion of form and size of viewed objects, contraction of the visual field.
Keratitis 31: Pain in the eyeball, feeling of something in the eye, decreased vision, cloudy cornea, photophobia.

Pain in the eye socket

Pain in the socket unless caused by a minor injury is usually a serious sign.

Optic neuritis 32: Movement of eyeball is painful, usually sudden loss of vision, narrowed visual field, blind spots.

Exophthalmos (protrusion of the eyeball) 41: Lid lag showing an unusually large amount of the white of the eye, absence of blinking, throbbing eyeball. Occasionally pain which can be extreme.

Pain radiating from the eyeball

Bell's palsy 3a: Tortured, paralysed face with pain radiating to and from the eyes, distorting the face. The eye cannot close: smiling is impossible.
Migraine headache 13b: Pain radiating to or from an eye, double vision, intense headache, temporary partial blindness, photophobia, nausea and vomiting.
Iritis 26: Pain in the eye radiating to the temple, swollen, muddy iris, blurred vision, redness, tearing, photophobia.
Temporal arteritis 33: Sometimes double vision at the beginning, headache pain radiating to and from an eye, often sudden loss of vision, contraction of the visual field, pain in the temporal artery which becomes prominent and pulsating.
Early syphilis (secondary) 209: Pain radiates to the temples, swollen eyelids, contracted pupils, body rash, severe headaches, arthritic pains, enlarged lymph nodes.

Pain upon moving eyeball

Iritis 26: Pain in eye radiating to the temple, pain upon moving eyeball, swollen, muddy iris, blurring, redness, tearing, photophobia.
Optic neuritis 32: Usually sudden loss of vision, narrowed visual field, blind spots. Movement of eyeball may cause pain.

Photophobia (unusual intolerance for light)

Photophobia is a very common eye symptom in most eye disorders and by itself is not significant of any particular eye disease. This symptom is especially common

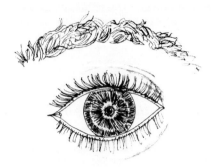

Highly contracted pupil

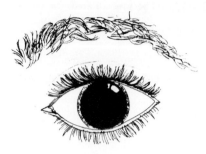

Dilated pupil. (*Julian A. Miller*)

in blondes and those with lightly pigmented eyes; these people are usually more disturbed by bright lights and glare.

Normal causes of photophobia are: 1) natural response to unusual light such as snow glare resulting in snow blindness; 2) exposure to bright sunlight for extended periods of time; 3) being in the dark for too long. In all these situations the eye soon corrects the problem itself. It can occur in psychoneurosis – hysterical photophobia is relatively common.

Meningitis 7: Overwhelming radiating headache, painful neck, red or purple spots over the body. Intolerance for sound and light, high erratic fever, vomiting.

Vitamin B₂ (riboflavin) deficiency 350: Impaired vision as well as intolerance for light, cloudy ulcerated cornea, burning feeling in the conjunctiva. Fissured tongue with reddish-purple edges, cracks in the corners of the mouth.

Measles 370: Intolerance for light, cold symptoms, high fever, cough, white spots with rosy areas inside the mouth, brownish-pink body rash.

reliable symptom. Addicts wear dark glasses not so much to hide the contracted pupils but because their eyes are light-sensitive.

Cluster headache 13c: Also throbbing headache which can radiate, pallor, sweating, prominence of veins and arteries.

Iritis 26: Pain in the eye, redness, blurred vision, tearing, photophobia, swollen muddy iris and contracted pupils.

Uraemia 207: Contracted pupils and double vision. Swelling of the face and ankles, diarrhoea, severe headache, scanty urine, nausea and vomiting, urine odour on the breath, uraemic frost, convulsions, finally coma.

Early syphilis (secondary) 209: Pain in eyes radiates to the temples, pupils are contracted, splotchy rash on the body, severe headache, enlarged lymph nodes, arthritic pains.

Typhus 392: Ten day high fever, severe headache, prostration, mottled rash with small red spots turning purple, contracted pupils, scanty, highly coloured urine, muscle tremors. Profuse sweating when fever breaks.

THE PUPILS
Contracted pupils

Usage of most habit-forming drugs (morphine, opium, heroin, even codeine) may contract the pupils; however, this is not a

Dilated pupils

Brain injury 10: Unequally dilated pupils, cold, clammy skin, bleeding from nose, mouth, ears. Headache, giddiness, vomiting, drowsiness, coma.

Glaucoma 23a and **23b:** In later stages

pupils may become dilated. In acute glaucoma, severe eye pain, rainbow around lights, hard eyeball, blurring, brow ache.

Shock 133: Great pallor, cold, clammy skin, cyanosis (lips, nails, fingertips), shortness of breath, sunken eyes, fast, weak pulse, anxiety state, coma.

Botulism 165: Dilated pupils, double and blurred vision, difficulty in talking, paralysis of the respiratory tract, difficulty breathing, extreme dryness of the mouth, cramps, vomiting, diarrhoea, extreme nausea.

Acute yellow atrophy 193: High fever with severe headache, jaundice, weakness, severe abdominal pain, black vomiting, apathy, confusion, bleeding under the skin and from the mouth, dilated pupils, foul breath, scanty, bloody urine, and rapid, feeble pulse. (Liver enlargement.)

Whitish pupils

Cancer of the retina 414: Whitish pupils and squinting are the first signs. Later, loss of vision and enlarged eyeball.

SQUINTING
Squinting

Often a habit pattern of many children; and often a consequence of blurring vision. By *itself* squinting is not a significant symptom.

TEARING (LACRIMATION)
Excessive tearing

Tearing is common to all inflammatory eye conditions; this symptom is never in itself definitive of a disorder. Any growth, inflammation, or dysfunction of the eye will usually cause it to tear, often profusely. Non-eye disorders such as hay

fever and vitamin B_2 (riboflavin) deficiency may also produce excessive lacrimation.

Dacryocystitis 24: Profuse tearing, pain, redness, and swelling below the eye and often conjunctivitis.

UNUSUAL VISUAL DISTURBANCES
Colour blindness

Colour blindness 39: Red and green are indistinguishable. In severe cases, no colour is distinguishable. Occurs mostly in males.

Cross-eye

Strabismus 20: Children: may lose useful vision in one eye. Adults: may be associated with double vision.

Hallucinatory visions

The so-called consciousness-expanding drugs such as LSD, and mescaline can create hallucinations which usually disappear after many hours. Occasionally they can continue for weeks or even months with disastrous mental stress.

Brain cancer 412: Severe headaches, vomiting, lack of balance sense, double vision, visual hallucinations, cloudy consciousness, drowsiness, lethargy.

Seeing floating spots

Floating spots 40: Occurs mostly after the age of fifty. The spots can be few in number or many. Although annoying and alarming, they are of no significance.

Seeing halos, rainbows around lights

Acute glaucoma 23b: Seeing rainbows around lights is the major symptom in acute glaucoma. Also severe eye pain,

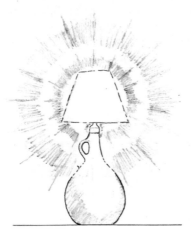

Halo around light. (*Julian A. Miller*)

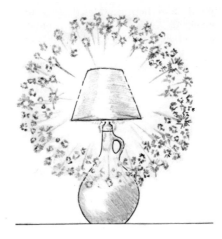

Sparks around light. (*Julian A. Miller*)

blurred vision, brow aches, dilated pupils, and hard eyeball.

Seeing shower of sparks

Detached retina 30: Seeing a shower of sparks, stars, or flashes of light followed later by a curtain being drawn across the eye.

Yellow vision

Seeing a yellow colouring on all objects is usually due to some form of poisoning.

Eye disorders resulting from side effects of commonly used drugs 35: The overuse of or unusual sensitivity to digitalis can induce yellow vision or seeing snowflakes.

Symptoms of the ear

Bleeding from the ear

Brain injury 10: In severe injury bleeding will occur from mouth, nose, and ears. Pupils are unevenly dilated. Confusion, intense headache, vomiting, coma.

Perforation of the eardrum 56: Agonizing pain, loss of hearing, hollow reverberation in the head, dizziness, possibly vomiting. Blood may appear in ear canal.

Boils in the ear

Boils in the ear canal 52: Along with boils there is pain, diminished hearing, and a feeling of fullness in the ear. Canal may be swollen or blocked with possible discharge.

Discharge from the ear

Chronic purulent otitis media 58b: Constant stream of pus, feeling of fullness in the ear, hearing loss, rarely earache.

Chronic secretory otitis media 58c: Severe earache, feeling of fullness in the ear, hearing loss, purulent discharge.

Mastoiditis 59: Begins as a sore throat and a moderate earache which soon becomes severe with tender, red area behind the ear. The discharge from the ear may be heavy.

Earache

Earache, slight to moderate, Earache, severe

Earache, slight to moderate

Boils in the ear canal 52: Pain, diminished hearing, feeling of fullness in the ear. Canal may be swollen or blocked.

External otitis 53: Moderate pain usually but can be severe.

Fungus-infected ear 54: Mild pain but strong itching in and around the canal. There may be grey or black particles in the ear.

Flying and earache 62: Earache is frequent among susceptible people especially when suffering from an upper respiratory infection.

Tonsillitis 70: Referred pain from the throat. High fever, difficulty swallowing, red, ulcerated, enlarged tonsils.

Tooth abscess (pulpitis) 91: Referred pain from an infected tooth.

Temporomandibular joint disorder 102: Mouth cannot be fully opened, severe pain at joint of the jaw and in the ear when speaking or chewing. The affected side of the face is sore.

Cancer of the tongue 436: Back of the tongue cancer will cause pain in the throat and ear.

Cancer of the pharynx (throat) 438: Pain in the throat, earache, difficulty swallowing, difficulty opening mouth, cough, swelling of neck lymph nodes.

Earache, severe

External otitis 53: Severe pain and high fever does occur on occasion. Usually there is no fever and mild pain.

Perforation of the eardrum 56: Agonizing pain, loss of hearing, hollow reverberation in the head, dizziness, possible vomiting. Blood may appear in canal.

Otitis media 58: Severe stabbing pain which may be constant or intermittent and may radiate over side of the head. Fullness in the ear, noises in the head, tenderness over the mastoid bone, high fever.

Mastoiditis 59: Very severe pain, high fever, redness behind the ear. Occasionally stiff neck, sore throat.

*

Fullness in the ear

Otosclerosis 50: Insidious loss of hearing, loss of low tones, noises in the ear, distortion of sound, increasingly soft-spoken voice, fullness.

Boils in the ear canal 52: Pain in the ear, diminished hearing, fullness, ear canal swollen or blocked. Possible discharge.

Blockage of the eustachian tube 57: Impaired hearing, fullness, crackling noise while swallowing, occasional dizziness, head noises, sense of fluid in ear.

Acute otitis media 58a: Fullness in the ear, severe stabbing pain, may be constant or intermittent and may radiate over the side of the head, ringing and noises in the head, tenderness over the mastoid bone, high fever.

Chronic purulent otitis media 58b: Discharge of pus, fullness in the ear, hearing loss, rarely earache.

Chronic secretory otitis media 58c: Fullness, hearing loss, discharge from the ear, sensation of fluid in the ear.

Ménière's syndrome 60: Mild deafness, loss of balance and vertigo main symptom, increasing noises in the head.

Growth in the ear

Chronic purulent otitis media 58b: A constant stream of pus can cause fatty tissues to grow around the eardrum (cholesteatoma); skin can grow through perforation into middle ear. If not removed can occasionally be fatal. Fullness and hearing loss.

Hearing distortion

Otosclerosis 50: Insidious loss of hearing, loss of low tones, distortion of sounds, noises in the head, fullness, increasingly soft-spoken voice.

Hearing loss

Many systemic febrile diseases will cause some deafness, particularly mumps. Flu, scarlet fever, and meningitis, as well as malaria, typhoid, and congenital or acquired syphilis can also cause hearing loss. This form of hearing loss is perceptive (nerve) deafness which cannot be restored. Patients suffering from these ailments should take extra precautions by putting themselves under a doctor's care early.

A pregnant woman who develops German measles (especially in the third month) runs a high risk of having her baby born deaf. (See *German measles in pregnancy* **244**.) Premature babies and very small babies have a higher incidence of deafness.

Perceptive hearing (nerve) loss 49: Loud voice, inability to hear high frequency sounds or such sounds as *p*, *k*, *t*, hard *g*. Other sounds may be heard normally.

Otosclerosis 50: Slow loss of hearing, loss of low tones, distortion of sounds, noises in the head, feeling of fullness in the ear, increasingly soft-spoken voice.

Wax in the ear 51: Most common cause of conductive hearing loss.

Boils in the ear canal 52: Diminished hearing, pain, feeling of fullness in ear. Canal may be swollen or blocked. Possible discharge.

Perforation of the eardrum (acute)

56: Agonizing pain, loss of hearing, hollow reverberation in the head, dizziness, possible vomiting. Blood may appear in canal.

Blockage of the eustachian tube 57: Impaired hearing, sensation of fullness in the ear, noises in the ear, crackling sounds when swallowing, occasional dizziness, sense of fluid in ear.

Chronic purulent and chronic secretory otitis media 58: Purulent discharge from the ear, hearing loss and sense of fullness. Pain mostly in chronic secretory otitis media.

Ménière's syndrome 60: Loss of balance, vertigo are the main symptoms. Mild deafness, sensation of fullness in ear, tinnitus, nausea and vomiting.

Paget's disease 267: Intermittent shifting bone pain, spontaneous fractures, grotesque enlargement of the head, height loss, impaired hearing.

Itching in the ear

Fungus-infected ears 54: Strong itching in and around ear canal. There may be grey or black particles in the ear. Some pain.

Lumps on the ear

Gout 334: Nodules of urate crystals on the ears and joints, pain and swelling of the big toe and joints, rapid pulse, scanty, dark urine.

Misshapen ears

Misshapen ears 55: Can be congenital, more often as a result of a blow or trauma. If untreated will develop into a cauliflower ear.

Noises in the ear (tinnitus)

Tinnitus (whistling, hissing, roaring or buzzing sounds in the ear) is a symptom of very many ear disorders. Other additional symptoms can help narrow down the ailment. The sounds vary from hissing to roaring or ringing from steady to intermittent. The intensity can change from day to day.

Unrelated diseases such as syphilis, high blood pressure, arterio-atherosclerosis, meningitis, allergic reactions, hysteria can also produce this symptom.

Tinnitus can appear as a side effect of many drugs and medications such as quinine, streptomycin, morphine, digitalis, too much aspirin, overindulgence in tobacco or alcohol. Some of these drugs are lifesavers in certain diseases; the side effects may be minor compared to their benefits.

Otosclerosis 50: Slow, insidious loss of hearing, loss of low tones, noises in the ear, distortion of sound, fullness, increasingly soft-spoken voice.

Perforation of the eardrum (acute) 56: Severe pain, loss of hearing, hollow reverberations in the head, loss of hearing. Blood in the ear canal.

Blockage of the eustachian tube 57: Impaired hearing, feeling of fullness in the ear, crackling noises while swallowing, sensation of fluid in the ear.

Acute otitis media 58a: Severe, stabbing pain may be constant or intermittent and may radiate over the side of the head, tinnitus. Note: Tinnitus is also common in chronic purulent and chronic secretory otitis media.

Ménière's syndrome 60: Loss of balance (vertigo) is the main symptom. Mild deafness, increasingly noises in the ear, nausea, vomiting.

Anaemia 332: Anaemic symptoms, palpitations, red, sore tongue. In severe cases, jaundice, numbness of limbs, tinnitus, thirst, poor memory, and shock.

Speaking too loudly

Perceptive hearing (nerve) loss 49: To compensate for his own voice which such a patient hears much more faintly, he will speak quite loudly. Presbycusis (a development of old age) accounts for much perceptive hearing loss. Ménière's syndrome if the disease persists will induce this symptom.

Certain medications are responsible for increasing deafness and thus for speaking too loudly. Examples are streptomycin and gentamicin (antibiotics), arsenic, mercury, mescaline, overdosage of aspirin. Heavy drinking can be a factor.

Noise pollution is surely one of the most common causes of permanent loss of hearing. Even a single loud blast can do great damage. There is no doubt that blaring rock music has caused considerable mischief.

Speaking too low

Conductive hearing loss 48: Speaking too low is often a symptom of conductive hearing loss due to the person hearing his own voice at amplified loudness. This symptom is often encountered wherever conductive hearing loss occurs such as otitis media, mastoiditis, blockage of the eustachian tube, boils or growths in the ear as well as the accumulation of wax.
Otosclerosis 50: Slow, stealthy loss of hearing, loss of low tones, noises in the ear, distortion of sounds, fullness, increasingly soft-spoken voice.

Swelling of the ear canal

Boils in the ear canal 52: Pain in the ear, diminished hearing, feeling of fullness in the ear, ear canal swollen and blocked. Possible discharge.

Tenderness behind the ear

Acute otitis media 58a: Primary symptom is severe, stabbing earache which may be constant or intermittent and which may radiate over the side of the head. Feeling of fullness in the ear, tinnitus, high fever, and tenderness over the mastoid bone.
Mastoiditis 59: Very severe pain, high fever, redness behind the ear, tenderness, occasional stiff neck, sore throat.

Symptoms of the nose

Bleeding nose (epistaxis)

A nosebleed rarely indicates a serious disease, even though it may be frightening in the young or in a young adult. However in the middle-aged it is quite often a sign of high blood pressure. Bleeding is occasionally seen in the common cold, scarlet fever, and flu. It may come on after a violent attack of hay fever, paroxysmal coughing, or severe sneezing. It can also be caused by over-enthusiastic nose picking. Some people have delicate vessels in the nose which can rupture from causes that would have no effect on others. Very rarely a nosebleed may be due to a malignant growth in the nose.

Brain injury 10: In severe trauma there is bleeding from the nose, mouth, and ears. The pupils are dilated (if unevenly this is a serious sign), skin is pale and clammy, drowsiness and coma.

Rheumatic heart disease and rheumatic fever 127: Nosebleeds are a frequent occurrence. Inflammation of the joints, rapid heartbeat, sweating, rash on the body, malaise.

Endocarditis 135: Bleeding from the nose and/or into the urine. There is usually fever, joint pains, anaemia, fatigue, red spots over the body.

High blood pressure 138: Nosebleed is a late symptom as are headache and dizziness. Bleeding is an attempt by the body to reduce the pressure.

Pernicious anaemia 323: Frequent nosebleeds, anaemic symptoms, palpitations, general body pain, pins-and-needles sensation, sore, beefy, red tongue, weight loss, jaundice, impotence and frigidity, difficulty in walking.

Aplastic anaemia 326: Symptoms of severe anaemia (pallor, shortness of breath), fatigue, brown pigmentation on pale, waxy skin, bleeding from the nose and mouth, and black-and-blue marks.

Vitamin K deficiency 354: Bleeding from the nose, gums, vagina, and stomach. Blood in the urine.

Typhoid fever 363: Sustained severe frontal or temporal headaches, sustained very high fever, slow doubled pulse beat, diarrhoea, rosy spots on abdomen, distended stomach, nosebleeds, coated tongue with red edges.

Leukaemia 415: Prolonged general bleeding from nose, gums, mucous membranes, under skin (small red-purplish spots). Acute anaemia, fatigue, deep malaise, great pallor. Children: (acute form) sore throat, rapid pulse, bruised body appearance. Adults: (chronic form) characteristic swollen lymph nodes, night sweats, weight loss.

Cancer of the pharynx (throat) 438: Nasal twang, nasal obstructions, pain in the nose, and bleeding from the nose.

Discharge from the nose

Common cold 63: Discharge and obstruction of the nasal passages are the major symptoms. Sneezing and laryngitis are very frequent.

Chronic rhinitis 64: Also obstructed nasal passages, postnasal drip, sore throat, intermittent headaches.

Hay fever and allergic rhinitis 65: Profuse watery discharge, tearing, violent sneezing, itching of nose and throat.

Sinusitis 66: Discharge is thick, yellow, continuous. Constant and recurrent headaches, postnasal drip, occasional swelling around eyes, chills and fever.

Nasal polyps 69: Excessive discharge, obstruction of air passages of the nose, loss of smell, headaches.

Acute bronchitis 103: Major symptom is the cough, at first dry and unproductive, later painful with heavy, purulent phlegm (white to yellowish). The cough is worse at night. The disease commences as a head cold. The fever may be high and prolonged.

Congenital syphilis 211: Infants: sniffles, blisters on the face, buttocks, soles and palms, symptoms of meningitis, curved shinbones. Later, saddle-backed nose and deformed teeth.

Cystic fibrosis 407: Failure of the infant or child to grow normally, ravenous appetite, greasy, foul-smelling stools, chronic cough, rapid breathing, wheezing, running nose, irritability, and thin, protuberant abdomen.

Itching nose

Overgrowth of hair in the nostril is a common cause of itching.

Hay fever and allergic rhinitis 65: Also itching of throat, profuse nasal discharge, tearing, violent sneezing.

Loss of smell (anosmia)

Both a cold and chronic rhinitis can temporarily dull the sense of smell. When the symptom is more prolonged and quite persistent it is more often due to *Sinusitis* **66** or *Nasal polyps* **69**.

The taste of food is actually a combination of smell and taste; the tongue can only distinguish sweetness, salt, and bitterness. A loss of smell also means a considerable loss of taste. (For *Loss of taste*, see *Symptoms of the tongue*.)

Adenoiditis 71: Breathing through the mouth, nasal speech, nasal obstruction, lowered mental ability, snoring, open-mouthed, lethargic face.

Misshapen nose

Congenital syphilis 211: Infants: blisters or rash on face, buttocks, palms, and soles, sniffles, symptoms of meningitis, curved shinbones, later saddle-backed nose and deformed teeth.

Hypothyroidism 339: Children: possible goitre, mental and physical retardation, puffy hands and feet, coarse face, flat and thick nose, dry skin becoming wrinkled, subnormal temperature, cold intolerance, pot-belly, apathy.

Nasal speech

Adenoidits 71: Breathing through the mouth, snoring, lowered mental ability.

Quinsy 72: Nasal twang, swelling of throat, severe pain on the affected side, difficulty in opening mouth, fever. This is a *Medical Emergency*.

Polio 374: High fever, severe headache, sore throat and muscle pain. Stiff neck is a vital sign. In serious cases, prostration, extreme weakness, twitching muscles, paralysis of the arms and legs. Difficulty in speaking and nasal voice are early signs of brain stem involvement.

Cleft lip and cleft palate 397: Besides the physical manifestation, other symptoms are inability to suck or swallow, dental problems, nasal voice, and possible ear infection.

Cancer of the pharynx (throat) 438: Nasal twang, nasal obstruction, pain in the nose and throat, nosebleed, difficulty swallowing.

Obstructed nose (mouth breathing)

Common cold 63: Obstruction, running nose, sneezing, irritated throat.
Chronic rhinitis 64: Constant nasal discharge, mouth breathing, postnasal drip, sore throat, intermittent headaches.
Deviated septum 67: Obstructed nostril and postnasal drip.
Nasal polyps 69: Obstruction, excessive nasal discharge, loss of smell, headache.
Adenoiditis 71: Mouth breathing is the primary symptom, nasal speech, obstruction, lowered mental ability, snoring.
Cancer of the pharynx (throat) 438: Nosebleeds, pain in the nose and throat, nasal twang, difficulty swallowing.

Pain in the nose

Neuralgia (tic douloureux) 4: Sharp jabs of pain run along the trigeminal or fifth cranial nerve from forehead to nose, lips, or tongue.
Cancer of the pharynx (throat) 438: Nasal twang, nasal obstruction, nosebleeds, pain in nose and throat, difficulty swallowing.

Postnasal drip

Chronic rhinitis 64: Obstructed and running nose, mouth breathing.
Deviated septum 67: Also clogged nostril.
Postnasal drip 68: Hawking, constant clearing of the throat. Coughing in some cases, occasional choking sensation in others.

Red nose

Rosacea 294: The nose is red and bulbous, face is flushed with redness along longitudinal centre of the face, pimples, dandruff.

Sneezing

Sneezing can be due to irritation. A change of temperature, strong sunlight, the presence of a foreign body in the nasal cavities, and fumes or emanations from some plants and from many chemicals, can all induce fits of sneezing.

However, sneezing is most commonly a symptom of a cold, of hay fever or of asthma.

Snoring

Snoring is due to the vibration of the soft palate or elongated uvula, which is often caused by sleeping on the back with the mouth open and breathing partly through the mouth and partly through the nose. Any obstruction in the nose will increase the likelihood of snoring. In children, many cases of snoring are due to enlarged tonsils and adenoids.

Extremely obese persons and the elderly have a greater tendency to snore; it is also a common feature in drunkenness and in patients under anaesthesia. Normally, snoring is harmless but annoying to the listener (the subject is never aware of it). If he is kept from lying on his back, he will stop.

Snoring, however, may be a grave sympton when the subject is in a coma.

Brain injury 10: If the patient is unconscious and snoring this is a serious sign. There will usually be bleeding from the mouth, nose, or ears.
Nasal polyps 69: Obstruction, excessive nasal discharge, loss of smell, headache, occasionally snoring.
Adenoiditis 71: Breathing through the mouth, nasal speech, lowered mental ability.
Stroke 139: Snoring reflects the gravity of the stroke if the patient is in a coma.

Symptoms of the breath, lips and mouth

THE BREATH
Bad breath (halitosis)

Bad breath is a symptom in a wide variety of disorders ranging from the innocuous to the quite serious. Certain foods will cause odoriferous breath such as onions, garlic, alcoholic beverages, etc. Many drugs will induce bad breath, as will infected gums and smoking. Putrefaction in the mouth or the nasopharynx (decay of food particles, tooth decay) will also produce this symptom. *Cancer of the lungs* **411**, *œsophagus* **429**, *tongue* **436**, *mouth* **437**, *pharynx (throat)* **438**, and *larynx* **439** all have as one of their symptoms foul breath. *Bad breath, Bad breath and bleeding gums, Bad breath and cough*

Bad breath

Postnasal drip 68: Hawking, constant clearing of throat, bad breath, particularly when condition is chronic.

Tonsillitis 70: The chronic form producing constant nasal discharge. Low fever, low energy level.

Adenoiditis 71: Due to mouth breathing. Snoring.

Gangrenous stomatitis 81: Dead black tissue on gums and mucous lining inside the mouth, bad breath. This is a *Medical Emergency*.

Traumatic stomatitis 82: Pain in the mouth, excessive salivation, bad breath.

Tongue disorders (chronic) 87: Enlarged, flabby tongue with indented teeth marks, foul taste in the mouth, bad breath.

Chronic gastritis 156: Constipation, vomiting with blood, blood in stools, burning, boring pain often radiating from abdomen to chest and back, sallow complexion, furry, red-rimmed tongue, bad taste in mouth, foul breath, heartburn, flatulence. Patient is morose, depressed.

Cirrhosis of the liver 191: Nausea, vomiting, flatulence, loss of weight. Later, severe jaundice, emaciation, foetid breath, ascites (abdomen distended from accumulation of liquid), spider angiomas (red spots with red lines radiating out), puffiness of legs and feet, enlarged vein on abdomen, general bleeding, bleeding into the stools. In men, enlarged breasts, atrophy of the testicles, loss of pubic hair, and impotence.

Acute yellow atrophy 193: Severe headache with high fever, jaundice, weakness, severe abdominal pain, black vomit, apathy, confusion, bleeding under the skin and from the mouth, dilated pupils, scanty, bloody urine, and rapid, feeble pulse. (Liver enlargement.)

Diphtheria 358: Sore throat, false membrane in throat, foul mouth odour, fever, difficulty swallowing. In severe cases, prostration, difficulty breathing.

Bad breath and bleeding gums

Trench mouth 77: Major symptoms are painful, bleeding gums, excessive salivation, bad breath. Ulceration in the mouth, and the appearance of a dirty-grey membrane.

Periodontitis (pyorrhoea) 101: Pus discharged from gums between the teeth will cause foul breath. The gums are usually bleeding, eroded, and have pockets.

Bad breath and cough

Acute bronchitis (foetid bronchitis) 103: Painful cough brings up foetid phlegm.

Bronchiectasis 105: The cough produces an extremely foul-smelling sputum. Very strong halitosis, cyanosis, shortness of breath, and great fatigue.

Pulmonary tuberculosis 112: Variable foul breath depending on state of cavitation in lungs. Other symptoms: cough, bloody sputum, drenching sweats, great loss of vitality and energy, shortness of breath.

Lung abscess 115: Cough brings up bloodstained and particularly foul-smelling phlegm. The lung is gangrened. There is also shortness of breath, prostration, and chills and fever.

Empyaema 119: Sharp pain in the side, dry cough, chills and fever, deep malaise, emaciation, and foul breath.

Lung cancer 411: Chest pain, coughing, wheezing, shortness of breath becoming worse. Chest pain behind breastbone can be stabbing or dull. Weight loss, fatigue, hoarseness, and night sweats.

*

Sweetish breath

Acute infectious hepatitis 187 and **Serum hepatitis 188:** Jaundice, dark urine, light-coloured stools, red, itching wheals, tenderness in liver area, sickly sweet, foetid breath, gastrointestinal upset.

Diabetes 332: Excessive thirst, urination,

and hunger, weight loss, weakness, sweet, fruity breath, blurred vision, pins-and-needles sensation in the legs, leg cramps, skin and vaginal infections, impotence.

Urine breath

Uraemia 207: Very scanty urine, urinous odour on breath, uraemic frost, parts of the body become swollen, severe headaches, impaired or double vision, contracted pupils, nausea, vomiting, diarrhoea, convulsions, coma.

Acute kidney failure 208: Scanty urine, breathing difficulties, urine breath, lethargy, dry skin and mucous membranes, vomiting, diarrhoea, convulsions.

THE LIPS
Blue lips (cyanosis of the lips)

Chronic bronchitis 104: Paroxysmal cough, wheezing, breathlessness, barrel chest, and cyanosis of the lips and fingernail beds.

Hypoxia 122: Palpitations, shortness of breath upon exertion, headache, giddiness, difficulty concentrating, poor judgement, malaise, weakness, blue lips.

Shock 133: Great pallor, cyanosis of lips, fingernail beds, earlobes, and tips of fingers, cold, clammy skin, fast, weak pulse, shortness of breath, sunken eyes, dilated pupils, anxiety state, finally coma.

Cleft lip

Cleft lip and cleft palate 397: Besides the obvious physical malformation there is the inability to suck or swallow, dental problems, possible ear infection, and nasal voice.

Cracked and reddened lips (chapped)

Cheilitis, inflammation of the lips, will occur when they are exposed to severe weather, or may be due to an individual's hypersensitivity to the colouring matter in lipstick and occasionally in toothpaste. Hypersensitivity to fingernail polish is another frequent cause. This will occur when a woman has the habit of resting her chin on the palm of her hand so that the fingernails touch the lips.

Gingivitis (pellagra gingivitis) 100: Cracked and reddened lips, gums, scalded feeling on gums and on the tongue which is very red, smooth, and ulcerated.

Vitamin B$_2$ (riboflavin) deficiency 350: Weakness, tongue is swollen and the edges inflamed, chapped lips, cracked corners of the mouth, cloudy, ulcerated cornea, dry, red, scaly skin around the nose, ear, and scrotum.

Lesions on or around lips

Perlèche 76: Corners of the mouth are an intense red, fissured, and ulcerated. Area is burning and painful.

Herpes labialis 80a: Fever blisters, or cold sores, which burst and become crusty sores, form on or around lips.

Early syphilis 209: Hard, painless ulcer on genitalia or around mouth. Later (second stage), varying widespread body rash, ulcers in the mouth, severe headaches, sore throat, arthritic pains, eye disorders.

Skin cancer 409: A white or dark red, hard area which suddenly begins to ulcerate into a hard, crusted sore. The lower lip is a common site.

Cancer of the lip 435: A scaled ulcer where the skin meets the lip, bleeds easily. Can also be in the form of a fissure, hardened nodule, irregular, raised horny surface, or a blister, all of which eventually ulcerate and bleed.

THE MOUTH
Bleeding from the mouth

Brain injury (concussion) 10: When head wound is severe, bleeding from nose, ears, mouth, dilated or uneven

pupils (a more serious sign), drowsiness, confusion, vomiting, and coma.

Acute yellow atrophy 193: Severe headache with jaundice, high fever, weakness. Severe abdominal pain, black vomit, apathy, confusion, bleeding under the skin and from the mouth, dilated pupils, scanty, bloody urine and rapid, feeble pulse. (Liver enlargement.)

Aplastic anaemia 326: Severe anaemic symptoms, bleeding from nose and mouth, brown pigmentation of the skin, black-and-blue marks.

Purpura 328: Tiny red spots on the body turning purple and later becoming black-and-blue marks, bleeding from mouth and mucous membranes at slightest injury, pain in the abdomen and joints, slow clotting of blood.

Yellow fever 379: High fever, flushed face, prostration, severe headache, pain in the back and limbs, scanty urine. After intermission, jaundice, vomiting of black blood and bleeding from mucous membranes.

Cancer of the thyroid 417: Goitre, hoarseness, difficulty swallowing, vocal paralysis, expectorating bloody mucus, choking attacks, weight loss.

Cancer of the mouth 437: Begins as soft, whitish patch inside mouth which thickens until hard. Can be irregular protrusion (felt by the tongue), fissured, or ulcerated. May or may not bleed. Stiffness of jaw muscle. Pain is a late sign.

Cracks in the corners of the mouth

Perlèche 76: Intense red areas at corners of the mouth which may become fissured and ulcerated. Area is burning and painful.

Vitamin B$_2$ (riboflavin) deficiency 350: Cracks in corners of the mouth, cloudy or ulcerated cornea, photophobia, burning sensation in the eye, impaired vision.

Dry mouth

The most common normal cause of dry

mouth is fear, experienced by all in the normal course of living at one time or another. Hysteria and some forms of neurosis can also inhibit salivation. Excessive smoking will do the same. Such drugs as atropine and belladonna, used for gastro-intestinal disorders, for relief of muscle spasms, and for dilation of the pupils are known producers of this symptom.

Most acute infections and diabetes have dry mouth as one of their less significant symptoms.

Thrush 78: White patches, which later become shallow ulcers, form over entire mucous lining of the mouth, including inner lips, tongue and gums. Mouth is dry.

Shock 133: Dry mouth, extreme pallor, cold, clammy skin, cyanosis of lips, fingernails, and tips of fingers, shortness of breath, dilated pupils.

Botulism 165: Extreme dryness of mouth, double or blurred vision, fixed, dilated pupils, difficulty breathing or talking, cramps, diarrhoea, nausea, vomiting, paralysis of the respiratory tract.

Mumps 375: Pain, swelling of the salivary glands under jaw and in the neck, difficulty opening mouth or swallowing acidic food, scanty (dry mouth) or profuse salivation. Furred tongue.

False membrane in the mouth

also see **Throat** *in* **Symptoms of the neck, throat, and larynx**

Trench mouth 77: Painful, bleeding gums, bad breath, ulcers in the mouth, difficulty talking or swallowing. False membrane is dirty greyish in colour.

Gangrene of the mouth

Gangrenous stomatitis 81: Grey or black tissue appears on mucous lining of the mouth. Externally the cheeks become red and swollen, then black. Pain and fever. This is always a *Medical Emergency*.

Lesions of the mouth (inflammation, sores, spots, tumours)

Lesions of the mouth, Whitish lesions in the mouth

Lesions of the mouth

Perlèche 76: Corners of the mouth become intensely red, then fissured and ulcerated. Area is burning and painful.

Trench mouth 77: Ulceration and false membrane on mucosa of the mouth. Other symptoms are excessive salivation, bad breath, bleeding gums, difficulty talking or swallowing.

Aphthous stomatitis (canker sores) 79: Blisters with red margins inside the mouth, erupting into egg-shaped ulcers. They appear singly or in batches.

Tumours of the mouth 85: Lesions that show no sign of healing in five days may be cancerous.

Mucocoele 88a: Small, round, bluish translucent tumour inside the mouth.

Gingivitis 100: Various different lesions from such systemic causes as diabetes, which produces polyps between teeth and severe gum inflammation; leukaemia: enlarged, discoloured, and painful gums; scurvy: blue-black spots on gums and mouth; pellagra: ulcerated lesions on gums and mouth with a bright red, smooth tongue and cracked lips. Pregnancy may cause enlargement of the gums and formation of pseudo tumours.

Early syphilis 209: First stage: hard ulcer on genitalia. Second stage: varying rash over the body, ulcers in the mouth which produce greyish ooze, severe headache, arthritic pains, sore throat, eye disorders.

Vitamin B complex (niacin) deficiency (pellagra) 351: Loss of appetite and weight, weakness, red spots on the body which turn large, brown, and scaly, the tongue margins, gums, and mucous membranes become inflamed and scarlet, excessive salivation. Later, bloody diarrhoea, poor memory, and emotional instability.

Whitish lesions in the mouth

Thrush 78: White patches like milk curds appear inside the cheeks, lips, on the gums, tongue, or palate and later become shallow ulcers.

Herpetic stomatitis 80: Patient is sick and feverish. White plaques and ulcers inside mouth, inflamed gums, painful mouth conditions.

Oral lichen planus 83: Bluish-white lines in mucosa of mouth and/or inside of lips. There may be white patches as well. Mouth feels itchy and rough. Pain in the erosive form.

Leukoplakia 84: Whitish growths inside mouth, usually on tongue and cheeks, occurring mostly in middle-aged and elderly men. These patches are leathery, sometimes fissured and ulcerated. They can have a yellowish cast. Pain is a late sign.

Measles 370: Koplik's spots: rosy area with white centres inside of cheeks (an early sign of measles). Later, brownish-pink rash all over body. The disease starts with cold symptoms, high fever, cough, photophobia.

Cancer of the mouth 437: Often begins as a soft whitish growth or patch which thickens and hardens. May or may not bleed. Tongue will feel an irregular protrusion or fissured ulcer. Stiffness or spasm in jaw muscle. Pain is a late sign.

*
Pain in the mouth

Aphthous stomatitis (canker sores) 79: Very painful blisters inside mouth which erupt into egg-shaped ulcers (white centre on red).

Herpetic stomatitis 80: Painful white plaques and ulcers inside mouth, inflamed gums. Patient is sick and feverish.

Stomatitis traumatica 82: Excessive salivation, bad breath as well as pain.

Oral lichen planus 83: Bluish-white lines in mucosa of the mouth, mouth feels itchy and rough. Pain in the erosive form.

Gingivitis (leukaemia form) 100:

Gums enlarged, painful, discoloured, and bleeding.

Vitamin B complex (niacin) deficiency (pellagra) 351: Weakness, loss of weight, red, symmetrical spots on skin which turn brown and scaly, inflamed gums, mucous membranes of mouth become scarlet and painful, excessive salivation. Later, bloody diarrhoea.

Cancer of the mouth 437: Often begins as a soft whitish patch or growth inside the mouth which thickens and hardens. The tongue can feel the irregular protrusion and fissured ulceration. The patch may or may not bleed. The jaw muscles become stiff. Pain is a late sign.

Palate, cleft

Cleft lip and cleft palate 397: Besides the obvious physical malformation, other signs are the inability to suck or swallow, dental problems, possible ear infection, and nasal voice.

Paleness around the mouth

Scarlet fever 359: Face flushed except for the telltale paleness around the mouth, sore throat, vomiting, high fever, heavy, white, furry tongue turning raspberry, greyish-yellow false membrane in the throat and mouth. Body rash which blanches in squeezed spots. Later, flaking and peeling of the skin and dark red lines on the skin folds.

SALIVATION (PTYALISM)

Salivation, excessive, Salivation and difficulty swallowing

Salivation, excessive

In the absence of a physical disease excessive salivation can be brought on by deep emotion, shock, or chronic worry. It can also appear for no reason at all, usually in high-strung, middle-aged people. It is also one of the minor disturbances of pregnancy, occasionally a symptom of high blood pressure, and frequently characteristic of excessive smoking.

The following drugs, either swallowed or applied externally, can induce salivation: pilocarpine (used in glaucoma), mercury, iodides, bromides, antimony, and copper salts.

Epilepsy 2: Dusky face, muscular twitching, jerking of arms and legs, clenched hands, incontinence, drooling, and convulsions.

Encephalitis 8: High fever, pounding headache, drowsiness, stupor, stiff neck, excessive salivation.

Trench mouth 77: Also bleeding gums, bad breath, ulceration in mouth.

Stomatitis traumatica 82: Heavy salivation from mechanical injury (eg, ill-fitting dentures, jagged tooth), bad breath, and pain in the mouth.

Ulcer of the oesophagus 147: Radiating pain behind breastbone, heartburn, loss of weight, excessive salivation, diarrhoea.

Staphylococcus gastroenteritis 164: Nausea, vomiting, cramps, diarrhoea, excessive salivation, sweating. In severe cases, prostration and shock.

Minor disorders of pregnancy 235: Slight shortness of breath, backache, headache, varicose veins, haemorrhoids, dyspepsia, excessive salivation.

Vitamin B complex (niacin) deficiency (pellagra) 351: Loss of appetite, weight, red spots on body turning brown and scaly. Margins of the tongue and mucous membrane turn scarlet, inflamed gums, excessive salivation. Later, bloody diarrhoea.

Salivation and difficulty swallowing

Tongue disorders 87: Ulcerated tongue, thick saliva, difficulty swallowing.

Mumps 375: Painful swelling of the salivary glands below the ear, difficulty opening mouth or swallowing acidic food. Saliva can be scanty or excessive, never normal. Furred tongue.

Rabies 378: There is first depression, irritability changing to excitability and wildness, profuse salivation, drooling, swallowing impossible, collapse, coma.

Cancer of the oesophagus 429: Difficulty swallowing, distress in the throat, heavy salivation, cough, loss of voice, flatulence, thirst, emaciation, weight loss, foul breath.

*

Swelling inside mouth

Gingivitis (leukaemia form) 100: Enlarged gums that are also painful and discoloured. Considerable swelling.

Yawning

Tetanus 361: Stiffness of jaw, neck, yawning, difficulty swallowing. Later, permanent grin as jaws become fixed and agonizing. General muscle spasms.

Symptoms of the tongue

The tongue, like the eyes, will frequently leave a telltale clue to disorders elsewhere. Very often it is a barometer of the state of health of the body.

Normally the tongue is pink, moist, and clean. A slightly fissured or slightly furred tongue is usually of no significance. Some people have a coated tongue all their lives, while with others, a coated tongue may be an indication of serious disease. A coloured tongue may be due to medication or food.

Pain can be due to drinking hot beverages, or taking hot spices (often unremembered), or can result from excessive smoking, perforation from a fishbone, or the like. The practice of keeping an aspirin over a painful tooth can result in a burnlike effect on the mucosa and tongue.

Abnormalities of taste (loss of taste, perverted taste, foul taste)

The taste of food is really a combination of smell and taste. The normal taste buds on the tongue (several thousands of them) can only distinguish salt, sweet, sour, and bitter. In an upper respiratory infection one or both of these senses may be lost. Many abnormalities are due to *Tongue disorders* **87**.

Loss of taste: *Migraine headache* **13b** can often block off taste and smell; *Bell's palsy* **3a** can paralyse parts of the tongue; any cancer inside the mouth can obstruct the taste buds. Many forms of glossitis (*Tongue disorders* **87**) can impair taste, as can the *Common cold* **63**.

Perverted taste: For some unknown reason pregnancy can, on many occasions, distort this sense. Brain lesions can induce taste hallucinations and delusions. In some instances hysteria can produce alterations from the normal.

Foul taste: Most local conditions of the mouth can cause an unpleasant taste such as *Dental caries* **89**, *Tooth abscess* **91**, *Gingivitis* **100**, *Periodontitis* (*pyorrhoea*) **101**, *Trench mouth* **77**, *Herpetic stomatitis* **80** and *Gangrenous stomatitis* **81** and almost all forms of mouth cancer. The varying diseases of the tongue can cause this condition (*Tongue disorders* **87**).

Many gastrointestinal disorders present this symptom, notably *Chronic gastritis* **156**, *Hypertrophic pyloric stenosis* in adults **169** and *Stomach cancer* **430**. Infections of the respiratory tract, particularly *Bronchiectasis* **105**, lung cavitation from *Pulmonary tuberculosis* **112**, and *Lung abscess* **115**, usually develop a bad taste in the mouth but this is overshadowed by far more significant symptoms.

Black tongue

Black hairy tongue 87d: Elongation of

papillae of the tongue, causing tickling or gagging sensation. Black discoloration of the tongue. Note: after extensive therapy with an antibiotic which kills off all the bacterial flora in the mouth, a fungus infection can take over which can blacken the tongue. This discoloration will disappear on its own.

Bluish tinge of the tongue

A bluish tinge to the tongue can be due to poor blood circulation, heart disease, and any impairment of respiration, notably asthma. Any form of cyanosis can also appear on the tongue as well.

Brown tongue

Any oxygen-liberating mouthwash or long therapy with antibiotics can produce a brown tongue, usually with a furred surface. Brown tongue is occasionally seen in late stages of serious fever and can be a serious sign, especially if the tongue is also dry and tremulous.

Coated tongue

A coated tongue quite often is not very significant; it can indicate that the subject sleeps with his mouth open, or that he has not eaten for a long while, or some minor digestive disturbance. On some occasions it can indicate a more serious condition.

Acute gastritis (simple) 155: Burning pain and pressure in the stomach, loss of appetite, coated tongue, nausea and vomiting, occasionally headache and vertigo.
Scarlet fever 359: Vomiting, high fever, sore throat, heavy, white-coated, furred tongue with enlarged red papillae (white strawberry tongue). The coat soon peels leaving a bright red strawberry colour. A greyish-yellow false membrane appears on the throat and mouth. Body rash which blanches on squeezed spots. Later, skin peels, flakes. Face flushed except for paleness around the mouth.

Typhoid fever 363: Flu-like symptoms at first. Frontal or temporal headaches which are severe and sustained. Very high fever, nosebleeds, slow but double pulse beats, diarrhoea, distended stomach, white-coated (sometimes brown) tongue with red edges.

Fissured tongue (only significant if fissures are deep)

Leukoplakia 84: White or yellowish-white patches on inside of mouth or on tongue, becoming leathery and thickened. On tongue they may be fissured and ulcerated. Pain is a late symptom.
Scrotal tongue 87b: Surface of tongue lined with deep, haphazardly wandering grooves starting from the centre.
Vitamin B$_2$ (riboflavin) deficiency 350: Weakness. Cracks appear on the corners of the mouth, cloudy or ulcerated cornea, photophobia, conjunctivitis, impaired vision.

Furred tongue

This symptom is seen in all fevers, in indigestion, and in most mouth disorders.

Chronic gastritis 156: Furry and red-rimmed tongue. Burning pain and pressure in pit of stomach which may radiate to chest or back; frequently vomiting with blood, blood in stools, bad taste in mouth, flatulence. Patient is depressed.
Acute nephritis 197: Scanty but bloody urine, puffiness of face, swelling of ankles, sharp loss of appetite, nausea and vomiting.
Diabetes (ketoacidosis, diabetic coma) 332: Breathing is rapid, deep, and hungry, severe dehydration, dizziness, furry tongue, poor skin tone, abdominal pain, sunken eyeballs, nausea, vomiting, stupor, shock, finally, coma.
Mumps 375: Painful swelling of the salivary glands, furred tongue, difficulty opening mouth or swallowing acidic foods. Either dry mouth or profuse salivation.

Glossy tongue

Occurs often in elderly people with atrophy of the papillae of the tongue.

Pernicious anaemia 323: Pallor, weakness, shortness of breath, palpitations, tingling, numbness of hands and feet, sore tongue which is smooth, beefy, and red, loss of appetite, weight loss, yellowish-lemon colour of skin. In severe cases there may be heart failure, impotence, frigidity, nausea, vomiting, and mental confusion.

Large tongue (swollen tongue)

A large tongue may be congenital; or, it may be swollen from a bite (ordinary chewing of food or in an epileptic seizure), from an injury from a fishbone, from an aspirin kept in the mouth to reduce a toothache, or as the result of insidious mercury poisoning. A reaction to animal serum can cause tongue enlargement.

Tongue disorders 87: In some chronic forms of glossitis the tongue becomes enlarged and flabby, showing teeth marks. A not too rare form of glossitis can make the tongue swell so that chewing, swallowing or speaking is difficult; occasionally, breathing may be obstructed, causing a *Medical Emergency.*

Indigestion (chronic) 154: In the chronic state the tongue is not very large but remains uncomfortable. It is pale and flabby and shows marks of teeth.

Late syphilis 210: In one of the complications called gumma (development of a soft ulcerating tumour), a tumour may develop anywhere in the body and grow from pinhead to tennis ball size. If it shows up on the tongue it will enlarge it and can turn cancerous.

Acromegaly and gigantism 336: Abnormal tallness, enlarged skeleton, increased size in hands, feet, face, tongue jaws protrude, overgrowth of internal organs, mental deterioration, joint pains, severe headaches.

Hypothyroidism 339: Cretinism in children; in adults, mental apathy, thinking process slowed, obesity, puffiness of hands and face, enlarged tongue, dry, sandpapery skin, dull, falling hair, cold intolerance.

Magenta tongue

Vitamin B₂ (riboflavin) deficiency 350: Weakness, edges of the tongue are reddish-purple and fissured. Cracks usually appear at the corners of the mouth, cloudy or ulcerated cornea, photophobia, impaired vision, conjunctivitis.

Painful tongue

Neuralgia (tic douloureux) 4: Inflammation of the facial nerve running from forehead to the nose, mouth, or tongue.

Leukoplakia 84: White or yellowish-white patches appear on the tongue and elsewhere in the mouth; they are leathery, thickened, can be fissured and may become ulcerated. Pain is a late symptom.

Glossodynia 87a: May be due to local origin, systemic disorders, and psychiatric conditions. This condition is particularly sensitive to hot or spicy foods.

Ranula 88: This cyst on the underside of the tongue is translucent, containing a clear viscous fluid, and is usually painless until it becomes inflamed.

Gingivitis (pellagra gingivitis) 100: Cracked, reddened lips, scalded feeling in the tongue which is very red and smooth, ulcerated lesions in the mouth.

Pernicious anaemia 323: Anaemic symptoms, sore, red tongue, pins-and-needles sensation as well as pain in varying parts of the body, palpitations, weight loss, jaundice, difficulty walking, impotence or frigidity, nausea.

Trichinosis 386: The embryo of this parasite has a special penchant for the muscles at the base of the tongue, making it painful and tender. Swelling and pain in different parts of the body. Profuse sweating. Shortness of breath if severe.

Cancer of the tongue 436: Starts with irritation on the tongue or sides of it, then a slight growth appears and area is mildly painful. As tumour progresses hard nodules, ulcers appear with severe pain. Cancer in back of tongue will cause pain in throat as well.

Pale tongue

Anaemia 322: Pallor everywhere, of the skin, under eyelids, gums, fingernails. The tongue is pale, large, flabby, and shows teeth marks. Other signs are vertigo, rapid, pounding heartbeat, tinnitus, loss of libido, longitudinally ridged fingernails.

Scarlet tongue (bright red tongue, raspberry tongue, strawberry tongue)

Chronic gastritis 156: Pain in the stomach mild to acute, mild nausea, loss of appetite, constipation, distension of the stomach, bad taste in the mouth, foul breath and furred tongue.

Sprue 180: Diarrhoea three to four times daily, faeces fatty, light-coloured and foul. Stomach distended while rest of body emaciated, small bleedings under the skin, sore red tongue, flatulence, apathy. In children, retarded growth, spontaneous fractures.

Pernicious anaemia 323: Anaemic symptoms, palpitations, pins-and-needles sensation in hands, feet, and elsewhere, sore, red tongue, weight loss, difficulty walking, impotence, frigidity, nausea.

Diabetes 332: Excessive urination, thirst, hunger; weight loss, weakness, sweet, fruity breath, blurred vision, pins-and-needles sensation in the extremities, leg cramps, skin and vaginal disorders, red, sore, dry tongue.

Vitamin B complex (niacin) deficiency (pellagra) 351: Weakness, headaches, loss of weight, red spots on skin turning brown and scaly. The mucous membranes and margins of the tongue becoming scarlet, inflamed gums, diarrhoea, later becoming bloody, poor memory and emotional instability.

Scarlet fever 359: High fever, sore throat, vomiting, heavy, white, furry tongue with enlarged red papillae. The white coat soon peels revealing a bright red strawberry colour, yellowish-grey membrane forms in mouth. A rash appears – tiny, densely packed dots over the body. Face is flushed except for pallor around mouth.

Speech difficulties (stuttering, scanning)

Stuttering occurs in most children between ages two and four. Parents should not be overly concerned and should not draw attention to this condition. The child's mind may be faster than his speech development but he will soon catch up. Nagging him or shaming him will only increase his tension. This symptom should be ignored and an attempt made to understand the cause. As the child grows older or relaxes the speech defect will disappear.

Parkinson's disease 1: Slowness of all action, mask-like face, drooling, rigid, stooped posture, spastic gait, tremors at rest which diminish upon movement, slurred, slow speech.

Multiple sclerosis 6: Intention tremor, general tremor, spastic walk, disturbances of vision, paralysis or palsy of the eyeball, monotone voice, scanning speech (slow pronunciation of syllable by syllable).

Tonguetie 86: Interference in articulation of speech.

Minimal brain dysfunction 404: Visual perception errors, learning disabilities, attention span disorders, lack of concentration, hyperactivity, restlessness, emotional instability, poor coordination and occasional loss of balance.

Tremor of the tongue

A state of anxiety can cause tremor of the tongue and lips along with tachycardia, sweating, and indigestion. Cocaine and opium will induce tremors of hands, lips, and tongue upon withdrawal from these drugs. Toxaemia from uraemia will produce tremors of the hands, lips, and tongue. This symptom is often a feature of alcoholism.

Cirrhosis of the liver 191: Nausea, vomiting, flatulence, weight loss, jaundice, emaciation, massive collection of fluids in abdominal cavity, spider angiomas, feminizing changes in men, impotence, nosebleeds, and tremors of the tongue.

Late syphilis (paresis) 210: Tremor of tongue and lips, severe headaches, degeneration of memory and mind, increasingly slovenly habits.

Ulcers and tumours of the tongue

A jagged tooth will cause an ulcer which will heal rapidly upon repair of the tooth or its extraction. Ulcers also occur in chickenpox and indigestion.

Leukoplakia 84: Whitish growth inside the mouth, cheeks, or on tongue, usually among middle-aged and elderly men. These patches are leathery, sometimes fissured and ulcerated with a yellowish cast. Pain is a late sign.

Tumours of the mouth 85: Any ulcer on the tongue or mouth which does not show signs of healing within five days might be cancerous.

Ranula 88: A large cystic tumour on underside of the tongue, translucent, filled with clear viscous fluid. Neither painful nor cancerous.

Late syphilis 210: Soft ulcerating tumour (gumma) on the tongue; can also appear elsewhere in the body. This ulcer may become hard but then may break down into a deep cavity. It is not painful and usually does not increase in size. The gumma will respond to antisyphilitic treatment.

Histoplasmosis 393: Ulcers on the nose, ear, legs, pharynx, larynx, and the extremities. Irregular fever, emaciation, anaemia, swollen lymph nodes, nausea, vomiting, diarrhoea with black stools and debilitation.

Cancer of the tongue 436: Tumour usually preceded by area of irritation on the tongue or its sides, then slight growth, slightly painful. As the tumour progresses it becomes hard, ulcerous, and painful. Cancer at back of the tongue will produce pain in the throat and ear.

White raised tongue (geographical tongue)

Geographical tongue (benign migratory glossitis) 87c: Irregularly outlined pink to red and white, unhardened patches on a whitish tongue devoid of normal papillae. The configuration of patches changes constantly from day to day. So named because the raised area appears like a mountain range on a relief map.

Yellow tongue

Yellow tongue is really an extension of jaundice. Other signs of yellow tones should be observed and checked.

Symptoms of the gums, jaws, and teeth

THE GUMS
Bleeding gums

Bleeding gums, Bleeding gums as part of general bleeding

Bleeding gums

Very hard bristles on the brush, too vigorous or too frequent brushing may cause the gums to bleed.

Trench mouth 77: The gums are painful, spongy, and will bleed at the slightest touch. Greyish or yellowish membrane over mucosa of the mouth. There may be sores on the mucosa. Swallowing or talking can be painful.

Gingivitis 100: Gums inflamed in a band where they meet the teeth; gums are swollen and bleed at slightest touch. In the scurvy form of gingivitis, blue and purplish spots will appear on the gums and elsewhere in the mouth.

In pellagra gingivitis, ulcers will appear on the gums and in the mouth, the tongue is bright red and smooth with a scalded feeling. Red, cracked lips.

In pregnancy gingivitis, tumours appear on swollen, bleeding gums.

Periodontitis (pyorrhoea) 101: Bleeding gums, large pockets in the gums, and loosening teeth.

Bleeding gums as part of general bleeding

Aplastic anaemia 326: Pallor, shortness of breath, fatigue, palpitation, brown pigmentation on pale, waxy skin, bleeding from nose and gums, black-and-blue marks.

Purpura 328: Small reddish-blue spots on skin, bleeding from mucous membranes and gums on slight injury. Pain in the abdomen and joints, slow clotting of blood from cuts or wounds, black-and-blue marks.

Haemophilia 329: Bleeding from slight injury to any part of the body, including the gums.

Vitamin C deficiency (scurvy) 352: Weakness, bleeding under the skin (small red-purplish spots), bleeding from mucous membranes, gums; loose teeth, easily broken bones, skin rash. In infants, loss of appetite and weight, irritability, very painful and swollen legs.

Vitamin K deficiency 354: General bleeding: gums, nose, vagina, blood in urine and stools.

Leukaemia 415: Fatigue, malaise, pallor, general bleeding from the nose, gums, and in the skin (pinpoint red to purplish spots). Easy bruising, sore throat, weight loss, night sweats, rapid pulse, joint pains.

*

Bleeding socket

Complications in tooth extraction 94: Bleeding in varying degrees from a few hours to a prolonged period. Occasionally pain and swelling of the socket.

Gangrene of the gums

Gangrenous stomatitis 81: Black or grey tissues appear on gums and mucous lining of the mouth. The external cheeks become swollen, red, glazed, and then black. This is a *Medical Emergency*.

Painful gums

Neuralgia (trigeminal neuralgia) 4: Sharp jabs of pain along course of the nerve from head to face (lips, nose, tongue, or gums).

Trench mouth 77: Gums are painful, spongy, bleed at the slightest touch. Grey or yellowish membrane on the mucosa of the mouth. Sores may appear in the mouth.

Herpetic stomatitis 80: Patient is sick and feverish, pain in the gums, white plaques and ulcers inside the mouth.

Complications in tooth extraction 94: General pain which can become severe in 'dry socket'. There may be swelling and bleeding.

Tooth eruption and impaction of wisdom tooth 98: Pain in the gum around the area and swelling.

Gingivitis (leukaemia form) 100: The gums are inflamed, swollen, bleeding and discoloured. The entire mouth may also be inflamed.

Pocket in gums

Gingivitis 100: Pockets between gums and teeth, bleeding, swollen gums.

Periodontitis (pyorrhoea) 101: Formation of large pockets between gums and teeth, causing pus in the gums and loosened teeth,

Receding gums

Periodontitis (pyorrhoea) 101: Large gum pockets also cause gums to recede. Teeth are loosened; chewing often difficult.

Swollen gums (inflamed)

Herpetic stomatitis 80: Fever, inflamed gums, white plaques and ulcers appear on the mucous membranes of the mouth producing a foul taste. In a child, pain may be so severe as to keep him from taking food.

Tooth abscess 91: Also steady relentless ache. Tooth is sensitive to the touch; heat makes it worse.

Complications in tooth extraction 94: Swollen gums, bleeding of the socket.

Tooth eruption and impaction of wisdom tooth 98: Impacted wisdom tooth can cause toothache, also pain, swelling, and inflammation of the surrounding gum area.

Gingivitis 100: Very red gums, bleeding at slightest touch. Diabetic gingivitis: swollen gums, abscess and polyps between the teeth. Leukaemia gingivitis: gums are painful, swollen, discoloured, and bleeding. Pellagra gingivitis: gums are swollen, bleeding, ulcerated, lips reddened and cracked, tongue glossy and bright red.

Vitamin B complex (niacin) deficiency (pellagra) 350: Loss of appetite and weight, weakness, red spots on body turning brown and scaly, mucous membranes and margins of the tongue becoming scarlet, swollen gums, excess salivation, diarrhoea later becoming bloody. Poor memory and emotional instability.

Tumours, ulcers, and boils on the gums

Trench mouth 77: Gums are painful, spongy, and bleed at the slightest touch. Grey or yellowish membrane on the mouth mucosa. Sores may appear in the mouth.

Tooth abscess 91: A steady relentless ache, swelling of the face near the tooth, tooth very sensitive to the touch, swollen gums and gumboil. Heat makes it worse.

Gingivitis 100: Diabetic gingivitis: severe gum inflammation, abscesses and growth of polyps between the teeth.

Pellagra gingivitis: reddened, cracked lips, bright red glossy tongue feeling as if it's been scalded, ulcerated lesions on gums and mouth. Pregnancy gingivitis: enlarged gums with tumours.

THE JAWS
Pain in the jaw

Quinsy 72: Large swelling in the affected side of the mouth, severe pain at the site and back of the jaw, tension in jaw muscles. Often inability to open the jaw; swallowing is difficult. The soft palate and the uvula are swollen, as are the lymph nodes in the neck. This is a *Medical Emergency*.

Temporomandibular joint disorder 102: Mouth cannot be opened fully, severe pain at joint of the jaw in speaking or chewing. The affected side of the face is sore.

Mumps 375: Pain and swelling of the salivary glands below the ear. Difficulty in opening mouth or swallowing acidic foods. Either scanty or profuse salivation, dry mouth, furred tongue.

Cancer of the pharynx (throat) 438: Pain or difficulty in eating or swallowing, discomfort in the throat, difficulty opening mouth or coughing. Pain may radiate to side of face, swelling of neck lymph nodes.

Protruding jaw

Acromegaly and gigantism 336: Enlarged skeleton, abnormal tallness, increase in size of hands, feet, face, and internal organs, protruding jaw, loss of libido, mental deterioration, sweating, joint pains.

Stiff jaw

Quinsy 72: Large swelling at the affected side of the mouth, severe pain at the site and back of the jaw, and difficulty swallowing. The soft palate and uvula are swollen, as are the lymph nodes in the neck. This is a *Medical Emergency*.

Tetanus (lockjaw) 361: Stiffness of the jaw and neck eventually becoming fixed, immovable, and agonizing. Difficulty swallowing, yawning, fixed grin, extremely painful muscle spasms all over body, restlessness, apprehension.

Cancer of the mouth 437: Begins as soft white patch or growth in the mouth which the tongue can feel as an irregular protrusion. Patch becomes thick, hard, fissured, and ulcerated. May or may not bleed. Stiffness or spasm of the jaw muscles. Pain is a late development.

THE TEETH
Bruxism (grinding the teeth)

Bruxism 99: Usually occurs during sleep. Continuous grinding can injure the pulp, loosen the teeth, and eventually kill a nerve.

Cavity in tooth

Dental caries 89: General decay of a tooth. If pulp is involved, varying degrees of pain.

Deformed teeth

Congenital syphilis 211: Infants: rash or blisters on face, buttocks, soles, palms, symptoms of meningitis, curved shinbones, nose sniffles. Later, saddle-backed nose and deformed teeth.

Vitamin D deficiency (rickets) 353a: Infants: restlessness, softening and thinning of headbones, bow legs, badly formed teeth. Child cannot walk, stand, or sit at the proper age. Later, scoliosis (curvature of the spine).

Discoloured teeth

This is not a sign of a disorder. A tooth or teeth can become discoloured by certain medications, by too much smoking and occasionally by too much brushing, which can wear away the enamel in some parts of the tooth exposing the yellow dentine underneath. Teeth worn out from long usage due to old age will also expose parts of the dentine.

Impacted tooth

Tooth eruption and impaction of wisdom tooth 98: An unerupted wisdom tooth that remains inside the gum and jawbone or may erupt partially. Pain and swelling in the surrounding gum area.

Injured tooth

Broken or chipped tooth 95: If pulp is exposed (often not apparent to the patient), the tooth will become infected causing pulpitis and abscess.

Loose teeth

Periodontitis (pyorrhoea) 101: The large pockets in the gums between the teeth will cause bleeding and loosen the teeth from their sockets.

Vitamin C deficiency (scurvy) 352: Weakness, bleeding gums, bleeding into the skin and mucous membranes, easily broken bones, loose teeth. In infants, loss of appetite and weight, swollen and violently painful legs, irritability.

Malocclusion (bad bite)

Malocclusion 93: Imperfect meshing of upper and lower teeth. Contact between grinding surfaces is poor.

Sensitive teeth

Overuse of the toothbrush or too frequent brushing can rub off some of the tooth enamel making the teeth sensitive.

Pulpitis 90: Sharp, stabbing or throbbing pain; pain is often difficult to pinpoint. The tooth is particularly sensitive to cold.

Tooth abscess 91: Infection in the root of the tooth causing a steady gnawing ache and swelling of the face near the offending tooth. The tooth becomes so tender it cannot occlude with the opposing tooth without excruciating pain. Swelling of gums. Gumboil in chronic cases. Pain is worsened by heat.

Tooth abrasion 92: Loss of tooth substance at the gum margins from faulty brushing (horizontally instead of vertically), from keeping pins or nails between the teeth, or from habitual chewing of tobacco or smoking a pipe. V-shaped notches at border of teeth and gums.

Teething

The eruption of primary teeth in infants usually causes more discomfort and pain than the eruption of permanent ones. Signs of teething are drooling, and the biting, chewing, and gumming of anything the infant can put in his mouth. Teething does not cause a child to run a fever.

Toothache

A toothache can sometimes occur from filling a cavity too near the pulp or overheating from the drill.

Dental caries 89: A cavity that has been allowed to go too far into the dentine so that the nerve is exposed.

Pulpitis 90: Sharp stabbing or throbbing pain. The ache is often difficult to pinpoint. Application of cold will increase the pain.

Tooth abscess 91: A steady relentless ache, swelling of the face near the offending tooth. Tooth very sensitive to the touch; swollen gums; gumboil in chronic cases. Heat makes it worse.

Tooth eruption and impaction of wisdom tooth 98: Impacted wisdom tooth can cause toothache, also pain, swelling, and inflammation of the surrounding gum area.

Minor disorders of pregnancy 235: Slight breathlessness, varicose veins, haemorrhoids, excessive salivation, dyspepsia, headache, backache, or toothache.

Tooth decay

Dental caries 89: A disease process which destroys a part of the hard substance of the tooth. If allowed to go too far will affect the pulp.

Tooth abrasion 92: Loss of tooth substance at the margins of the gums (especially from horizontal brushing) causing V-shaped notches. This is a hard decay rather than a soft decay like caries.

Symptoms of the neck, throat, and larynx

THE NECK
Enlarged lymph nodes (lumps) in the neck

also see **Symptoms affecting the whole body)**

Quinsy 72: Large swelling on the affected side of the mouth, severe pain at site and at the back of the jaw muscles. Often subject is unable to open the jaw. Difficulty swallowing; the soft palate and uvula are swollen. This is a *Medical Emergency*.

Lymphadenitis 331: Enlarged lymph nodes in neck and elsewhere in the body are palpable and tender; the overlying skin may become red and tender as well and may even abscess.

Scarlet fever 359: High fever, sore throat, body rash which later peels and flakes, flushed face except around mouth, lymph nodes of the neck enlarged.

German measles 371: Light rosy rash over the body, swollen lymph nodes under jaw and neck. In adults, lassitude, slight stiffness of the joints.

Infectious mononucleosis 377: Fever, sore throat, headache, painful swelling of lymph nodes in neck and in armpit and groin, weakness, fatigue, occasional jaundice.

Hodgkin's disease and other lymphomas 416: Painless enlarged lymph nodes in the neck (often the size of an orange). If only on one side, Hodgkin's, if on both, other lymphoma. Later all body lymph nodes are affected. Itchy skin, anaemia, weakness, weight loss, persistent, recurrent fever, swelling of legs, difficulty breathing.

Cancer of the thyroid 417: Slow development of the thyroid tumour. Later hoarseness, difficulty swallowing and breathing, sensation of fullness in the neck. Vocal paralysis, weight loss, expectorating bloody mucus and coughing up blood.

Cancer of the pharynx (throat) 438: Pain or difficulty in eating or swallowing. Pain may radiate to side of the face, earache, difficulty opening mouth or coughing, swelling of lymph nodes in neck, nasal twang, nosebleed.

Prominence of blood vessels in the neck

Cluster headache 13c: Prominence of veins and arteries in neck and temples, radiating, throbbing headache to nose, mouth, neck, or eyes.

Oedema of the lungs 116: Breathing is difficult, laboured, and rapid, asthmatic wheezing, bloody cough, cyanosis, cold extremities, anxiety, and oppression in the chest.

Heart failure 126: Severe shortness of breath on exertion, swelling of ankles, jugular and other veins become pronounced, some loss of memory and mental faculties.

Pericarditis 136: Accumulation of fluid in chest and abdomen, pain in chest, moderate fever, distension of veins in the neck.

Stiff and/or painful neck

Causes of stiff neck run from insignificant to grave. In a serious disease it is never the only symptom but is the one complained of most.

Sleeping in an awkward or cramped position; exposure to cold (the subject will awaken in the morning with a stiff neck); a neck boil; injuries of the neck (including strains, dislocations, and fractures); unnatural twisting of the neck such as backing up a car or unusual exercise; a slipped disc in upper part of the spine; and occasionally tonsillitis, scarlet fever, typhoid, diphtheria, and arthritis can all bring about this condition.

Meningitis 7: Stiff neck usually appearing as a result of radiating headache pain. High irregular fever, small, uneven red-purplish spots, vomiting, convulsions, often coma.

Encephalitis 8: Radiating headache pain, stiff neck, drowsiness, stupor, convulsions, vomiting.

Stiff neck 271: Painful stiff neck, abnormal twisting of head to a side, difficulty moving head.

Whiplash 272: Stiffness, pain in the neck ranging from mild to agonizing. Pain can radiate to the hands causing tingling and numbness. Pounding headache, disturbed vision.

Tenanus 361: Stiffness of the jaw and neck, difficulty swallowing. Later, jaw and neck become fixed and painful, agonizing general muscular spasms, fixed grin, great apprehensiveness.

Polio 374: High fever, severe headache, sore throat, stiff neck a vital sign, muscle pain. In serious cases prostration, extreme weakness, twitching muscles, paralysis of arms, legs, or different parts of the body.

Swelling on the neck

Hypothyroidism 339: Children: occasional goitre, severe mental and physical retardation, 'good', undemanding child, puffy hands and feet, coarsening of face, dry skin becoming wrinkled, subnormal temperature 35·5°C, 96°F or less, flat nose, scanty hair. Adults: apathy, slower thinking process, weak muscles, slow heartbeat, obesity, puffiness of hands and around the eyes, gravelly, low-pitched voice, discoloured fingernails, dry, cool, sandpapery skin, brittle, falling hair, low temperature.

Hyperthyroidism 340: Goitre, fast and very heavy heartbeat, profuse sweating, great weakness, skin hot and moist, nervousness, irritability, increased appetite but loss of weight, tremors, bulging eyes, overactivity, sensation of excessive warmth.

Goitre 341: Only symptom is appearance of a goitre. If large, will cause swallowing and breathing difficulties.

Mumps 375: Painful swelling of the salivary glands below the ear or under the jaw, difficulty in opening the mouth and in swallowing acidic foods. Saliva may be scanty or profuse, furry tongue.

Cancer of the thyroid 417: Goitre, hoarseness, difficulty swallowing, vocal paralysis, expectoration of bloody mucus, choking attack, weight loss.

THE THROAT
Clearing the throat

Tics 11: Clearing the throat as well as swallowing and other body gestures such as grimacing, shaking the head, and jerking the thigh are nervous habits.

Postnasal drip 68: Hawking and occasional coughing.

Laryngitis 74: Also hoarseness. In severe form difficulty swallowing, fever, and sore throat.

Cancer of the larynx 439: Major sign is continuous or intermittent hoarseness, sticky mucus in throat needs constant clearing. Later, continual cough, earache, voice changes, difficulty breathing.

Difficulty in swallowing (dysphagia)

This is a widespread symptom due to a great variety of ailments ranging from nervous origins to obstruction. There are people who have never been able to swallow well or normally. A doctor can usually help remedy this condition.

Dysphagia may be due to a cleft palate, dry mouth (not enough saliva to lubricate swallowing), lead poisoning and alcoholism (both of which affect the nerve causing pain in the process of swallowing).

Difficulty in swallowing, Difficulty in swallowing and fever, Difficulty in swallowing and hoarseness, Difficulty in swallowing plus regurgitation or vomiting, Difficulty in swallowing and weight loss

Difficulty in swallowing

Trench mouth 77: False membrane in the throat, painful, bleeding gums, bad breath, ulcers in the mouth, painful swallowing.

Tongue disorders 87: Tongue is ulcerated, painful, may swell, making chewing and swallowing or speaking painful. Thick saliva.

Aneurysm 142: An aneurysm in the chest will produce a metallic cough, difficulty swallowing, high pulse, paroxysmal pain radiating to both shoulders, shortness of breath.

Benign tumour of the oesophagus 150: Difficulty swallowing a major symptom; pressure in the oesophagus – the larger the tumour, the greater the pressure.

Globus hystericus 152: No physical cause. Both liquid and solid food are swallowed by the subject with difficulty, leaving him with a feeling of a lump left in the throat. Another sign is general nervousness.

Goitre 341: A large goitre in the neck which can interfere with breathing and swallowing.

Cancer of the pharynx (throat) 438: Pain or difficulty in eating or swallowing, difficulty in opening the mouth or coughing. Pain may radiate to a side of the face. Additionally there are earache, swelling of the lymph node of the upper neck, nasal twang, and nosebleed.

Difficulty in swallowing and fever

Tonsillitis 70: High fever, pain in the tonsils, tonsils enlarged, spotted with amber and white streaks, painful swallowing.

Quinsy 72: Inability to open mouth, nearly impossible to swallow, large swelling in affected side of the throat, pain radiating to neck, high fever. This is a *Medical Emergency.*

Pharyngitis 73: Dry, fiery-looking, burning throat, feeling of lump in throat especially when swallowing, white spots in the throat.

Laryngitis (severe) 74: Hoarseness and constant urge to clear the throat. Pain in the throat.

Diphtheria 358: Sore throat, false membrane in throat, high fever, foul mouth odour. In severe cases prostration, difficulty swallowing, difficulty breathing, paralysis of the palate.

Tetanus 361: Stiffness of the jaw and neck, apprehensiveness. Later, jaw and neck become fixed, swallowing impossible, agonizing muscular spasms all over the body, fixed grin. There is usually fever, which may be quite high.

Polio 374: High fever, severe headaches, sore throat. In severe cases stiff neck, muscle pain, twitching, difficulty swallowing, nasal voice, prostration, extreme weakness, paralysis of arms, legs, or different parts of the body.

Rabies 378: The healed bite remains reddened; depression, irritability leading to excitability and wildness, drooling, swallowing becomes impossible, collapse and unconsciousness.

Difficulty in swallowing and hoarseness

Laryngitis 74: In the severe form difficulty in swallowing, hoarseness, pain in the throat.

Cancer of the thyroid 417: Goitre, hoarseness, vocal cord paralysis, expectorating bloody mucus, weight loss, difficulty swallowing, choking attacks.

Cancer of the larynx 439: Major sign is persistent hoarseness. Sticky mucus in throat necessitates constant clearing. Later, continual cough, difficulty swallowing, difficulty breathing, earache.

Difficulty in swallowing plus regurgitation or vomiting

Zenker's diverticulum of the oesophagus 145: Chief complaint is difficulty in swallowing. First few swallows are comfortable but condition becomes progressively worse until swallowing is impossible. Persistent gurgling sound from pouch in the oesophagus while eating or drinking, regurgitation, night cough, loss of weight.

Achalasia of the oesophagus 146: Swallowing is painful, food is often regurgitated. Pain behind breastbone and often in entire abdominal area radiating out to the jaw, back, and neck. Pain can mimic heart attack.

Hiatus hernia 148: Difficulty in swallowing is a late symptom. Earlier there is radiating pain from behind breastbone. Other signs are heartburn, vomiting of blood, insidious bleeding into the stools, pallor.

Acute gastritis (erosive) 155: Severe pain in the stomach, collapse, very fast pulse, cyanosis, excessive thirst, clammy skin, rigidity and tenderness in the abdomen.

Botulism 165: First signs are dizziness, fatigue, followed by blurred or double vision. Mouth becomes dry, swallowing or speaking becomes very difficult, vomiting and diarrhoea can be extreme, obstruction of the breathing passages is prevalent.

Difficulty in swallowing and weight loss

Oesophagitis 148: Difficulty in swallowing accompanied by heartburn, severe pain behind breastbone, loss of appetite and weight.

Hodgkin's disease and other lymphomas 416: Painless enlarged lymph nodes growing to any size, anaemia, backache, swollen legs, difficulty breathing and swallowing. Later, severe itching, weakness, weight loss and persistent, recurring fever.

Cancer of the oesophagus 429: Difficulty swallowing, vague pressure beneath the breastbone, rapid weight loss, dehydration, salivation, cough, flatulence, loss of voice, anaemia, fever, foul-smelling breath.

*

False membrane in throat

Diphtheria 358: High fever, sore throat, foul mouth odour, growth of sticky false membrane in throat, mouth, and even nose which can obstruct breathing. In severe cases prostration, cyanosis, closure of the throat, and paralysis of the palate, nerves of the eyes, larynx and other areas.

Scarlet fever 359: High fever, sore throat, vomiting, false membrane in mouth and throat, white, furry tongue later becoming raspberry. General body rash, blanching on squeezed spots. Later, skin peels and flakes. Face flushed but area around mouth remains pale.

Inflamed throat

Tonsillitis 70: Severe pain in tonsil area and in back of jaw. Tonsils enlarged, very red, flecked with amberish-white spots. Difficulty swallowing, high fever.

Pharyngitis 73: (May be strep sore throat.) Dry burning throat, feeling of lump in throat, difficult, painful swallowing, white spots in throat, fever may be high.

Sore throat

Sore throat, Sore throat and fever

Sore throat

Early syphilis 209: First stage: ulcer on penis or genitalia. Second stage: widespread varying body rash, mouth ulcers, severe headache, arthritic pains, sore throat, eye disorders.

Late syphilis (tabes dorsalis) 210: Crises (pain and spasms) in throat and/or stomach, 'lightning' pain occurring episodically all over the body, loss of balance when eyes are closed.

German measles 371: Rash (light rose in colour) all over the body, swollen lymph nodes under jaw and neck. In adults, lassitude, slight headache, joint stiffness.

Leukaemia 415: General bleeding from gums, nose, under skin (small red-purplish spots). Deep fatigue, malaise, pain in the joints, severe anaemia with great pallor. Children (acute form): sore throat, bruised body appearance, rapid heartbeat. Adults (chronic form): characteristic enlarged lymph nodes, night sweats, difficulty breathing, weight loss.

Cancer of the tongue (back of the tongue cancer) 436: Pain in throat and in the ear.

Cancer of the pharynx (throat) 438: Pain or difficulty eating or swallowing, general discomfort in throat, difficulty opening mouth or coughing, earache. Pain in throat may radiate to side of face, lymph nodes of neck may swell, nosebleeds.

Cancer of the larynx 439: Most common, major and early symptoms are hoarseness, difficulty breathing and swallowing, bad breath, sticky mucus in throat requiring constant clearing, sore throat, and pain in the ear.

Sore throat and fever

Tonsillitis 70: Severe pain in tonsil area and in back of the jaw. Tonsils enlarged, very red, flecked with amberish-white spots. Difficulty swallowing, high fever.

Quinsy 72: Inability to open mouth, nearly impossible to swallow, large swelling in affected side of throat, pain radiating to neck, high fever. This is a *Medical Emergency*.

Pharyngitis (strep throat) 73: Dry, burning throat, feeling of a lump in the throat, difficult, painful swallowing, white spots in throat, fever may be high.

Laryngitis (severe) 74: Hoarseness, constant urge to clear throat. Pain in throat.

Diphtheria 358: False membrane in throat, high fever, foul mouth odour, difficulty swallowing. In severe cases, prostration, difficulty breathing.

Scarlet fever 359: High fever, vomiting, white furry tongue later becoming raspberry, false membrane in throat, general body rash, blanching in squeezed spots. Face flushed but pale around mouth.

Polio 374: High fever, severe headache, stiff neck (important sign), sore throat. In serious cases muscle pain and twitching, severe weakness, paralysis of various parts of the body.

Infectious mononucleosis 377: Fever, headache, sore throat, painful swelling of lymph nodes in the neck, armpits, and groin, weakness; jaundice occurs in some cases.

*

Sticky mucus in throat

Pharyngitis (chronic) 73: Mucus very heavy, difficult to clear away, swelling in back of throat, nausea from mucus.

Laryngotracheobronchitis (croup) 107: Begins with cold symptoms, high fever, gasping breath, cyanosis, sticky, tenacious phlegm, croupy cough, hoarseness.

Cancer of the larynx 439: Persistent hoarseness (weeks), sticky mucus requiring constant clearing. Later, continual cough, difficulty breathing, earache.

Swollen throat

Quinsy 72: Large swelling on affected

side of throat and neck. Severe pain at site, impossible to swallow, high fever, inability to open mouth. This is a *Medical Emergency.*

Pharyngitis (chronic) 73: Swelling throat, mucus heavy, sticky, difficult to clear away, nausea from mucus.

Diphtheria 358: High fever, sore and swollen throat, false membrane in throat, foul mouth odour. In severe cases, prostration, difficulty breathing.

Scarlet fever 359: High fever, vomiting, white tongue becoming raspberry, false membrane in throat, general body rash, face flushed except around mouth.

Tickle in the throat

The *Common cold* **63** and *Hay fever* **65** will cause a tickle in the throat. The swallowing of something hard or sharp can often leave the throat with a sensation of scratchiness or irritation or even of something caught in the gullet. Eating something bland like cooked rice and occasional sips of water will help alleviate the symptom. If the sensation persists for more than a day a physician should be seen.

Ulcer in the throat

Histoplasmosis 393: Ulcers on the larynx and pharynx or on the ear, nose, legs, and extremities. Irregular fever, emaciation, anaemia, swollen lymph nodes, nausea, vomiting, diarrhoea with black stools, debilitation.

White spots on the throat

Tonsillitis 70: Chills, high fever, pain in the tonsillar region, in the back of the jaw, or in the neck. Painful swallowing, enlarged tonsils with amberish-white streaks.

Pharyngitis 73: Dry, burning throat, feeling of a lump in the throat, difficult and painful swallowing. Fever may be high.

THE LARYNX
Hoarseness

The causes of hoarseness run the gamut from trivial to grave. Clergyman's throat, singer's nodes, hoarseness from shouting too loud and too long are common forms of the condition. Many upper respiratory infections such as measles, the common cold, flu, quinsy, and diphtheria have hoarseness as a symptom. Other bases for this voice change are polyps and fibrous nodules in the larynx, enlarged thyroid, and some forms of hysteria. Hoarseness, from whatever cause, which does not disappear after a week should be checked by a doctor. (The examination is simple and easy.)

Laryngitis 74: Both acute and chronic. The cardinal symptom is hoarseness and a constant urge to clear the throat. In severe form there is fever, pain in the throat, difficulty in swallowing.

Benign growths on the vocal cords 75: Hoarseness and other changes of the voice.

Laryngotracheobronchitis (croup) 107: Begins with cold symptoms, high fever, gasping breath, cyanosis, sticky, tenacious phlegm, croupy, non-productive cough, hoarseness and loss of voice. Patient is anxious and frightened.

Aneurysm (chest) 142: Constant or paroxysmal pain in the chest radiating to both shoulders, to the back, and to the neck. Shortness of breath, husky voice, metallic cough, and difficulty swallowing.

Hypothyroidism 339: Adults: goitre, slower thinking process, slow heartbeat, obesity, puffiness in hands and around the eyes, dry, cool, sandpapery skin, dull, falling hair, gravelly voice, discoloured fingernails, subnormal temperatures.

Leprosy 368: Red and/or brown patches on skin with whitish centres, open sores, hoarseness, loss of feeling in various parts of the body. Growing, hard nodules on face and body, atrophy of muscles, loss of fingers and toes.

Lung cancer 411: Chronic cough with blood, pain in chest, wheezing, shortness of breath, hoarseness, persistent fever, night sweats, weight loss.

Cancer of the thyroid 417: Goitre, difficulty swallowing, vocal paralysis, expectorating bloody mucus, choking attacks, weight loss.

Cancer of the oesophagus 429: Difficulty swallowing, some pressure or pain under the breastbone, emaciation, dehydration, thirst, cough, heavy salivation, and flatulence. Later, anaemia, loss of voice, fever, and foul breath.

Cancer of the larynx 439: Major sign is hoarseness either continuous or intermittent, persisting beyond three weeks. Sticky mucus in throat needs constant clearing. Later, continual cough, earache, difficulty breathing.

Impaired speech
also see **Speech difficulties** p105

Multiple sclerosis 6: Secondary symptoms are monotonous voice, difficulty putting syllables together, spastic gait, tremors of the hands, impaired vision.

Tonguetie 86: Tongue attached to floor of mouth too close to the tip causing speech impairment.

Stroke 139: Loss of equilibrium sense and memory, confusion, dizziness, paralysis, impairment of vision and varying degrees of speech deterioration.

Minimal brain dysfunction 404: Children: lowered mental ability, stuttering, hyperactivity, restlessness, emotional instability, poor coordination.

Symptoms of the chest

BREATHING
Difficulty in breathing

Difficulty in breathing, Difficulty in breathing, asphyxiating attacks, Difficulty in breathing and cough

Difficulty in breathing

Heart failure 126: Respiration is harsh (variation between rapid and slow breathing). Prominent jugular vein, and swelling of tissues around ankles and legs.

Acute kidney failure 208: Failure to urinate or very scanty output, particles in the urine, nausea, vomiting, diarrhoea, drowsiness, convulsions, twitching, urine odour on breath, dry skin and dry mucous membrane.

Diabetes (ketoacidosis, diabetic coma) 332: A late complication before stupor, shock, and coma. Earlier, severe dehydration, deep, rapid, hungry breathing, dizziness, nausea, vomiting, abdominal pain, excessive thirst and excessive urination.

Goitre 341: A large goitre in the neck can interfere with breathing and swallowing.

Vitamin B₁ (thiamine) deficiency 349: Fatigue, appetite and weight loss, prickly numbness in the hands, feet, and elsewhere, cramp in the leg, difficulty walking, rapid heartbeat, difficulty breathing, swelling due to excess fluid in the tissues, and emotional instability.

Hodgkin's disease and other lymphomas 416: Painless enlarged lymph nodes, anaemia, backache, swollen legs, difficulty breathing and swallowing. Later, severe itching everywhere, weight loss, weakness, and persistent, recurring fever.

Cancer of the pharynx (throat) 438: Usually no early symptoms. If they do occur they include nosebleeds, nasal twang, difficulty breathing, throat pain which may radiate to a side of the face, and bad breath.

Difficulty in breathing, asphyxiating attacks

Laryngotracheobronchitis (croup) 107: Children: gasping, strident breathing, cough, sticky tenacious phlegm, high fever. In severe cases, cyanosis. Patient is anxious and frightened. Danger of choking. This may be a *Medical Emergency.*

Asthma 108: Breathing is wheezing, gasping, laboured, near suffocation level at times, distended chest, sweating, face flushed or pale. In severe cases, cyanosis. Later, coughing with heavy phlegm.

Oedema of the lungs 116: Breathing is difficult, laboured, and rapid, asthmatic wheezing, cyanosis, bloody cough, cold extremities, pallor and sweating. Patient is anxious with a feeling of oppression in the chest.

High altitude lung oedema 116a: Noisy, laboured breathing, bloody cough, cyanosis, and prostration.

Pneumothorax (intense) 120: Shortness of breath, breathing very difficult, severe and sharp pains in the chest which are worse upon inhaling. Pain may go to the shoulder, hacking cough, no phlegm. Patient appears anxious.

Hyperventilation 121: Fast heartbeat, rapid, deep breathing, oppression in the chest, blackout, numbness in the extremities.

Botulism 165: In early period, difficulty in breathing, later paralysis of the respiratory tract. Symptoms appear 18–36 hours after eating contaminated food. Extreme dryness of mouth, double or blurred vision, fixed, dilated pupils, nausea, vomiting, cramps, and diarrhoea.

Anaphylactic shock 292: Obstructed breathing may cause asphyxiation, giant hives, swelling all over the body, rapid pulse, and shock.

Diphtheria 358: Sore throat, false membrane in the throat, high fever, difficulty swallowing and breathing, danger of asphyxiation, paralysis of the palate, and foul breath.

Cancer of the thyroid 417: Goitre, hoarseness, difficulty swallowing, vocal cord paralysis, choking attacks and weight loss.

Difficulty in breathing and cough

Laryngotracheobronchitis (croup) 107: Children: gasping, strident breathing, croupy cough, phlegm is sticky, tenacious, high fever. In severe cases, cyanosis, patient is anxious and frightened. This may be a *Medical Emergency*.

Asthma 108: Breathing is wheezing, gasping, laboured, near suffocation at times, chest distended, sweating, flushed or pale face. In severe cases, cyanosis. Later, coughing with heavy phlegm.

Oedema of the lungs 116: Breathing is difficult, laboured and rapid, asthmatic wheezing, cyanosis, cough is bloody, ex-

tremities are cold, pallor, sweating. Patient is anxious with a feeling of oppression in the chest.

High altitude lung oedema 116a: Noisy, laboured breathing, bloody cough, cyanosis, prostration.

Pneumothorax 120: Shortness of breath and difficulty in breathing, severe, sharp pains in chest which are worse on inhaling. Pain may go to shoulder, hacking cough, no phlegm. Patient appears anxious.

Lung cancer 411: Chronic bloody cough, wheezing, acute shortness of breath, hoarseness, pain in chest, night sweats, sunken eyeballs, constant fever.

Cancer of the larynx 439: Major sign is hoarseness that persists beyond two weeks. Sticky mucus in the throat requiring clearing and hawking. Later, continual cough, difficulty in breathing, earache.

Shortness of breath

Breathlessness is always an important symptom and must never be ignored, except when it is due to normal non-disease factors such as running, heavy exercise, fear, excitement, sexual intercourse, mountain climbing, remaining in high altitudes, and excessive smoking. Breathlessness is also a symptom in uraemia and acute kidney failure but other symptoms in these kidney disorders are more expressive. A slight shortness of breath can occur as one of the early symptoms of pregnancy.

Shortness of breath and cough, Shortness of breath and bloody cough, Shortness of breath and fatigue, Shortness of breath and fever, Shortness of breath and pain in the chest or abdomen, Shortness of breath and pain in the chest or abdomen and cough, Shortness of breath and palpitation or rapid heartbeat, Shortness of breath upon slight exertion

Shortness of breath and cough

Chronic bronchitis 104: A progressively worsening disease, wheezing breath, shortness of breath, violent, paroxysmal cough, barrel chest, cyanosis.

Bronchiectasis 105: Shortness of breath can be extreme, cyanosis, anaemia, great fatigue. In advance cases, cough is copious with foul-smelling phlegm.

Laryngotracheobronchitis (croup) 107: Children: gasping, strident breathing, croupy cough, sticky, tenacious phlegm, and high fever. Danger of choking. In severe cases, cyanosis. The patient is anxious and frightened. This may be a *Medical Emergency*.

Aspiration and lipoid pneumonias 111: Plus fever.

Emphysema 113: Shortness of breath even upon slight exertion, difficulty in exhaling, hard, tiring cough, producing small amounts of thick phlegm, barrel chest, lessened vital capacity.

Pneumoconiosis 117: Plus wheezing.

Pleurisy 118: In dry pleurisy: considerable shortness of breath, knife-like pain in the chest worsened by breathing and coughing and often felt in the shoulder, neck, and abdomen. In wet pleurisy: rapid, shallow breathing, pain in the chest on breathing, turning, or twisting, cough, and lowered vital capacity.

Pneumothorax 120: Shortness of breath, difficulty breathing, severe sharp pains in the chest becoming worse on inhaling (the pain may go to the shoulder), hacking cough but no phlegm. Patient appears anxious.

Heart failure 126: Growing shortness of breath upon exertion, paroxysm of rapid and slow breathing, wheezing dry cough, swelling around ankles and legs, very rapid heartbeat on slight exertion, prominence of jugular vein.

Aneurysm (arterial) 142: When this disease strikes the chest section of the aorta, breathlessness is the major symptom. Often rapid pulse, metallic cough, and difficulty in swallowing.

Cystic fibrosis 407: Infants, children: ravenous appetite, emaciation, bulky, fatty, foul-smelling stools, chronic cough, rapid breathing, protruding abdomen.

Shortness of breath and bloody cough

Foreign body in the bronchi 106: Breathlessness is severe, cyanosis, heavy cough with bloodstained, foul-smelling phlegm, high fever.

Pneumonia 109: Shaking chills, high fever, pain in the chest, painful cough with rusty phlegm, rapid pulse.

Pulmonary tuberculosis 112: Irritating to severe cough producing blood-stained phlegm, deep fatigue, loss of weight and appetite. Drenching night sweats, pain in the chest, and loss of some vital capacity.

Lung abscess 115: Also repeated severe chills, high fever, painful cough with bloodstained, foul phlegm, drenching sweats, and great malaise.

High altitude lung oedema 116a: Noisy, laboured breathing, bloody cough, cyanosis, and prostration.

Coccidioidomycosis 394: Pain in the lungs, cough often with bloody phlegm, shortness of breath, weakness, cyanosis, weight loss.

Lung cancer 411: Chronic cough (later with blood), pain in the chest, wheezing, acute shortness of breath, hoarseness, night sweats, persistent fever, sunken eyeballs.

Shortness of breath and fatigue

Bronchiectasis 105: Shortness of breath can be extreme, cyanosis, anaemia, great fatigue. In advanced cases, cough is present with copious, foul-smelling phlegm.

Pulmonary tuberculosis 112: Irritating to severe cough producing blood-stained phlegm, deep fatigue, loss of weight and appetite, drenching night sweats, pain in the chest, loss of some vital capacity.

Congenital heart disorders 128: Breathlessness is the characteristic symptom, cyanosis, easy fatigue.

Dietary deficiencies in pregnancy 236: Also anaemia and fatigue.

Haemolytic anaemia 324: All the

anaemia symptoms (pallor, breathlessness, fatigue), jaundice, dizziness, fainting, weak, rapid pulse, rapid breathing,
chills, fever, and aches in the extremities
and the abdomen.

Polycythaemia 327: Bluish-red itching
skin, bleeding in the gastrointestinal tract
causing bloody or tarry stools, fatigue,
dizziness, constant dull headache.

Obesity 347: (Over twenty per cent
overweight) In severe cases, shortness of
breath and fatigue, aching back and feet.
Arthritis is frequent.

Lung cancer 411: Chest pain, cough,
wheezing, foul breath, shortness of
breath. Later, cough is persistent, shortness of breath more acute, pain in the
chest becomes stabbing or dull behind
the breastbone, drenching night sweats,
weight loss, hoarseness and fatigue.

Shortness of breath and fever

Foreign body in bronchi 106: Severe
breathlessness, cyanosis, heavy cough
with bloodstained, foul-smelling phlegm,
high fever.

Pneumonia 109: Shaking chills, high
fever, pain in the chest, painful cough
with rusty phlegm, rapid pulse.

**Aspiration and lipoid pneumonias
111:** Plus cough.

Lung abscess 115: Repeated severe
chills, high fever, painful cough, drenching sweats, great malaise. Phlegm is
bloodstained and foul.

**Rheumatic heart disease and rheu-
matic fever 127:** Breathlessness occurs
in severe cases, as well as cough and chest
pains. Inflammation of the joints, sweating, rapid heartbeat, St Vitus's dance,
skin rash, loss of appetite, pallor.

Pericarditis 136: After the disease has
progressed, shortness of breath is a distinctive symptom. Severe pains in the
chest and moderate fever.

Sunstroke 313a: Headache, dizziness,
no sweating, flushed, hot, dry skin, very
high temperature, fast pulse and rapid
breathing.

Malaria 381: Teeth-chattering chills,
high fever, drenching sweats, severe head-

ache, vomiting, diarrhoea, rapid pulse.

Trichinosis 386: Swollen eyelids, high
fever, pain and swelling in all muscles,
profuse sweating, diarrhoea. In severe
cases, shortness of breath.

Shortness of breath and pain in the chest or abdomen

Atelectasis 114: Severe shortness of
breath, cyanosis, pain on side of chest
affected, weakness, rapid heartbeat,
shock.

Angina pectoris 124: Severe pain in
chest lasting only for minutes, usually
brought on by exercise or effort; a bout
of breathlessness, pallor, cold sweat,
palpitations.

Coronary thrombosis 125: Intense
vice-like chest pains, unrelieved and prolonged, considerable shortness of breath,
cold sweat, pallor, rapid heartbeat, pain
can radiate to arm, neck, or jaw. Great
fear of death.

Pericarditis 136: After the disease has
progressed, shortness of breath is a
distinctive symptom. Severe pain in the
chest, moderate fever.

Pulmonary embolism 140: Shortness
of breath is a major symptom; it is acute
with accompanying cyanosis. Chest
pains and rapid heartbeat.

Cardiac neurosis 144: Breathlessness
is the predominant sign but the condition
never worsens with effort. Fast heartbeat,
vague pains in the chest of the non-
radiating type, great anxiety and fatigue.

**Rupture and/or foreign body in the
oesophagus 153:** Also severe chest pains
and shock.

**Massive haemorrhage in peptic ulcer
159:** Profuse blood in vomit, persistent
blood in the stools, rapid, thready pulse,
pallor, collapse, irregular pain, dizziness
and shock.

Shortness of breath and pain in the chest or abdomen and cough

Pleurisy 118: In dry pleurisy: considerable shortness of breath, knife-like pain

in chest worsened by breathing or coughing and often felt in shoulder, neck, and abdomen. In wet pleurisy: rapid, shallow breathing, pain in chest on breathing, turning or twisting, cough, and lowered vital capacity.

Pneumothorax 120: Shortness of breath, difficulty breathing, severe, sharp pains in chest which worsen on inhaling (pain may go to shoulder), hacking cough, no phlegm. Patient appears anxious.

Reumatic heart disease and rheumatic fever 127: Inflammmation of the large and small joints especially at the ankles, knees, and wrists. Rapid heartbeat, St Vitus's dance, malaise, pallor, sweating, failure to gain weight, skin rash, loss of appetite. In severe cases, shortness of breath, cough, and chest pain.

Perforation in peptic ulcer 160: Patient is breathless and ashen grey. Sudden agonizing pain in stomach, rigid abdomen, pain in tips of the shoulders, rise in pulse and temperature.

Late syphilis (cardiovascular syphilis) 210: Also agonizing paroxysmal pain in chest radiating out to both sides, metallic cough, high pulse.

Coccidioidomycosis 394: Pain in the lungs, cough often with bloody phlegm, shortness of breath, malaise, weakness, cyanosis, weight loss.

Lung cancer 411: Chronic cough (later with blood), pain in chest, wheezing, acute shortness of breath, hoarseness, night sweats, persistent fever, sunken eyeballs.

Shortness of breath and palpitation or rapid heartbeat

Hypoxia 122: Also cyanosis of the lips, palpitation, giddiness, headache, difficulty in concentration, poor judgement, malaise, and nausea.

Angina pectoris 124: Severe pain in the chest lasting only a few minutes usually brought on by exercise or effort. A bout of breathlessness, pallor, cold sweat, and palpitations.

Heart failure 126: Shortness of breath is a major symptom, may come on gradually or suddenly, accompanied by a wheezing cough. This symptom becomes noticeable usually upon some minor exertion, like walking up a flight of stairs. At a later stage, occurs even at rest, often awakening patient from sleep. Palpitations, swelling of ankles, prominent neck veins, diminishment of mental vigour, poor memory.

Rheumatic heart disease and rheumatic fever 127: Breathlessness is a sign in severe cases. Inflammation of the joints, sweating, and rapid heartbeat.

Shock 133: Great pallor, cold, clammy skin, cyanosis (lips, nails, fingertips), sunken eyeballs, fast, weak pulse, anxiety state and coma.

Pulmonary embolism 140: Shortness of breath is a major symptom. It is acute with accompanying cyanosis. Also, chest pains and rapid heartbeat.

Aneurysm (arterial) 142: When this disease occurs in the chest section of the aorta, breathlessness is the indicative symptom. Often rapid pulse, metallic cough, difficulty in swallowing.

Cardiac neurosis 144: Shortness of breath is the predominant sign, but the condition never worsens with effort. Fast heartbeat, vague pains in the chest of the non-radiating type, great anxiety and fatigue.

Sunstroke 313a: Headache, dizziness, no sweating, skin flushed, hot, and dry, very high temperature, fast pulse and rapid breathing.

Anaemia 322: Anaemic symptoms (pallor, breathlessness, fatigue), red, burning tongue, palpitations, vertigo. In severe cases, jaundice, numbness of the limbs, unusual thirst, poor memory and shock.

Shortness of breath upon slight exertion

Chronic bronchitis 104: A progressively worsening disease, wheezing breath, violent, paroxysmal coughing, barrel chest, cyanosis.

Emphysema 113: Shortness of breath on slight exertion, difficulty exhaling, hard, tiring cough producing small amounts of thick phlegm, barrel chest.

Lung abscess 115: Also repeated severe chills, high fever, painful cough, drenching sweats, great malaise, phlegm is bloodstained and foul.

Pneumoconiosis 117: Also coughing and wheezing.

Hypoxia 122: Also cyanosis of lips, palpitation, giddiness, headache, difficulty in concentration, poor judgement, malaise, nausea, and night blindness.

Heart failure 126: Growing shortness of breath on exertion as the disease progresses, paroxysm of rapid and slow breathing, wheezing, dry cough, swelling around ankles and legs, very rapid heartbeat on slight exertion, prominence of jugular vein.

Chronic nephritis 197: Breathlessness on slight exertion, excessive late night urination, blood in urine, puffiness of face, ankles, abdomen, anaemia, impaired vision from bleeding into retina.

*

Stertorous breathing (snoring)

Snoring (stertorous breathing) under normal circumstances is a sign of profound sleep when sleeping on one's back; it can also be indicative of adenoids, nasal polyps or anything that may block the nasal passages. Deep coma will also cause snoring.

Stroke 139: Basic symptom is paralysis of some part of the body. If in coma breathing is stertorous. Symptoms experienced while conscious are loss of equilibrium, loss of speech and memory, confusion, disturbance of vision, vomiting.

Diabetes (ketoacidosis, diabetic coma) 332: Breathing rapidly, deeply, hungrily, severe dehydration, dizziness, poor skin tone, nausea and vomiting, abdominal pain, excessive thirst and urination, sunken eyeballs, stupor, shock, and finally coma.

THE COUGH

Contrary to popular belief coughing is not a deleterious or pernicious act; mostly it serves a useful purpose in keeping the respiratory tract free of excessive and harmful secretions. However, the body can at times react to disease in a panic with paroxysms of coughing that serve no purpose but to fatigue the patient. That is the only time coughing should be suppressed.

A cough can often be only a psychological habit. Coughs that appear for the first time in a young adult quite often indicate the beginning of tuberculosis and should be acted on quickly. A cough that appears for the first time in a middle-aged man may often indicate bronchial carcinoma. A cough which appears first on lying down at night often indicates *Bronchiectasis* **105**. Heavy smokers usually have an early morning cough.

Dry cough without phlegm (unproductive cough), Coughing up phlegm (productive cough), Coughing up bloody phlegm, Coughing up bloody phlegm with pain in the lungs

Dry cough without phlegm (unproductive cough)

Aspiration and lipoid pneumonias 111: Plus shortness of breath and fever.

Empyema 119: Short dry cough, pain on side of chest, chills, fever, emaciation, sweating, clubbing of fingers, great malaise.

Pneumothorax 120: Slight cough. Severe, sharp pain in chest, worse when inhaling, and may radiate to shoulder; difficulty in breathing, breathlessness, anxiety.

Heart failure 126: Wheezing cough, shortness of breath on exertion, swelling around ankles and legs, very rapid heartbeat on slight exertion, paroxysm of rapid and slow breathing.

Aneurysm (chest) 142: Metallic cough, fast pulse, sharp pain radiating to both shoulders, shortness of breath.

Zenker's diverticulum of the oesophagus 145: Night cough, chief complaint is difficulty in swallowing, regurgitation, loss of weight.

Measles 370: Begins like a cold, then high fever, harsh, hacking cough, bloodshot, burning eyes, photophobia, red spots with white centres on the inside of the cheeks, brownish-pink rash over the body consisting of elevated spots which run into each other. Rash disappears in a few days.

Cystic fibrosis 407: Infants, children: failure to gain weight, emaciation, ravenous appetite, chronic cough, rapid breathing, protruding stomach, bulky, greasy, foul-smelling stools.

Coughing up phlegm (productive cough)

Postnasal drip 68: Hawking, constant clearing of the throat, coughing may occur, phlegm is in small amounts if noticeable. In chronic conditions bad breath is common.

Acute bronchitis 103: Commences as a head cold. Major symptom is a cough which is first dry and unproductive but later becomes painful with profuse, heavy, purulent, white to yellowish phlegm. Cough is worse at night. Mild sore throat. Fever may be high and prolonged.

Chronic bronchitis 104: Violent paroxysmal cough until phlegm is raised. Shortness of breath especially on exertion, cyanosis of the lips and fingernail beds from insufficient oxygen, barrel chest development, very low chest expansion.

Bronchiectasis 105: Regular periodic cough with foul-smelling phlegm, foul breath, shortness of breath, anaemia, easy fatigue.

Laryngotracheobronchitis (croup) 107: Children: at first croupy, unproductive cough, later with sticky, tenacious phlegm. Breathing is gasping, strident, high fever. In severe cases, cyanosis. Patient is anxious and frightened. This may be a *Medical Emergency.*

Asthma 108: Gasping, wheezing breathing, near suffocation at times, distended chest; later, heavy coughing with profuse, tenacious phlegm.

Atypical pneumonia 110: Coughing is incessant and paroxysmal with copious phlegm, moderate fever, prolonged fatigue in long convalescence.

Emphysema 113: Hard, tiring cough bringing up small amounts of thick, heavy phlegm, shortness of breath on slight exertion, barrel chest, cyanosis, and lessened vital capacity.

Pneumoconiosis 117: Early stage of all dust-inhalant diseases is usually manifest by coughing without phlegm. When the disease has progressed seriously, there may be phlegm and even bloody phlegm coughed up. The cough is wheezing. Shortness of breath is a slowly developing symptom.

Whooping cough 357: Crowing cough with heavy, gagging phlegm, vomiting, cold symptoms, loss of appetite.

Cancer of the oesophagus 429: Difficulty swallowing, some pressure or pain under the breastbone, rapid loss of weight, emaciation, dehydration, thirst, cough, heavy salivation, and flatulence. Later, anaemia, loss of the voice, fever, and foul breath.

Coughing up bloody phlegm

Foreign body in the bronchi 106: Heavy cough with bloodstained, foul phlegm, gagging, very laboured breathing, high fever, cyanosis.

Oedema of the lungs 116: Also very difficult, laboured breathing that is asthmatic and wheezing, sense of oppression in chest, cold extremities. Patient is pale, sweating, and anxious.

High altitude lung oedema 116a: Bloody cough, laboured, noisy breathing, weakness, cyanosis, prostration.

Histoplasmosis 393: Cough with bloody phlegm appears in the severe form, also weight loss, drenching sweats, extreme fatigue, black stools, emaciation, ulcerations on nose, ear, pharynx, enlarged lymph nodes on the body.

Cancer of the larynx 439: Major sign

is hoarseness, persisting over two weeks, sticky mucus in throat. Later, continual cough, occasionally with blood; earache and difficulty in breathing.

Coughing up bloody phlegm with pain in the lungs

Pneumonia 109: Painful cough with rusty or bloodstained phlegm, severe, shaking chills, high fever, pain in chest, rapid breathing, rapid heartbeat.

Pulmonary tuberculosis 112: Irritating to severe cough producing a bloodstained phlegm, deep fatigue, loss of weight and appetite, drenching sweats, pain in chest, loss of some vital capacity.

Lung abscess 115: Painful cough with phlegm that is bloodstained and foul, repeated severe chills, high fever, great malaise, breathlessness on exertion.

Pulmonary embolism 140: Also acute shortness of breath, pain in lungs, rapid heartbeat, cyanosis.

Coccidioidomycosis 394: Cough, often with blood, pain in lungs, deep malaise. In the serious, progressive form: weight loss, cyanosis, shortness of breath.

Lung cancer 411: Chronic bloody cough, pain in chest, wheezing, night sweats, acute shortness of breath, persistent fever, sunken eyeballs, distended veins in neck, hoarseness.

HEARTBEAT
Extra beat (extrasystole, premature beat, skipped beat)

This is a premature contraction of the heart. The heart seems to miss a beat while the next one is a very heavy thump. In some people the sensation may be an alarming flip-flop in the heart. This symptom is rarely serious, occurring more often in normal hearts than in diseased ones. Premature beats can occur occasionally or regularly for short periods or long. In the absence of any other signifi-cant symptom they are best disregarded. The causes may be an excess of coffee, alcohol, cigarettes, intense emotion, in short too much of anything. But often there is no cause at all.

Heart block 134: In this disorder there is not a premature beat but a missing beat after every second or fifth one. Dizziness, faintness especially on sudden change of position, as in jumping out of bed or suddenly standing up.

Diphtheria 358: High fever, difficulty swallowing, false membrane in the throat. In severe cases, difficulty in breathing, missing beat due to heart block.

Irregular beat (cardiac arrythmia)

Rheumatic heart disease and rheumatic fever 127: An irregular and fast beat is a major symptom. Other important indications are migratory pain in the joints which are swollen and red, tenderness over the heart, rash over the body, nosebleeds, St Vitus's dance, pallor. (The doctor can hear a unique heart rhythm called the gallop rhythm.)

Atrial fibrillation 132: The beat seems very irregular and rapid, changing in amplitude as well. Pallor and weakness.

Endocarditis (bacterial) 135: Although the heartbeat is decidedly irregular, the distinctive symptom is pain in the joints. Also anaemia, fatigue. Spots over the body are characteristic. There may be clubbing of the fingers, unexplained initial fever, bleeding from the nose and often into the urine.

Pericarditis 136: Acute form of this disease is painful, tender chest, accumulation of fluids in chest and abdomen. Neck veins may be distended. Fever is moderate. In extreme cases, shortness of breath. (The doctor can hear the friction-rub sound through his stethoscope, the qualifying indication. Often he can also hear the unique gallop rhythm.)

Pulmonary embolism 140: Heartbeat is irregular and rapid. Also breathlessness, pain in lungs, and cyanosis.

Typhoid fever 363: Continuous severe frontal or temporal headaches, sustained very high fever, diarrhoea, slow double pulse beat, stupor, rosy spots on abdomen, nosebleeds, distended abdomen.

Palpitations

Palpitation is a blanket description that covers a multitude of varying heartbeat symptoms from unduly fast to irregular to forceful. Usually it means that the subject is acutely aware of his heart, most often because it is beating heavily. Although there is no pain it is a distinctly unpleasant sensation.

Almost any illness can induce this symptom. It is more likely to be significant of some nervous disorder or degenerative condition. In true heart ailments, palpitation is usually a minor complaint as opposed to the more demanding ones of shortness of breath and pain.

For many people the heart is used as a 'whipping boy' to express their problems – for them any unpleasant stimulation can set it off. Some people are heart listeners and magnify its beat especially while in bed. Palpitation in itself is not so much a symptom of disease as it is a symptom of the stress of living. Children rarely complain of palpitation.

Many drugs and substances can induce this heartbeat disorder, such as coffee, tea, alcohol, atropine, belladonna, adrenalin, inhalation of various gases. Extra exertion in some people can induce palpitation most especially if they are out of condition. Other known causes are being in a room heated by a gas fire, dyspepsia, flatulence, fear, shock, anger, high emotion, trauma, and most especially the swallowing of air (see *Table 12*). An extra or missing beat can make one unpleasantly aware of the heart.

There are some real disorders with palpitation as a main symptom. They are listed below.

Hypoxia 122: Breathlessness on exertion, headache, giddiness, poor judgement, cyanosis of lips, difficulty in concentrating, malaise and nausea.

Postgastrectomy syndrome 161: Sweating, dizziness ranging in intensity from lightheadedness to fainting, palpitations, explosive diarrhoea.

Menopause 221: In some women no symptoms at all but for most, hot flushes, chills, sweating, headache, fatigue, frequent urination, giddiness, palpitation, loss of appetite, insomnia, dyspepsia, nausea, nervous irritability, emotional instability, crying jags and periods of depression and anxiety.

Anaemia 322: Anaemic symptoms, red, sore tongue, vertigo. In some cases, jaundice, numbness of limbs, poor memory, excessive thirst, palpitations, shock.

Pernicious anaemia 323: Anaemic symptoms, pain in varying parts of the body, pins-and-needles sensation in hands and feet, beefy, red, sore tongue, weight loss, jaundice, palpitations, difficulty in walking, impotence and frigidity.

Hypoglycaemia 333: Weakness, dizziness, palpitation, shaking, sweating, blurring of vision, headache, poor concentration, irrational or psychotic behaviour, blackouts, convulsions, coma.

Hyperthyroidism 340: Goitre, rapid heartbeat, profuse sweating, nervousness, increased appetite but loss of weight, hyperactivity, bulging eyes, weakness.

Phaeochromocytoma 346: Pounding headache, sweating, tremulousness, flushing, nausea and vomiting. (High blood pressure.)

Vitamin B₁ (thiamine) deficiency 349: Loss of appetite and weight, prickling numbness in hands, legs, or feet, emotional instability, alarming palpitations, difficulty in breathing, swelling and fluid in the tissues.

Rapid heartbeat (tachycardia)

also see **Palpitations** p127

The symptom of tachycardia can indicate conditions ranging from the utterly harmless to disorders of a life-threatening nature. Rapid heartbeat occurs normally from exercise, sexual intercourse, excitement, fear; it is often a sign of over-response to many drugs and substances such as belladonna, tobacco, and amyl nitrite. Other drugs having this effect are scopolamine, epinephrine, benzedrine, quinine, and oxalates.

Tachycardia appears in most fevers and is a frequent symptom of menstruation, pregnancy, menopause, obesity; it is common after a heavy meal and is especially noticeable upon mild exertion of the unfit. Pain can induce rapid heartbeat. Such disorders as gastritis, peptic ulcer perforation, and pancreatitis have tachycardia as one of their many symptoms. Peristent rapid heartbeat among the elderly usually indicates some form of heart disease. Patients recovering from diphtheria and flu quite often show considerable tachycardia for weeks.

The normal heartbeat for the average male ranges between 65 and 72 beats per minute at rest, for the average female 70 to 80. General range for the middle-aged is between 70 and 75; for the elderly, 50 to 65. In children: first year, 115 to 130; second year, 100 to 115; third year, between 90 and 100; up until age 7, 85 to 90; up until age 15, between 80 and 85.

Tachycardia ranges between 100 to 250 (or more) beats per minute for the adult. *Rapid heartbeat, Rapid heartbeat, extreme, Rapid heartbeat plus fatigue or weakness, Rapid heartbeat plus jaundice, Rapid heartbeat with pain in the chest or abdomen*

Rapid heartbeat

Stroke 139: In grave cases, rapid heartbeat, high fever, rapid, stertorous breathing and recurrent coma. The main symptom is paralysis. Also, loss of equilibrium sense, confusion, speech or memory failure, vertigo, and frequently vomiting.

Phlebitis 141: White leg. Swelling of the leg which may feel heavy and sensitive. Pain may be severe. Surface veins become prominent and the area affected on the leg may become discoloured. The fever is low grade and the pulse is rapid.

Acute kidney infection 200: Fast pulse,

kidney pain which may radiate out, scanty, cloudy urine, painful, urgent, frequent urination, chills, fever and headache.

Physical allergy (hypersensitivity to cold) 290: Rapid pulse, hives, and loss of consciousness.

Anaphylactic shock 292: Rapid pulse, giant hives on the body, body swelling, obstructed breathing and shock.

Gout 334: Painful swollen joint of the big toe (other joints can also be affected), lumps in the ears and joints, scanty, darkish urine and fast pulse.

The plague 365: Sudden onset. Chills, high fever, rapid pulse, stupor and prostration. Important sign is development of buboes in the groin and under the arms (inflamed lymph nodes ranging from crab apple to apple size). These may suppurate and drain. Also minute bleeding points on the skin which turn black. Final stages are shock and coma.

Typhus 392: High fever, severe headache, prostration, bloodshot eyes, flushed face, body rash with pinpoint bleeding in the centre of spots which turn purple. Rapid, weak pulse, stupor which may change to coma, muscular twitching, and highly coloured, scanty urine.

Rapid heartbeat, extreme

Rapid heartbeat (tachycardia) 130a: Usually a result of some other disorder (an infectious fever, kidney, anaemia, poisoning from insect or snake bite or some drug). If the beat is very rapid there can be nausea and weakness, pallor, and even fainting. In extreme cases, shock. There is no pain. Seen mostly in the young adult, it may last for minutes, hours, even days.

Aneurysm 142: Heartbeat very rapid and throbbing, metallic cough, shortness of breath, pain radiating to the back from either stomach or chest depending upon location of the aneurysm.

Hyperthyroidism 340: Goitre, staring appearance, extreme nervousness, tremor of the fingers, sweating, diarrhoea.

Rapid heartbeat plus fatigue or weakness

Atelectasis 114: Also severe shortness of breath, pain on one side of the chest, weakness, cyanosis, shock.

High blood pressure 138: A fast beat is not always a dependable sign of the disease but it is more commonly than not. Other symptoms may be throbbing headache, dizziness, and fatigue.

Cardiac neurosis 144: Fast pulse is always a dominant sign, but it is rarely irregular as it might be in true heart disease. Chest pains are never worsened by exertion. There is shortness of breath, great anxiety, fatigue.

Diabetes (insulin shock) 332: Weakness, sweating, trembling, hunger, rapid pulse. If severe, fainting and coma.

Leukaemia 415: General bleeding from gums, nose, under the skin (small red spots), anaemia with great pallor, pain in the joints, fatigue, malaise. In a child: (acute) sore throat, bruised body appearance, rapid heartbeat. In an adult: (chronic) characteristic enlarged lymph nodes, weight loss, night sweats.

Rapid heartbeat plus jaundice

Chronic relapsing pancreatitis 167: Severe abdominal pain may be continuous or intermittent, nausea, vomiting, chills, jaundice, rapid heartbeat and weight loss. Stools are fatty, frothy and foul smelling.

Gallstones 194: Biliary colic, agonizing pain from upper abdomen radiating in waves to the back, shoulder or pelvis, mild jaundice, flatulence, fast pulse.

Cholecystitis 195: Biliary colic, agonizing pain from upper abdomen radiating to the back, shoulder or pelvis, mild jaundice, fever, flatulence, belching, fast pulse.

Morning sickness 243: Nausea and vomiting from mild to pernicious. In extreme cases, severe loss of weight, jaundice, and rapid heartbeat.

Haemolytic anaemia 324: Anaemic symptoms, jaundice, faintness, dizziness, weak, rapid pulse, chills and fever, aches in the abdomen and extremities.

Relapsing fever 369: Chills, high fever, rapid heartbeat, severe headache, vomiting, muscle and joint pain, profuse sweating and rash turning to rose-coloured spots. Jaundice may appear. The distinguishing feature of this disease is that the fever abates, dropping to normal, and then reappears within a week.

Rapid heartbeat with pain in the chest or abdomen

Pneumonia 109: Heartbeat and breathing are rapid. Pain in the chest, chills, fever, painful cough with rusty phlegm.

Hyperventilation 121: Fast heartbeat, oppression in the chest, numbness in the extremities, fainting.

Angina pectoris 124 and **Coronary thrombosis 125:** Severe pain and distress in the chest may radiate to the arm, jaw, or shoulder. If the attack lasts a few minutes it is angina, if longer, coronary thrombosis. Also rapid heartbeat, pallor, shortness of breath, shock.

Rheumatic heart disease and rheumatic fever 127: Inflammation of the large and small joints, especially at the ankles, knees, and wrists. Rapid heartbeat, St Vitus's dance, malaise, pallor, sweating, failure to gain weight, skin rash, appetite loss. In severe cases, shortness of breath, cough, and pain in the chest.

Pulmonary embolism 140: The major symptom is acute shortness of breath with accompanying cyanosis, chest pains, and rapid, erratic heartbeat.

Perforation in peptic ulcer 160: Agonizing pain in the abdomen which is rigid and tender, fever, vomiting of blood, great pallor, pain in the shoulder tip, and rapid heartbeat.

Childbed fever 247: Fast pulse, high fever, chills, vomiting and abdominal pains.

Salt deficiency 356: Stomach cramps, loss of skin elasticity, severe drop in urination, twitching muscles, very faint but rapid pulse, finally convulsions.

*

Slow heartbeat (*bradycardia, brachycardia*)

Bradycardia ranges under fifty beats per minute (see *Slow heartbeat* **130**). This symptom is more suggestive of bounding good health than an illness. Slow heartbeat is characteristic of athletes and well-exercised people.

However, a slow heartbeat is found in some patients suffering from jaundice and a few infectious diseases. It is also fairly common in convalescence from a long and serious disease.

Poisoning from opium (or any of its derivatives) can cause the heart to slow down. Also barium, tetraethyl lead, carbon monoxide, and food poisoning can have this effect.

Hypopituitarism 337: Children: stunted growth and dwarfism. Adults: easily fatigued, scanty menstruation, diminished libido, diminished pubic and underarm hair, loss of appetite and weight, apathy, slow, feeble pulse, intolerance for cold.

Hypothyroidism 339: Adults: goitre, mental apathy, slowed thinking process, slow heartbeat, obesity, drowsiness, puffiness of hands and face, especially around the eyes; gravel voice, subnormal temperature and cold intolerance.

GENERAL
Misshapen chest

Chronic bronchitis 104: Chest becomes barrel-shaped because of narrowing of air passages, violent paroxysmal cough until phlegm is raised. Breathlessness especially on exertion, wheezing breath. In extreme cases, cyanosis.

Asthma 108: Chest becomes distended, breathing is gasping, laboured, wheezing, face is pale, flushed, or cyanotic depending on severity of attack. Later, heavy coughing with tenacious phlegm.

Emphysema 113: Breathing difficulties cause barrel-like chest, shortness of breath

on exertion, difficulty in exhaling, a hard, tiring cough bringing up a small amount of thick, heavy phlegm. Loss in vital capacity.

Pain in the chest

Pain in the chest does not always mean a heart attack. There are a considerable number of ailments that have this symptom which are not related to heart disease. Often chest pains can be quite innocuous, such as those induced by coffee or tobacco (occasionally seen in sensitive individuals). The pain is seldom severe, usually dull and not very definable.

In *Hyperventilation* **121**, the symptoms can be alarming – tightness and an oppressive, suffocating feeling in the chest with a fast heartbeat and ensuing panic. The patient can even faint. This is not a serious disease except for swimmers.

Chest pains need very careful evaluation in terms of type, quality, and location.

Pain in the chest caused by heart and circulatory disorders, Pain in the chest resembling heart attack, Pain in the chest, respiratory

Pain in the chest caused by heart and circulatory disorders

Angina pectoris 124 and **Coronary thrombosis 125:** The pain is constricting and vice-like over the heart; the patient usually describes it with a clenched fist. Most often the pain will radiate into the shoulder, down the arm and to the wrist, usually on the left side but not infrequently on the right; it can go to the jaw as well. If the attack lasts only a few minutes, it is angina; if it lasts for a more prolonged time (more than half hour), then the patient is having a coronary thrombosis, in which case the pain is more intense. Other signs of heart attack are pallor, shock, cyanosis, shortness of breath.

Characteristically the heart attack patient will lie quite still, not restlessly rolling around. Another differentiating sign is that the standard medication of nitroglycerine for angina sufferers will not relieve the intense distress if the patient is having a heart attack.

There may also be nausea and vomiting.

Rheumatic heart disease and rheumatic fever 127: Pain and tenderness around the heart. Significant symptom may be irregular, rapid heartbeat. Pain in the joints which often swell up. Rash is occasionally encountered (red and purple spots over the body). Nosebleeds, chorea (St Vitus's dance), sweating, loss of appetite, fever.

Endocarditis (bacterial) 135: Pain around the heart is not overwhelming, irregular temperature, bleeding from nose, mouth, and into the urine. Red spots all over the body, pronounced anaemia, clubbing of the fingers.

Pericarditis 136: Pain in the chest is severe, lancinating, but the distinguishing feature of this condition is that changing position can relieve it. Veins in neck may be prominent; later, shortness of breath. (The physician notes the characteristic symptom of accumulation of fluids in abdomen or chest. Friction rub is heard on the stethoscope.)

Pulmonary embolism 140: Pain in the lung area, but the major symptom is shortness of breath. Cyanosis and shock when disease is severe. (Stethoscope will reveal the crackling sounds in the lungs known as rales and the gallop rhythm of the heart.)

Aneurysm 142 and **Cardiovascular syphilis 210:** Agonizing, paroxysmal pain radiating to both shoulders, back, and neck. Shortness of breath, husky voice, metallic cough. Swallowing becomes difficult.

Pain in the chest resembling heart attack

Pain related to the heart
- Sustained, vice-like, agonizing.

- Pain is *usually* in upper third of the sternum.
- Pain is always worsened by exertion.
- Pain most often radiates from the heart.
- Pain does not worsen when moving the shoulder.
- Pain is never altered by breathing.
- Pain is very rarely relieved by vomiting or belching or passing of gas.

Pain not related to the heart
- Spasmodic, stabbing, dull, or boring.
- Pain is often at lower end or below the sternum or under left nipple.
- Pain is unlikely to be worsened by exertion. In cardiac neurosis, exertion can often relieve it.
- Pain can sometimes radiate from the heart but more often towards the heart.
- In many disorders pain will worsen when moving the shoulder.
- In many disorders breathing will exacerbate the pain.
- In chest pains due to indigestion relief is usual upon eructation of gas or vomiting.

Neuritis 3: The neck or spine can produce a radiating pain similar to that of a heart attack but this one goes towards the heart, not away from it. Pain is not increased by effort.

Cardiac neurosis 144: The patient usually complains of tenderness of the heart, or pain that is short, stabbing or vague (none of which is characteristic of a heart attack). His pain is never worsened by exertion (occasionally actually helped by it). He might have all the other symptoms such as sweating, pallor, extreme anxiety. A doctor can always make the diagnosis.

Achalasia of the oesophagus 146: Radiating pain from behind breastbone mimicking heart attack. Distinguishing symptoms are difficulty swallowing and regurgitation, which are never symptomatic of heart attack. Pain does not worsen with effort.

Ulcer of oesophagus 147: Pain under breastbone radiating to the back appears soon after eating (can be mistaken for heart attack). Heartburn, belching, vomiting which is frequently bloody, excessive salivation, loss of weight, diarrhoea.

Oesophagitis 148: Severe pain behind the breastbone often mistaken for heart attack pain. Difficulty in swallowing, heartburn, and loss of weight from long illness.

Hiatus hernia 149: From soreness to deep ache behind the breastbone often radiating to the left shoulder (classic for heart attack). But unlike heart attack, pain does not worsen with exertion. Pain occurs soon after eating. Earliest symptom is heartburn; most important symptom, vomiting blood. There can be insidious, unnoticed bleeding into bowels and stools causing symptoms of anaemia. Later, difficulty in swallowing.

Indigestion 154: Nausea, flatulence, air pressing against the heart which may cause heartburn, sometimes severe enough to simulate heart pains. The distress is never overwhelming and is not worsened by exertion.

Cholecystitis 195: An acute gallbladder attack can often simulate a heart attack. The pain is severe and writhing, emanating from lower sternum or mid-abdomen; it is deep seated and often spasmodic; it can radiate to the back or shoulders. Sweating is profuse, heartbeat rapid, jaundice, fever. Jaundice never appears in true heart attack.

Bursitis 263: On some occasions bursitis pain can radiate from the shoulder into the breast (the wrong direction for heart attack). Movement of the shoulder exacerbates the pain, a symptom which should distinguish it from heart pains.

Cancer of the oesophagus 429: Some pressure or pain under the breastbone, rapid weight loss, emaciation, dehydration, thirst, cough, heavy salivation, and flatulence. Later anaemia, loss of voice, fever, and foul breath.

Pain in the chest, respiratory

Pain that occurs from coughing or breathing is almost always due to some respiratory disease.

Pneumonia 109: Ache in lungs or chest area. Begins with shaking chills, high fever, painful cough with rusty phlegm, rapid breathing, rapid heartbeat.

Aspiration and lipoid pneumonias 111: Fever, chest pains, shortness of breath, and cough.

Pulmonary tuberculosis 112: Pain in chest with cough producing bloodstained phlegm. Severe fatigue, drenching sweats, loss of vital capacity, weight loss.

Atelectasis 114: Pain on one side of the chest, severe shortness of breath, rapid heartbeat, weakness, cyanosis, shock.

Pleurisy 118: Sudden pains, occasionally mild, more often sharp, stabbing. Shortness of breath, cough. All symptoms worsened by heavy breathing or cough.

Empyema 119: Sharp pain on affected side of chest, short, dry cough, chills, fever, sweating, pallor, emaciation, clubbing of fingers, great malaise.

Pneumothorax 120: Severe sharp pain in chest, worse when inhaling, may go to shoulder. Shortness of breath, hacking cough producing no phlegm. Patient appears anxious.

Lung cancer 411: Chest pains, wheezing, acute shortness of breath, chronic bloody cough, night sweats, hoarseness, persistent fever, sunken eyeballs.

Symptoms of the digestive system

THE ABDOMEN
Distended abdomen

In the female the possibility of pregnancy should not be overlooked. Also, fibroid tumours of the uterus and distension of the fallopian tubes due to the presence of menstrual fluid or pus can cause swelling of the lower abdomen.

Distended abdomen, Distended abdomen and constipation, Distended abdomen and diarrhoea, Distended abdomen, infant and child

Distended abdomen

also see **Lump or mass in the abdomen**

Aneurysm (abdominal) 142: Palpable throbbing in the abdomen, pain in the back and abdomen which may be excruciating. Later, very high pulse.

Chronic gastritis 156: Pain in the stomach, appetite loss, constipation, bad taste in mouth, foul breath and furred or red-tipped tongue.

Obstruction in peptic ulcer 158: Bloody vomiting is the major symptom, appetite and weight loss, foul belching and dehydration.

Peritonitis 179: Pain severe enough to cause shock; distended abdomen, acute nausea, persistent vomiting, dehydration,

rapid heartbeat. Progressive toxaemia, sunken eyes, hollow cheeks, and anxiety.

Cirrhosis of the liver 191: Jaundice, enlarged, palpable liver, swollen abdomen, red dots with red lines on the skin, swelling of feet and legs, emaciation, enlarged abdominal vein, haemorrhoids. In men, feminizing characteristics: enlarged breasts, atrophy of testicles and loss of pubic hair.

Chronic nephritis 198: Swelling of stomach and ankles, bloody urine, excessive late night urination, breathlessness at slight exertion, impaired vision and anaemia.

Cancer of the ovary 423: Abdominal swelling and pain, pelvic mass, backache, changes in bowel and urinary habits and enlarged, painful breasts.

Stomach cancer 430: Heartburn, abdominal distension, rapid satiation at meals, sudden distaste for certain foods (especially meat), gradual weight loss and anaemia. Often the first sign is sudden pain, vomiting blood, and black, tarry stools.

Distended abdomen and constipation

Intestinal obstruction 170: Intermittent cramping pain around navel, heavy vomiting, constipation, diminished urine output. If obstruction persists, dehydration, thirst, sunken features, total suppression of urine, fever, fast pulse, shock.

Irritable colon 172: Chronic constipation frequently alternating with diarrhoea, occurring mostly in the mornings. Variable epigastric pain usually in the upper left quadrant, abdominal distension with anaemia.

Diverticulitis 173: General distress in distended abdomen becoming painful and tender especially in the lower left quadrant. In severe cases, malaise, chills, and fever. In chronic cases, constipation alternates with diarrhoea.

Distended abdomen and diarrhoea

Acute gastroenteritis 162: Tenderness in lower quadrants of distended abdomen, nausea and vomiting, cramps, diarrhoea.

Ulcerative colitis 171: Major symptom is diarrhoea (may be bloody) 10 to 20 times daily, cramps, distension of abdomen and tenderness in lower quadrants; anaemia.

Irritable colon 172: Chronic constipation frequently alternating with diarrhoea occurring mostly in the morning, variable epigastric pain usually in upper left quadrant, abdominal distension.

Diverticulitis 173: General distress in distended abdomen, becoming painful and tender especially in lower left quadrant. In severe cases, malaise, chills, fever; in chronic cases, constipation which may alternate with diarrhoea.

Sprue 180: Flatulence then diarrhoea, stools fatty, light-coloured, frothy, and foul-smelling. Red, sore tongue, distended abdomen, emaciated body, some bleeding under the skin. In children, retarded growth, deformities of bone, spontaneous fractures.

Typhoid fever 363: Very high fever, sustained, severe frontal headache, slow double pulse beat, diarrhoea, rosy spots on distended stomach, nosebleeds, stupor.

Distended abdomen, infant and child

Megacolon 175: Enlarged abdomen, severe constipation, and retarded growth.

Coeliac disease 181: A recurrent childhood disease, it is characterized by persistent diarrhoea, protuberant stomach, thin body, retarded growth, low appetite, weight loss and fretfulness.

Nephrosis 199: Distention of abdomen, puffiness of face, swelling of ankles, anaemia.

Hypothyroidism 339: Children: goitre, severe retardation, puffy hands and feet, coarse face, subnormal temperature, pot-belly, dry, wrinkled skin, flat nose.

Low birth weight 396: Infants: inactivity, weakness, irregular breathing, large head, prominent eyes, protruding abdomen, small genitals, slow to gain weight.

Colic 401: Infants: excessive, prolonged crying, fretfulness, diarrhoea, vomiting, passing of gas, distended abdomen.

Cystic fibrosis 407: Emaciation despite ravenous appetite, greasy, foul stools, cough, rapid breathing, protruding stomach.

*

Enlarged vein on the abdomen

Cirrhosis of the liver 191: Jaundice, enlarged, palpable liver, abdomen distended with enlarged veins, red lines radiating out of red spots on skin, swelling of ankles, feet, emaciation, foetid breath, haemorrhoids. In men, enlarged breasts, atrophy of testicles and loss of pubic hair, impotence.

Lump or mass in the abdomen
also see **Distended abdomen**

Regional enteritis 168: Pain and sausage-shaped mass in lower right quadrant, diarrhoea.

Hypertrophic pyloric stenosis 169: Infants: palpable lump in abdomen, projectile vomiting, constipation, loss of weight, dehydration.

Diverticulitis 173: Abdominal distress becoming painful in lower left quadrant with distended abdomen. Occasionally a mass is felt in lower left quadrant. In severe cases chills, fever and malaise. In the chronic form, constipation alternating with diarrhoea.

Ovarian tumour 227: Frequently asymptomatic. Low abdominal pains, irregularities in menstruation. Often masculinization such as deep voice and hairiness.

Malignant tumours of the nervous system 413: Infants, children: swollen lymph nodes are usually the first sign. Palpable mass in the abdomen, discoloration and pain around the eyes, rapid weight loss, anaemia, and fever. There may be urine obstruction and respiratory distress.

Cancer of the kidney 427: Abdominal mass, back pain, and blood in the urine are the classic triad of symptoms. Also weight loss and anaemia.

Wilms' tumour 428: Children: first sign is a large abdominal mass on one side of the abdomen, frequent appearance of blood in the urine. Later, pain, anaemia, loss of weight.

Pain or cramps in the abdomen

Pain in the abdomen can range in cause from a mild stomach upset to cancer of the stomach. It is therefore important to evaluate all the other symptoms. For easier diagnosis, pain in the abdomen has been further subdivided into the following categories:
Pain in the abdomen, Severe pain in the abdomen, Pain in the abdomen and diarrhoea, Pain in the abdomen a:..! weight loss, Pain in the abdomen and vomiting, Pain in the abdomen and vomiting blood, Severe pain in the abdomen and vomiting, Pain in the abdomen, vomiting and fever, Pain in the abdomen, vomiting and jaundice

Pain in the abdomen

Indigestion 154: Mild abdominal distress, heartburn, flatulence, nausea.

Diverticulitis 173: Abdominal distress becoming painful in lower left quadrant with distended abdomen. Occasionally a mass is felt in the lower left quadrant. In severe cases chills, fever and malaise. In the chronic form constipation alternating with diarrhoea.

Meckel's diverticulum 174: Pain, tenderness, and rigidity in lower left quadrant, bleeding into stools.

Cholangitis 196: Severe jaundice, chills, and high fever, profuse sweating, pain in the upper right abdomen and clay-coloured stools.

Late syphilis (tabes dorsalis) 210: Crises (spasms and pain) in throat and stomach, 'lightning' pain occurring episodically in different parts of the body, loss of balance when eyes are closed.

Haemolytic anaemia 324: All the anaemic symptoms (pallor, breathlessness, fatigue), jaundice, dizziness, fainting, weak, rapid pulse, rapid breathing, fever, and aches in the extremities and the abdomen.

Purpura 328: Crop of tiny red spots on skin later turning purple and black, bleeding from mucous membranes on slightest injury. Pain in abdomen, joints, slow clotting of blood, blood in the stools.

Salt deficiency 356: Stomach cramps, loss of skin elasticity, severe drop in urine output, twitching muscles, faint, rapid pulse, convulsions.

Bilharziasis 383: Swelling of the face, limbs, and genitalia. Also skin rash and abdominal pain.

Severe pain in the abdomen

Aneurysm (stomach) 142: Throbbing and great pain in the abdomen or back, shortness of breath and metallic cough.

Perforation in peptic ulcer 160: Sudden agonizing, writhing pain in the abdomen is the prime symptom. Patient is ashen grey. Vomiting may occur and will increase with peritonitis.

Pain in the abdomen and diarrhoea

Postgastrectomy syndrome 161: Cramps after meals, pain in abdomen, explosive diarrhoea, sweating, palpitations.

Infected food gastroenteritis 163: Violent cramps, nausea, and vomiting, diarrhoea, chills and fever. Symptoms usually occur 12 hours after intake of contaminated food. In severe form, dehydration, kidney failure, and shock.

Staphylococcus gastroenteritis 164: Strong cramps, nausea, vomiting, diarrhoea, salivation, sweating. Symptoms usually appear from two to four hours after intake of contaminated food. In severe form, blood and mucus in the stools, prostration and shock.

Ulcerative colitis 171: Major symptom is diarrhoea (sometimes bloody), often 10 to 20 times a day; mild to severe abdominal cramps, futile, urgent efforts at defecation, tenderness in lower quadrants, distension of abdomen, anaemia.

Irritable colon 172: Chronic constipation occasionally alternating with diarrhoea. Variable epigastric pains usually in upper left quadrant, distended abdomen, headache and insomnia.

Cholera 364: Constant, voluminous, watery diarrhoea, massive dehydration, severe abdominal cramps, violent vomiting, intense thirst, sunken eyes, clammy, wrinkled skin.

Bacillary dysentery 366: Constant diarrhoea, blood and mucus in the stools, thirst, urgent need to defecate without effect, vomiting, dehydration.

Amoebic dysentery 382: Pain on right side of the abdomen, run-down body, severe diarrhoea, purulent, bloody stools, weight loss, prostration.

Tapeworm 390: Abdominal cramps, diarrhoea, loss of appetite, exhaustion. Segment of worm seen in stools.

Cancer of the colon and rectum 434: Discomfort in the rectum not relieved by bowel movement, narrowing of stools, alternating constipation and diarrhoea, painful defecation, anaemia. Later, there will be persistently bloody stools, excessive gas, cramping pain, and weight loss.

Pain in the abdomen and weight loss

Regional enteritis 168: Mid-abdominal cramps, diarrhoea, anaemia, malnutrition, migratory arthritis, anal abscess, and weight loss.

Adrenal insufficiency (Addison's disease) 344: Weakness, piebald skin or bronzing, black freckles, weight loss, craving for salt, dizziness, fainting, abdominal pain and vomiting, nervous disorders, intolerance for cold, dehydration.

Amoebic dysentery 382: Pain on right side of abdomen, run-down body, severe diarrhoea, purulent, bloody stools, weight loss, prostration.

Roundworm 388: Vague colicky pain in abdomen, weight loss, fatigue.

Cancer of the pancreas 431: Boring pain in the upper abdomen extending to the back, indigestion, jaundice, brown urine, clay-coloured stools, weight loss.

Cancer of the colon and rectum 434: Discomfort in rectum not relieved by bowel movement, narrowing of stools, alternation of constipation and diarrhoea, painful defecation, anaemia. Later, persistently bloody stools, excessive gas, cramping pain, and weight loss.

Pain in the abdomen and vomiting

Achalasia of the oesophagus 146: Radiating pain from behind the breastbone mimicking heart attack. Distinguishing symptoms are difficulty swallowing, regurgitation (never symptomatic of a heart attack). Pain never worsens with exertion.

Acute gastritis (simple) 155: Pain and pressure at the pit of the stomach, nausea, vomiting, coated tongue.

Acute gastroenteritis 162: Nausea, vomiting, distension of the stomach, diarrhoea, tenderness in the lower quadrants, rapid pulse, weakness, possible shock.

Diverticulitis 173: Abdominal distress settling as pain in the lower left quadrant, occasional vomiting, distended abdomen. In chronic form, constipation alternating with diarrhoea. In severe form, chills and fever.

Diabetes (ketoacidosis, diabetic coma) 332: Pain in abdomen, nausea and vomiting, breathing rapidly, deeply, hungrily, severe dehydration, dizziness, poor skin tone, excessive thirst and urination, sweet, fruity breath, furry tongue, sunken eyeballs, stupor, shock, and finally coma.

Adrenal insufficiency (Addison's disease) 344: Weakness, piebald skin or bronzing, black freckles, weight loss, craving for salt, dizziness, fainting, abdominal pain and vomiting, nervous disorders, intolerance for cold, dehydration.

Bacillary dysentery 366: Constant diarrhoea, blood and mucus in the stools, thirst, urgent need to defecate without effect, vomiting, dehydration.

Pain in the abdomen and vomiting blood

Acute gastritis (erosive) 155: Severe stomach pain, collapse, very fast pulse, cyanosis, difficulty swallowing, excessive thirst, blood in stools, possible vomiting of blood. Stomach may be rigid and tender; skin is cold and moist.

Peptic ulcer 157: Pain in pit of stomach is burning, boring, relieved only by food and antacids. Frequent vomiting with blood, black stools.

Stomach cancer 430: Prolonged indigestion, upper abdominal distress after meals, early satiation at meals, inexplicable distaste for certain foods, notably meat and especially red meat, vomiting of blood, anaemia, black, tarry stools. Occasionally first sign may be sudden pain in stomach.

Severe pain in the abdomen and vomiting

Acute gastritis (erosive) 155: Severe pain in the stomach, fast heartbeat, excessive thirst, vomiting, collapse.

Perforation in peptic ulcer 160: Sudden, agonizing, writhing pain in the abdomen is the prime symptom. Patient is ashen grey. Other symptoms are shortness of breath and cough. Vomiting may occur and will increase with oncoming peritonitis.

Staphylococcus gastroenteritis 164: Strong cramps, nausea, vomiting, diarrhoea, excessive salivation, sweating within two to four hours after intake of contaminated food. In severe form, blood and mucus in stools, prostration and shock.

Botulism 165: Appears 18–36 hours after intake of contaminated food. Begins with lassitude, dizziness, then nausea and vomiting (which can be extreme), severe cramps, difficulty in breathing, double vision, blurred vision, dilated, fixed pupils, paralysis of respiration.

Acute pancreatitis 166: Severe writhing pain high in abdomen, often extending to the back, severe vomiting, frequent jaundice, cyanosis, feeble, rapid pulse, shock.

Peritonitis 179: Abdominal pain is so severe as to cause prostration and even shock. Abdominal area rigid and distended. Persistent vomiting. Patient is very sick, anxious, with sunken eyes and hollow cheeks, rapid heartbeat, hiccups, thirst, dehydration.

Gallstones 194: Biliary colic, accompanied by agonizing cramps coming in waves radiating to the back and right shoulder or back. Mild jaundice, nausea, and vomiting, flatulence, belching, and rapid heartbeat.

Cholecystitis 195: Biliary colic, agonizing, writhing cramps coming in waves radiating to the back and right shoulder or pelvis. Mild jaundice, nausea, vomiting, flatulence, belching, and rapid heartbeat.

Inguinal hernia (groin) 255: (Strangulated hernia only) Sudden bulge in the groin, severe pain in abdomen, vomiting, collapse, fainting.

Cholera 364: Constant voluminous, watery diarrhoea, massive dehydration, ·

severe abdominal cramps, violent vomiting, intense thirst, sunken eyes, clammy, wrinkled skin.

Pain in the abdomen, vomiting and fever

Infected food gastroenteritis 163: Severe cramps, nausea and vomiting, diarrhoea, chills and fever. Usually symptoms occur twelve hours after intake of contaminated food. In severe form, dehydration, kidney failure, and shock.

Regional enteritis 168: Pain and sausage-shaped, palpable mass in lower right quadrant, diarrhoea, vomiting, fever. Skin dry, scalp shrunken, anal fistula.

Intestinal obstruction 170: Cramping pain at navel, vomiting greyish then brown, always constipation, distended stomach, heartburn, diminished urine. If obstruction persists, total suppression of urine, thirst, sunken features, high fever, rapid pulse, anxious face, dehydration and shock.

Appendicitis 178: Discomfort around navel becoming painful in lower right quadrant. Tenderness and rigidity in that area, nausea and occasional vomiting. If fever becomes higher, pain may be severe. If appendix ruptures, peritonitis follows.

Childbed fever 247: High fever, chills, fast pulse, low abdominal pain, vomiting, vaginal discharge.

Pain in the abdomen, vomiting and jaundice

Chronic relapsing pancreatitis 167: From mild to writhing pain high in abdomen, vomiting, often jaundice, fast pulse, fatty, frothy stools, weight loss.

Acute yellow atrophy 193: High fever, severe headache, jaundice, severe abdominal pain, black vomiting, apathy, confusion, bleeding under the skin and from the mouth, dilated pupils, foul breath, scanty, bloody urine and rapid, feeble pulse.

Toxaemia of pregnancy (preeclampsea) 246: Puffiness of the body, large gain in weight, severe headache, visual disturbances, dizziness, vomiting, amnesia, and jaundice. Pain in the upper abdomen.

Cancer of the pancreas 431: Boring pain in the upper abdomen extending to the back, indigestion, jaundice, brown urine, clay-coloured stools, weight loss.

Cancer of the gallbladder 432: Pain in upper right abdomen near the centre, jaundice, progressive weakness, weight loss. There may be vomiting.

Cancer of the liver 433: Severe pain and pressure in the abdomen, dull ache on right side of the mid-abdominal area, vomiting, jaundice, constipation, anaemia, weight loss.

*

Rigidity of the abdomen

Acute gastritis (erosive) 155: Severe pain in the stomach, collapse, very fast pulse, cyanosis, difficulty swallowing, excessive thirst, clammy skin. Possible vomiting, often of blood.

Perforation in peptic ulcer 160: Sudden agonizing pain in stomach, rise in pulse and temperature, shortness of breath; patient is ashen grey.

Meckel's diverticulum 174: Pain in lower left quadrant, blood in stools.

Appendicitis 178: Begins as discomfort in navel area soon becoming acute, constant pain in lower right quadrant with rigidity in the area. Nausea, occasional vomiting, rapid pulse. If fever goes higher, pain becomes more severe with danger of rupture and peritonitis.

Peritonitis 179: Severe abdominal pain to point of prostration or shock. Abdomen rigid, distended, persistent vomiting, rapid pulse, dehydration, thirst, scanty urine, hiccups. Patient appears very anxious and very sick.

Tenderness in the abdomen

Acute gastroenteritis 162: Tenderness in lower quadrants, distended abdomen, nausea, vomiting, cramps and diarrhoea.

Acute pancreatitis 166: Tenderness in pit of stomach, writhing pain high in abdomen, severe vomiting, cyanosis, feeble, rapid pulse, shock.

Ulcerative colitis 171: Major symptom is diarrhoea (possibly bloody) 10 to 20 times a day. Moderate to severe cramps, tenesmus, tenderness in lower quadrants, distended abdomen, anaemia.

Diverticulitis 173: Pain in lower left quadrant of the abdomen; distension of the abdomen, nausea and occasional vomiting. In severe form, chills and fever; in the chronic form, constipation alternating with diarrhoea.

Appendicitis 178: Tenderness and rigidity in lower right quadrant. Begins as discomfort in navel region soon becoming severely painful in indicated area. Nausea, occasional vomiting. If fever goes higher, pain increases and rupture of appendix and peritonitis may be imminent.

Acute infectious hepatitis 187 and **Serum hepatitis 188:** Tenderness and palpability of the liver, jaundice, dark urine, red, itching wheals, weakness, headache, nausea and vomiting. In severe cases, clay-coloured stools.

Throbbing in abdomen

Aneurysm (abdominal) 142: Throbbing with or without great pain in the abdomen and/or in the back, shortness of breath, cough.

THE ANUS
Abscess in anus

Regional enteritis 168: Diarrhoea, malnutrition, anaemia, migratory arthritis, mid-abdominal cramps, weight loss, fistulas and abscesses around anus. Later, palpable mass and pain in lower right quadrant, vomiting, skin dry, scaly, shrunken.

Anal fistula 185: Sore rectum, uncontrolled seepage from the anus.

Bleeding from the anus

Haemorrhoids 182: Painful defecation, bleeding into the stools (blood is bright red, never dark), itching anus.

Itching anus

Haemorrhoids 182: Painful defecation, bleeding into stools (blood is bright red, never dark), itching anus.

Anal pruritus 186: Severe itching around anal area.

Threadworm 389: Severe, painful itching, restless sleep, poor appetite, failure to gain weight, worms visible in stools.

Pain in anus

Haemorrhoids 182: Painful defecation, bleeding into stools (blood is bright red, never dark), itching anus.

Anal fissures 183: Sharp, knife-like pain during defecation.

Proctitis 184: General pain in rectum and anus, tenesmus.

Lymphogranuloma venereum 217: Transient small pimple around genitalia, enlarged lymph nodes in groin. In severe cases very enlarged penis or vulva. Tumours from stems in labia; growths can occur around anus of both sexes. Inflammation of anus, narrowing (stricture) of rectum. Fever, aches in joints, skin rash.

Minor disorders of pregnancy 235: Haemorrhoids, varicose veins, indigestion, headache, backache, slight shortness of breath, excessive salivation.

DEFECATION
Abnormal stools

Abnormal stools, clay-coloured, Abnormal stools, varied

Abnormal stools, clay-coloured

Acute infectious hepatitis 187 and **Serum hepatitis 188:** Stools are light, clay-coloured. Other symptoms are jaundice, dark urine, red, itching wheals, weakness, tenderness in liver area, headache, gastrointestinal upsets.

Cholangitis 196: Clay-coloured stools, jaundice, severe chills, high fever.

Cancer of the pancreas 431: Pain in the upper abdomen extending to the back, indigestion, jaundice, brown urine, clay-coloured stools, weight loss.

Abnormal stools, varied

Chronic relapsing pancreatitis 167: Fatty, frothy, foul stools, pain in the upper abdomen ranges from mild to raging, vomiting, fast pulse, chills, occasional jaundice.

Sprue 180: Stools fatty, light-coloured, frothy, and foul, distended abdomen, emaciation, bleeding under the skin. Children: retarded growth, deformities of bone and muscle, spontaneous fractures.

Coeliac disease 181: Infants, children: stools are loose, foul, and fatty. Persistent diarrhoea touched off by upper respiratory infection. Distended abdomen, thin body. Child is fretful, weak, with retarded growth.

Bacillary dysentery 366: Blood, pus, and mucus in stools, constant diarrhoea, dehydration, abdominal pain, thirst, vomiting, tenesmus.

Infant diarrhoea 402: Large number of watery stools which are foul-smelling, often greenish containing blood and mucus; vomiting and fever.

Cystic fibrosis 407: Infants, children: failure to grow normally, ravenous appetite, greasy, foul-smelling stools, chronic cough, rapid respiration, wheezing, running nose, irritability, thin and protuberant stomach.

Cancer of the colon and rectum 434: Narrowing of stools. Discomfort in rectum not relieved by defecation, painful defecation. Constipation followed by diarrhoea, anaemia. Later, persistent bleeding into stools, gas, cramps, weight loss.

*

Alternating constipation and diarrhoea

Irritable colon 172: Chronic constipation often alternating with diarrhoea (mostly in the mornings), epigastric pain usually in upper left quadrant, distended abdomen, headaches, loss of appetite, and fatigue.

Diverticulitis 173: Abdominal distress settling to pain in lower left quadrant, distended abdomen. In severe cases, chills, fever; later, constipation alternating with diarrhoea.

Cancer of the colon and rectum 434: Discomfort in rectum not relieved by bowel movement, narrowing of stools, constipation followed by diarrhoea or vice versa. Pain on defecation, anaemia. Later, persistent bleeding into stools, excessive gas, cramping pain, loss of weight.

Blood in the stools, black stools (melaena)
also see **Diarrhoea, bloody** p142

This is not the same as bloody diarrhoea; this is blood discovered after a bowel movement. The colour is bright red (from anus or rectum) to black (from stomach or intestines).
Blood in the stools, Blood in the stools and abdominal pain

Blood in the stools

Massive haemorrhage in peptic ulcer 159: Profuse blood in vomit, bloody stools, heavy sweating, collapse and shock.

Haemorrhoids 182: Bleeding piles, blood bright red, never dark, painful defecation, itching anus.

Cirrhosis of the liver 191: Loss of weight, flatulence, foul breath and abdominal distension. Later, severe jaundice, emaciation, spider angiomas (red spots with red lines radiating out), puffiness of the feet and legs, enlarged vein in the abdomen, general bleeding, blood in the faeces. In men, atrophy of the testes.

Polycythaemia 327: Bleeding in the gastrointestinal tract causing bloody, tarry stools, bluish-red skin, dizziness, shortness of breath, itching, constant dull headache.

Vitamin K deficiency 354: General bleeding from nose, gums, vagina, blood in urine and stools.

Histoplasmosis 393: Ulcers on the ear, nose, legs, pharynx, larynx, and the extremities. Irregular fever, emaciation, anaemia, and swollen lymph glands. Vomiting, diarrhoea with black stools, debilitation.

Blood in the stools and abdominal pain

Hiatus hernia 149: Insidious, unnoticed bleeding into stools, pain radiating out from behind breastbone, heartburn, pallor.

Acute gastritis (erosive) 155: Blood in stools, vomiting of blood, severe pain in pit of stomach, fast heartbeat, cyanosis, thirst, rigid stomach, collapse.

Peptic ulcer 157: Tarry stools, vomiting, frequently with blood, steady boring, burning pain in pit of stomach relieved by food and antacids.

Staphylococcus gastroenteritis 164: Symptoms begin two to four hours after eating contaminated food – nausea, vomiting, cramps, diarrhoea, and sweating. In severe cases, prostration, blood in the stools, and shock.

Intestinal obstruction 170: Intermittent mid-abdominal pain, vomiting becoming brown, constipation, distension of the abdomen and heartburn. If the disease persists, fast pulse, cold extremities, anxious, sunken features, thirst, complete suppression of the urine, high fever, dehydration and shock.

Meckel's diverticulum 174: Rigidity of the abdomen, pain in the lower left quadrant, bloody stools.

Purpura 328: Small red spots which often run together, bleeding from the mouth and mucous membrane on slight injury, pain in the abdomen and joints, slow clotting of the blood, black-and-blue marks and traces of blood in the stools.

Stomach cancer 430: Prolonged indigestion, upper abdominal distress after meals, rapid satiation at meals, inexplicable distastes for some foods, notably meat and especially red meat, black, tarry stools, bloody vomiting, anaemia, progressive weight loss. Occasionally first sign is sudden abdominal pain.

*

Change in bowel habits

Any change in bowel habits for anyone of middle-age and beyond which lasts for more than ten days should be reason enough to visit a doctor. It may be a functional condition but it may also be the first signs of cancer.

Cancer of the ovary 423: Abnormal swelling, pelvic mass, backache, changes in bowel and urinary habits, vaginal bleeding frequent, enlarged, painful breasts, accumulation of fluid in abdomen.

Cancer of the colon and rectum 434: Discomfort in rectum not relieved by defecation, narrowing of stools, constipation followed by diarrhoea, pain on defecation, anaemia. Later, persistent bleeding into stools, gas, cramps, loss of weight.

Constipation
also see **Alternating constipation and diarrhoea** p142

Many healthy people do not move their bowels every day. Evacuations can occur every two days and still be compatible with good health. There are many causes outside of direct disease. Worry and anxiety or a highly nervous disposition can dispose one towards constipation. See *Table 11, How to avoid constipation.*

The following can contribute to constipation:
• Insufficient consumption of liquids or roughage. This is particularly noted in dieters. Excessive loss of water can be due to diabetes or to heavy perspiration

from extremely hot weather or extensive exercise.

● Weakness of the anal muscles may be due to pregnancy, obesity, old age or leading too sedentary a life.

● Excessive use of laxatives making the body dependent upon their use.

● Pain from fissures and haemorrhoids.

● Habitual disregard to the call of defecation quite common in busy people who do not take time out at the required moment.

● Constipation from lead poisoning can be identified by a blue line on the gums.

Constipation, Constipation and abdominal pain

Constipation

Hypertrophic pyloric stenosis 169: Infants: projectile vomiting, lump in the abdomen, dehydration and loss of weight.

Megacolon 175: Infants, children: major symptom is constipation. Also abdominal distension from faecal impaction, and retarded growth.

Constipation 176: The only symptom is constipation without discomfort or pain, except for mental distress over this condition.

Cystocoele and rectocoele 225: Females: in rectocoele, constipation is the major symptom.

Minor disorders of pregnancy 235: Slight breathlessness, excessive salivation, dyspepsia, variable headaches, backache, toothache, and constipation.

Cancer of the cervix 421: Irregular menstrual periods, bleeding discharge from the vagina and bleeding after intercourse or exertion. Later, yellowish discharge, pain in the lower back, erratic urination, nausea, vomiting, constipation and weight loss.

Constipation and abdominal pain

Chronic gastritis 156: Pain in the stomach, appetite loss, distension of the stomach, bad taste in the mouth, foul breath, and furred or red-tipped tongue.

Intestinal obstruction 170: Intermit-

tent cramping pain around the navel, heavy vomiting, distended abdomen. If obstruction persists then high fever, suppression of urine, fast pulse, thirst, sunken features, anxiety, dehydration and shock.

Irritable colon 172: Chronic constipation after alternating with diarrhoea, epigastric pain in upper left quadrant of the abdomen, distended abdomen, appetite loss, and fatigue.

Cancer of the uterus 422: Vaginal bleeding between menstrual periods or after menopause. Major sign is malodorous, watery discharge from vagina, erratic urination, constipation, pain in lower back and abdomen radiating to hips and thighs.

Cancer of the pancreas 431: Pain in pancreatic region extending to the back, indigestion, jaundice, brown urine, clay-coloured stools, weight loss, and constipation.

Cancer of the liver 433: Nausea, vomiting, pressure in abdomen, dull ache in area of the liver, jaundice, anaemia, constipation, weight loss.

Diarrhoea

Besides disease, dietary indiscretions such as eating unripe fruit, or taking such foods that are known to disagree with some people (eggs, strawberries, shellfish, even drinking very cold liquids) can be the cause of diarrhoea. Other factors are eating under great stress or excitement, antibiotics, all arsenic and mercury compounds, saccharin (for some individuals), aspirin (for many people), gold salts, barium and bismuth.

Diarrhoea, Diarrhoea, bloody, Diarrhoea and vomiting, Diarrhoea and vomiting leading to shock or coma

Diarrhoea

Postgastrectomy syndrome 161: Cardinal symptom is explosive diarrhoea shortly after meals. There is also sweating, palpitations, lightheadedness and fainting.

Sprue 180: Diarrhoea, stools fatty, light-coloured, frothy, and foul. Red, sore tongue, distended abdomen, emaciation, bleeding under the skin. In children, retarded growth, deformities of bone and muscle, and spontaneous fractures.

Coeliac disease 181: Children: recurrent disease, persistent diarrhoea touched off by upper respiratory infection. Stools are loose, fatty, and foul; protuberant abdomen, thin body. Child is fretful, weak, with retarded growth.

Toxic hepatitis 189: Jaundice, itchy skin, rash, diarrhoea, and collapse.

Hyperthyroidism 340: Nervousness, sweating, intolerance for heat, muscle weakness, fatigue, weight loss, scanty menstruation, diarrhoea, hot, moist skin, hand tremors, rapid pulse, pounding heart, bulging eyes, and hyperactiveness.

Blood poisoning 360: Shaking chills, irregular fever, intense headache, severe diarrhoea, periods of profuse sweating, red rash, small purplish, haemorrhagic points under the skin, and collapse.

Traveller's dysentery 367: Diarrhoea, usually without other symptoms.

Tapeworm 390: Abdominal cramps, diarrhoea, exhaustion, and loss of appetite.

Diarrhoea, bloody

Staphylococcus gastroenteritis 164: Two to four hours after eating contaminated food, vomiting, cramps, often bloody diarrhoea, salivation, sweating. In severe form, prostration and shock.

Ulcerative colitis 171: Major symptom is bloody mucus evident in diarrhoea occurring 10–20 times daily (also watery and foul-smelling), cramps in abdomen, distension and frequent urge to defecate. Later, anaemia and weight loss.

Vitamin B complex (niacin) deficiency (pellagra) 351: Loss of weight, weakness, red spots on the body turning brown and scaly, the mucous membranes and tongue margins becoming scarlet, inflamed gums, salivation and diarrhoea later becoming bloody. Also poor memory and emotional instability.

Typhoid fever 363: Constant severe frontal and/or temporal headache, sustained very high fever, distended abdo-

men, slow double pulse beat, nosebleeds, rosy spots on abdomen, bloody diarrhoea and stupor.

Bacillary dysentery 366: Constant diarrhoea which is bloody, purulent and full of mucus, abdominal pain, thirst, vomiting, dehydration, tenesmus.

Amoebic dysentery 382: Body is run-down, severe diarrhoea, bloody, purulent stools, abdominal pain on right side, prostration, weight loss.

Histoplasmosis 393: Ulceration on ear, nose, pharynx, vomiting, diarrhoea, black stools, emaciation, enlarged lymph nodes. In chronic form, bloody cough, drenching sweats, extreme fatigue, weight loss.

Infant diarrhoea 402: Diarrhoea of watery, foul-smelling stools containing blood and mucus. Stool colour is often green. Fever and vomiting.

Cancer of colon and rectum 434: Discomfort in rectum not relieved by bowel movement, change of bowel habits, narrowing of stools, constipation followed by diarrhoea. Pain on defecation, anaemia. Later, persistent bleeding into stools, excessive gas, cramps, loss of weight.

Diarrhoea and vomiting

Acute gastroenteritis 162: Vomiting, cramps, distended abdomen, and diarrhoea.

Infected food gastroenteritis 163: Twelve hours or more after eating, vomiting, cramps, diarrhoea, chills and fever. In severe form, kidney failure, dehydration, and shock.

Regional enteritis 168: Considerable diarrhoea, pain in lower right quadrant which can wax and wane, vomiting, fever, sausage-shaped mass in lower right quadrant, anal fistula, dry, scaly, shrunken skin.

Flu 376: Diarrhoea and vomiting are characteristic of intestinal flu and are accompanied by the other flu symptoms such as chills, high fever, backache, great weakness, prostration, and the usual cold symptoms.

Histoplasmosis 393: Ulceration on the

ear, nose, and pharynx, vomiting, diarrhoea, black stools, emaciation, and enlarged lymph nodes. In the chronic form, bloody cough, drenching sweats, extreme fatigue, and weight loss.

Colic 401: Infants: prolonged crying, fretfulness, gas, diarrhoea, and vomiting.

Diarrhoea and vomiting leading to shock or coma

Staphylococcus gastroenteritis 164: Symptoms occur two to four hours after intake of contaminated food. Stomach cramps, nausea, vomiting, sweating, occasionally excessive salivation. In severe cases, blood and mucus in the stools, prostration and shock.

Botulism 165: 18–36 hours after eating contaminated food, symptoms appear: lassitude, dizziness, then extreme nausea, vomiting, cramps, diarrhoea, speaking and breathing difficulties, double or blurred vision, dilated fixed pupils, paralysis of the respiratory tract.

Uraemia 207: Severe headache, drowsiness, twitching, blurring and double vision. Contracted pupils may herald coma. Also urinous breath odour, urea frost on body. In children: body puffiness, including the face.

Acute kidney failure 208: Vomiting, scanty urine, urinous breath odour, difficulty breathing, drowsiness, twitching and convulsion. Victim may finally lapse into coma.

Cholera 364: Constant voluminous, watery diarrhoea, massive dehydration, severe cramps in the stomach and legs, violent vomiting, intense thirst, sunken eyes, clammy, wrinkled pain. Victim may finally lapse into coma.

*
Difficulties in defecation (rectal tenesmus)

Rectal tenesmus is the ineffectual straining at stools, often with an urgent feeling to do so without results. Impacted faeces will cause tenesmus – this disorder can be easily remedied by a doctor, although in many of its aspects it simulates cancer

of the rectum. Eating unripe fruit is another cause. Tenesmus can also be due to arsenic, calomel, and cantharides as well as to most of the powerful purgatives.

Ulcerative colitis 171: Major symptom is diarrhoea 10–20 times daily, abdominal cramps with distension, frequent tenesmus, anaemia.

Proctitis 184: Tenesmus, general pain in rectum and anus.

Cystocoele and rectocoele 225: Females: in rectocoele, tenesmus and occasionally vaginal pain.

Bacillary dysentery 366: Constant diarrhoea (the urge to defecate continues after there's nothing left to expel except blood and mucus), abdominal pain, dehydration, thirst, nausea and vomiting.

Cancer of the colon and rectum 434: Narrowing of the stools, abdominal discomfort not relieved by bowel movement, rectal bleeding, anaemia, difficult defecation, constipation followed by diarrhoea. Later intestinal obstruction causing gas, weight loss, and pain.

Worms in the stools

Threadworm 389: Severe anal itching and pain, restless sleep, failure to gain weight, white worms visible in stools.

GENERAL
Distaste for certain foods

Stomach cancer 430: Prolonged indigestion, upper abdominal distress after meals, rapid satiation at meals, inexplicable distaste for certain foods, notably meat and especially red meat, fatigue, bloody vomiting, black, tarry stools. Occasionally first sign may be sudden abdominal pain.

Flatulence and belching

Eructation of gas is not always due to a stomach disorder; often the cause is swallowing air, aerophagia. (See *Table 12,*

How to avoid swallowing air.) Air swallowing is characteristic among high-strung and neurotic personalities. If a subject can belch at will, one may safely assume he is an air swallower.

Ulcer of the oesophagus 147: Radiating pain behind the breastbone, eructation, vomiting frequently bloody, diarrhoea, weight loss.

Hiatus hernia 149: Pain radiating out from behind the breastbone simulating a heart attack; heartburn, insidious bleeding into the stools causing anaemia and pallor.

Indigestion 154: Belching, heartburn, nausea, low grade abdominal distress.

Obstruction in peptic ulcer 158: Vomiting is the major symptom, distended abdomen, foul belching, dehydration, weight loss.

Sprue 180: Diarrhoea, fatty, frothy, light-coloured stools, brown pigmentation of the skin, pallor, anaemia, red, sore tongue, apathy, bleeding under the skin, distended stomach and emaciation. In children, retarded growth, deformities and spontaneous fractures.

Gallstones 194 and **Cholecystitis 195:** Agonizing pain coming in waves from upper abdomen and radiating to the back, shoulders, and pelvis. Mild jaundice, nausea, rapid heartbeat, vomiting, both belching and flatulence.

Colic 401: Infants: prolonged crying, fretfulness, diarrhoea, vomiting, passing of gas, distended abdomen.

Cancer of the oesophagus 429: Difficulty swallowing, distress or pain in chest, heavy salivation, cough. Rapid loss of weight, loss of voice, flatulence, thirst and emaciation, foul breath.

Cancer of the pancreas 431: Pain in upper abdomen extending to the back, indigestion, jaundice, brown urine, clay-coloured stools, weight loss.

Cancer of the colon and rectum 434: Discomfort in rectum not relieved by bowel movement, narrowing of stools, constipation followed by diarrhoea, pain on defecation, anaemia. Later, persistent bleeding into stools, excessive gas, cramps, loss of weight.

Heartburn (*pyrosis*)

Heartburn is a burning sensation in the oesophagus felt behind the breastbone. When it is severe it is frequently mistaken for a heart attack. Heartburn is not characteristic of any disease and can occur in healthy individuals, but it can also be a significant symptom in several grave disorders. Nervous people, those under great stress, and air swallowers (see *Table 12*) often suffer from heartburn.

Ulcer of the oesophagus 147: Pain radiating from behind the breastbone, diarrhoea, loss of weight.

Oesophagitis 148: Difficulty swallowing accompanied by heartburn, pain behind the breastbone, loss of appetite and weight.

Hiatus hernia 149: Heartburn is the earliest sign. Severe pain behind the breastbone that can radiate to the left shoulder, bloody vomiting, insidious bleeding into the stools.

Indigestion 154: Heartburn, nausea, flatulence, belching, abdominal distress.

Chronic gastritis 156: Constipation, distension of the stomach, loss of appetite, bad taste in mouth, tongue furred and red at tips and edges, foul breath. Pain in stomach may be mild to acute. In chronic cases, sallow complexion and irritability.

Stomach cancer 430: Prolonged indigestion, loss of appetite, upper abdominal distress, rapid satiation at meals, inexplicable distaste for some foods, notably meat and especially red meat. Fatigue, anaemia, progressive weight loss, bloody vomiting, black, tarry stools. Occasionally first sign may be sudden stomach pain.

Indigestion (*dyspepsia*)

The features of impaired digestion (dyspepsia) are acidity, eructation of gas, vague abdominal distress, heartburn, nausea and occasionally vomiting. The causes of dyspepsia run from mild (the majority) to grave.

Dietary causes: Dyspepsia can be brought on by badly cooked or unpalatable foods, hasty eating, insufficient food, eating when overly fatigued or chilled. The abuse of alcohol, coffee, tea, and tobacco can also induce indigestion.

Physical causes: Bad teeth, mouth diseases, extended constipation, and too sedentary a life, as well as tuberculosis, anaemia, diseases of the heart, liver, kidneys.

Mental and emotional causes: Overwork, prolonged mental strain, disastrous love affair (any emotional trauma), hysteria, anxiety, hypochondria, and shock.

The digestive system is often used as a scapegoat for the ills and resentments encountered in the course of life.

Periodontitis 101: Bleeding gums is the prominent sign. Swallowing of pus from infection between teeth and gums will cause stomach distress, as well as general ill-health.

Indigestion 154: Belching, heartburn, abdominal distress, nausea, stomach acidity, occasional vomiting.

Chronic gastritis 156: Loss of appetite, oppression in the epigastrium, nausea is common. Vomiting and pain are not prominent signs.

Appendicitis (chronic) 178: Occasionally the appendix may not be in its usual place causing new or additional symptoms often characteristic of dyspepsia especially when the discomfort can be relieved by antacids. There may be belching, heartburn, nausea, vomiting. Suspicion should be aroused if there is fever.

Gallstones 194 and **Cholecystitis 195:** Agonizing upper abdominal pain coming in waves radiating to the back, right shoulder, and pelvis, jaundice, nausea, occasional vomiting, rapid heartbeat, belching and flatulence.

Hydronephrosis 204: Recurring nagging or spasmodic pain in the kidneys, pus in the urine, dyspeptic symptoms.

Menopause 221: Hot flushes, sweating, frequent urination, headaches, dizzy spells, depression, anxiety, irregular periods, dyspeptic symptoms.

Minor disorders of pregnancy 235: Dyspeptic symptoms, headache, backache, slight shortness of breath, varicose veins, haemorrhoids, toothache, salivation.

Stomach cancer 430: A history of indigestion which begins abruptly in middle age (more often in men) and does not respond to ordinary treatment for dyspepsia should arouse suspicion. If there is early loss of weight and anaemia, the suspicion is generally justified. Identification is further confirmed by presence of bloody vomiting, black, tarry stools, prolonged indigestion, early satiation at meals. Occasionally the first sign may be sudden abdominal pain.

Nausea

also see **Vomiting** p147

Nausea and vomiting are usually joint symptoms. However, there are instances of nausea without vomiting. Almost everyone has experienced nausea, more commonly termed as 'feeling sick'. In some diseases vomiting may not occur but nausea remains a significant symptom as in *Morning sickness (pregnancy)* **243**, *Gallstones* **194**, *Chronic gastritis* **156**. Nausea is a frequent symptom in the early stages of heart failure, TB, and many renal diseases; it can appear as the presenting symptom without other signs at first in stomach cancer. But generally nausea is a transient symptom, either a response to many medications or a result of eating foods which are contaminated or which disagree with the individual.

Ménière's syndrome 60: Mild deafness, loss of balance, vertigo, tinnitus, nausea and occasionally vomiting.

Pharyngitis (chronic) 73: Swelling of the throat, heavy, sticky mucus that is difficult to clear away.

Mountain sickness 122a: Severe headaches, impairment of judgement and concentration, cyanosis, shortness of breath on exertion, rapid heartbeat, weakness, nausea and restlessness.

Rapid heartbeat 130a: Nausea, weakness, palpitation, pallor, often shock.

Indigestion 154: Heartburn, flatulence, abdominal distress, frequent nausea.

Acute gastritis (simple) 155: Pain or pressure at pit of the stomach, loss of appetite, fullness in stomach, nausea, vomiting and coated tongue.

Postgastrectomy syndrome 161: Cardinal symptom is explosive diarrhoea shortly after meals, sweating, palpitations, light-headedness and fainting.

Diverticulitis 173: Pain in the lower left quadrant of the abdomen, distension of the abdomen, nausea, and occasional vomiting. In severe form, chills and fever. In the chronic form, constipation alternating with diarrhoea.

Peritonitis 179: Very severe abdominal pain causing shock, distension of the abdomen, acute nausea, persistent vomiting, rigid abdominal wall, dehydration, rapid heartbeat, fever, thirst, sunken eyes and hollow cheeks, anxiety.

Pernicious anaemia 323: Anaemic symptoms, palpitations, pain all over the body, pins-and-needles sensation, sore, beefy, red tongue, jaundice, nausea, difficulty walking, impotence and frigidity.

Vitamin D toxicity 353b: Loss of appetite, weakness, excessive urination, yellow deposits under the skin, kidney failure, weight loss, nausea.

Rapid satiation at meals

Stomach cancer 430: Prolonged indigestion, upper abdominal distress after meals, rapid satiation at meals, inexplicable distaste for some foods, notably meat and especially red meat. Fatigue, progressive loss of weight, bloody vomiting, anaemia, black, tarry stools. Occasionally first sign may be sudden abdominal pain.

Vomiting
also see **Vomiting** *classifications under*
Pain or cramps in the abdomen

Vomiting actually means return of food from the stomach; regurgitation is not true vomiting since it is food that has not yet reached the stomach and has not gone beyond the oesophagus. Almost all oesophageal disorders are regurgitative: Zenker's diverticulum, achalasia, ulcers, oesophagitis, hiatus hernia, benign tumour, varices and cancer of the oesophagus. Nausea, almost always a concomitant of vomiting, is not common at all in disorders of the oesophagus.

Vomiting is characteristic in almost all serious infectious diseases, noted particularly in *Meningitis* **7**, *Encephalitis* **8**, *Whooping cough* **357**, *Scarlet fever* **359**, *Cholera* **364**, and *Yellow fever* **379**.

Vomiting is also a feature of all kidney and urinary disorders, such as *Acute nephritis* **197**, *Uraemia* **207**, and *Acute kidney failure* **208**.
Vomiting, Vomiting blood, Vomiting and headache

Vomiting

Brain injury 10: Vomiting, dilated or uneven pupils, sometimes bleeding from the mouth, nose, and ears, drowsiness, coma.

Motion sickness 61: Great nausea, vomiting, greenish pallor, cold sweat, difficulty breathing, mental prostration.

Coronary thrombosis 125: Severe crushing pain in the chest, shortness of breath, pallor, fear of impending death. Occasionally vomiting.

Chronic relapsing pancreatitis 167: Varying, usually severe, pain in the upper abdomen of varying duration. Nausea, vomiting, jaundice, chills, rapid heartbeat, weight loss, and fatty, frothy, foul-smelling stools.

Hypertrophic pyloric stenosis 169: Infants: symptoms appear about four months after birth. Projectile vomiting, constipation, lumps in the abdomen, dehydration and weight loss.

Cirrhosis of the liver 191: Loss of weight, flatulence, foul breath, distension of the abdomen. Later, severe jaundice, emaciation, spider angiomas (red spots with red lines radiating out), puffiness of the legs and feet, enlarged vein in the abdomen, general bleeding and bleeding into the faeces. In men, atrophy of the testes.

Morning sickness (pregnancy) 243:

Vomiting can range from mild to pernicious. In rare cases, weight loss, jaundice, and rapid pulse.

Orchitis (mumps orchitis) 253: Swelling of the testes and scrotum accompanied by great pain. Chills, fever, vomiting, and hiccups. In mumps orchitis, swelling of the salivary glands as well.

Cancer of the cervix 421: Bloody discharge from the vagina, irregularity of menstrual periods, bleeding after intercourse or exertion. Later, yellow vaginal discharge, pain in lower back, constipation, vomiting and weight loss.

Vomiting blood

Varices of the oesophagus 151: Massive vomiting of blood, anaemia and shock.

Acute gastritis (erosive) 155: Severe pain in the stomach, collapse, very fast pulse, cyanosis, difficulty swallowing, thirst, possible vomiting of blood and blood in the stools.

Peptic ulcer 157: Boring pain in the abdomen between the end of the breastbone and the navel relieved by intake of food; bloody vomiting and tarry stools.

Obstruction in peptic ulcer 158: Vomiting is the major symptom; distended abdomen, foul belching, dehydration.

Massive haemorrhage in peptic ulcer 159: Profuse blood in vomit, persistent blood in stools, heavy perspiration, irregular pain, collapse and shock.

Perforation in peptic ulcer 160: Writhing abdominal pain, vomiting, rigid abdomen, fast heartbeat, high temperature and ashen grey face.

Acute yellow atrophy 193: Jaundice, black vomiting, severe headache, intense abdominal pain around the liver, foetid breath, emotional instability and coma.

Stomach cancer 430: Abdominal distension, heartburn, rapid satiation at meals, sudden distaste for certain foods (especially meat), gradual weight loss and anaemia. Often the first signs are sudden abdominal pain, vomiting blood, and black, tarry stools.

Vomiting and headache

Brain tumours 9: Vomiting is a most important symptom. Severe headache, dizziness, lethargy, drowsiness, disorders of personality and mental deterioration.

Migraine headache 13b: Vomiting is a basic symptom together with nausea, visual disturbances, and severe headache.

Acute glaucoma 23b: Headache, diminished vision, eyeballs becoming hard as stone (an important sign), blind spots, dilated pupils, vomiting.

Stroke 139: Paralysis of the limbs and/or eyeballs, severe headache, vomiting, impairment of vision, confusion and coma.

Acute yellow atrophy 193: Jaundice, black vomiting, severe headache, intense abdominal pain around the liver, foetid breath, emotional instability and coma.

Acute nephritis 197: Appetite loss, headache, vomiting, bloody or cloudy but scanty urine, puffiness of ankles and face, mild kidney ache, furred tongue.

Uraemia 207: Severe headache, vomiting, blurring and double vision, urinous breath odour, urea frost, diarrhoea, muscular twitching, contracted pupils and potential coma. In children, body swelling including the face.

Phaeochromocytoma 346: Pounding headache, vomiting, sweating, palpitation, tremulousness and flushing. (High blood pressure.)

Relapsing fever 369: Chills and high fever, rapid heartbeat, severe headache, vomiting, muscle and joint pains, rash on the trunk and extremities, profuse sweating. Jaundice may appear.

Brain cancer 412: Headaches, vomiting, faulty vision. Any symptom becomes possible, including one-sided muscular weakness, loss of balance, visual hallucination, cloudy consciousness, obtuseness, lethargy, and irrational behaviour.

Symptoms of the urinary tract

THE URINE

The urine is a barometer of many diseases in the body; it gives us clues by its colour, quantity, absence, odour, sediment, by failure to control its egress, or by its urgency for voiding.

Normally about a quart and a half is excreted during the waking hours in four to six occasions daily. In healthy individuals the colour is straw and the odour aromatic.

Colour and odour of the urine

Foul odour: Infection in kidneys or bladder.
Sweet and fruity: Diabetes.
Odour of overripe apples: Diabetic acidosis, faulty metabolism, or starvation.
Fishy: Some inflammation of the bladder.
New-mown hay: Diabetes.
Pale colour: Diabetes insipidus, or too much liquid has been imbibed.
Green or blue: Due to some medication or food, not a morbid sign.
Orange or deep yellow: Insufficient fluid in body, possibly jaundice, or high fever.
Greenish-yellow: Possibly jaundice.
Brown or black: Jaundice, poisoning from mercury or lead, possibly bleeding.
Milky white: Presence of fat globules indicating faulty metabolism.
Smoky: Blood or pus mixed with the urine. A red cast indicates blood.
Cloudy or opaque: May be phosphates in normal urine or pus from infection.

Frothy: May indicate bile in the urine (possible kidney disorder).
Casts in the urine: Probably some kidney disease.
Long, thin, white threads: Disorder of the urethra.

Blood in the urine (haematuria)

Blood in the urine is always a significant symptom and must never be ignored.
Blood in the urine, Blood in the urine and painful urination

Blood in the urine

Endocarditis 135: Small purplish-red spots all over the body, chills, fever, pain in the chest and joints, fatigue, clubbing of the fingers, nosebleeds, loss of appetite and enlarged, painful spleen. Blood in the urine may be minute or gross.
Acute nephritis 197: Urine is scanty and smoky, puffy face, swelling of the ankles, severe headache, sharp loss of appetite, nausea, vomiting, furred tongue.
Chronic nephritis 198: Also excessive urination (often late at night), anaemia, impaired vision, puffiness of face, swelling of ankles, distended stomach, breathlessness on slight exertion. (Rise in blood pressure.)

149

Kidney stones 202: Excruciating on and off kidney pains radiating to groin, sweating, chills, nausea and vomiting, may be shock.

Vitamin K deficiency 354: General bleeding everywhere, nose, gums, vagina; blood in urine and stools.

Cancer of the kidney 427: Primary symptom is blood in the urine. Pain in ribs and spine, palpable mass in the kidney region, anaemia.

Blood in the urine and painful urination

Stones in the bladder 203: Frequent, painful passage of purulent and bloody urine.

Cystitis 205: Painful, urgent, frequent urination with scanty output, night urination. In severe cases, blood in the urine.

Benign tumours of kidneys and bladder 206: Primary sign is blood in urine.

Prostatitis 249: Occasional show of blood at beginning or end of painful, difficult urination. Bladder frequently cannot be fully emptied. Severe pain radiating to testicle, pain between scrotum and anus. Often chills and fever.

Enlarged prostate 250: Males: occasional show of blood at the beginning and end of painful, difficult urination. Bladder cannot be fully emptied. Possible impotence. Straining at urination ending up dribbling. Low back pain.

Cancer of the prostate 424: Males: progressively increasing difficulty in urination, increasing frequency, diminished stream, inability to empty bladder. Later, low backache, impotence, and painful urination. Blood in urine most important symptom.

Cancer of the bladder 426: At first, painless passing of blood in the urine (major sign). Later, painful and increasingly frequent urination.

Wilms' tumour 428: Children: first sign is a large abdominal mass on one side of the abdomen, frequent appearance of blood in the urine. Later, pain, anaemia, loss of appetite and weight.

*

150

Cloudy urine

Acute kidney infection 200: Urine is scanty and smelling of decay. Painful, urgent, frequent urination, pain radiating from kidney, high pulse, chills and fever.

Chronic kidney infection 201: Pain radiating from kidney, painful, urgent, frequent urination, excessive late night urination. (Rising blood pressure.)

Stones in the bladder 203: Blood in the urine which is cloudy from pus and albumin. Painful, frequent urination.

Hydronephrosis 204: Pus in urine, recurrent, nagging, spasmodic pain in the kidney, dyspepsia.

Cystitis 205: Painful, urgent, frequent urination, burning in the urethra, scanty, purulent urine.

Gonorrhoea 212: Dripping white or yellow discharge from the urethra of both sexes, cloudy urine, frequent, urgent, painful urination, redness at mouth of the urethra.

Dark urine

Acute infectious hepatitis 187 and **Serum hepatitis 188:** Jaundice, light-coloured stools, dark urine, red, itching wheals, sweetish, foul breath, weakness, tenderness in liver area, headache, stomach upsets.

Cholangitis 196: Severe jaundice, high fever, profuse sweating, pain in upper right abdomen, clay-coloured stools.

Cancer of the pancreas 431: Boring pain in the upper abdomen extending to the back, indigestion, jaundice, dark brown urine, clay-coloured stools, weight loss.

URINATION
Difficulty in empyting bladder

Cystocoele and rectocoele 225: (Female) Cystocoele: incontinence in urinating. Rectocoele: difficulty defecating, pain in vagina.

Prostatitis 249: Males: difficult, painful urination, with blood at beginning or end of act, pain on sitting, chills and fever.

Enlarged prostate 250: Males: also difficult, burning urination, straining ending up dribbling. Blood in urine occasionally.

Cancer of the prostate 424: Males: progressively increasing difficulty in urination, diminished stream, increased frequency, inability to empty bladder. Later, painful urination, low backache, and blood in urine (an important sign).

Difficulty in urination

Difficulty in urination can mean straining, dribbling weakness of the stream.

Multiple sclerosis 6: Impaired vision, sudden temporary blindness or blurring, tremor of the hands, spastic gait, difficulty in speech, both retention of urine and slight incontinence.

Acute kidney infection 200: Pain in enlarged, tender kidney radiating to the groin, fast pulse, chills, fever, vomiting, foul-smelling urine. Frequent, painful urination if bladder is involved.

Cystitis 205: Strangury, constant need to urinate, painful burning sensation in urethra particularly at end of the act, pus in the urine.

Nonspecific urethritis 213: Strangury, plus discharge from men. In older women, senile urethritis and vaginitis due to oestrogen deficiency.

Enlarged prostate 250: Males: low back pain, bouts of impotence, difficult, burning urination requiring straining, ending up dribbling and never fully completed. Occasional blood in the urine and pain when sitting.

Cancer of the prostate 424: Males: progressive difficulty in urination, diminished stream and increasing frequency, inability to empty bladder. Later, painful urination, low back pain and blood in the urine (most important symptom).

Excessive urination
also see **Night urination**

Besides disease, excessive urination can occur after pregnancy, from the use of diuretic drugs, and from eating water melon or other foods high in water content.

Migraine headache 13b: Headache radiating to the eye, vision difficulties, dizziness, nausea, vomiting, chills, considerable urination.

Diabetes 332: Excessive urination, thirst, hunger, weight loss, weakness, sweet, fruity breath, blurred vision, red, sore tongue, leg cramps, pins-and-needles sensation, impotency. In diabetic keto-acidosis complication: rapid, deep, hungry breathing, severe dehydration, dizziness, abdominal pain, nausea and vomiting, excessive urination, stupor, shock and coma.

Diabetes insipidus 338: The main symptom is massive excretion of urine (several gallons daily), awakening at night to urinate, severe dehydration, thirst.

Primary aldosteronism 345: Excessive urination, thirst, muscle weakness, fatigue, numbness, tingling.

Vitamin D toxicity 353b: Loss of appetite and weight, nausea, weakness, yellow deposits under the skin, kidney failure, considerable urination.

Loss of bladder control (incontinence)

A child learns bladder control by the time he is two years old. If he is incontinent beyond that age he could be under tension, be of neurotic temperament, or have a congenital anomaly of the urinary tract. Spinal column injuries can make a patient incontinent.

Epilepsy (grand mal) 2a: Premonitory period may be heralded by nausea, flashing lights or disorder of smell or taste. At seizure, loss of consciousness, contracted muscles, eyeballs rolled upwards, twitching of muscles and limbs, foaming at the mouth, incontinence and then deep coma.

Multiple sclerosis 6: Impaired vision (sudden temporary blindness or blurring), tremors of the hand, spastic gait, difficulty in speech. Both retention of urine and slight incontinence.

Cystocoele and rectocoele 225: Females: incontinence especially on sneezing, coughing, laughing; difficulty in defecation and completely emptying the bladder, vaginal pains.

Night urination (nocturia)
also see **Excessive urination**

Chronic nephritis 198: Excessive night urination, blood in urine, puffiness of face and ankles, great distension of the abdomen, poor vision (from bleeding into the retina), anaemia, shortness of breath on exertion. (Rise in blood pressure.)

Chronic kidney infection 201: Excessive night urination which is painful, urgent, and frequent, scanty, cloudy urine, pain in kidney. (Rise in blood pressure.)

Cystitis 205: Painful, urgent, frequent urination but with scanty output. In severe cases blood in the urine.

Prostatitis 249: Urgent, frequent, painful urination with an occasional show of blood at the beginning and end of the act. Severe pain between the scrotum and anus, flu-like chills and fever.

Enlarged prostate 250: Urgent, painful, frequent urination, night urination. Bladder cannot be completely emptied. Occasionally blood in the urine, impotence or premature ejaculation which may be painful, pain in prostate region and low back, discomfort in sitting.

Diabetes insipidus 338: Massive excretion of urine (several gallons daily). Awakening at night to urinate, severe dehydration, extreme thirst.

Pain in the kidney

Acute nephritis 197: Urine is bloody or cloudy and scanty, puffiness of face and ankles, mild ache in the kidneys, head-

ache, loss of appetite, nausea, vomiting and furred tongue.

Acute kidney infection 200: Pain radiating from kidney to groin, painful, urgent, frequent urination, scanty, cloudy urine, high pulse, deep malaise, headache, chills and fever, nausea and vomiting.

Chronic kidney infection 201: Pain, radiating from kidney, cloudy urine, painful, frequent, urgent urination mostly late at night. (Rising blood pressure.)

Kidney stones 202: Excruciating on and off kidney pain radiating to groin, sweating, chills, blood in urine, shock.

Hydronephrosis 204: Spasmodic, naggaing kidney pain, pus in urine, indigestion.

Hyperparathyroidism 342: Cardinal sign is formation of kidney stones with all' its characteristic symptoms such as blood in urine, excruciating on and off pain in the small of the back radiating to abdomen, groin, and genitalia, nausea, sweating, chill, and shock.

Vitamin A deficiency 348a: Retarded growth in children, night blindness, cloudiness or ulceration of the cornea, horny skin.

Pain on urination
also see **Blood in the urine** *and* **Painful urination**

Some of the causes can be simple – a long, jolting car or motorcycle ride, a straddle injury, vaginal tampons, 'honeymoon cystitis'. When pain is intermittent, tension can be the cause (often some form of sex guilt). For the most part, however, painful urination is due to infection in the urinary system.

Acute kidney infection 200: Pain in the kidney radiating to the abdomen and groin. Urination is frequent, urgent, urine is scanty, cloudy, burning, and smelling of decay. Also chills, headache, fast pulse, fever, nausea and vomiting.

Chronic kidney infection 201: Excessive late night urination, pain on urination and in the kidneys, cloudy, pussy urine. (Rise in blood pressure.)

Stones in the bladder 203: Frequent urination, pain experienced mostly at the end of the act, blood and pus in the urine.

Gonorrhoea 212: Urgent, frequent, burning urination, whitish or yellowish discharge from male or female urethra (or vagina).

Trichomoniasis 214: Females: painful urination, yellowish-green discharge, offensive vaginal odour, itching vulva. Males: painful, burning urination, discharge from penis can be scanty or profuse, later becoming creamy.

Gonorrhoeal arthritis 262: Burning sensation in the joints with bony lumps around the joints in the hands, painful urination, rash and fever. Prostatitis in males, lower abdominal pain, vaginal discharge in women.

Scanty urination (oliguria)

The dwindling down of urinary output can be a very serious sign and must be checked by a doctor at once. Less than a pint a day is considered dangerous. This condition is found in cases of dehydration, haemorrhage, severe burns, toxaemia of pregnancy, septic abortion, peritonitis, reaction to blood transfusion, postoperative reaction, and in poisoning from pesticides, fungicides, phosphorus, carbon tetrachloride, and even sulfa drugs.

Acute yellow atrophy 193: High fever, severe headache, jaundice, severe abdominal pain, black vomiting, apathy, confusion, bleeding under the skin and from the mouth, dilated pupils, foul breath, scanty, bloody urine and rapid, feeble pulse.

Acute nephritis 197: Low urine output with a show of blood and albumin, swelling of face and ankles, headache, sharp loss of appetite, nausea, vomiting, furred tongue. (Rise in blood pressure.)

Acute kidney infection 200: Urine scanty, cloudy, with odour of decay; pain in kidney radiating to groin, pain on

urination, fast pulse, chills, fever, headache.

Cystitis 205: Painful, urgent, frequent urination, scanty, purulent urine.

Uraemia 207: Very scanty urine, urinous odour on breath, uraemic frost, swelling of parts of the body, severe headaches, impaired or double vision, contracted pupils, nausea, vomiting, diarrhoea, convulsions, coma.

Acute kidney failure 208: Very scanty urine output, urinous odour on breath, breathing difficulties, lethargy, twitching, nausea, vomiting, diarrhoea, convulsions.

Gout 334: When kidneys are involved: inflamed, painful swelling of big toe and other joints, rapid pulse, dark, scanty urine, lumps in ear and around joints (urate crystals).

Salt deficiency 356: Stomach cramps, loss of skin elasticity, scanty urine, muscle twitching, faint, rapid pulse, finally convulsions.

Yellow fever 379: High fever, flushed face, prostration, severe headache, pain in back and limbs, scanty urine. After intermission of the disease then jaundice, vomiting with black blood, bleeding from mucous membranes.

Typhus 392: Ten day high fever, severe headache, prostration, mottled rash with red spots turning purple, highly coloured, scanty urine, contracted pupils, muscle tremors, flushed face, profuse sweating when fever breaks, delirium, coma.

Total arrest of urination (anuria, kidney failure)
also see **Scanty urination**

This is always a *Medical Emergency.*

Infected food gastroenteritis 163: Symptoms occur twelve or more hours after eating. In milder form only nausea and vomiting, cramps and diarrhoea; in severe form, urinary suppression, dehydration, and shock.

Intestinal obstruction 170: Cramping abdominal pain, vomiting, constipation, abdominal distension, anxiety. In severe, persistent cases there is thirst, dehydration, total suppression of the urine and shock.

Acute kidney infection 200: Pain in the kidney radiating to the lower abdomen and groin. Urination is frequent, urgent, painful, urine is scanty, cloudy, with an odour of decay. Also chills, fever, nausea, vomiting, and fast pulse. In severe cases, total arrest of urination.

Urgent, frequent urination

This is not necessarily the same as excessive urination.

Urgent, frequent urination, Urgent, frequent, bloody urination

Urgent, frequent urination

Acute kidney infection 200: Scanty, cloudy, purulent urine with decaying odour, urgent, painful, frequent urination, pain in the enlarged kidney radiating to the groin, fast pulse, chills and fever, headache, nausea, vomiting, deep malaise.

Chronic kidney infection 201: Painful, excessive night urination, pain in the kidneys which may radiate, cloudy, purulent urine. (Rising blood pressure.)

Cystitis 205: Painful, urgent, frequent urination, scanty, purulent urine.

Gonorrhoea 212: Urgent, burning, frequent urination, whitish-yellow discharge from penis or urethra and vagina.

Menopause 221: Hot flushes, sweating, headaches, dizzy spells, depression, anxiety, indigestion, irregular menstrual periods, urgent, frequent urination.

Prolapsed uterus 224: Dragging sensation in lower abdomen, backache while standing or upon exertion, frequent urination.

Detection of pregnancy 234: Missed period, larger, more sensitive breasts and nipples, urgent, frequent urination.

Urgent, frequent, bloody urination

Stones in the bladder 203: Blood and pus in the urine, painful, frequent urination.

Prostatitis 249: Painful, urgent, frequent urination with occasional show of blood at beginning and/or end of the act. severe pain between scrotum and anus.

Enlarged prostate 250: Urgent, burning, frequent urination requiring straining with terminal dribbling, inability to completely empty the bladder, low back pain, painful sitting, bouts of impotence and premature ejaculation. Occasionally show of blood at beginning or end of urination.

Cancer of the prostate 424: Males: progressive difficulty in urination, diminished stream, increase of frequency, inability to empty bladder. Later, painful urination, low backache, blood in urine (most important sign).

Cancer of the bladder 426: Painless passing of blood in urine (major sign). Later, painful urination becoming more frequent and urgent.

*

Weakened stream (slow stream)

Enlarged prostate 250: Males: difficult, burning urination requiring straining, ending up dribbling, never fully emptying bladder. Often blood in urine, pain when sitting.

Cancer of the prostate 424: Males: progressive difficulty in urination, weakened stream, great frequency, inability to empty bladder, impotence. Later, blood in urine (most important sign).

Symptoms of the genital system common to both men and women

Blisters on the genitalia

also see **Sores, tumours, ulcers on genitalia**

Herpes simplex virus 2 212a: Painful blisters appear on the penis and on interior of the vagina or exterior genitalia of the female. They can also show up on the buttocks and thighs of both sexes. Occasionally, enlarged lymph nodes and fever. The disease will reappear from time to time.

Enlarged genital organs

Lymphogranuloma venereum 217: Small transient blister or pimple in genitals, enlarged lymph nodules in the groin, very enlarged penis or vulva, tumours on stems in clitoris, labia, and around anus of both sexes, stricture of rectum. Fever, chills, headache, vomiting, ache in joints, skin rash.

Enlarged lymph nodes in the groin

The most common cause is infection of the foot.

Early syphilis (secondary) 209: From one to six months after the disease has been contracted, a widespread, varying rash appears. Also ulcers in the mouth, arthritic pains, sore throat, and possible disorders of the eyes.

Herpes simplex virus 2 212a: Painful blisters appear on the penis and interior of the vagina or exterior genitalia of the female. They can also show up on the buttocks and thighs of both sexes. Occasionally, enlarged lymph nodes and fever. The disease reappears from time to time.

Lymphogranuloma venereum 217: Small blister or pimple in genital area healing quickly. In severe form, very enlarged penis or vulva, tumours on stems in clitoris, labia, and around anus of both sexes, stricture of rectum. Fever, chills, headache, vomiting, ache in joints, skin rash.

The plague 365: Large egg-sized lymph nodes in the groin (buboes), chills, very high fever, rapid heartbeat, black spots on skin, buboes may burst and suppurate, stupor and finally coma.

Infectious mononucleosis 377: Feeling unwell for weeks or months. Low daily fever, daily recurring headaches and sore throat. The major symptom is painful swelling of the lymph nodes under the jaw and swelling of the lymph nodes under the arms and in the groin.

Itching of the genitalia

Nonspecific urethritis 213: Discharge from urethra heavy to watery, pain in the groin, penis, vulva; itching in urethra.

Trichomoniasis 214: Females: itching of the urethra and vagina. Greenish-yellowish vaginal discharge accompanied by offensive odour. Burning urgency in urination. Males: the discharge may be profuse or scanty, thin or creamy.

Crab louse 311: Small blue spots and severe itching in pubic area. Nits attached to skin at base of hair roots. The lice can be seen.

Diabetes 332: Excessive thirst, urination, hunger, weight loss, genital itching, sweet, fruity breath, blurred vision, leg cramps, pins-and-needles sensation in the extremities, impotence, red, sore tongue, skin and vaginal infections.

Loss of libido

Most of the time loss of libido is due to psychological and psychiatric conditions.

Anaemia 322: Anaemic symptoms, palpitation, red, sore tongue, vertigo, loss of libido, fingernails ridged longitudinally and spoon-shaped, lustreless hair. In severe cases, jaundice, numbness of limbs, thirst, poor memory, and shock.

Acromegaly and gigantism 336: Enlarged skeleton, abnormal tallness, increase in size of hands, feet, internal organs, coarsening of the face, protruding jaw, loss of libido, sweating, severe headache, joint pains, mental deterioration.

Hypopituitarism 337: Children: stunted growth and dwarfism. Adults: scanty menstruation, easy fatigue, diminished libido, thinning of pubic and underarm hair, loss of appetite and weight, apathy, slow, feeble pulse, intolerance for cold.

Loss of pubic hair

Cirrhosis of the liver 191: Atrophy of the testicles, impotence, frigidity, jaundice, distension of the stomach with enlarged veins, red dots on skin with red lines radiating out, swelling of feet and ankles, emaciation, loss of pubic hair.

Hypopituitarism 337: Children: stunted growth and dwarfism. Adults: scanty

menstruation, easy fatigue, diminished libido, thinning of pubic and underarm hair, loss of appetite and weight, apathy, slow, feeble pulse, and intolerance for cold.

Adrenal insufficiency (Addison's disease) 344: Easy fatigue, bronzing of skin, weight loss, nausea, vomiting, abdominal pain, dizziness, fainting, dehydration. Also black freckles, piebald skin, loss of pubic hair.

Smallness of genitals

Low birth weight 396: Infants: weakness, inactivity, irregular breathing, large head, prominent eyes, protruding abdomen, small genitals, slow to gain weight.

Sores, tumours, ulcers on genitalia

Early syphilis 209: Hard, painless ulcer on penis or vulva or around mouth. In second stage, varying widespread body rash, ulcers in mouth, severe headaches, sore throat, arthritic pains, eye disorders.

Chancroid 215: Blisters or red pimples over genitalia which can form into dirty-looking, painful ulcers. They can heal easily or become sloughing, proliferating outwards and inwards and bleeding easily. In men, there may be constriction of the penis from tightening of the foreskin, causing painful erection.

Granuloma inguinale 216: Pimples, blisters, nodules turning into beefy red ulcers which ooze. Granular tissue appears in the area which is not painful but bleeds easily. Ulcers heal and proliferate at the same time. There is a sour, pungent odour around the genitalia.

Lymphogranuloma venereum 217: Quick healing pimple or blister in the genital area. Later, enlarged lymph nodes in the groin. In the severe form, very enlarged penis or vulva, tumours appear on stems in clitoris, labia and around anus of both sexes, stricture of the rectum. Fever, headache, vomiting, skin rash.

Unpleasant genital odour

also see **Vaginal odours** p164

Poor hygiene in the genital area (especially in uncircumcised males) or any infection of the vagina (*Vaginal inflammation* **222**, *Trichomoniasis* **214**) will produce an unpleasant odour.

Granuloma inguinale 216: Pimples, blisters, nodules turning into beefy, red, oozing ulcers. Granular tissue appears in the area which is not painful but bleeds easily; ulcers heal and proliferate at the same time. There is a sour, pungent odour around the genitalia.

Symptoms special to women

THE BREASTS
Dimpling

Breast cancer 420: Painless hard lump which is not easily movable, most commonly in upper outer quadrant. There may be thickening and dimpling of skin, possibly retraction of the nipple or discharge. Occasional pain, swelling and ulceration of the lump may occur.

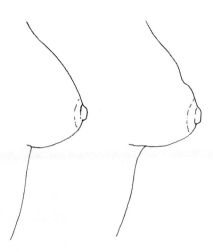

Normal breast and dimpling of breast.
(*Julian A. Miller*)

Discharge from nipples

Clear fluid or milk in normal circumstances; a clear fluid will occasionally be discharged from a benign cyst.

Breast cancer 420: Painless hard lump, not easily movable; there may be thickening, dimpling of the skin, possible retraction of or discharge from nipple. Discharge may be clear or bloodstained. At times the lump may be painful and ulcerate.

Enlarged nipples (swollen nipples, sensitive nipples)

Detection of pregnancy 234: Also enlarged, fuller, heavier breasts, missed period and urinary frequency. (For other signs of pregnancy see *Table 16*.)

Heavy breasts

Heavy breasts is most usual among women who breast-feed their children.

Contraception 233: The 'pill' can cause general puffiness, bleeding, dizziness, nausea and vomiting, heavy or sore breasts.

Detection of pregnancy 234: Enlarged nipples and fuller, heavier breasts, missed period, urinary frequency.

Cancer of the ovary 423: Swelling and pain of the abdomen, palpable pelvic mass, backache, changes in bowel and urinary habits, possible vaginal bleeding, enlarged, painful breasts. In children, precocious puberty.

Lump in the breast

Benign cystic tumour in the breast 228: Hard lumpy mass which often grows larger during menstrual time and then shrinks, or after applications of warm, moist heat. Nevertheless should be seen by a doctor.

Breast cancer 420: Painless hard lump not easily movable, most commonly in upper outer quadrant of the breast. There may be thickening and dimpling of the skin, possibly retraction of the nipple or discharge. Occasionally pain and ulceration of the lump.

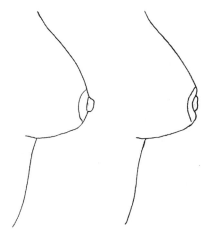

Normal breast and retracted nipple. (*Julian A. Miller*)

Pain in the breast

Pain in the breast is not a common symptom. Occasionally it is encountered at puberty and during the early months of taking the contraceptive 'pill'. In the first few months of pregnancy there may be a tingling in the breasts rather than pain. In breast cancer pain is a rare sign.

Premenstrual tension 219: Irritability, nervousness, headache, puffiness of the body, occasionally pain in the breasts.

Retraction of the nipple

Breast cancer 420: (See under *Lump in the Breast*.)

GENERAL
Cramps, pain in lower abdomen

Painful menstruation 220: Mild to severe pain in lower abdomen often radiating to the thighs, low backache, bleeding can be copious or scanty, malaise, sweating.

Prolapsed uterus 224: Dragging sensation in the lower abdomen, backache while standing or upon exertion, frequent urination (see *Early warning signals*).

Ovarian tumour 227: Most often without symptoms. Most common complaints are low abdominal discomfort, abdominal distension and palpable mass. Often abnormal menstrual periods. Occasionally early cessation of menstruation and appearance of masculine characteristics (deep voice, hairiness, etc).

Contraception 233: The IUD (intrauterine device) can on some occasions cause cramps in lower abdomen and bleeding.

Miscarriage 242: Cramps (usually severe), heavy bleeding from vagina with passage of clots.

Tubal pregnancy 245: Missed period, severe one-sided abdominal pain, heavy bleeding.

Abruptio placentae 248: Lower abdominal pain and bleeding.

Inguinal hernia 255: Pain in the groin, lump behind the pubic hair which may disappear upon lying down. In strangulated hernia, pronounced bulging, severe pain, vomiting and collapse.

Gonorrhoeal arthritis 262: Joints are red, hot, inflamed and aching, bony lumps may appear in joints of a hand, urethritis, rash, fever, pain in the lower abdomen more severe on one side, tenderness around ovaries, vaginal discharge.

Hot flushes

Menopause 221: Hot flushes, chills, sweating, fatigue, frequent urination, giddiness, palpitations, irritability, emotional instability, depression, crying bouts and anxiety.

Masculinization

Pituitary and adrenal tumours can frequently cause masculinzation.

Ovarian tumour 227: Most often without symptoms. Common complaints are low abdominal discomfort, distension of abdomen and appearance of a palpable mass in ovarian area, abnormal menstrual periods. Some tumours may cause early cessation of menstruation as well as masculinizing characteristics, such as deep voice, hairiness, etc.

MENSTRUATION
Bleeding after menopause

Menopause is not necessarily a distinct occurrence; it can be incomplete with occasional persistent periods. Supplementary oestrogens administered after menopause can often induce bleeding. Any bleeding after menopause should be investigated by a doctor.

Cervicitis 223: Inflammation of the cervix of the womb causing discharge and bleeding, particularly after intercourse. Occasionally ache in pelvis.
Fibroid tumours 226: These tumours can occur at any age and are usually quite large. Bleeding can be heavy, often to the point of anaemia.
Ovarian tumour 227: Low abdominal pain, abdominal distension and appearance of a palpable mass in that area. After menopause these tumours will cause bleeding. Masculinization may also occur.

Cancer of the cervix 421: Slightly bloody vaginal discharge; later, vaginal bleeding, pain in the lower back, various urinary problems, weight loss.
Cancer of the uterus 422: Vaginal bleeding, malodorous discharge. Later, urinary difficulties, general pains in the lower back or lower abdomen.
Cancer of the ovary 423: (Benign ovarian tumours occur six times more frequently than malignant ones. The symptoms are similar.) Pain in lower abdomen and low back, enlarged abdomen, mass in the pelvis and vaginal bleeding. Growing tumours will press upon the intestinal and urinary tracts causing symptoms in these systems.

Excessive menstrual flow (menorrhagia)

Heavy bleeding during menstruation can be brought on by many infectious diseases such as the flu, scarlet fever, measles, malaria, smallpox, diphtheria, leukaemia, purpura, high blood pressure (particularly when nearing menopause), chronic alcoholism, cirrhosis of the liver, emphysema, hyperthyroidism, and myxoedema.

A single excessive period can be due to some violent exercise, violent emotion, fright, or even excessive sexual intercourse.

Heavy bleeding may also be due to an IUD (intrauterine device).

Cervicitis 223: Heavy menstruation, ache in pelvis and low back, vaginal discharge, bleeding after intercourse.
Fibroid tumours 226: Pressure against the bladder can cause difficult, painful urination as well as heavy bleeding in the vagina.

Irregular periods

Menopause 221: Menstruation is first irregular, then completely absent. Hot flushes, chills, sweating, frequent urination, headaches, giddiness, palpitation, emotional instability, depression, anxiety, crying bouts.

Cushing's disease 343: Weight gain on the trunk, back and face (moon face), excessive hair growth, acne, easy bruising, irregularity or absence of menstrual periods, bones fracture easily, muscular weakness.

Cancer of the cervix 421: Bleeding discharge from vagina, irregularity of menstrual periods, bleeding after intercourse or after exertion. Later, yellowish discharge from vagina, pain in lower back, urinary problems, nausea, vomiting, constipation, weight loss.

Cancer of the uterus 422: Vaginal bleeding, malodorous vaginal discharge. Later, urinary difficulties, general pain in the lower back and lower abdomen.

Missed periods (amenorrhoea)

Early menopause is often an overlooked cause. Also, birth control pills frequently cause missed periods.

Absence of menstruation 218: Failure to menstruate at monthly periods, possibly tumour.

Ovarian tumour 227: Premature cessation of the period, low abdominal pain. Masculinization frequent.

Detection of pregnancy 234: A missed period under normal conditions means pregnancy. Further indications are enlargement of the breasts and nipples, urinary frequency. (See *Table 16* for additional signs.)

Tubal pregnancy 245: Missed periods, severe one-sided abdominal pain, heavy intraperiod bleeding.

Painful periods (dysmenorrhoea)

Painful menstruation is frequently due to some infection but more often arises from some long-standing anxiety, the wear and tear of living, or from an inadequate or troubled sex life. The likelihood of this condition's occurrence can be increased by a sedentary existence, insufficient exercise, and constipation.

Painful menstruation 220: Mild to severe cramps in lower abdomen sometimes running down the thighs and legs, low backache. Some women may have a copious flow, others scanty. Many feel quite sick, appearing pale and sweating.

Premature menstruation

Cancer of the ovary 423: (Benign ovarian tumours occur six times more frequently than malignant ones. The symptoms are similar.) Pain in the lower abdomen and lower back, enlarged abdomen, mass in the pelvis, vaginal bleeding. Growing tumours will press on the intestinal and urinary tract causing changes of bowel and urinary habits. In children these tumours can cause precocious puberty.

Premenstrual tension

This condition begins a week or so before the period and ends a few hours after the commencement of flow.

Premenstrual tension 219: Irritability, nervousness, headaches, emotional changes, occasional breast pain, puffiness around the abdomen or elsewhere.

Frigidity 230: Neurotic patterns, or painful sexual intercourse, constriction of the mouth of the vagina, inability to achieve orgasm, drying up of the precoital fluid and repugnance for sex.

Scanty bleeding during period

Possibly due to lactation but more likely a result of some glandular malfunction, some metabolic disorder such as diabetes, obesity, malnutrition, and quite often a result of emotional upset (love affair, divorce, nervous shock).

Hypopituitarism 337: Children: stunted growth and dwarfism. Adults: scanty menstruation, easily fatigued, diminished libido, thinning of pubic and underarm hair, loss of appetite and weight, apathy, slow, feeble pulse, and intolerance of cold.

Hyperthyroidism 340: Enlarged goitre, nervousness, sweating, intolerance of heat, muscle weakness, fatigue, weight loss, scanty menstruation, diarrhoea, hot, moist skin, hand tremors, rapid pulse, pounding heart, bulging eyes, and hyperactivity.

Pelvic mass (pelvic lump)

If fallopian tubes are distended from pus or menstrual fluid, a pelvic mass can be produced.

Fibroid tumours 226: Difficult, painful urination and heavy bleeding from vagina are common. When these tumours grow large enough, the mass can be noticeable.

Ovarian tumour 227: Pain and distension of abdomen with appearance of a mass in the pelvis. Some tumours may cause cessation of menstruation and development of masculine characteristics. (Benign ovarian tumours occur six times more frequently than malignant.)

Cancer of the ovary 423: Abdominal swelling and pain, lump in the pelvic area, backache, change in bowel and urinary habits, enlarged, painful breasts, occasionally vaginal bleeding. In children, precocious puberty.

SEXUAL PROBLEMS
Failure to achieve orgasm

Orgasm for a woman is as natural as it is for a man and as desirable although not nearly as certain. Failure to achieve orgasm is due, above all, to social and psychogenic reasons. The non-orgasmic woman is not necessarily frigid; she might even enjoy sex but her response may be stifled or inhibited. Such a woman often learns to accommodate herself to this situation but the inevitable results are harmful: the injury she does herself (anxiety, deep frustration, resentments) probably equals the injury she inflicts upon her partner, eroding their relation-

ship, casting doubts upon his masculinity, and not infrequently reducing him to impotence. Women who cannot achieve orgasm need professional help.

Frigidity 230: Neurotic patterns of living, premenstrual tensions, painful intercourse, painful spasm and closure of the vagina, inability to reach orgasmic levels, drying up of precoital fluid, repugnance for sex.
Painful sexual intercourse and vaginal spasm 231: Lack of precoital fluid, vaginismus, inflamed remains of hymen, cystitis, cervicitis, trichomoniasis infection.
Orgasmic failure in women 232: Repugnance for the male partner, aversion for sex, fear, prudery, painful intercourse.

Frigidity
*also see **Failure to achieve orgasm***

The causes of frigidity are rarely physical; they are overwhelmingly social and psychogenic, engendered by shame, repugnance for sex or for the partner, memories of traumatic sexual experiences, a frustrating sexual partner, fear of pregnancy, fear of disease, anxiety, lovelessness – all of which can induce or contribute to this condition.

Multiple sclerosis 6: Tremors, spastic gait, disturbances of bladder control, impaired vision, difficulty in speech, frigidity.
Pernicious anaemia 323: Anaemic symptoms, palpitation, general pain everywhere, pins-and-needles sensation in hands, feet, and elsewhere, weight loss, jaundice, difficulty walking, frigidity (and impotence), nausea.

Painful sexual intercourse

Besides disease, there are a number of other causes that will produce painful intercourse, such as the inflamed remains of the hymen, a scar remaining from a childbirth injury, an ill-fitting diaphragm, and haemorrhoids and anal fissures, both of which can be extremely painful and make intercourse difficult.

Vaginal inflammations 222: Vaginal discharge, itching, occasional pain during intercourse.

Cervicitis 223: Heavy menstruation, ache in pelvis and lower back, vaginal discharge, pain on intercourse, bleeding afterwards.

Prolapsed uterus 224: Dragging sensation in the lower abdomen, backache while standing or upon exertion, frequent urination. If male penetration is too deep, it will reach the affected tilted uterus causing pain. (See *Early warning signals.*)

Frigidity 230: Neurotic patterns, contraction of the mouth of the vagina, inability to achieve orgasm, drying up of precoital fluid, and repugnance for sex.

Painful sexual intercourse and vaginal spasm 231: Spasm and closure of the outer third of the vagina may be due to psychoneurotic causes. (See *Failure to achieve orgasm.*) Absence of precoital fluid (vaginal lubrication) normally produced during intercourse can be a factor.

Sterility in women

Sterility is due either to some structural defect in the generative organs or to unknown causes in the absence of any generative defect. In very many occasions the basis for sterility is a psychological determinant.

Sterility in women 229: Obstruction of the egg's passage, blockage of the fallopian tubes, ovarian cysts or tumours, hormonal imbalance interfering with ovulation, ingestion of some known sterilizing drugs such as quinine, scopolamine (used in many non-prescription tranquillizers), barium, ergot, and many others. A high level of acidity in the vagina will kill the sperm; polyps on the cervical canal and fibroid tumours will block the entrance preventing the sperm from reaching the egg. A pattern of ectopic pregnancies in which fertilization of the egg takes place elsewhere than in the uterus can be a major factor in sterility. Lastly, the effects of x-ray radiation will destroy ovarian function.

THE VAGINA
Vaginal bleeding

Vaginal bleeding, Vaginal bleeding and discharge, Vaginal bleeding and urinary disorders

Vaginal bleeding

Contraception 233: The intrauterine device (IUD) can cause bleeding and cramps among a small percentage of its users; the contraceptive pill on some occasions will cause bleeding, nausea, vomiting, sore breasts and dizziness.

Miscarriage 242: Passage of clots (bits of tissue), cramps in lower abdomen, bleeding can be heavy.

Tubal pregnancy 245: Heavy bleeding, missed period, severe one-sided abdominal pain.

Placenta praevia and abruptio placentae 248: Abdominal pain is absent in placenta praevia but bleeding occurs in both disorders.

Vaginal bleeding and discharge

Cervicitis 223: Bleeding and some discomfort after intercourse, vaginal discharge, ache in pelvis and low back, heavy periods.

Cancer of the cervix 421: Bloody discharge from vagina, bleeding after intercourse or after exertion, irregular menstruation. Later, yellow discharge, pain in lower back, urinary aberrations, nausea, vomiting, weight loss.

Cancer of the uterus 422: Vaginal bleeding, between menstrual periods or after menopause, malodorous watery discharge (significant of this disease), urinary irregularities, constipation, pain in the lower back and abdomen radiating to the thighs.

163

Vaginal bleeding and urinary disorders

Benign tumours of the uterus can cause bleeding. Dysfunctional bleeding (hormonal) can occur at any time.

Fibroid tumours 226: Pain and bleeding in the vagina, difficult urination.
Vitamin K deficiency 354: General bleeding of the nose, gums, vagina, blood in the stools and in the urine.
Cancer of the cervix 421: Bloody discharge from the vagina, bleeding after intercourse or after exertion, irregular menstruation. Later, yellow discharge, pain in the lower back, urinary aberrations, nausea, vomiting, and weight loss.
Cancer of the uterus 422: Vaginal bleeding between menstrual periods or after menopause, malodorous watery discharge (significant of this disease), urinary irregularities, constipation, pain in lower back, abdomen radiating to the thighs.
Cancer of the ovary 423: Abdominal swelling and pain, appearance of a pelvic mass, change in bowel or urinary habits, often vaginal bleeding, enlarged, painful breasts. In children, precocious puberty.

*

Blisters in the vagina

Herpes simplex virus 2 212a: Painful blisters appear inside vagina and often on exterior of genitalia. They can also show up on buttocks and thighs of both sexes. Occasionally enlarged lymph nodes in groin and fever. This disease will recur from time to time.

Vaginal discharge

Normally the vaginal secretion should do no more than moisten the vagina; if it does more, that is to the extent of staining the underclothing, then it is due to some disorder (with the exception of wetness from unsatisfied sexual needs).

Gonorrhoea 212: Whitish or yellowish discharge, frequent, burning, urgent urination.
Trichomoniasis 214: Greenish or yellowish discharge, itching vulva, offensive vaginal odour.
Vaginal inflammations 222: White discharge, itching vagina.
Cervicitis 223: Bleeding or discomfort after intercourse, varying discharge, ache in pelvis and lower back, heavy periods.
Prolapsed uterus 224: Cervix protrudes from vagina, pain on walking, discharge.
Gonorrhoea 212: Whitish-yellow discharge, burning urination, urethritis, may be pain in lower abdomen.
Cancer of the cervix 421: Bloody discharge, irregular menstrual bleeding, bleeding after intercourse or exertion. Later, discharge turns yellow, pain in lower back, urinary aberrations, constipation, nausea, vomiting, weight loss.
Cancer of the uterus 422: Bleeding between periods and after menopause, malodorous watery discharge (significant sign of this disease), urinary irregularities, constipation, pain in lower back, abdomen radiating to the thighs.

Itching in vulva

One of the symptoms of diabetes is itching in the vulva.

Trichomoniasis 214: Itching vulva, green or yellowish discharge from urethra or vagina, offensive vaginal odour, burning urgency of urination.
Vaginal inflammations 222: Fungus infection may develop if the subject has been taking a broad spectrum of antibiotics, thus killing off the bacteria and leaving the field to the fungus. White discharge and considerable itching.

Vaginal odours

A number of disorders causing vaginal odours are discussed under *Vaginal inflammation* **222**.

Trichomoniasis 214: Green or yellow discharge, itching, offensive vaginal odour, burning, urgent urination.
Cancer of the uterus 422: Bleeding between periods and after menopause, malodorous, watery discharge (signifi-

cant sign of this disease), urinary irregularities, constipation, pain in lower abdomen radiating to the thighs.

Pain in vagina

Prolapsed uterus 224: Pain on walking, cervix protrudes from vagina, vaginal discharge. (See *Early warning signals.*)

Cystocoele and rectocoele 225: Cystocoele: urinary incontinence, difficulty in completely emptying bladder. Rectocoele: Problems in defecation, pain in vagina.

Fibroid tumours 226: If tumour is large

will cause pain and bleeding, difficulty in urination.

Protrusion from vagina

Prolapsed uterus 224: Cervix protrudes from vagina, pain on walking. (See *Early warning signals.*)

Cystocoele and rectocoele 225: Cystocoele will also cause urinary incontinence and difficulty in emptying bladder. Rectocoele will also cause problems in defecation and pain in the vagina. Another form called urethrocoele will cause pouch-like protrusion of the urethral wall.

Symptoms special to men

Discomfort on sitting

Prostatitis 249: Difficult, painful urination, difficulty in emptying bladder, show of blood at beginning or end of the act, pain on sitting, chills, fever.

Enlarged prostate 250: Difficult, burning urination, difficulty emptying bladder, requiring strain and ending up dribbling. Occasionally blood in urine.

Cancer of the prostate 424: Progressively increasing difficulty in urination, diminished stream, increasing frequency, inability to empty bladder. Later, painful urination, pain on sitting, low backache; blood in urine is the most distinctive sign.

Feminization

The development of some female qualities may arise from hormone-producing tumours of the adrenal glands (such as *Cushing's disease* **343**), of the pituitary gland, and of the testes. Heavy dosage of x-rays on the groin can destroy testicular hormones. Castration is a well-known cause of this condition (if occurring early in life).

Cirrhosis of the liver 191: Jaundice, abdominal distension with enlarged veins, emaciation, enlarged breasts, atrophy of the testes, impotence.

Cancer of the testis 425: Development of a scrotal mass which can be hard or soft, increasing in size. Occasionally a dull ache and/or pain in the small of the back, urinary difficulties. In a child, precocious puberty; in an adult, feminization.

Lump in the pubic area

Inguinal hernia 255: Pain in the groin on effort often radiating to the scrotum. A lump is felt behind the pubic hairs either small or as large as an egg. The lump might disappear upon lying down. In strangulated hernia (constricted), sudden pronounced bulging, severe pain, collapse, fainting, vomiting.

Pain in prostate region

Prostatitis 249: Severe pain between scrotum and anus radiating to the testes, swelling of the prostate gland, difficult, painful, frequent urination, flu-like chills and fever, pain on sitting. Blood appears in the urine occasionally at the beginning and end of the act.

Enlarged prostate 250: Pain between scrotum and anus and in low back. Frequent show of blood in urine and semen, bouts of impotence and premature ejaculation, difficult, painful urination requiring straining with dribbling at the end, inability to fully empty the bladder.

Gonorrhoeal arthritis 262: General arthritic aches, festering of a single joint which becomes painful, red, and hot (knee, wrist or ankle). Urethritis is always present with painful urination. Also rash and high fever. Prostatitis.

Cancer of the prostate 424: Progressive difficulty in urination, increasing frequency and diminished stream, inability to empty bladder, impotence. Later, painful urination, pain in prostate region and low back. Blood in urine is the major sign.

THE PENIS
Blisters on the penis

Herpes simplex virus 2 212a: Painful blisters appear on the penis. May also show up on buttocks and thighs of both sexes. Occasionally enlarged lymph nodes in groin and fever. The disease will reappear from time to time.

Chordee

Chordee is a downward, painful curvature of the penis on erection. It usually occurs during the early stage of *Acute urethritis* **213** and is accompanied by profuse urethral discharge.

Constriction of the penis

Chancroid 215: Blisters and red pimples over the genitalia forming dirty-looking, painful ulcers which can either heal quickly or begin sloughing and proliferate outwards and inwards. These ulcers bleed easily. Penis is constricted from tightening of the foreskin.

Phimosis and circumcision 258: The foreskin envelops the penis so tightly that it causes constriction and very painful erection.

Discharge from penis

Gonorrhoea 212: Whitish-yellow discharge, burning urination.

Nonspecific urethritis 213: From watery to heavy pussy discharge, itching in urethra. Pain in head of penis, in urethra, in the testes, and in the groin.

Trichomoniasis 214: Discharge from penis, urgent, burning urination.

Pain in the penis
*also see **pain on urination** p152*

Venereal diseases which produce varying lesions on that organ often (but not always) will cause some pain. (See *Venereal Diseases, Part II.*) An injury on the penis, a violent act of intercourse, or some form of leukaemia can cause a haematoma (a swelling or tumour filled with blood) which is painful.

All prostate disorders will cause referred pain in the penis. Any cancer that attacks the penis will cause considerable pain.

Stones in the bladder 203: Painful, purulent, frequent urination, blood in the urine. Especially painful after a jolting ride.

Cystitis 205: Painful, urgent, frequent urination, scanty, purulent urine.

Gonorrhoea 212: Whitish-yellowish discharge.

Nonspecific urethritis 213: Pain in urethra and glans penis, also in the testes. From watery to heavy discharge and itching in the urethra.

Phimosis and circumcision 258: The foreskin envelops the penis so tightly that it causes constriction and painful erection.

SEXUAL PROBLEMS OF THE MALE
Impotence

Impotence means the inability of a man to perform the sexual act. Specifically it is his incapacity to become erect and remain so at the indicated moment. An impotent man may have sperm that are viable and healthy and is therefore not sterile, just as a sterile man may not be impotent.

Potency varies in healthy men from time to time. All men at some time or another experience temporary impotence for various reasons – fatigue, anxiety, fear, overexcitement, heavy drinking. An abnormally small penis (not only a physical but a psychological condition), overexposure to x-ray, and any major chronic disease will diminish a man's potency. (See *Impotence* **257**.) Although impotence is primarily a psychogenic disorder, there are a number of diseases that are also responsible.

Multiple sclerosis 6: Tremor of hands, spastic gait, disturbance of bladder control, impaired vision, difficulty in speech, impotence.

Cirrhosis of the liver 191: Jaundice, abdominal distension with enlarged veins, red spots on the skin, emaciation, enlarged breasts, atrophy of the testicles, loss of pubic hair, impotence.

Prostatitis 249: Severe pain in region between anus and scrotum, painful sitting, flu-like chills and fever, great urinary frequency. Blood may appear in urine at beginning or end of the act. Impotence is usual.

Enlarged prostate 250: Pain in the region between the anus and the scrotum, also in low back. Pain on sitting, bouts of impotency and premature ejaculation. Difficult, burning urination requiring straining and ending up dribbling without being able to fully empty bladder. Occasional blood in urine and semen.

Pernicious anaemia 323: Anaemic symptoms, palpitations, general body pain, pins-and-needles sensation in hands, feet, and elsewhere, red, sore tongue, weight loss, jaundice, difficulty walking, impotence (frigidity), nausea.

Diabetes 332: Excessive thirst, hunger, urination, weight loss, weakness, sweet, fruity breath, blurred vision, pins-and-needles sensation, leg cramps, skin disorders, impotence.

Leukaemia 415: Deep chronic fatigue, strong malaise, pallor, general bleeding from nose, gums, under skin (pinpoint spots turning from red to purple), weight loss, night sweats, rapid pulse, joint pains, impotence.

Cancer of the prostate 424: Progressive difficulty in urination, increasing frequency and diminished stream, inability to empty bladder, impotence. Later, painful urination, pain in prostate region and lower back. Blood in the urine is the major sign.

Precocious puberty, male

Cancer of the testis 425: Hard or soft mass palpable in the scrotum, ache or pain in the testes, backache, precocious puberty in boys and feminization of adult men.

Premature ejaculation

This is another form of impotence with mostly the same reasons and causes. In premature ejaculation the man achieves erection but is unable to maintain it long enough to effect proper sexual intercourse. For this condition there are even fewer physical causes than for impotence, there being no lack of ability to become erect but only the inability to maintain this state – distinctly a psychogenic problem.

Sterility in men

Sterility does not mean that the man is impotent; he may easily be a sexually effective man. (See *Sterility in men* **256**.)

Undescended testicle 251: Absence of one of the testicles from the scrotum. Pain in the undescended testicle. If condition is not corrected early sterility may result if the other testicle is malfunctioning.

Orchitis (mumps orchitis) 253: Swelling of both the testes and the scrotum, great pain, chills and fever, hiccups, vomiting, swelling of the salivary glands. If both testes are affected there may be sterility.

THE TESTICLES AND SCROTUM
Atrophy of the testicles

Cirrhosis of the liver 191: Jaundiced, enlarged liver, distension of the abdomen with enlarged veins, small red spots on skin with red lines, emaciation, swelling of the ankles, feet, enlarged breasts, loss of pubic hair, atrophy of one or both testicles, impotence.

Mass or lump in the scrotum

Scrotal cysts 252: Varying mass or lumps in the scrotum.
Cancer of the testis 425: A scrotal mass which can be hard or soft but which always increases in size, often presenting a dull ache. There may be pain in the small of the back. In a child, precocious puberty; in an adult, feminization.

Pain in the testicles or scrotum

Nonspecific urethritis 213: Pain in the glans penis, urethra, testicles, perineum. Itching in the urethra and discharge.
Undescended testicle 251: Absence of testicle in scrotum, pain, possible sterility.
Orchitis (mumps orchitis) 253: Swelling and pain in the testicle and scrotum,

chills, fever, hiccups, vomiting, often swelling of salivary glands.
Epididymitis 254: Sickening pain in testicle, swelling of the scrotum, chills and fever.
Inguinal hernia 255: Lump behind pubic hair, pain in groin often radiating to the testicles. Lump (may be as large as an egg) often disappears when lying down. Exertion can worsen the condtion.
Cancer of the testis 425: Scrotal mass which can be hard or soft but always increasing in size often presenting a dull ache. There may be pain in the small of the back. In a child, precocious puberty; in a man, some feminization.

Swelling of the testicles and scrotum

A hydrocoele or variocoele can cause enlargement of the scrotum (see *Scrotal cysts* **252**).

Orchitis (mumps orchitis) 253: Swelling of the testes and scrotum, pain in the testes, chills, fever, hiccups, vomiting.
Epididymitis 254: Sickening pain in the testicles, swelling of the scrotum, chills and fever.

Undescended testicle

Undescended testicle 251: Absence of testicle in scrotum, pain in the undescended testicle; if not corrected, sterility.

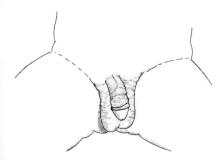

Normal male genitalia.

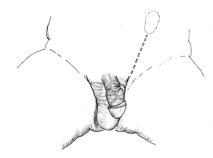

Undescended testicle. (*Julian A. Miller*)

Symptoms of the hair and skin

THE HAIR
Baldness (alopecia)

There are many types of baldness ranging from small patches to total body denudation. Male pattern baldness is inherited; it may start in youth but more often in middle-age. Other permanent forms of baldness are due to senility and drugs such as thallium, gold salts, ergot, lead, and morphine, and to exposure to x-rays. (See *Baldness* **299**.)

Temporary baldness may result from ringworm. Hair curlers cause patchy spots, reversible in early stages; however, further abuse will cause permanent loss of hair. Dyes, bleaching, hair straightening, continual traction from certain types of hair styles (ponytail) can cause temporary baldness; occasionally the condition can become permanent.

Fevers ranging upwards from 39·4°C, 103°F will cause temporary loss of hair which will usually grow back after the illness is over.

Leprosy 368: Onset is insidious. Red and brown patches with white centres on the skin. Small hard nodules on face, feet, and legs. Loss of feeling in various parts of the body. Hoarse voice, hair loss (notably the eyebrows and lashes), wasting of the bones, open sores, deformity, loss of fingers and toes, muscle atrophy.

Dandruff

Rosacea 294: Redness along the longitudinal centre of the face, bulbous red nose, pimples, dandruff, occasionally ulceration of cornea of the eye.

Dandruff 316: The only symptom (mild and chronic) is the flaking, small, white, snowlike particles from the scalp.

Excess hair (hirsutism)

Although this is usually a benign symptom it can on occasion indicate a serious glandular disorder. In women any suppression of the ovarian function can frequently engender hair growth. Thus, at menopause some women will grow hair on the face, and some women when pregnant will grow excess hair (temporarily).

Cushing's disease 343: Weight gain in face, back, and trunk, excess hair growth, acne, easy bruising, muscle weakness, easily broken bones; in women, loss of menstrual periods.

Falling hair

Certain forms of chronic poisoning may be associated with falling hair such as boric acid, ergot, lead, morphine, and x-ray.

Allergic drug reactions 289: Heparin,

an anti-blood-clotting drug, will cause falling hair.

Hypothyroidism 339: Children: mental and physical retardation, short stocky body, coarse face, broad flat nose, potbelly, puffy hands and face, scanty hair, subnormal temperature. Adults: slower thinking, apathy, puffy eyelids, weak muscles, slow pulse, obesity, dull, falling hair, discoloured fingernails, subnormal temperatures.

Vitamin A toxicity 348b: Loss of appetite, pain in joints, irritability, severe pressure headaches, retarded growth in children, falling hair.

Lifeless hair

The hair can often be a reflection of the condition of the rest of the body. When the hair becomes dull and lifeless, it is frequently indicative of some more basic disorder. One should look for other symptoms when the hair has become suddenly lustreless and dead.

Anaemia 322: Anaemia symptoms, palpitations, sore, red tongue, vertigo, loss of libido, lifeless hair, fingernails longitudinally ridged and spoon-shaped. In severe cases, jaundice, numbness of limbs, excessive thirst, poor memory, shock.

THE SKIN
Abnormal skin colour

Vitiligo 298: Patches of skin have no colour at all.

Aplastic anaemia 326: Severe anaemic symptoms, brown skin pigmentation, bleeding from nose and mouth, black-and-blue marks.

Polycythaemia 327: Bluish-red itching skin, constant dull headache, dizziness, fatigue, shortness of breath, and blood in the stools.

Adrenal insufficiency (Addison's disease) 344: Easily fatigued, weakness, bronzing of the skin, weight loss, nausea, vomiting, abdominal pain, craving for salt, nervous disorders, freckles, piebald skin, loss of hair, dizziness, fainting.

Leprosy 368: Red or brown patches on skin with whitish centres, loss of feeling in these patches and elsewhere, growing hard nodules on face and body. Also muscle atrophy, open sores, hoarseness, loss of fingers and toes.

Black-and-blue marks

Aplastic anaemia 326: Severe anaemic symptoms, brown pigmentation of skin, bleeding from nose and mouth, black-and-blue marks.

Purpura 328: Small red spots turning purple, later becoming black-and-blue marks; on slight injury, bleeding from mouth and mucous membrane; pain in abdomen and joints, slow clotting of blood.

Adrenal insufficiency (Addison's disease) 344: Easily fatigued, weakness, bronzing of skin, weight loss, nausea, vomiting, abdominal distress, nervous disorders, craving for salt, dehydration, freckles, loss of hair, piebald skin, dizziness, fainting.

Blackened skin

Black skin usually means gangrene – the skin is dead and can never be revived.

Gas gangrene 362: Upon pressure at the wound site, gas bubbles will escape with a crackling sound. Skin around the wound is first dark, then turning black. In severe cases, prostration and coma.

Blackheads and whiteheads

Acne 293: The skin break-out is on the face with pimples, blackheads, whiteheads, large cystic masses, plus scars and pittings. The face is usually oily and flabby.

Blisters, large (bullae)

Large blisters ranging from 1cm, ½in in diameter to a plum in size are called bullae. Besides the listings below, they are characteristic of burns, scalds, and jellyfish stings.

Pemphigus 297: Large water blisters all over the body, anaemia, itching.

Impetigo 302: Red patches turning to water blisters around mouth, nostrils, on scalp and arms, a condition similar to that caused by ringworm. The blisters enlarge, burst, exuding a straw-coloured fluid, and form yellowish, itching crusts.

Chilblains 313: The part of the body affected becomes red, swollen and itching. May blister and go on to frostbite.

Sunburn 314: Skin angry red, painful and itching, peeling. In severe cases, blisters, chills, fever, headaches.

Blisters, small (vesicles)

Vesicles are small blisters ranging from pinhead to tackhead size. They can be caused by vaccination, gnats, mosquito and other insect bites, as well as by disease and some of the disorders listed below.

Congenital syphilis 211: Symptoms appear about a month after birth: sniffles, blisters on face, buttocks, palms and soles, saber shins (curved shinbones), meningitis, saddle-backed nose; possibly loss of vision and deformed, peg-like teeth.

Herpes simplex virus 2 212a: Painful blisters on penis and vagina. Also may appear on external genitalia, thighs, and buttocks; swollen lymph nodes (groin), fever.

Contact dermatitis 286: Usually small blisters (may become large) which rupture, ooze, and crust; redness, swelling, and itching over contact site.

Allergic drug reactions 289: Blister can appear from iodides.

Shingles 303: Usually begins with mild, flu-like symptoms, then a rash around the waist or chest or neck which turns into a line of small painful blisters going around the body on one side. Can also go around an eye. Blisters dry and crust.

Herpes simplex 304: Tingling, itching around corners of the mouth; then blisters break out which dry and form yellowish crusts.

Ringworm 307: Intensely itching, red, ringed eruption of blisters on body or scalp growing larger and scaly around the edges. Healing in centre while infection spreads at periphery.

Athlete's foot 308: Itching and redness of skin on the toes. In severe cases, skin becomes decomposed. Also scaly cracking areas with white patches that can blister.

Scabies 309: Pimples, blisters, tiny, with radiating, jagged, grey lines, intense itching. Itch mite can be seen best with a magnifying glass.

Chicken pox 372: Itching eruptions changing from body rash to pimples to teardrop blisters and finally to scabs. In adults, chills, headache, backache.

Smallpox 373: Begins with high fever, violent frontal headaches, intense muscle pain; convulsions in children. Then large crop of small, reddish spots changing to pimples, to purulent blisters, and finally to foul-smelling scabs.

Body odour

This symptom is due to the activity of bacteria in the sweat after excretion. It has been particularly noted in uraemia and pneumonia. Usual sites are under the arms, the feet, and groin (See *Body odour* **319.**)

Boils and carbuncles

Boils and carbuncles 301: A boil is a hard, red, hot, tender and painful lump; a carbuncle is larger or made up of multiple boils and breaks, exuding pus. Possible toxicity.

Diabetes 332: Excessive thirst, hunger and urination. Weight loss, weakness, blurring of vision, numbness, tingling, leg cramps, impotence, boils, and vaginal fungus.

Clammy cold skin

Shock 133: Great pallor, cyanosis (lips, nails, earlobes, fingertips), fast, weak pulse, shortness of breath, sunken eyes, dilated pupils, anxiety, coma.

Acute gastritis (erosive) 155: Severe pain in the stomach, very rapid pulse, collapse, cyanosis, difficulty swallowing, excessive thirst, possibly vomiting of blood.

Heat exhaustion 313b: Clammy, moist skin, profuse sweating, headache, dizziness, nausea, faintness. Temperature normal or slightly elevated. Possible muscle cramps.

Cholera 364: Onset is sudden and extreme, constant diarrhoea, great dehydration, voluminous rice-water stools, violent vomiting, intense thirst, cyanosis, cramps in the stomach and legs, total collapse.

Corns and calluses

Corns and calluses 317: Hard corns are located on toes, pea-sized with hard core; soft corns are found between the toes, kept soft by moisture; may be inflammation and infection underneath corn. Callus is an area of thickened skin, usually painless. Corns will ache on pressure.

Cracked skin

Athlete's foot 308: Skin around toes is cracked, reddened, with occasional white patches and blisters. Considerable itching.

Crusting of the skin

Contact dermatitis 286: Blisters which rupture, ooze, and crust; redness and swelling at contact site.

General neurodermatitis 291: Scaly red patches on elbows, knees, neck, and face, hardening of skin, bloody crusts, intense itching.

Impetigo 302: Red patches turning to watery blisters around mouth, nostrils, on scalp and arms, a condition similar to that caused by ringworm. Blisters enlarge and burst, exuding straw-coloured liquid. Yellowish crust forms, itching.

Shingles 303: Begins with mild flu-like symptoms, then a rash around the body (one side only) followed by a line of small blisters. Can also go around the chest, neck or an eye. Blisters dry, leaving crusts.

Herpes simplex 304: Tingling, itching area around corners of the mouth (most usual site) which then breaks out in blisters. They dry leaving yellowish crusts.

Chicken pox 372: From itchy red eruptions on the skin over body, to pimples, to blisters, and finally to crusting. In adults also headache, chills and backache.

Smallpox 373: Begins with high fever, violent frontal headache, severe muscle pain; convulsions in children. Then large crop of small, reddish spots all over body changing to pimples, to purulent blisters and finally to foul-smelling crusts.

Darkened skin

Gas gangrene 362: Upon pressure, gas bubbles emerge from the wound with a crackling sound. Skin around wound going from dark to black. Later, prostration and coma.

Dry skin

Acute kidney failure 208: Total arrest of urination or very scanty output. Visible particles in the urine, vomiting, diarrhoea, drowsiness, breathing difficulties, convulsions, twitching, urinous breath odour and dry mucous membrane.

Sunstroke 313a: Very hot, dry, flushed skin, headache, dizziness, *no* sweating, high fever, very fast pulse, rapid breathing.

Hypothyroidism 339: Children: mental and physical retardation, short stocky body, coarse face, broad flat nose, potbelly, skin rough and dry, subnormal temperature. Adults: slower thinking process, apathy, skin dry, cool, and rough, puffy eyelids, weak muscles, slow pulse, obesity, subnormal temperature.

Flabby skin

Acne 293: On face. Pimples, blackheads, whiteheads, large cystic masses, scars, pittings, oily flabby skin.
Salt deficiency 356: Stomach cramps, considerable drop in urinary output, muscles twitching, faint, rapid pulse, finally convulsions.

Freckles, red, brown, or black

Freckles are caused by exposure to the ultraviolet rays from the sun or from artificial sources. Blond and red-haired people are most susceptible. Once they occur they are usually permanent. Liver spots (they have nothing to do with the liver) are brown, can become numerous and merge into irregular shapes. They are characteristic of ageing people with fair skins, but can also appear in over-exposure to sunlight, in pregnancy, and as reactions to some skin oils and medications.

Adrenal insufficiency (Addison's disease) 344: Weakness, bronzing of skin, weight loss, vomiting, loss of hair, craving for salt, dizziness, dehydration, freckles.

Gas bubbles emanating from a wound

Gas gangrene 362: Upon pressure bubbles will emerge from oozing wound with accompanying crackling sound. Dark skin around wound will turn black. Collapse, coma.

Hardening of the skin

General neurodermatitis 291: Scaly red patches on elbows, knees, neck, and face, bloody crusts, intense itching, hardening of skin around lesions.
Scleroderma 321: First swelling of skin which becomes mottled, red and shiny, condition starting at hands and feet then proceeding to the rest of the body. Skin becomes hard, leathery, rigid, face becomes mask-like, hands claw-like.
Vitamin A deficiency 348a: Retarded growth in children, night blindness, cloudy or ulcerated cornea, kidney inflammation, horny skin.

Hot moist skin

Hyperthyroidism 340: Goitre, fast heartbeat, hot, moist skin, nervousness, overactivity, increased appetite but loss of weight, bulging or staring eyes, overheated body. (High basal metabolism.)

Itching

Itching in a specific area is listed under that category such as anal, rectal, vaginal. *Itching without rash, Itching with rash, Itching rash with blisters* (see Blisters, large and Blisters, small), *Intense itching rash, Itching red spots over entire body*

Itching without rash (pruritis)

Pruritis actually means itching without visible lesions on the skin. Local or general itching when it is due to disease is usually more intense and persistent. Itching usually accompanies jaundice and may be a symptom of diabetes, anaemia, leukaemia, many forms of carcinoma, gout, and of all fungal skin infections as well as a reaction to certain foods and drugs. It can be a symptom of psychoneurosis and is frequently noted in pregnancy.

Acute infectious hepatitis 187 and **Serum hepatitis 188:** Jaundice is the main symptom. Dark urine, clay-coloured stools, loss of appetite, general itching with or without rash, weakness, muscle ache, tender, palpable liver, gastrointestinal upset, headache.
Toxic hepatitis 189: Jaundice, general itching, nausea, vomiting, collapse.
Hodgkin's disease and other lymphomas 416: Painless enlarged lymph

174

nodes in the neck (often the size of an orange). If only on one side, it is Hodgkin's; if on both sides, other lymphoma. Later, all lymph nodes are affected. Other symptoms are itchy skin, anaemia, weakness, weight loss, persistent, recurrent fever, swollen leg, difficulty breathing.

Itching with rash
see also **Rash**

Acute infectious hepatitis 187 and **Serum hepatitis 188:** Jaundice is the main symptom. Fever, headache, loss of appetite, dark urine, clay-coloured stools, fatigue, palpable liver causing tenderness in abdomen and general itching with or without rash.

Contact dermatitis 286: Usually small blisters (may become large) which will rupture, ooze, and crust. Redness and swelling at the contact site.

Serum sickness 288: Itching wheals, fever may range from mild to high, swelling of lymph nodes near injection site, inflamed joints.

Pityriasis rosea 306: First a single, large, round, red patch which is raised and scaly (similar to condition due to ringworm). A multitude of itching smaller patches all of which appear five to ten days later. Never above the neck or below the knees.

Athlete's foot 308: Cracked skin around toes, red and white spots, itching. In severe cases, blisters.

Chilblains 313: The cold extremity is red, swollen and itching. May go on to blisters and frostbite.

Lupus erythematosus 320: Patchy, butterfly-shaped red rash on cheek and bridge of nose, also occurring elsewhere. As old patches heal, new ones form which scale and itch. In the systemic lupus erythematosus form there are joint pains, pleurisy, collapsed lung, heart failure, nephritis, fever, anaemia, and emaciation.

Polycythaemia 327: Bluish-red skin, dizziness, fatigue, constant dull headache, itching, breathlessness, bleeding

into gastrointestinal tract evidenced by bloody or tarry stools.

Intense itching rash

Hives 285: Large and small wheals with intense itching.

Physical allergy 290: Large and small wheals limited to the area of exposure. In extreme cases rapid pulse and loss of consciousness.

General neurodermatitis 291: Red scaly patches on elbows, knees, neck, and face, bloody crusts, intense itching, hardening of the skin.

Anaphylactic shock 292: Giant hives all over the body, obstructed breathing with asthmatic attack, swelling over the entire body and rapid pulse.

Lichen planus 296: Pimple-like, violet lesions from pinhead to tackhead size with a flat and angular space. The lesions gleam and tend to coalesce. Severe itching.

Ringworm 307: Red, ringed eruptions of blisters on body or scalp which grow larger with scaling around outer edges and healing in the centre. Infection spreads on the periphery. Intense itching.

Scabies 309: Pimples, blisters, extending into tiny, jagged, grey lines, up to 1cm, ⅜in in length. Intense itching of blister and lines.

Lice infestation 310: Severe itching, tiny red bite marks, occasionally swollen lymph nodes, small wheals. Lice, nits are visible. Nits attached to hair and clothing.

Crab louse 311: Severe itching, small pale blue spots in pubic region, nits attached to skin at base of hair root. Lice can be seen.

Itching red spots over entire body

Chicken pox 372: From widespread itching red spots to raised pimples to tear-drop blisters and finally to scabs. In adults, also chills, headache, backache.

Smallpox 373: Begins with high fever, violent frontal headache, intense muscle pain, convulsions in children; crops of itching small reddish spots which become first pimply then purulent blisters, and finally foul-smelling crusts.

Jaundice

Jaundice is a yellow or greenish-yellow tinting of the skin. This coloration can also appear in the white and conjunctivae of the eyes and in the urine. Jaundice manifests itself in the colour of stools as greyish-white or clay-coloured. Jaundice is always a serious or significant symptom, except in *Gilbert's disease* **190**.
Mild jaundice, Mild jaundice and vomiting, Severe jaundice, Severe jaundice and vomiting

Mild jaundice

Gilbert's disease 190: Only symptom is mild jaundice.
Allergic drug reactions 289: Chlorpromazine can induce jaundice and liver damage.
Anaemia 322: Anaemic symptoms, vertigo, palpitations, red, sore tongue. In severe cases, mild jaundice, numbness of limbs, excessive thirst, poor memory, shock.
Pernicious anaemia 323: Anaemic symptoms, palpitations, general body pain, sore, red tongue, pins-and-needles sensation in hands, feet, and elsewhere, weight loss, difficulty walking, nausea, impotence and frigidity.
Haemolytic anaemia 324: Anaemic symptoms, faintness, dizziness, weak, rapid pulse, chills, fever, aches in extremities and abdomen.
Sickle cell anaemia 325: Severe anaemic symptoms, arthritic pain, poor physical development (long arms and legs, short trunk), severe general body pain. In infants, painful, swollen hands and feet.
Infectious mononucleosis 377: Painful swelling of lymph nodes in neck, armpit, and groin, weakness, fatigue, low fever, and occasional mild jaundice.
Mental retardation 403: Infants: abnormally sized head at birth, low birth weight, jaundice, slow general development.

Mild jaundice and vomiting

Acute pancreatitis 166: Writhing pain high in the abdomen often extending to the back. Jaundice, severe vomiting, cyanosis, feeble, rapid pulse, shock.
Chronic relapsing pancreatitis 167: Pain from mild to raging, nausea, vomiting, fast pulse, fatty, frothy stools, often jaundice.
Gallstones 194: Biliary colic, agonizing pain in waves from upper abdomen to back and radiating to shoulder or pelvis. Mild jaundice, vomiting, rapid heartbeat, flatulence, belching.
Cholecystitis 195: Agonizing pain in waves from upper abdomen radiating to back and shoulders or pelvis. Mild jaundice, vomiting, rapid heartbeat, indigestion.
Morning sickness (pregnancy) 243: Nausea and vomiting from mild to pernicious. In extreme cases, loss of weight, mild jaundice, and rapid heartbeat.
Toxaemia of pregnancy (preeclampsia) 246: Puffiness of body, weight gain, severe headaches, visual disturbances, dizziness, vomiting, jaundice, amnesia.
Relapsing fever 369: Chills, high fever, rapid heartbeat, severe headache, vomiting, muscle and joint pains, profuse sweating, and rose-coloured rash on the trunk and the extremities. Jaundice may appear.

Severe jaundice

Acute infectious hepatitis 187 and **Serum hepatitis 188:** Yellowing of skin and eyes, dark urine, light-coloured stools, red, itching wheals, great weakness, enlarged, tender liver, severe headache, gastrointestinal upsets.
Cirrhosis of the liver 191: Severe jaundice, enlarged palpable liver, abdominal distension, red dots with red lines emanating out on skin, swelling of feet and legs, enlarged abdominal veins, foetid breath, internal haemorrhoids, emaci-

ation. In men, feminizing characteristics, enlarged breasts, atrophy of the testicles, impotence.

Cholangitis 196: Jaundice, high fever, severe chills, clay-coloured stools.

Cancer of the pancreas 431: Boring pain in upper abdomen extending to the back, indigestion, jaundice, brown urine, clay-coloured stools, weight loss.

Severe jaundice and vomiting

Toxic hepatitis 189: Yellowing of the skin and whites of the eyes, rash, nausea, vomiting, diarrhoea, collapse.

Acute yellow atrophy 193: Severe jaundice, black vomiting, painful, palpable liver, severe headache, foetid breath, emotional instability, coma.

Yellow fever 379: High fever, prostration, severe headache, pain in back and limbs, flushed face, scanty urine. Jaundice appears on the second attack with vomiting of black blood and bleeding from the mucous membrane.

Cancer of the gallbladder 432: Pain in upper right abdomen near centre, may be vomiting, progressive weakness. Loss of appetite, jaundice.

Cancer of the liver 433: Nausea, vomiting, pressure in the abdomen, constipation, dull ache in area of liver, jaundice, anaemia, weight loss.

*

Lines on the skin

Scabies 309: Tiny lines on the skin can be as long as 1cm, ⅜in caused by the itch mite. Also pimples, blisters, itching.

Lymphangitis 330: Red lines or streaks going upwards on arms or legs. Swelling of lymph nodes, chills, high fever (38·9°–40·5°C, 102–105°F), general aching, headache.

Scarlet fever 359: HIgh fever, sore throat, vomiting, white furry tongue turning raspberry. There may be a yellowish-grey false membrane in the mouth and throat. Also body rash, darkened lines on the skin folds and flushed face except for pallor around the mouth.

Lumps in the skin

Gout 334: Extreme pain in big toe joint, inflammation and pain in the joints, rapid pulse, nodules of urate crystals (tophi) on the ear and in various joints.

Leprosy 368: Red and brown patches on skin with white centres, loss of feeling in these patches and elsewhere, growing hard nodules on face and body, muscle atrophy, open sores, hoarseness, loss of fingers and toes.

Skin cancer 409: Pearly raised nodules that slowly erode and ulcerate; growing inwards and outwards.

Breast cancer 420: (See *Symptoms special to women*)

Moles

Moles and birthmarks 315: Moles range from pale and colourless to dark brown or black (the majority). They can be hairy, flat or raised, and may be found anywhere on the body.

Malignant melanoma 410: Any dark mole which changes in any way (eg, begins to grow or bleed). The disease is rare.

Peeling

Sunburn 314: Very red skin, painful, itching, and finally peeling. In severe cases blisters, chills, fever, headache.

Scarlet fever 359: Vomiting, sore throat, high fever, white, furry tongue later turning raspberry, greyish false membrane on throat and mouth. Body rash which blanches at squeezed spots. Later skin peels, flakes, face flushed except for paleness around mouth.

Pimples

Allergic drug reactions 289: (Chlorine, iodine, fluorine.) Can produce acne-like skin eruptions.

Acne 293: Crops of pimples, blackheads, whiteheads on face, large cystic masses, scars and pittings, flabby, oily skin.

Rosacea 294: Flush or redness along

longitudinal centre of the face, bulbous red nose, pimples, dandruff.

Lichen planus 296: Papule-like violet lesions which are flat and angular, from pinhead to tackhead size. They glisten. The lesions coalesce to form larger ones. Severe itching.

Scabies 309: Tiny, grey, ragged lines, pimples, blisters, severe itching. The mite can be seen more easily with a magnifying glass.

Cushing's disease 343: Weight gain on face (moon face), trunk, and back. Excess hair growth, acne, easy bruising, muscle weakness, bones easily fracture. In women, loss of menstrual periods.

Rash

The number of skin and systemic diseases that can cause a rash is formidable. Rash is too vague a word for identification; it generally means any eruption on the skin. Medically it refers to some form of redness but its general meaning has no specification of precise colour. An attempt has been made here to narrow down this symptom by characterizing the type. (Itching rash appears under *Itch*)
Rash turning to blisters, Rash, measles-like spots, Rash, red spots turning purple or black (pinpoint bleeding), Rash of varying character over the body, Rash of varying character in a localized area

Rash turning to blisters

Impetigo 302: Red rash turning to watery blisters around mouth, nostrils, scalp, and arms simulating the condition due to ringworm. Blisters enlarge, break, exude straw-coloured fluid and form yellowish itching crusts.

Shingles 303: Begins with mild flu-like symptoms; then a rash forms on one side around the waist, sometimes around the chest, neck, or an eye; then followed by a line of small painful blisters. Blisters dry, crust, and heal with scars.

Chicken pox 372: Spotty rash becoming raised, itching pimples which then turn

to blisters and finally crust. All stages can exist at the same time. In adults it is more severe, with headache, backache, chills, and high fever.

Smallpox 373: High fever, violent frontal headache, intense backache, muscle pain, and rapid pulse. Convulsions in children. Crops of small reddish-pink spots appear, turning to pimples and then to blisters (which will not collapse when pricked). The fluid in the blisters becomes pustular; they finally dry into foul-smelling scabs and crusts. Unlike chicken pox, only one stage is present at a time.

Rash, measles-like spots

Measles 370: Begins with cold symptoms, high fever, cough, photophobia, then rosy areas with white centres inside cheek, brownish-pink spots all over the body.

German measles 371: Begins with slight sore throat, then light rosy-coloured rash all over body, swollen lymph nodes behind ear and at back of neck, stiffness of joints. In adults, lassitude and headache.

Dengue fever 380: Chills, high fever, pain in back of eyeballs, pain in muscles and joints severe enough to cause prostration, measles-like rash over body.

Roseola 399: Children: high fever up to 40·5°C, 105°F. When fever drops, rash appears on chest, abdomen, less on face and extremities. Frequently the rash can assume spots that are larger and more irregular than the more typical measles-like eruptions.

Chicken pox 372 and **Smallpox 373:** (See *Itching rash over entire body*)

Rash, red spots turning purple or black (pinpoint bleeding)

This usually indicates bleeding under the skin.

Meningitis 7: Breaking out in red to

purple spots all over body, irregular fever, intense headache, stiff neck, vomiting, delirium.

Endocarditis 135: Small red-purplish spots over the body, unexplained fever, chills, pain in the chest and joints, fatigue, clubbing of fingers, loss of appetite, enlarged, painful spleen and bleeding from nose and into the urine.

Sprue 180: Diarrhoea, fatty, frothy, clay-coloured stools, red, sore tongue, distended stomach, emaciation. Children: retarded growth, bone and muscle deformity, spontaneous fractures.

Purpura 328: Crops of small red spots turning purple, later becoming black-and-blue marks, bleeding from mouth and mucous membranes on slight injury. Pain in abdomen and joints, slow clotting of blood.

Vitamin C deficiency 362: Weakness, bleeding gums, red spots turning purple on skin, bleeding under skin, loose teeth, easily broken bones. In infants, loss of appetite and weight, irritability, legs are very painful.

Blood poisoning 360: Shaking chills, severe headache, irregular fever, profuse sweating, skin rash with minute and extensive haemorrhage points turning black and blue, severe diarrhoea, collapse.

The plague 365: Chills, very high fever, rapid heartbeat, buboes (egg-sized lymph nodes in the groin) which suppurate and burst, small red spots on skin which turn black.

Typhus 392: Ten day high fever, intense headache, prostration, mottled rash over body with small red spots inside turning blue, contracted pupils, highly coloured, scanty urine, twitching muscles, furry white tongue, profuse sweating when fever breaks. If not cured, stupor, delirium, coma.

Rash of varying character over the body

Rheumatic heart disease and rheumatic fever 127: Rash is not the most significant symptom. In this disease it is a reddened area which spreads and coalesces. Major symptoms are inflamed joints, rapid heartbeat, easily fatigued, failure to gain weight, malaise, sweating, St Vitus's dance in children in the age range of 10–13.

Early syphilis (secondary) 209: (From one to six months after the disease has been contracted.) Widespread varying body rash, dusky red splotches, ulcers in the mouth, enlarged lymph nodes, severe headache, arthritic pain, sore throat, possible eye disorders.

Congenital syphilis 211: Infants: red spots or blisters all over the infant's body, sniffles, curved shinbones, later saddle-backed nose and deformed teeth.

Allergic drug reactions 289: Barbiturates and sulfa drugs cause varying skin eruptions and rashes.

Psoriasis 295: Small, red, slightly raised patches covered with dry silvery scales, tiny bleeding points under the scales. Patches coalesce to form larger ones.

Scleroderma 321: Skin swells, becomes mottled, red, and shiny, then hardens, turning leathery and rigid. This begins at hands and feet and spreads to rest of the body. Face becomes mask-like, hands can become claw-like.

Vitamin B complex (niacin) deficiency (pellagra) 351: Loss of appetite and weight, weakness, red spots turning brown and scaly, margins of tongue and mucous membranes turning scarlet, excess salivation. Later, diarrhoea becoming bloody, poor memory, and emotional instability.

Scarlet fever 359: Vomiting, high fever, sore throat, white, furry tongue later turning raspberry, grey false membrane in mouth and throat. General body rash, blanching when squeezed. Later, skin peels and flakes. Face flushed except for paleness around mouth.

Bilharziasis 383: Smarting redness at the site of the worm entry, abdominal pains, swelling of the face, legs, and genitalia, anaemia, chronic fatigue, general malaise.

Toxoplasmosis 385: Chills, high fever, inflammation of the heart muscle, body rash, swollen lymph nodes, severe headache, and hepatitis.

Rash of varying character in a localized area

Rosacea 294: Redness along longitudinal centre of the face, bulbous red nose, pimples, dandruff.

Erysipelas 300: Raised rash on face and head ranging in colour from dull red to scarlet with advancing margins, chills, high fever, intense headache, swollen face, swollen lymph nodes.

Bedsores 318: Red, shiny unfeeling skin; later, large, ugly ulcers and sores in the area of involvement – the pressure points of the buttocks, heels, elbows, shoulder blades.

Typhoid fever 363: Flu-like symptoms, severe sustained frontal headaches, continuous very high fever, stupor, distended stomach, diarrhoea, double pulse beat, nosebleed, rosy spots mostly on abdomen which disappear in a few days.

Relapsing fever 369: Chills, high fever, rapid heartbeat, severe headache, vomiting, muscle and joint pains, profuse sweating, rose-coloured rash on the trunk and the extremities. Jaundice may appear.

Scaling skin

Regional enteritis 168: Diarrhoea, nausea, vomiting, fever, sausage-shaped mass in lower right quadrant, variable pain, fistula or abscess around anus, dry scaly skin.

Psoriasis 295: Slightly raised red patches covered with dry silvery scales. Tiny bleeding points underneath. Patches coalesce to form larger ones.

Pityriasis rosea 306: Begins with single large, red, scaly patch similar to that caused by ringworm; five to ten days later, a multitude of smaller ones (which itch) appear all over body except above neck or below knee.

Ringworm 307: Red, ringed eruption of blisters on scalp or body which grow larger, with scales on outer edges. While centre heals, infection spreads at outer periphery. Intense itching.

Athlete's foot 308: Skin around toes be-

comes red, cracked, and scaly with occasional white spots and blisters. Considerable itching.

Lupus erythematosus 320: Red, itching, butterfly-like patches which scale on face, bridge of nose, and elsewhere. As old patches heal, new ones form. In the SLE form (systemic lupus erythematosus), there are joint pains, possible complications of lung, heart, and kidneys. Patient is usually emaciated, anaemic, and feverish.

Vitamin B$_2$ (riboflavin) deficiency 350: Weakness, dry, scaly, red skin around the nose, ears, scrotum. Cloudy, ulcerated cornea, impairment of vision, photophobia, burning sensation in the conjunctiva, chapped lips, and cracks in the corners of the mouth.

Scars and pittings

Acne 293: Pimples, blackheads, whiteheads appear on face. Later, cystic masses, scars and pittings. Face is oily and flabby.

Sores and ulcers

(For ulcers that appear on the genitalia – syphilis, chancroid, granuloma inguinale – see *Sores, tumours, ulcers on genitalia*, p156.)

Late syphilis 210: Soft ulcers (gummas) over the skin, tongue, testes, and liver which are very slow to heal.

Acne 293: Lesions on face and neck, crops of pimples, blackheads, whiteheads, large cystic masses which can ulcerate, scars, pittings, oily, flabby face.

Bedsores 318: Red shiny skin on buttocks, heels, elbows, and shoulder blades, later becoming large ugly sores and ulcers.

Lymphadenitis 331: Enlarged, swollen, painful lymph nodes. Skin over the lymph nodes becomes tender and may abscess.

Leprosy 368: Red and brown patches on skin with whitish centres, loss of feeling in these patches as well as elsewhere, growing hard nodules over face and body, hoarseness, open sores and ulcers, loss of fingers and toes.

Histoplasmosis 393: Black stools, diarrhoea, vomiting, ulcers on nose, ear, lips, and even the pharynx. Emaciation, enlarged lymph nodes. In severe cases, bloody cough, loss of weight, extreme fatigue, drenching sweats.

Skin cancer 409: Any raised area that is white or red and hard which suddenly begins growing into a hard crusted ulcer. Lower lip is a common site.

Spider markings (spider angiomas)

This symptom is a red spot with red lines radiating from it. Common in pregnancy.

Cirrhosis of the liver 191: Jaundice, enlarged liver, distension of the abdomen, swelling of feet and legs, enlarged vein on abdomen. Vascular spiders are seen over face, neck, arms, and upper trunk. Also haemorrhoids, foul breath. In men there may be feminizing characteristics (enlarged breasts), atrophy of the testicles, and loss of pubic hair.

Tiny blue spots

Crab louse 311: Tiny pale blue spots in the pubic area which itch intensely. The crab louse can be seen. Its nits are attached to the hair roots.

Tiny red spots

Lice infestation 310: Tiny red bites, small wheals, severe itching, occasionally swollen lymph nodes. Lice, nits can be seen. Nits are attached to hair and clothing.

Visible parasites

The itch mite that causes scabies will leave tiny grey lines on the skin. Lice cause tiny red bite marks which itch severely anywhere on the body. The crab louse is found only in the pubic hairs causing tiny, pale blue, itching spots.

Warts

Warts 305: Greyish, firm growths, painless, insensitive, ranging in size from pinhead to tackhead.

Wheals

A wheal is a transient, itching elevation of the skin which is round and reddish with a white centre.

Hives 285: Large or small wheals with intense itching.

Serum sickness 288: Wheals may be large or small with considerable itching.

Physical allergy 290: Wheals, sometimes rapid pulse. Loss of consciousness frequent when persons allergic to cold suddenly submerge in cold water.

Anaphylactic shock 292: Giant wheals and swelling over entire body, obstructed breathing, rapid pulse, shock.

Lice infestation 310: Tiny red bite marks, severe itching, occasionally enlarged lymph nodes, small wheals, lice and nits can be seen. Nits are attached to hair and clothing.

White patches on the skin

Vitiligo 298: Loss of pigmentation in patches of skin that is not affected by sunlight.

Athlete's foot 308: Skin around toes is red and cracked with white patches. Blisters may form. Considerable itching.

Frostbite 312: The part of the body that is frozen becomes dead white, numb, and slightly swollen. Pain on rewarming.

Adrenal insufficiency (Addison's disease) 344: Easily fatigued, weakness, bronzing of the skin, irregular milk-white patches, weight loss, vomiting, abdominal pain, craving for salt, nervous disorders, fainting, dizziness, dehydration, freckles.

Yellow deposits on the skin

Xanthelasma (xanthoma) 38: Flat or slightly raised painless nodules on eyelid or around eye may be the result of high blood cholesterol. Additional yellow deposits may appear on elbows, knees, heels, and palms.

Vitamin D toxicity 353b: Loss of appetite and weight, nausea, weakness, excessive urination, kidney failure, whitish-yellow calcium deposits in the skin.

Symptoms of the bones, joints, muscles, and extremities

ANKLE
Pain and weakness

Sprained ankle 280: Weak, collapsing, painful, swollen ankle.

Swelling

Heart failure 126: Swelling of ankles and legs, jugular vein prominent, laboured breathing, judgement and memory poor.
Acute nephritis 197: Swelling of ankle, puffiness of face, scanty and bloody urine, sharp loss of appetite, nausea, vomiting, furred tongue. (Hypertension.)
Chronic nephritis 198: Swelling ankles, puffiness of face, distended abdomen, scanty, bloody urine, breathlessness on slight exertion, excessive late night urination, anaemia.
Nephrosis 199: Swelling ankles, puffiness of face, distended abdomen, anaemia.
Sprained ankle 280: Weak, collapsing, painful swollen ankle.

BACK
Lump in the back

Cancer of the kidney 427: Blood in urine, pain in ribs and spine, palpable mass in kidney region, anaemia.

Pain in the back
Pain in the back, Pain in the lower back, Pain in the lower back, men, Pain in the lower back, women

Pain in the back

Backache is one of the most common complaints. It can be due to overuse of muscles resulting from an unaccustomed exertion or exercise, a product of sheer fatigue, or quite often can be an expression of psychogenic problems such as depression, anxiety, or most likely frustration. Diseases that will occasionally have backache as a symptom are peptic ulcer, pancreatitis, pneumothorax. Postmenopausal women frequently suffer from back pains.

Acute bronchitis 103: Pain in muscles and back, racking, painful cough, yellowish, purulent, heavy phlegm.
Minor disorders of pregnancy 235: Slight shortness of breath, dyspepsia, headache, backache, varicose veins, haemorrhoids.
Osteoporosis of the spine 266: Chronic aching spine, round shoulders, height loss, fragility of bones, spontaneous fractures.
Obesity 347: (twenty per cent above normal weight). In severe cases, shortness of breath, aching back and legs, arthritis.

Chicken pox 372: Itching rash on body first becoming pimply, then blistering, and finally crusting. In adults, also chills, headache, backache.

Smallpox 373: High fever, violent frontal headache, intense backache, muscle pain, rapid pulse, and convulsions in children. Crops of small reddish-pink spots appear, turning first to pimples and then to blisters (which will not collapse when pricked). The fluid in the blisters becomes pustular and they finally dry into foul-smelling scabs and crusts. Unlike chicken pox, only one stage at a time.

Flu 376: Chills, high fever, severe head pains, back and muscle aches. Great weakness and prostration. Excessive fatigue and sweating, dry or hacking cough, cold symptoms, flushed face. Intestinal flu has additionally diarrhoea and vomiting.

Yellow fever 379: Fever, flushed face, prostration, severe headache, pain in back and limbs, scanty urine. After intermission: jaundice, vomiting with black blood, bleeding from mucous membranes.

Hodgkin's disease and other lymphomas 416: Painless, enlarged lymph nodes growing to any size, anaemia, backache, swollen legs, difficulty breathing and swallowing. Later, severe itching, weakness, weight loss, and persistent, recurrent fever.

Cancer of the kidney 427: The classic triad of symptoms are backache, abdominal mass, and blood in the urine. Also weight loss and anaemia.

Cancer of the pancreas 431: Pain in upper abdomen extending to the back, indigestion, jaundice, brown urine, clay-coloured stools, weight loss.

Pain in the lower back

Aneurysm 142: Extension of severe chest pain to lower back, high pulse, shortness of breath.

Low back pain 268: Unable to straighten up after bending down. Chronic pain in small of back.

Slipped disc 269: Pain in small of back, pain radiating to buttocks and back of thigh and below the knee to the ankle.

Pain in the lower back, men

Enlarged prostate 250: Difficult, burning urination, not able to fully empty bladder requiring strain and ending up dribbling. Occasional show of blood in urine. Bouts of impotence.

Cancer of prostate 424: Progressively difficult urination, diminished stream and increasing frequency. Inability to empty bladder. Impotence. Later, painful urination, low backache and blood in urine (most important sign).

Cancer of the testis 425: Scrotal mass which can be soft or firm but increasing in size. Sometimes a dull ache in scrotum, often pain in small of the back. Difficulty in urination. In a child, precocious puberty; in an adult, feminization.

Pain in the lower back, women

Painful menstruation 220: Mild to severe cramps in lower abdomen, lower back, and thighs; bleeding from scanty to copious, malaise, sweating.

Cervicitis 223: Ache in pelvis and low back, heavy menstruation, vaginal discharge, bleeding after intercourse.

Prolapsed uterus 224: Backache while standing or on exertion, frequent urination, dragging sensation in lower abdomen, protrusion from vagina.

Cancer of the cervix 421: Bloody discharge from vagina, irregularities of menstrual cycle, bleeding after intercourse or on exertion. Later, discharge becomes yellow, low back pain, urinary aberrations, vomiting, constipation, weight loss.

Cancer of the uterus 422: Bleeding between menstrual periods or after menopause. Malodorous watery discharge from vagina (a significant symptom), urinary aberrations, constipation, pain in lower back or abdomen radiating to hip and thighs.

Cancer of the ovary 423: Abdominal

swelling and pain, large pelvic mass, low backache, change in bowel and urinary habits, occasionally vaginal bleeding, enlarged painful breasts; in children, precocious puberty.

BODY SIZE
Decrease in body size (height loss)

Osteoporosis of the spine 266: Chronic aching spine, round shoulders, fragility of bones, height loss.

Paget's disease 267: Intermittent shifting bone pain, spontaneous fractures, grotesque enlargement of the head, height loss, impaired hearing.

Hypopituitarism 337: Premature ageing, low libido, fatigue, apathy, weight loss, loss of pubic hair, slow pulse. In children, stunted growth. Body properly proportioned but small.

Enlarged skeleton

Acromegaly and gigantism 336: Abnormal tallness, increased size of hands, feet, and internal organs, protruding jaw, loss of libido, mental deterioration, headaches, joint pains.

BONES
Deformity of the bones or muscle

Sprue 180: Diarrhoea three to four times daily, flatus, fatty, light-coloured frothy stools, red, sore tongue, distended stomach, emaciated body, small amount of bleeding under the skin (small purple or black spots). Children: retarded growth, bone and muscle deformities, spontaneous fractures.

Congenital syphilis 211: Infants: curved shinbones, rash or blisters on face, buttocks, palms, or soles, nose sniffles. Later, saddle-backed nose, deformed teeth.

Vitamin D deficiency 353a: Infants: restlessness, softening and thinning of head-bones, bow legs. Infant cannot walk, stand, or sit at proper age. Older infants: badly formed teeth, scoliosis, and lordosis. Adults: progressive weakness, rheumatic pains in pelvis, limbs, and spine.

Leprosy 368: Red or brown patches with white centres on skin, loss of feeling in these patches and elsewhere as well, hard nodules over face and body which increase in size, atrophy of muscles, open sores, hoarseness, loss of fingers and toes.

Pain in the bone

Osteomyelitis 265: Deep pain in the bones and adjacent joints, overlying muscles are swollen, rigid, and painful. High fever, sweating.

Paget's disease 267: Intermittent shifting bone pain, spontaneous fractures, grotesque enlargement of head, impaired hearing.

Malignant tumours of the nervous system 413: Rapid weight loss, distended stomach, loss of strength. Metastasis is usually to the bones causing bone pain. Discoloration around the eyes, loss of strength, anaemia, lymph node swelling.

Bone cancer 418: Pain in the affected bone, enlargement of diseased limb. Vulnerable areas are thighs, upper arms, hips, and legs.

Multiple myeloma 419: Deep-seated, boring pain in the bone, often extreme, worsens with exercise. Spontaneous fractures, severe anaemia. Bones most often affected are thighs, pelvis, and upper arms.

Spontaneous fractures (fragility of bone)

Sprue 180: Diarrhoea three to four times daily, flatus, fatty, light-coloured, frothy stools, red, sore tongue, distended stomach, emaciation, bleeding under the skin (black or purple spots on the skin).

Children: retarded growth, bone and muscle deformities, spontaneous fractures.

Osteoporosis of the spine 266: Back pain, chronic ache in spine, round shoulders, loss of height.

Paget's disease 267: Intermittent shifting bone pain, fragility of bones, grotesque enlargement of head, impaired hearing.

Cushing's disease 343: Weight gain on face, back, and trunk, excess hair growth, easy bruising, loss of menstrual periods, muscle weakness, easy bone fracture.

Multiple myeloma 419: Deep-seated, boring pain in bone which can be intense, pain worsens with exercise, spontaneous fractures, severe anaemia. Bones most often affected are thighs, pelvis, upper arms.

ELBOW
Pain in the elbow

Bursitis (tennis elbow) 263: An acute inflammation of the bursa at the outer side of the elbow, causing pain and swelling. The pain can radiate to the forearm.

EXTREMITIES OF THE BODY
Burning, itching redness of an extremity

Frostbite 312: Advance warning of oncoming frostbite is a tingling, numbing sensation in a toe, finger, earlobe or the nose. The skin becomes red to violet-red, burning, itching, and swelling may develop. Later, the frostbitten extremity becomes all white.

Chilblains 313: The affected extremity develops an itching, burning sensation. Later it becomes red and swollen. Blisters may form and break. In really cold weather, may become frostbitten.

186

Coldness in extremities

Oedema of the lungs 116: Cold extremities, difficulties with breathing which may become rapid, wheezing, laboured, and asthmatic. Cyanosis, coughing with bloodstained phlegm, oppression in chest. Patient is anxious, pale, and sweating.

Hyperventilation 121: Numbness or coldness in extremities, fast heartbeat, fast, deep breathing, feeling of oppression in chest area, fainting.

Peripheral vascular disease (Buerger's disease) 137: Affected foot is cold and very sensitive to cold, cramps and numbness in legs, intermittent limping.

Cardiac neurosis 144: Vague non-radiating pain in chest, coldness in extremities, shortness of breath, slight giddiness, fatigue, great anxiety.

Intestinal obstruction 170: In persistent cases besides mid-abdominal pain there is constipation, vomiting which turns brown, and rectal bleeding. Later, increased vomiting, high fever, thirst, total suppression of the urine, anxious, sunken features, fast pulse, dehydration, collapse, and shock.

Chilblains 313: The affected part becomes red with itching and swelling. Later, blisters form. If not treated may go on to frostbite.

Freezing of an extremity

Frostbite 312: Part of the body affected becomes dead-white, numb, slightly swollen. No pain except on warming.

Chilblains 313: Not quite frozen but cold enough for the affected part to become red, itch, and swell. Later, blisters will form. If not treated can go on to frostbite.

Numbness

Neuritis 3: Pain, numbness begins in fingers or toes spreading to arms and legs. Area is red and swollen.

Multiple sclerosis 6: Numbness of limbs, weakness in one or several limbs often to the point of paralysis. Tremors of the hands, unsteady gait, poor judgement, short attention span, periods of apathy or euphoria, impaired vision, difficulties in speech, urinary incontinence.

Peripheral vascular disease 137: Leg cramps, numbness in the leg, intermittent limping. Foot is cold and affected by cold. When foot is lowered, toes and foot become red, when raised they turn white.

Frostbite 312: Part of the body affected goes dead-white, numb, becomes slightly swollen. Pain on warming.

Anaemia 322: Anaemia symptoms, palpitation, vertigo, sore, red tongue, fingernails longitudinally ridged and spoon-shaped, loss of libido, lifeless hair. In severe cases, jaundice, numbness of the limbs and loss of their control, poor memory, thirst.

Pernicious anaemia 323: Anaemic symptoms (pallor, weakness, shortness of breath), palpitations, nosebleeds, numbness, sore, red tongue, appetite and weight loss, yellow-lemon skin colour. In severe cases, cardiac failure, difficulty walking, and impotence or frigidity.

Diabetes 332: Excessive hunger, thirst, urination, numbness, pins-and-needles sensation.

Primary aldosteronism 345: Fatigue, muscle weakness, numbness, tingling in varying areas of the body, excessive urination, thirst.

Vitamin B₁ (thiamine) deficiency 349: Loss of appetite and weight, prickling or numbness in the extremities, emotional instability, alarming palpitations, difficulty breathing, swelling and fluid in the tissues.

Leprosy 368: Red and brown patches with whitish centres on the skin. Loss of feeling in these patches and elsewhere as well, hard nodules over face and body which increase in size, atrophy of muscles, open sores, hoarseness, loss of fingers and toes.

Pins-and-needles sensation (tingling)

Pernicious anaemia 323: Anaemic symptoms plus general body pain, sore, red tongue, weight loss, jaundice, pins-and-needles sensation in hands, feet, and elsewhere, nausea, difficulty walking, impotence or frigidity.

Diabetes 332: Excessive hunger, thirst, and urination, numbness, pins-and-needles sensation in the extremities, weight loss, leg cramps, skin and vaginal infections, weakness, fruity breath, blurred vision, red, sore, dry tongue, impotence.

Primary aldosteronism 345: Fatigue, muscle weakness, numbness, tingling, excessive urination, thirst.

Vitamin B₁ (thiamine) deficiency 349: Loss of appetite and weight, prickling or numbness in the extremities, emotional instability, alarming palpitations, difficulty breathing, swelling and fluid in tissues.

THE FEET
Enlarged feet

Acromegaly and gigantism 336: Overgrowth of hands, feet, face, and lower jaw, low, husky voice, severe headache, excessive sweating, pain in the joints, loss of libido, and impairment of mental ability

Flatfeet

Flatfeet 281: Early fatigue in walking, pain in arch of foot often radiating to the calf or lower back.

Painful arch

Flatfeet 281: Early fatigue in walking, pain in the arch often radiating to the calf or lower back.

Painful sole of the foot

Plantar wart 283: Walking is painful. Wart is yellowish, translucent thickening of skin on sole of the foot is surrounded and covered by callus; it is sensitive to pressure and weight.

Hookworm 387: Anaemia, black stools, pallor, great hunger, malnutrition, ex-

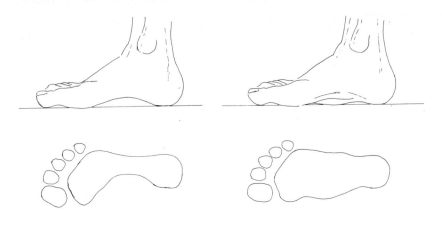

Normal foot and footprint and flatfoot and footprint. (*Julian A. Miller*)

treme fatigue, weakness, shortness of breath.

Swollen feet

Cirrhosis of the liver 191: Swelling of feet and legs, jaundice, abdominal distension, red spots with radiating lines on skin, emaciation, enlarged vein on abdomen, foul breath, haemorrhoids. In men, enlarged breasts, atrophy of the testicles, loss of pubic hair, impotence.

Sickle cell anaemia 325: Severe anaemic symptoms, general body pain, jaundice, arthritis, poor physical development (long arms, legs, short trunk). In infants, painful swelling of hands and feet.

Hypothyroidism 339: Children: mental and physical retardation, short, stocky body, coarse face, broad, flat nose, pot-belly, low body temperature. Adults: slower thinking process, apathy, puffy eyelids, weak muscles, obesity, low body temperature, slow pulse.

Ulcers and infections of the foot

There are numerous and varied causes for ulceration and/or infection of the foot: diabetes, gummas (soft ulcers) occurring in tabes dorsalis (late syphilis), leprosy, and spread of fungus infection of the foot (athlete's foot). Foot ulceration may occur among paraplegics and among those who have been treated with an excessive amount of x-ray radiation for a plantar wart condition.

Peripheral vascular disease 137: Cramps and numbness in the affected feet; one of them may develop an ulcer; intermittent limping.

Ingrown toenail 284: Edges of nail overlaid with tissue which can become granulated, infected, and pustular.

FINGERS

Clubbed fingers

Although this condition does rarely occur for no reason, perhaps as part of a familial pattern, it is mostly a symptom of disease. A minor degree of clubbing is often seen in emphysema, chronic bronchitis, pleurisy, late in tuberculosis, and pulmonary abscess. It is always seen in congenital heart disease when cyanosis is also present.

Empyaema 119: Sharp pain in affected side of the chest, short, dry cough, chills,

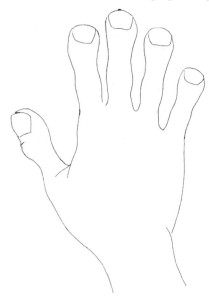

Clubbed fingers. (*Julian A. Miller*)

fever, clubbing of fingers, sweating, emaciation, great malaise.
Endocarditis 135: Pain in the joints, fever, chills, tiny red spots turning purple on the body, bleeding from nose and into the urine, anaemia, clubbing of fingers, deep fatigue.

Disorders of the fingernails

The condition of the fingernails reflects many ailments of the body, most particularly skin disorders. Horizontal furrows usually follow acute diseases, forming at the time of occurrence and growing out gradually, often lingering long after the disease has passed (five to six months later). Nails respond sensitively to trauma – a hammer blow on the nail can often cause it to discolour and fall off; biting the fingernails can cause a short, ragged nail, warts around the edges, and infection.

● Black-and-blue or red spots under nail: Injury.

● Brittleness and fragility: May be due to ringworm, but cause is often unknown. May be due to too much wetting and drying. More common in women. The use of nail polish and nail polish remover could be a factor.
● Cross-ridged: Excessive manicuring; cuticles being pushed back too often.
● Cyanotic nails and beds: *Chronic bronchitis* **104**; also cyanosis of the lips, paroxysmal cough and breathlessness.
● Discoloured: Injury; *Hypothyroidism* **339**; *Psoriasis* **295**.
● Disintegration of nail, split and cracked: *Psoriasis* **295**; *Ringworm* **307**.
● Greyness: *Ringworm* **307**.
● Linear haemorrhage (small) under nail: *Endocarditis (subacute)* **135**; *Trichinosis* **386**; injury, and on occasion no reason at all.
● Loss of lustre: *Ringworm* **307**.
● Loss of nail: Injury, overexposure to x-ray, *Syphilis (severe secondary)* **209**.
● Pitting: *Psoriasis* **295** (an early sign); all kinds of skin disorders.
● Pockets on fingernail sides, oozing pus: May develop in anyone who keeps hands in water for long periods of time, such as fishermen, housewives, cleaning women, others. This bacterial infection often needs medical attention.
● Red half moons: Some cases of *Heart failure* **126**.
● Separation from nail bed: *Psoriasis* **295**.
● Spoon-shaped (curvature opposite of normal) and longitudinally ridged: *Anaemia* **322**.
● White: Varying degrees of abnormal whiteness appear in *Cirrhosis of the liver* **191**, *Heart failure (chronic)* **126**, *Pulmonary tuberculosis* **112**, *Diabetes* **332**, and *Rheumatoid arthritis* **259**.

Loss of deformity of fingers

Rheumatoid arthritis 259: Early stage: pain or burning sensation in the joints, swelling and stiffness in mornings. Later stages: deformity of finger joints, lumpy nodules around inflamed joints.
Degenerative joint disease 261: Aching, burning, and swelling of the

joints, morning stiffness, bony lumps around the joints in the hand, pain after vigorous exercise, joint aches in inclement weather.

Leprosy 368: Red and brown patches with whitish centres, loss of feeling in these patches and elsewhere as well, hard nodules on face and body which increase in size, atrophy of muscles, open sores, deformity and loss of fingers and toes, hoarseness.

THE HANDS
Enlarged hands

Acromegaly and gigantism 336: Overgrowth of hands, feet, face, and jaws. Low husky voice, severe headache, excessive sweating, pain in the joints, loss of libido and impairment of mental ability.

Palsy

Morphine and cocaine will cause palsy of the hands especially on withdrawal.

Parkinson's disease 1: Hand palsy, slow, shuffling steps, posture rigid and stooped, unblinking eyes (staring), expressionless face, drooling.

Mutliple sclerosis 6: Intention tremor of hands and head as well, also general muscle tremor, unsteady gait, vision and voice disturbances, urinary incontinence, impotence and frigidity.

Puffiness of the hands

Sickle cell anaemia 325: Severe anaemic symptoms, general pain, jaundice, long arms and legs but short trunk, arthritis. In infants, painful swelling of hands and feet.

Hypothyroidism 339: Children: mental and physical retardation, short, stocky body, coarse face, broad, flat nose, potbelly, skin rough and dry, subnormal temperature, goitre. Adults: slower thinking process, apathy, skin dry, rough,

and cool, puffy eyelids and hands, weak muscles, slow pulse, obesity, subnormal temperature.

HIP
Dislocation of the hip

Congenital dislocation of the hip 275: Infants: buttocks and thighs are asymmetrical; if walking, child moves in an odd waddling gait. Adults: pain and sciatica, femur bone in an odd position.

Pain in the hip

Congenital dislocation of the hip 275: Adults: pain and sciatica, femur bone in an odd position.

Legg-Perthes' disease 276: Mild pain in the hip, usually in the groin, noticeable limp, limitation of motion. Often only sign is pain in the knee.

Vitamin D deficiency 353a: Adults, chiefly women: rheumatic pain in pelvis, limbs, and spine, progressive weakness (osteomalacia).

JOINTS
Bad weather ache in the joints

Degenerative joint disease 261: General ache, burning or swelling in the joints, morning stiffness, bony lumps around joints in the hands. Pain after vigorous exercise.

Gonorrhoeal arthritis 262: General ache, burning or swelling in the hands, then moving to a large joint, rash, fever, inflammation of the urethra. Pain in lower abdomen, vaginal discharge in women, prostatitis in men.

Deformity of the joints

Haemophilia 329: Uncontrolled bleeding at slight injury, deformity of joints due to bleeding into them.

Inflammation of the joints

Inflammation of the joints with fever, Inflammation of the joints with low-grade fever, Inflammation of the joints without fever

Inflammation of the joints with fever

Rheumatic heart disease and rheumatic fever 127: First the larger, then the smaller joints at ankles, knees, and wrists become red and swollen, ranging from tender to painful. Rapid heartbeat, St Vitus's dance, malaise, pallor, sweating, failure to gain weight in child, loss of appetite, skin rash.

Endocarditis 135: The three most dominant symptoms are pain in joints, uneven fever, crops of tiny red to purplish spots all over body. Blood in the urine on occasion as well as nosebleeds.

Juvenile rheumatoid arthritis 260: Pain, burning, stiffness in the joints, swelling and hotness around the joints, high fever, iritis.

Gonorrhoeal arthritis 262: Burning and pain around the joints, general ache in bad weather, rash, fever, inflammation of the urethra. In men, prostatitis; in women, pain in lower abdomen, usually more on one side, and vaginal discharge.

Tuberculosis of the joints and bones 264: Joint swelling but neither pain nor hotness, limitation of movements. If in leg, then weakness, stiffness, limp; if in back, changes of normal posture, rigid spine. If in hip, 'night cries'; that is, child cries out in sleep but does not wake up. Rise in temperature, night sweats.

Osteomyelitis 265: Deep pain in bone and affected joints, high fever (up to 40°C, 104°F), overlying muscles are rigid, painful, swollen, and festering.

Serum sickness 288: Itching wheals, occasionally mild to high fever, swelling of lymph nodes around injection, inflamed joints.

Lupus erythematosus 320: Red, butterfly-like patches on cheek, bridge of nose, and elsewhere. As old patches heal new ones form. Also scaling, itching, emaciation, anaemia, fever. In the SLE (systemic lupus erythematosus) form: joint pains; other complications are usual, such as collapsed lung, heart failure, pleurisy, nephritis.

Relapsing fever 369: Chills, high fever, rapid heartbeat, severe headache, vomiting, muscle and joint pains, profuse sweating, and a rose-coloured rash on the trunk and the extremities. Jaundice may appear.

Dengue fever 380: Sudden appearance of chills, high fever, severe headache. The distinctive symptom is pain in the back of the eyes. Pain in the muscles and joints of such severity as to cause prostration. There is intermission of the disease, then return with rash and lowered fever.

Leukaemia 415: General bleeding from gums, skin (tiny red spots turning purple), nose. Fatigue, great pallor, malaise, fever, anaemic symptoms. Children (acute form): sore throat, bruised body appearance, rapid pulse. Adults (chronic form): characteristic enlarged lymph nodes, night sweats, weight loss, joint pains.

Inflammation of the joints with low-grade fever

Phlebitis 141: White, sensitive, swollen leg, pain in the joints, surface leg veins prominent, rapid pulse, low-grade fever.

Regional enteritis 168: Migratory arthritis, anaemia, malnutrition, mild fever, abscesses around anus, weight loss, mid-abdominal cramps.

Early syphilis 209: Primary stage: hard ulcer on penis or genitalia of female. Secondary stage (weeks later): widespread varying rash on body, ulcers in the mouth, arthritis pains in joints, headaches, sore throat, eye disorders, fever is low grade or absent.

Rheumatoid arthritis 259: Pain or burning sensation in the joints, hotness or swelling around the joints, morning stiffness, sweating in palms and soles, varying fever, lumpy nodules around infected joints, swollen knees.

Sickle cell anaemia 325: Severe anaemic symptoms, may be fever, acute general body pain, jaundice, poor physical development (long arms and legs, short trunk). Infants: painful, swollen hands and feet.

Gout 334: Inflammation of the big toe joint, other joints as well. May be fever, chills. Rapid pulse, urate crystals (lumps) in ear or in joints.

Inflammation of the joints without fever

Degenerative joint disease 261: Pain not too severe, arthritic pain more pronounced on vigorous exercise; stiffness in morning without moderate exercise. Bony lumps around affected joints in the fingers, joints ache in bad weather.

Bursitis 263: Affected joint very painful on movement. Joint is hot, red, and swollen.

Purpura 328: Small red spots, which often run together, bleeding from the mouth and mucous membrane on slight injury, pain in the abdomen and joints, slow clotting of the blood, black-and-blue marks and traces of blood in the stools.

Acromegaly and gigantism 336: Overgrowth of hands, feet, face, and jaws, low, husky voice, severe headache, excessive sweating, pain in the joints, loss of libido, and impairment of mental ability.

Vitamin A toxicity 348b: Loss of appetite, falling hair, irritability, severe pressure headaches, retarded growth in children, joint pains.

Vitamin D deficiency 353a: Adults: rheumatic pain in pelvis, limbs, and spine, developing weakness. Children: possibility of lordosis and scoliosis.

*

Lumps or nodules around a joint

Rheumatoid arthritis 259: Attacks of pain around a joint beginning in the fingers, morning stiffness, fever, sweating on the palms and soles, brittle nails, swelling of tissues around an affected joint. Later, bone shrinkage, muscle atrophy, deformed fingers, knobby swollen knees, and lumpy nodules around joints.

Degenerative joint disease 261: Pain not too severe, arthritic pain more pronounced on vigorous exercise; however, stiffness in the morning without some moderate exercise. Bony lumps around affected finger joints, which ache in bad weather.

Gonorrhoeal arthritis 262: Burning and pain around the joints, followed by single festering joint, general ache in bad weather, rash, fever, inflammation of the urethra. In men, prostatitis; in women, pain in lower abdomen, usually more on one side, and vaginal discharge.

Gout 334: Inflammation of the big toe joint, other joints as well. Often fever and chills. Rapid pulse and urate crystals (lumps) in ear or joints.

KNEE
Collapsing knee (locked knee)

Legg-Perthes' disease 276: Limp, mild pain in the hip, pain in the leg. Often only pain in the knee.

Trick knee 279: Knee can collapse suddenly and lock. Usually a result of something floating in the joint or a cartilage injury such as a football knee.

Painful knee (swollen knee)

Rheumatoid arthritis 259: Attacks of pain around a joint, beginning in the fingers; morning stiffness; fever, sweating on the palms and soles, brittle nails, swelling of tissues around an affected joint. Later, bone shrinkage, muscle atrophy, deformed fingers, knobby, swollen knees, and lumpy nodules around joints.

Bursitis 263: Bursitis in the knee is called 'housemaid's knee'. The knee becomes swollen (in front only), hot, red, and painful especially on movement.

LEGS AND THIGHS

Blisters on the thigh

Herpes simplex virus 2 212a: Blisters appear on the penis and the interior of the vagina. Blisters may also show up on the buttocks and thighs.

Bow-legs

Vitamin D deficiency 353a: Infants: restlessness, softening and thinning of head bones, badly formed teeth, bow-legs, child cannot walk, stand, or sit at proper age. In older children, lordosis and scoliosis.

Limping

Peripheral vascular disease 137: Affected foot is cold and affected by cold; cramps, numbness in the leg, intermittent limping.

Tuberculosis of the joints and bones 264: Weakness of leg, stiffness, limp, swelling of joint (but no pain or heat), rise in temperature, night sweats.

Legg-Perthes' disease 276: Mild pain in the hip, occasionally the pain may only be manifest in the knee. Noticeable limp.

Pain (cramp) in the thigh and leg

also see **Cramps in the muscles**

Pain in the leg is often a complaint without known cause of highly nervous people; it is also a lesser symptom in measles, scarlet fever, and smallpox. *Pain (cramp) in the thigh and leg, Severe pain in the thigh and leg*

Pain (cramp) in the thigh and leg

Common cold 63: Vague aches in the back and legs, running, obstructed nose.
Legg-Perthes' disease 276: Leg pain, limp, mild pain in the hip. Often only pain in the knee.

Flatfeet 281: Early fatigue in walking for some, occasionally night cramps in the leg, pain in the arch of the foot radiating to the calf.

Diabetes 332: Excessive thirst, hunger, urination; weight loss, weakness, boils, vaginal fungus, blurring, numbness, tingling, leg cramps, and impotence.

Obesity 347: (Overweight by twenty per cent.) Aching back and legs. In severe cases, shortness of breath, arthritis.

Vitamin C deficiency 352: Weakness, bleeding gums, bleeding into the skin and mucous membrane, loose teeth. Infants: swelling, painful legs.

Vitamin D deficiency 353a: Adults: progressive weakness, rheumatism pain in pelvis, limbs, and spine. Children: lordosis and scoliosis.

Cholera 364: Onset is sudden and extreme, constant diarrhoea, great dehydration, voluminous rice-water stools, violent vomiting, intense thirst, cyanosis, cramps in the stomach and legs, and total collapse.

Yellow fever 379: High fever, flushed face, prostration, severe headache, pain in the back and limbs, scanty urine. After intermission, jaundice, vomiting with black blood, bleeding from mucous membrane.

Severe pain in the thigh and leg

Sciatica 5: Agonizing pain begins at buttocks and continues along the thighs to the ankles or outer aspect of the foot. Pain can abate and return. A sneeze, cough, or strain will worsen it.

Peripheral vascular disease 137: Leg cramps particularly when walking, limping, leg can collapse suddenly when walking, numbness of leg, foot is cold and sensitive to cold.

Phlebitis 141: Swelling with severe pain in the leg, white leg, surface vein prominent in leg with discoloration of the affected area.

Aneurysm (thigh) 142: Pulsation can be seen and felt in the thigh.

Late syphilis (tabes dorsalis) 210: Loss of position and balance, 'lightning pains' in episodes in ankles, knees, legs, and writsts, 'crises' (severe pains or spasms) in any part of the body.

*

Prominent vein in the leg

Phlebitis 141: Surface vein of the leg becomes prominent (as differentiated from varicose veins which are knotted and twisted). The vein may be discoloured. The leg becomes swollen, very painful, and white.
Varicose veins 143: Knotted torturous, discoloured veins, often ulcerated.
Minor disorders of pregnancy 235: Mild varicose veins, haemorrhoids, dyspepsia, backache, excessive salivation, headaches.

Swollen leg (oedema of the leg)
also see **Swelling, the ankle**

Heart failure 126: Oedema of ankles and legs, prominent jugular vein, shortness of breath, memory and judgement poor.
Phlebitis 141: Swelling of leg and thigh, leg feels weighted, is white and very painful, surface vein prominent and discoloured.
Aneurysm (thigh) 142: Throbbing artery in thigh can be seen and felt, swelling.
Cirrhosis of the liver 191: Oedema of feet and legs, jaundice, enlarged palpable liver, distension of the abdomen, foul breath, haemorrhoids. In men, enlarged breasts, atrophy of the testicles, impotence, loss of pubic hair.
Hodgkin's disease and other lymphomas 416: Painless, enlarged lymph nodes growing to any size, anaemia, backache, swollen legs, difficulty breathing and swallowing. Later, severe itching, weakness, weight loss, and persistent, recurrent fever.

Weakness in the leg

Peripheral vascular disease 137: Leg cramps, particularly when walking. Leg can collapse suddenly when standing or walking, numbness of leg, intermittent limping; leg is cold and affected by cold.
Phlebitis 141: Swelling with severe pain in leg, white leg, surface vein prominent with discoloration of the affected area.
Tuberculosis of the joints and bones 264: Swelling of the affected joints sometimes without heat or pain, limitation of movement, stiffening and weakening of leg, limp, rise in temperature, and night sweats. If pain in hip, child cries out in sleep without awakening.
Muscular dystrophy 405: Infants: difficulty standing or walking, waddling gait, frequent falls, mask-like face; loss of muscle control, first of the face, then the pelvis and legs.

White leg

Phlebitis 141: Swelling with severe pain in leg, white leg, surface vein is prominent with discoloration of the affected area.

MUSCLE
Muscular atrophy

The withering, wasting, or reduction of muscle occurs in many chronic diseases (tuberculosis, hookworm infestation, malaria, diabetes, amoebic dysentery, sprue, and others). Muscular atrophy may also be due to disuse from prolonged immobilization such as from a fracture of a long bone, and is a frequent consequence of old age. Injury to or disease of the periphery nerves can also cause wasting of muscle. Overuse of some drugs and chronic poisoning from arsenic, lead, petrol containing lead, mercury, ergot, and the sulfonamides can affect many nerves to the point of muscle degeneration.

Neuritis 3: Sensory nerves affected become painful along their course with tingling, numbness and loss of sense of touch. If motor nerves are affected (nerves involved in movement of muscles), the muscle becomes weak and, if not treated, shrunken and atrophied.

Peripheral vascular disease 137: Intermittent cramping of the leg upon physical exertion, numbness and coolness of the leg. Blood vessel blockage can bring on muscle degeneration and gangrene.

Vitamin B₁ (thiamine) deficiency 349: Fatigue, appetite and weight loss, prickly numbness of the hands and feet, emotional instability, cramp in the legs, difficulty walking, muscle degeneration, rapid heartbeat, difficulty breathing, swelling of the tissues.

Leprosy 368: Onset is insidious. Red and brown patches with white centre on the skin. Hard nodules on face, feet, and legs, loss of feeling in various parts of the body, wasting of bone, open sores, deformity, loss of fingers and toes, muscle atrophy.

Polio 374: High fever, severe headache, sore throat, and muscle pain. Stiff neck is a vital sign. Later, prostration, extreme weakness, muscles that are atrophying, twitch, and paralysis of arms and legs. Speech difficulties and nasal voice indicates brain stem involvement.

Muscular dystrophy 405: Duchenne type: child has difficulty in walking or standing, waddling gait. Muscle atrophy causes lordosis and scoliosis, cramping pains, difficulty in rising. Facioscapulohumeral type affects shoulders and upper arms, face becomes expressionless; disease begins at adolescence, later spreads to pelvis and legs.

Cerebral palsy 406: Infants, children: spasticity most common symptom, affecting legs more than the arms. Difficult articulation and swallowing, tremors, rigidity and lack of muscle control.

Loss of muscle control

Mountain sickness 122a: Above 5,000 metres, 17,000 feet climbers may suffer loss of peripheral vision, dimness, and muscular incoordination.

Muscular dystrophy 405: Infants: difficulty standing or walking, waddling gait, frequent falls, face mask-like; loss of muscle control, first of the face, then pelvis and legs.

Cerebral palsy 406: Infants: twitching limbs and muscles, spasticity, loss of sense of balance, loss of alertness, partial paralysis of the face, high-pitched crying, difficulty swallowing, vomiting, susceptibility to infections.

Cramps in the muscles (pain or soreness)

A muscular cramp is a sudden seizure of a muscle, so painful as to prevent movement. Most of the time this is due to overexertion. Heat cramps are caused by loss of body salt. Chronic strain such as that experienced by a salesman on his feet all day, or by a house painter, are other common causes, as well as dehydration from long fevers. Anxiety and stress are no small contributors to this disorder. Cramp is also common in gout and uraemia.

Cramps in the muscles (pain, soreness, or spasm), Cramps, ache or spasm in the muscles and headache

Cramps in the muscles (pain, soreness, or spasm)

Common cold 63: Cold symptoms, vague ache in most of the muscles.

Acute bronchitis 103: Pain in the muscles and in the back; racking, painful cough, cold symptoms, yellowish, heavy, profuse phlegm.

Osteomyelitis 265: Deep pain in bones and joints, very high fever, overlying muscle rigid, swollen, festering, and painful.

Vitamin B₁ (thiamine) deficiency 349: Fatigue, appetite and weight loss, prickly numbness of the hands and feet, emotional instability, cramps in the legs, difficulty walking, rapid heartbeat, difficulty breathing, swelling and fluid in the tissues.

Trichinosis 386: Swelling of face around eyes and forehead, high fever, pain and swelling in muscles, profuse sweating, diarrhoea. In severe cases, shortness of breath.

Cramps, ache or spasm in the muscles and headache

Acute infectious hepatitis 187: Jaundice is the main symptom. Fever, headache, loss of appetite, dark urine, clay-coloured stools, fatigue, general itching and palpable liver causing tender abdomen.

Tetanus 361: First real sign is stiffness of the jaw, difficulty opening the mouth and swallowing. Restlessness, apprehension, muscle stiffness and spasms, persistent, fixed grin, and yawning.

Relapsing fever 369: Chills, very high fever, severe headache, rapid heartbeat, pain in muscles and joints, profuse sweating. Recurrent attacks of the disease with high fever.

Smallpox 373: High fever, violent frontal headache, intense muscular pain, convulsions in children, large crop of small reddish spots becoming first pimply, then purulent blisters, and finally foul-smelling crusts.

Polio 374: High fever, severe headache, sore throat, stiff neck, great weakness, twitching muscles. In severe cases, prostration, paralysis of legs, arms, and other parts of the body. Difficulty in swallowing.

Flu 376: Mild cold symptoms, flushed face, chills and fever, severe headaches, aches in bones and muscles, prostration, fatigue, sweating.

Dengue fever 380: Chills, high fever, headache, pain in back of the eyeballs, severe pain in muscle and joints causing prostration.

*

Pulled or strained muscle

A muscle may be overstretched from a twist of the arm, from a slip, or from taking a wrong step which may strain a muscle that bolsters the ankle. Although walking is still possible it is painful. (A strain is never as bad as a sprain.) Treatment comprises resting the injured muscle, applying warm compresses, and providing protection with a bandage.

Swollen muscle

Osteomyelitis 265: Overlying muscle is rigid, swollen, and painful. Deep pain in the affected joint and bone, high fever, sweating.

Trichinosis 386: Sometimes there are no symptoms but more often there is swelling of the area around the eyes and forehead, high fever, pain and swelling of the muscles, profuse sweating, diarrhoea. In severe cases, shortness of breath.

Weakness of muscle

Weakness of a muscle and even atrophy can result from disuse, whether it be voluntary or due to disease or injury. All muscles of the body need to be used and exercised for proper tonicity.

Neuritis 3: Muscle condition within the area of inflammation can range from weakness to atrophy plus considerable pain along the path of the inflamed nerve. Often loss of sensation.

Peripheral vascular disease 137: Weakness in the leg musculature, limping, cramps and numbness in the leg. Leg is cold.

Cushing's disease 343: Weight gain on face, trunk or back, excessive hair growth, easy bruising, muscle weakness, easy bone fracture, loss of menstrual periods, development of diabetes.

Primary aldosteronism 345: Fatigue, muscle weakness, numbness and tingling, thirst, excessive urination.

Brain cancer 412: Severe headache, vomiting, faulty vision, one-sided muscular weakness, loss of sense of balance, visual hallucinations, cloudy consciousness, drowsiness, obtuseness, lethargy, disordered conduct, psychotic behaviour.

SHOULDER
Dislocation of the shoulder

Dislocation of the shoulder 274: Motion is painful, no normal roundness of shoulder, one arm seems shorter than the other.

Frozen shoulder

Frozen shoulder 273: Pain deep inside shoulder, can involve arm, chest, and back. The basic symptom is inability to move shoulder due to adhesion in the joints. The patient can't lie down. Pain is worse at night.

Pain in the shoulder

Perforation in peptic ulcer 160: Sudden agonizing pain in stomach, rigid abdomen, rise in pulse rate and temperature, patient is ashen grey and breathless. Pain in shoulder tip.

Bursitis (shoulder) 263: Affected joint very painful on movement. The joint is hot, red, and swollen.

Frozen shoulder 273: Pain deep inside shoulder, can involve arm, chest, and back. The basic symptom is inability to move shoulder due to adhesion to the joints. The patient can't lie down. Pain is worse at night.

Dislocation of the shoulder 274: Motion is painful, no normal roundness of the shoulder, one arm seems shorter than the other.

Round shoulders

Osteoporosis of the spine 266: Back pain, chronic aching spine, height loss, fragility of the bones.

Spinal curvature 270: Lateral curvature (scoliosis) and/or forward curvature (lordosis), and round shoulders.

Weak shoulder

Muscular dystrophy 405: Facioscapulohumeral type: shoulder and arms more affected than the legs, unable to raise arms above head, expressionless, mask-like face. After adolescence can spread to pelvis and legs.

SPINE
Disorders of the spine

Tuberculosis of the joints and bones 264: Swelling of the joints sometimes without pain, rigid spine, postural changes, fever, night sweats. Child may cry out at night without awakening.

Spinal curvature 270: Lateral curvature (scoliosis) and/or forward curvature (lordosis), and round shoulders.

Vitamin D deficiency 353a: Infants: restlessness, thinning and softening of the head bones, bow-legs, inability to walk, stand, or sit at proper age. Later scoliosis and lordosis may develop. Adults: progressive weakness and rheumatic pain in pelvis, limbs, and spine.

Inability to straighten up

Low back pain 268: Pain can range from sudden, acute, and agonizing to low-keyed and chronic. Onset can be dramatic, such as bending down and being unable to straighten up, or a slow-growing chronic pain in small of the back. Ache may occur once or it may be frequent and chronic.

Slipped disc 269: Early signs are stiffness, pain in lower back, may be pain in buttock, thighs, or calf. Occasionally a list to one side and often upon bending down, inability to straighten up.

THE TOES
Bump on the toe joint

Bunion 282: Walking is painful and impeded, large bump on outside of large toe joint, pain in the joint.

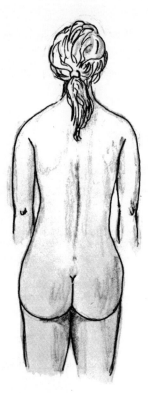

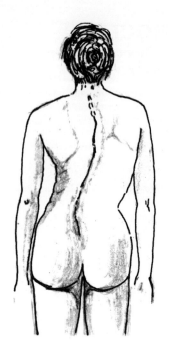

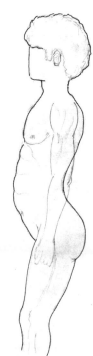

ABOVE LEFT: Normal spine.
ABOVE RIGHT: Scoliosis.
BELOW RIGHT: Lordosis or swayback.
(*Julian A. Miller*)

Pain in the toe

Bunion 282: Walking is painful and impeded, large bump on outside of large toe joint, pain in the joint.
Ingrowing toenail 284: Pain in toenail, difficulty walking, tender area.
Gout 334: Extreme pain in big toe joint, inflammation and pain in the joints, rapid pulse, nodules of urate crystals on the ear and in the joints, scanty, dark urine.

WALKING
Abnormal fatigue or pain in walking

Flatfeet 281: Early fatigue in walking

for some. Pain in arch of foot, radiating to the calf and lower back.

Pernicious anaemia 323: Anaemic symptoms, palpitations, general body pain, pins-and-needles sensation in hands, feet, and elsewhere, sore, red tongue, weight loss, jaundice, abnormal fatigue from walking, impotence and frigidity.

Vitamin B₁ (thiamine) deficiency 349: Loss of appetite and weight, prickling numbness of the hands, legs, and feet, heavy palpitation, difficulty breathing, swelling and fluid in the tissues, and emotional instability.

Waddling gait

Muscular dystrophy 405: Duchenne type: Strikes males only, child has difficulty in standing or walking, waddling gait, a weakness in the legs, frequent falls, lordosis, scoliosis, cramping pain in the muscle.

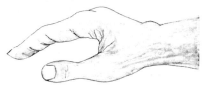

Lump on wrist. (*Julian A. Miller*)

THE WRIST
Lump on the wrist

Ganglion of the wrist 277: Painless lump or bump on the back of the wrist.

Pain in the wrist (swollen wrist)

Sprained or strained wrist 278: Reddish-blue bruise marks on the wrist, swelling with considerable pain. (Almost all sprained wrists in adults are fractures.)

Part 2
Diseases

1 The brain and nervous system

Linda Donelle Lewis

Besides being the source of our thoughts, the brain is also the body's computer. To build a computer that does the work of the human brain, the structure would have to be as long as Manhattan Island and as high as the Empire State Building. The complexity of the brain is beyond the scope of this book or any book, for that matter.

The brain has more than twelve billion cells, which function as batteries, resistors, transformers, and switches. If one considers that the average TV set has fewer than twenty-five resistors and trans-formers, one can begin to comprehend the awesome grandeur of that compact mass of matter, weighing little more than 1·4kg (3lb), that fills the skull.

The automatic part of the brain performs all the household functions of the body – organizing, planning, directing such activities as the efficient beating of the heart, the proper rate of breathing, and the thousands of other duties the body unceasingly demands. Our need for sleep is not so much to rest our bodies as to rest our brain. The body rarely needs more than an hour of rest, but parts of the brain require seven or eight.

What is so miraculous is that this incredible organ breaks down so infrequently, given its astronomical complexities. Things do go wrong, of course, although most of the time we really do not know why. But often the disorder can be alleviated or even cured.

Parkinson's disease 1

This chronic disease of the central nervous system is characterized by palsy, a rigidity of the muscles, and slowness. Although the cause of Parkinson's remains unknown, we have discovered that it is possibly a chemically induced disease, since poisoning by carbon monoxide and manganese or the heavy use of tranquillizers over an extended period of time can produce a similar picture.

Parkinson's is not contagious nor can it be inherited. It does not markedly affect the mind or the memory, although it can impede speech by the rigidity and slowness of the mouth and tongue.

One of its peculiar facets is the small number of patients with Parkinson's who also develop high blood pressure.

The danger: Parkinson's is not a killer, but it can make invalids of its victims. The disease is progressively degenerative, until the victim has difficulty in dressing, shaving, bathing, writing, getting in and out of a car or bed, and even eating. When it affects throat and neck muscles, the patient is in danger of malnutrition. The wasting away of muscles is another serious development.

Symptoms: Parkinson's is characterized by a slowness of all action. The face is immobile, with a wide-eyed, unblinking, often staring appearance. The mouth is partially open with a drooling of saliva. The patient's posture is rigid and stooped, at times simian, with the arms stiff and bent, held close to the sides. He walks with small, shuffling steps, his body pitched forward in a constant search for his centre of gravity. This posture may cause the patient to adopt a running gait to prevent himself from falling. The arm swing is decreased. Often he cannot stop himself unless he finds a wall or some obstruction to slow his headlong motion.

The hands exhibit a tremor, particularly at rest. The patient cannot stop the involuntary shaking of the fingers and thumbs except for a short time and only by great effort. The hand tremor disappears when asleep and intensifies under emotional stress and fatigue.

Treatment: Until recently there were only palliative medications, but within the past few years there has been a breakthrough with a new drug, L-dopa, which has helped more than two-thirds of the patients by controlling rigidity and tremor. In addition, a new surgical approach that involves cooling a part of the brain has shown some promise. With a battery of other drugs, the symptoms can either be alleviated or the full impact kept under reasonable control.

The patient should keep well exercised and active. For hands and fingers, squeezing a rubber ball several times daily is valuable; grimacing, face-twisting, smiling, can help frozen face muscles. The 'lion' pose from Yoga can loosen the face: the mouth is kept wide open, the tongue stuck out as far as possible, hands and fingers outstretched, muscles of the face and neck tense. The object is to make a sudden ferocious face as if trying to frighten someone. This pose is held for four seconds, then slowly relaxed. This exercise should be repeated many times.

For every muscular failing, the patient must invent his own exercise to help strengthen and control his movements. He should also engage in as many gross motor exercises as he is capable of doing. If he is able to go to a gym, all the better. Here he can take advantage of a stationary bicycle, pulleys, rowing machine, and bar-bells.

Exercising is his most important therapy.

If possible, a physiotherapist for those with frozen muscles will be helpful. Massage should be vigorous, and stretching is most important to keep the muscles and joints from stiffening and freezing up.

A positive determination and energetic effort by the patient to fight this crippling affliction can prevent his becoming an invalid.

Outlook: Although we cannot yet eradicate this disease, we can slow it down, thus affording many of its victims the opportunity of a hopeful life.

Epilepsy 2

Grand mal **2a**, *Petit mal* **2b**, and *Temporal lobe seizures* **2c**, also known as psychomotor seizures, are the three major forms of epilepsy, an age-old, worldwide malady. It is not a mental disorder but an affliction resulting from an abnormality of the central nervous system, in the form of convulsive seizures, or fits, that appear with episodic frequency. About one quarter of those suffering from this ailment show a specific cause such as brain tumour or brain injury. The rest show no known cause or origin. However, this disease does have a hereditary factor; some people can inherit a tendency for it. If two people who have epilepsy in their genes marry, their children have a better likelihood of being epileptic.

Except during the period of the attacks, the patient is normal both mentally and physically and can function like everyone else.

There are other diseases similar to epilepsy that have convulsive seizures, but in the non-epileptic variety the convulsions are somewhat different in character and disappear when the basic ailment disappears. They are not chronic. All central nervous system infections and disorders can produce convulsions, including meningitis, encephalitis, brain abscess, tetanus, rabies, neurosyphilis, strokes, eclampsia, and heat stroke, as well as almost any drug withdrawal and a large number of drugs and medications, such as camphor, strychnine, and lead.

Epilepsy may appear clearly defined in the brain wave test (electroencephalo-graph). The disease affects all ages but mostly the young.

The danger: A few of those suffering from epilepsy undergo some mental deterioration and become increasingly worse. A sinister development of epilepsy is called status epilepticus, in which one seizure follows on the heels of the other, without any cessation in between. Death can occur during this state.

Grand mal 2a

In grand mal (generalized major motor), the more important and more common form, the seizure may start with an aura – a premonition period – in which the patient undergoes some peculiar change. Warning signs might be nausea, lights flashing, a ringing in the ears, a disorder of smell or taste or sensation. The victim can smell sunshine, rain, or have a strange tingling or warmth in some part of his body. These premonitions can occur from several hours before the seizure to several seconds.

The seizure may be heralded by a loud shout (the epileptic cry) with the simultaneous loss of consciousness, followed by falling. All his muscles are tense, contracted; hands are clenched and eyeballs rolled upward. This condition lasts a few seconds, followed by a stage of muscular twitching, limbs and arms jerking, eyeballs rolling, and foaming at the mouth. He truly seems possessed. One of the embarrassing concomitants of this convulsion is incontinence (the escape of urine and faeces). The jerking movements diminish and the patient falls into a state of deep coma, from which he may awaken dazed, with headache and sore muscles; or if he is allowed to sleep, he may do so for a protracted period. The dark colour that had come over his face lightens. The attack lasts from two to five minutes.

Petit mal 2b

Petit mal is most common in children, with the seizure lasting between five and ten seconds, rarely more than half a minute. Spells begin and end abruptly with a sudden dimming of consciousness. The patient becomes pale and stares blankly or blinks his eyes rapidly. Whatever he is doing is suspended for the moment but is resumed as soon as the seizure is over. Petit mal rarely, if ever, affects anyone over twenty-one. The attack may occur several times a day in rapid succession.

Temporal lobe seizures 2c
(psychomotor seizures)

This variety is nowhere near as dramatic as grand mal. The patient usually does not fall, but he does not understand what is being said to him and is out of contact with his environment. He may stagger, wander, make unintelligible sounds, chew, or make purposeless movements. The patient may be stupefied, torpid, or he may be uncontrollably emotional and violent. The attack may last from two minutes to a half hour – occasionally for a whole day or so.

Treatment: The development of Dilantin, Mysoline, Zarontin together with phenobarbital has been a godsend to epileptics, keeping the disease under excellent control and considerably reducing the number of attacks. When attacks do occur the dangers of the patient hurting himself must be mitigated. Once it starts nothing can shorten the seizure. Emergency aid consists of putting the patient on his back or side, head lowered to prevent him from sucking vomitus into his lungs. All tight clothing should be loosened.

In many cases certain known incidents can trigger off a seizure such as exhaustion resulting from physical or emotional strain. Needless to say, such incidents should be avoided.

The patient should try to lead as normal a life as he can with only a few modifications, such as not driving a car or flying an airplane or doing whatever might jeopardize his life or the safety of the people around him. Every form of

recreation is open to him. He can enjoy almost every form of sport, including swimming (never alone).

Basically, he faces mainly a psychosocial problem of self-consciousness, often shame. Overprotection on the part of his family and too much of a show of concern can do the patient real harm. He must be made to face up to his difficulty and live within its demands. He must fight for his rights as a human being, regardless of his seizures. He must be made aware that sinking into some form of invalidism means defeat not only before the world but to his own self-prestige.

Prevention: For epilepsy of unknown origin, there is none; for those related diseases that cause convulsive seizures, early treatment of the underlying disorder can do much to prevent their occurrence. (See *Part 3, Early warning signals, Epilepsy* **2a**.)

Outlook: With the wise administration of many of the new medications now available, epileptic conditions can be checked and often permanently prevented. This containment depends on strict adherence to the medication schedule.

Further information on epilepsy may be obtained from The British Epilepsy Association, 3 Alfred Place, London WC1.

Neuritis 3

Neuritis is an inflammation of a nerve or nerves (polyneuritis) anywhere in the body. It is a general term denoting a disease process resulting from a number of causes

1. *Mechanical.* Such as a physical injury; pressure on a nerve while sleeping; a violent overexertion; a prolonged cramped position, such as holding a tool for a long time as in drilling or constantly bending down like an agricultural worker.

2. *Vascular.* An artery being shut off.

3. *Infectious.* Invading organisms that attack the nerves, such as in diphtheria or botulism.

4. *Poisoning*. Metallic poisons such as lead, arsenic, mercury, tin, zinc, bismuth, copper, manganese, as well as alcohol, carbon monoxide, carbon tetrachloride, and others. Toxic poisoning is a major cause of polyneuritis and can produce this disease not only by a sudden large dose but by insidious, tiny amounts absorbed over a long period of time.

5. *Metabolic Disorders*. Diabetes, gout, and others. Especially those diseases that cause nutritional deficiencies and most especially those that deplete vitamin B_1 (thiamine).

The danger: Neuritis is an agonizing ailment and if untreated can occasionally result in pain and atrophy and deformity of the muscles, an unpleasant contingency that can usually be avoided. When neuritis is accompanied by intense and unrelievable pain, the possibility of a malignancy should be investigated.

Symptoms: The sensory nerves (feeling, sensation) become painful along their course. A tingling, numbness, burning, and loss of sense of touch or an insensitivity to hot or cold are other characteristics.

If motor nerves (nerves attached to the muscles) are affected, the muscles become weak and often paralysed. If not treated, they become shrunken and atrophied.

In polyneuritis, the pain or numbness or tingling (pins-and-needles) usually begins at the fingers or toes and spreads into the arms and legs. Neuritis pain can vary from an unpleasant sharp prickling to an intense piercing or stabbing pain. Sometimes the pain appears to be more prominent at night; temperature changes may affect it.

The underlying symptoms of all other forms of neuritis are the symptoms of the contributing disease or cause.

Bell's palsy 3a

An inflammation of the facial nerve that controls facial expression, the basic cause of Bell's palsy is unknown. Long exposure to draughts on the face can precipitate an attack. This form of neuritis begins with a vague, unrelated mild ache near the ear and within a few hours or a day paralyses the face, distorting the side affected. The eye cannot close, creating additional hazards. Smiling is impossible, speech is impeded, and eating is difficult.

Treatment: The provoking disease should first be identified and treated. Treatment of neuritis itself includes bed rest, passive exercise, and warm baths with water kept at a constant temperature. When applying heat to the affected nerve, special care must be taken not to place the heat on naked skin, as numbness can lead to severe burns.

The pressure of clothes must be avoided and, above all, immobilization of an arm or leg should be scrupulously avoided, as immobilization can lead to freezing of the joints.

Immediate palliatives are aspirin, codeine, or other drugs the doctor might deem useful. After the acute stage of the neuritic attack is over, massage and electrical stimulation can be very beneficial. What is imperative is keeping up full movement of all joints involved through their full range of motility. This procedure should be started immediately, being careful to avoid any strong, violent action.

Diet should be high protein and well balanced. Supplementary vitamins are essential in neuritis that originates from poisoning or infectious and metabolic diseases. (Excessive amounts of vitamins A and D are potentially toxic to the human body.)

When the acute stage has abated, active exercises should supplant the passive form. The sooner the patient returns to active muscular exercise, the safer he is against the atrophying of the affected muscles.

Prevention: Alertness to and prompt treatment of the underlying affliction can appreciably help in the prevention of very unpleasant symptoms.

Outlook: With immediate treatment, the attacks tend to subside with the least amount of residual damage. In mild cases recovery is rapid, but if the causative disease is still there, recurrence is more than likely. Energetic determination to conquer this affliction by means of exercise and control of the causative disease most often results in effective cure.

Neuralgia 4
(tic douloureux, trigeminal neuralgia)

Although neuralgia means pain along the course of any nerve in the body, the most common of all neuralgias is tic douloureux, or trigeminal neuralgia, in which the head and face pain is among the worst known to man. Neuralgia does not produce atrophy or deformity of any part involved. The disease may occur at any age but most often after fifty. The cause of this nerve disorder is unknown.

The danger: The advent, course, and intensity of this disease is completely unpredictable.

Symptoms: The lightning-like, harrowing jabs of pain along the course of the nerve occur from the top of the head down the face, lasting only a minute or so, with periods between attacks stretching out to weeks or months. As the disease progresses, the in-between period may become shorter.

The pain of tic douloureux may be in the forehead, lip, nose, and tongue and gums, often interfering with eating.

A touch on the nose or lips can trigger it off, as can washing the face or a breath of cool air or eating or talking.

Treatment: Hot or cold applications on affected areas and aspirin or other pain-relieving drugs may help. A number of medical procedures have been successful, such as cutting the trigeminal nerve or injecting the nerve with alcohol. This is an effective procedure but may leave the patient with a strange, new indescribable sensation.

Some of the drugs currently in use are Dilantin, which is mildly effective, and Tegretol, which is more effective. Many doctors hesitate to use the latter, for it may cause anaemia.

Prevention: Since nothing is really known about the source of this ailment, knowledge of prevention is unavailable.

Outlook: If the patient does not elect one of the curative procedures, he can at least survive the attacks by using less drastic treatment. The objective is to keep the unpleasantness to a minimum during the course of this disease.

Sciatica 5

This is an inflammation along the sciatic nerve, the longest nerve in the body – from the buttocks down to the feet. It affects more men than women and mainly in the age range between thirty and fifty.

Sciatica is due to a number of causes, the most common one being pressure at the root of the nerve in the spine by a ruptured or slipped disc or by an arthritic condition. Also, anything that presses against the nerve outlet, such as engorged blood vessels or heavy bowels from constipation or a tumour or some infection of a nearby organ, will induce this disorder. The inactivity occasioned by a long car drive or lifting a heavy object the wrong way can precipitate sciatica (see *Table 15 – How to lift a heavy weight*).

The disease can be worsened by cold, dampness, and excessive muscular work during the acute period, as well as poor posture.

The danger: Actually no danger to life or longevity is posed by sciatica, but it can be a depleting disease because of its agonizing pain.

Symptoms: The basic symptom is pain, agonizing and torturous, which begins at the buttocks and continues along the line of the nerve. The pain often abates but usually returns.

If the disorder is due to spinal root involvement, the pain may be aggravated by a sneeze, cough, defecation, or any strain. If the fault is a ruptured or slipped disc, acquired frequently by lifting a heavy weight the wrong way, the pain may be sharp and stabbing.

The nerve becomes sensitive to touch all

along its course, hampering movements of the leg by increasing the pain. When the leg is straightened, the patient receives an extra sharp jab in the buttock.

Treatment: Bed rest on a firm mattress with a pillow under the knee, immobilization of the back or a back brace, and a pelvic support (a properly padded brace) are all helpful. Local heat is salutary, any kind of heat – a poultice, hot water bottle, electric pad, or diathermy – along with aspirin. In addition to these remedies, sciatica caused by a slipped or ruptured disc can be alleviated by the surgical removal of the disc.

Acupuncture has been somewhat successful.

Prevention: Lift heavy weights properly. Avoid poor posture. Proper posture, when sitting, means upright and relaxed, never on one buttock or on the edge of a chair.

Outlook: The underlying cause must be identified and treated before the sciatic nerve can be restored.

Multiple sclerosis 6

A chronic disease of the central nervous system, multiple sclerosis is characterized by a decline of muscle movement and co-ordination with final degeneration of nervous tissue. The entire body is affected. It strikes mostly between the ages of twenty and forty.

The cause remains a mystery. Theories abound explaining multiple sclerosis as infection by a virus, as induced by poisoning, the result of an injury or an abnormal blood-clotting factor, but as yet they remain only theories with no facts to sustain them.

The average longevity from onset is twenty years. Some patients live much longer, some have remission from the disease that can last twenty years or more, and some have frequent wasting attacks with a rapid downhill course. Multiple sclerosis is a bizarre and unpredictable ailment, still unyielding to our most intense medical efforts.

The danger: The course of this malady is extremely variable and quixotic. The major imperilment is muscular atrophy and invalidism.

Symptoms: The early symptoms, which can appear months or even years before the onset of the disease itself, are mild visual disturbances, fleeting palsy of the eyeball, unusual fatigability of an arm or leg, which can interfere with walking, unexplained and ill-defined trouble with bladder control or difficulty in urination, giddiness, and mild, inexplicable emotional upsets.

Then the disease does finally strike, the first definite symptom is a gradual failure of the muscles, worsening to jerky movements and eventually paralysis. An eye can go blind, a limb go numb. Often the first symptoms abate, disappear, and return months or years later, with an additional crop of new ones.

A peculiarity of this disease is the baffling periods of remission and then relapse. Symptoms appear, disappear, and return.

Tremor of the hand is a common sign. It is called intention tremor, which means that when the patient makes a purposeful movement, like picking up a cup, the hand that was not trembling before will begin to tremble.

The gait eventually becomes tight, weak, and unsteady as the disease worsens.

In men, impotence develops; in women numbness of the vagina. There are disturbances of bladder and bowel control and a tingling of the extremities or even of a whole side of the body. Judgement becomes poor and the patient can become either apathetic or euphoric. His attention span is limited.

As the illness progresses, problems of sight become serious, such as dimness of vision, partial blindness, double vision, ocular palsy, and inability to control the movement of the eyeball. There are also speech problems – a slurred voice and difficulty in connecting syllables.

Treatment: There is no specific medical therapy. Common sense suggests avoiding the usual pressures, such as fatigue, overwork, emotionalism. If legs or arms have been weakened or paralysed, massage can be very helpful. Exercise, retraining the muscles, and physical therapy have very considerable value in some degree of restoration of function.

Drugs have not proven useful. Occasionally, cortisone-like drugs are tried for an acute attack, but their effectiveness is low and their danger is quite high.

Prevention: (See *Part 3, Early warning signals, Multiple sclerosis* **6**)

Outlook: A positive psychological approach of the patient to this affliction cannot only postpone invalidism, it can often prevent it. Whatever each patient feels can help him should be tried. He must take an active attitude in combating the disease, for partial remission is common and total remission also occurs.

Since this disease usually does not occur in people born in the tropics, many desperate doctors have urged their patients to retire to this climate. There are no statistics to ascertain the value of this practice.

Meningitis 7
(spotted fever, epidemic meningitis, cerebrospinal fever)

An inflammation of the meninges (membranes covering the brain) by infection from bacteria, virus, or fungus usually emanating through the bloodstream from other parts of the body.

There are several varieties of meningitis with similar symptoms. The most common form is meningococcal meningitis, which is most prevalent in the epidemic form and is also known as spotted fever, cerebrospinal fever, epidemic meningitis. Tuberculous meningitis is obviously caused by the tubercle germ and affects children between one and five. The pneumococcal, staphylococcal, and influenzal meningitis are non-epidemic but strike mainly children.

The staphylococcal form is of particularly grave concern because the germ has the greatest resistance to antibiotics and requires extremely rigorous care on the part of the doctor in order to find the right combination of germicidal drugs for each particular patient.

Meningitis can be one of the complications of middle-ear infection (otitis media) or mastoiditis or any sinus or tonsil infection or even a scalp injury that becomes infected. Any septic blood condition may carry the infection to the brain.

Contagion: Like a cold, meningitis can be spread by coughing or sneezing from a carrier. The carrier may not even have active disease, that is, he is harbouring the germ but has not become sick; he can even be in good health and still spread the disease – for months and as long as a year.

During epidemics, as many as thirty per cent of the exposed public can contract the disease. The great epidemics of the past no longer afflict us, but smaller outbreaks do occur in schools, prisons, and army camps.

The danger: This is a *Medical Emergency*. Not too long ago, the fatalities from meningitis ran as high as 90 per cent; today the incidence stands at 4 per cent, but it still remains a deadly ailment, which if untreated will kill up to 90 per cent of its victims. Severe cases, especially those untreated or treated too late, can leave harsh residue, such as varying degrees of blindness, deafness, paralysis, and mental retardation. Occasionally meningitis can develop so rapidly that it can kill the patient within several hours. Any sign or hint of possible meningitis should mean an instant call for help.

Symptoms: Meningitis occasionally begins with deceptive mildness, like a cold, but suddenly shows its hand with high and erratic fever. Septicaemia, or invasion of the bloodstream by bacteria, sets in quickly. The accompanying headache is overwheming, unremitting, and radiating. The distinctive, characteristic sign is severe headache with a stiff and painful neck. Vomiting is common.

Often there is intolerance to light and sound. In children particularly, there can be twitching, convulsions, delirium, and vomiting. Confusion, weakness, delirium, and often coma are additional developments.

Another identifying symptom of acute meningococcal meningitis is a rash – small, irregular purplish or reddish spots all over the body. There may also be fever blisters around the lips.

The tuberculous form of meningitis is quite difficult to control and needs constant alert medical attention.

The doctor will need to take a sample of the spinal fluid to determine the form and type of meningitis.

Treatment: Intravenous injections of penicillin sulphonamides and other antibiotics are the basic drugs to control meningitis. In the desperately ill patient, cortisone therapy can be a lifesaver.

Meningitis is a highly contagious disease and must be given extreme care. All discharges and tissues must be burned. The patient should be kept in some form of isolation. He needs plenty of fluids and nourishing food. To ensure rest, occasionally sedation is employed. Aspirin is a useful drug to treat the headache and fever.

The sickroom should be dark and quiet. For the patient's comfort, his eyes should be protected from bright lights and noise kept to an absolute minimum. In comatose or semi-comatose patients, tube feeding may be necessary; nourishment must be kept up.

Before the patient is pronounced cured, more spinal taps are necessary to make sure that none of the germs are still in his body.

Prevention: An alert parent can save a child's life, and a doctor should be called for at any sign of a sudden high fever, a stiff neck, a severe headache, and pinpoint haemorrhages under the skin. Speed in diagnosis and treatment is the single most important factor in avoiding harsh complications or even death.

It may be considered necessary to treat all contacts as an outbreak. Only those caring for the patient approach him, all others must stay away from the area of the sick bed. Everything used by the patient must be burned or sterilized.

A child or an adult who has an inner-ear infection or mastoiditis should take special pains to protect himself against this disease by seeing a doctor at once and following his instructions closely. Meningitis strikes mainly in cold weather and therefore care should be taken during this season. (See *Part 3, Early warning signals, Meningitis* **7**.)

Outlook: Meningitis is no longer the dread malady of the past, but it is still a dangerous disease. With prompt diagnosis and immediate therapy, the outlook is very favourable.

Encephalitis 8
(sleeping sickness)

Encephalitis is caused by a virus and produces inflammation of the brain substance. Occasionally it may be a complication of flu, measles, chicken pox, whooping cough, or meningitis. Encephalitis is contagious.

There are several forms of this disease: St Louis, western equine, eastern equine, and a few others. Encephalitis is also known as sleeping sickness, but it should not be confused with African sleeping sickness, an even worse disease, which is transmitted by the tsetse fly.

Encephalitis is more common in epidemic form than in sporadic cases.

The danger: Encephalitis has a high mortality and morbidity (incidence) rate. Much depends on the virulence of the disease and the age of the patient – the very young and the very old are the most susceptible. Some of the more pernicious forms can cause death within a few hours.

Generally, no permanent damage is sustained; a small percentage of patients suffer a residual burden for the rest of their lives, in the form of diminished mental acuity or some other degeneration of character and behaviour.

Symptoms: Infants: The disease strikes suddenly with a high fever, ranging from 39·4° to 41°C, 103° to 106°F and lasting about two days, usually accompanied by convulsions and bulging fontanelles (spaces between the bones in the head). The fever diminishes in about a week.

Older children and adults: The fever is high, about 39·4°C, 103°F, and usually drops to normal about the tenth day. The headache is most severe, pounding, and unremitting. A common symptom is drowsiness to stupor. In more severe cases, coma, delirium and convulsions, weakness of eyes and muscles, persistent hiccups, and excessive salivation may occur. The characteristic symptoms of brain disease, stiff neck and vomiting, may be present.

Treatment: There is no specific treatment of any value. The medical profession can only recommend alleviatory measures. Bed rest, keeping the patient quiet, keeping his bowels normal, cold compresses to the head and intravenous feeding if the patient is in a coma. If complications interfere with breathing, the doctor may be obliged to perform an emergency tracheotomy.

Convalescence is usually quite prolonged. After apparent recovery, the patient should be kept from school or work for a minimum of a month.

Prevention: Various vaccines for different forms of encephalitis exist, but, unfortunately, they are not generally available. The best preventive advice is to stay away from areas or homes where there has been an outbreak or an incidence of this disease. (See *Part 3, Early warning signals, Encephalitis* **8**.)

Outlook: Most people recover from encephalitis without permanent damage.

Brain tumours 9

There are a variety of brain tumours and much depends on the location of the growth. Both benign and malignant tumours are serious disorders. They can occur at any age but more often appear in young adulthood and middle age.

The danger: Brain tumour is not a common disease; it can even be classified as rare. A pounding headache almost surely is not being caused by a brain tumour.

However, brain tumours have a high fatality rate. Although everyone is aware of how deadly these tumours can be, it does not mean that everyone who develops a brain tumour is going to die – not at all. Most people survive and are even cured. An interesting and curious note is that two per cent of all autopsies held for various causes of death showed some form of brain tumour which has shown no symptoms.

Symptoms: Contrary to general belief, headache is not always the first symptom. Quite often it is preceded by slow progressive disturbances in balance, sight and smell, or unexplained weakness in the muscles of the extremities.

When headaches first appear they usually occur in the morning and are short-lived. Later, however, they become constant and very severe. (In many cases the headache is deceptively mild.) Anyone over twenty-five who has never suffered from headaches and then suddenly develops a severe persistent one should be checked. It does not mean he has a tumour, but this may be a characteristic sign.

Persistent nausea and vomiting are common to most far-advanced brain tumours. Swelling of the optic nerve may be seen. (Only a doctor can observe this sign.) Convulsions are a frequent additional symptom.

There may be indications of mental deterioration if the tumour is located where it can do such harm. Deterioration, however, may not be evidenced until late in the development of the tumour.

Disorder of personality, impairment of mental function, lethargy and drowsiness are late and serious signs of progression of this disease.

The doctor will want a medical history, make a detailed physical examination and take an x-ray of the skull, an encephalogram, and a brain scan besides examining the eyes, testing speech, hearing, memory, checking balance and coordination, and evaluating arm and leg strength.

Treatment: There are many forms of treatment, most of them drastic. The basic one, of course, is surgical excision of the tumour. This method is growing in efficiency with corresponding success, but the tumours deep inside the brain can rarely be cut out completely. Partial excision, however, does give the patient extra years before the tumour regrows.

Another form of treatment is irradiation by x-ray. There is also decompression (making a hole in the skull with placement of a shunt to relieve the pressure). This method was practised by the Egyptians 3,000 years ago.

All of these measures can preserve life and give the patient many years of normal functioning. Occasionally, none of these procedures are of any avail.

Prevention: (See *Part 3, Early warning signals, Brain tumour* **9**.)

Outlook: Hopeful. More and more brain tumours are being brought under control. Surgical skill is being perfected, thus presenting less danger for the patient.

Brain injury 10
(concussion, craniocerebral trauma)

Most blows on the head, even though some may render the victim unconscious, have no serious lasting effects, especially among children, whose recovery is little short of phenomenal.

The danger: The vast majority of head injuries heal without complications, but a few may cause lasting brain damage or death. Any blow on the head that causes unconsciousness or any of the symptoms listed below is a *Medical Emergency*. It should be immediately attended to by a doctor.

Symptoms: In the mild form there is headache, giddiness, and often unconsciousness for a brief time.

When the injury is more serious, there can be bleeding from the mouth, nose, ears; the skin becomes pale and clammy; the pupils dilated.

If unconsciousness is prolonged, if the pupils of the eyes are unequal, if there is frequent vomiting, or if the victim is continuously drowsy, lethargic, or confused, the injury is likely to be serious.

Treatment: The patient should be kept in bed in a darkened, quiet room with his head and shoulders elevated. If his extremities are cold, they should be kept warm. No stimulants of any kind should be administered. If the concussion is uncomplicated, the patient will regain consciousness and revive fully in a short time. In any event, a doctor must be called.

Prevention: Protective devices, such as helmets when riding a motorcycle and safety belts when riding in an automobile, may help.

Outlook: Good, especially with a doctor in attendance.

Tics 11
(muscle spasms)

A tic is a purposeless repetitive movement of a muscle or group of muscles, occurring mainly in children from the ages of six to fourteen. They can, however, occur at any age. Normally causes for all ages are fatigue, overexertion of a muscle, and anxiety. Basically, tics are involuntary nervous twitches, although sometimes they are the residue of an attack of encephalitis.

The danger: None, except the psychological damage of the underlying neuroses.

Symptoms: Tic appears in many forms, such as blinking of the eye, grimacing, shaking the head, clearing the throat, swallowing, jerking the thigh, shrugging the shoulder, pulling up the corners of the mouth, or a more complex series of tics always carried out in the same precise order, like shrugging the shoulder and then grimacing.

Tics are never seen when the subject is asleep.

There are usually other signs of the subject being nervous and highly geared in terms of behaviour, maladjustments, and other psychological signs. Anxiety intensifies the tic.

Treatment: The doctor, parent, or friend should attempt to discover the underlying cause of nervousness and try to remove or alleviate it – usually a very tall order. In any event, an effort should be made to improve the subject's general health. The subject should never be criticized for his tic, as it will only tend to exacerbate his nervousness and worsen his condition.

Nervous tics should be distinguished from chorea (St Vitus's dance), a symptom of *Rheumatic heart disease* **127**. The twitching in chorea is haphazard and dissimilar, whereas in nervous tic it is always precisely the same. Chorea is usually seen in a child with rheumatic fever; tic has no relationship to bodily disease.

Psychotherapy is helpful for tic, particularly when the child's problems are beyond his ability to handle. A severe tic is usually a sign that the child or adult cannot cope with his problems. In a way, the tic is a kind of safety valve. The use of tranquillizing drugs tends to mask the problem rather than help it.

In mild cases, where the child is extremely sensitive or going through a difficult phase, the tic will eventually disappear.

Outlook: Children survive their childhoods and their tics.

Hiccups 12

Hiccups are due to an irritation or temporary disturbance of the phrenic nerve to the diaphragm, or within it. Hiccups have been experienced by everyone. However, there is a form known as hysterical hiccups and a very dangerous type known as infective (epidemic) hiccups. The former, although long-lasting, is not dangerous. The only way to distinguish between the two is the epidemic character of the infective type.

The causes are many: indigestion, nervousness, exercising too soon after a big meal, faulty swallowing of food or food gone down the wrong way, alcoholism, hiatus hernia, pleurisy, pregnancy, even

some brain disorders, and often no known reason at all.

The danger: None, unless the hiccups are too prolonged or if the patient has just had an operation.

Symptoms: An involuntary inspirational spasm with a characteristic sound.

Treatment: To stop hiccups:

1. Take a deep breath, hold it, then blow out slowly.
2. Drink a glass of water without a break.
3. Apply pressure on the eyeballs.
4. Swallow crushed ice.
5. Place an icebag on the diaphragm just below the rib cage.
6. Breathe and rebreathe into a paper bag.

Most attacks of hiccups last less than an hour; should an attack go on for much longer, medical advice should be sought. A baby's hiccuping is natural and no effort should be made to restrain him in any way.

Outlook: Except for the infective (epidemic) hiccups, recovery is certain.

Headaches 13

Every human being at some time or another is subject to headaches – probably the most common affliction of man.

Headache is often a complaint of the body against a condition of the mind. However, the vast majority of headaches are without major or permanent significance. The one we all worry about, the brain tumour headache, is the least common of all. Few headaches, with the exception of those resulting from high blood pressure or the rare brain tumour, are sinister.

For source of further information, see note at end of this chapter.

Tension headache 13a

Tension headaches are usually related to some unpleasant or worrisome event or condition that causes chronic anxiety. These headaches can be chronic or transient. Prolonged anxiety can bring it on, as can strain resulting from long periods of driving or sitting at work. From a third to a half of all headaches fall into this group.

The danger: None.

Symptoms: Usually there is some prior warning such as visual disturbances, fatigue, nausea and weakness. A tension headache may start in one place and soon become generalized over the top of the head. It is a steady pressing ache; it can also be throbbing. It is not usually severe and often feels like a tight hat on the head.

The duration of tension headaches can run from minutes to hours; it may even go on for weeks at a time. During an attack, muscles in the jaw, in the temples, or at the back of the neck may become tense, with subsequent tenderness in the areas of attachment to the skull.

Emotional disturbances or increased anxiety always worsen the condition. The patient usually appears apprehensive and often depressed.

Treatment: Moist heat application, neck massage, and removal of the cause of anxiety if this is possible are helpful. Aspirin is occasionally effective. The most effective home treatment is a change of activity. If the sufferer has been sedentary for several hours, sitting at a desk or at a work bench, he should take a brisk walk or jog or some form of energetic full bodied activity, preferably out in the open.

Prevention: The body has limits – a driving personality may go beyond these limits.

Migraine Headache (sick headache) 13b

Migraine headaches occur as four distinct classes: classical migraine, common migraine, vascular headaches, and cluster headaches.

Classical migraine is a common affliction of women (eighty per cent), two-thirds of whom have a history of migraine

in the family. Most of these living at too fast a pace for make-up – either by overwor play. A sudden relaxation fro driving themselves can also brin attack. So can faulty resting or sleeping patterns.

Many sufferers of migraine show a clivity for certain foods that are high in tyramine or tyrosine. These are amino acids that can trigger migraine attacks in some vulnerable people. Tyramine is found in a wide variety of foods such as most cheeses, especially ripe and aged cheese, yeast, some wines, chicken liver, chocolate, and citrus fruits.

For some women nothing can prevent an attack, but for others changing the diet or habit patterns can prove very worth while.

The danger: There are usually no serious after-effects of migraine.

Symptoms: Although there are early forerunning symptoms, when the headache does come, it is sudden and harsh.

Premonitory symptoms include a tingling of limbs, seeing dazzling or scintillating light, often in elaborate coloured patterns, noises in the ear, and depression or violent change in mood. These may appear minutes or hours before the actual headache paroxysm.

The pain is throbbing, usually in the same location each time, but may change its area in the head, and frequently may radiate out of the eye. Nausea and vomiting are characteristic; often there is temporary or partial blindness, blind spots, double vision and drooping eyelid. Normal bright lights make the patient flinch; normal sounds seem over-loud. There is agonizing ache on the affected side of the head. No fever but occasionally such concomitant symptoms as chills, tremor, dizziness, and excessive urination occur. It is truly named the 'sick headache'. Duration: From two to forty-eight hours.

In common migraine, in which the premonitory symptoms are very similar, the patient may see flashing lights followed by severe headache with nausea and vomiting. This, in turn, is followed by a throbbing, severe headache, rejection of light, and the desire to go to a cool, quiet room.

Treatment: In severe cases highly effective but rather hazardous drugs are available, such as ergotamine (or some other derivative of ergot), which is injected into a muscle as close to the beginning of the attack as possible. Since these drugs are potentially dangerous, because of the side effect of shrinking the arteries in the head, their use should be the decision of the doctor. If the patient is pregnant or suffering from any blood vessel disease, these drugs are absolutely forbidden.

An ice pack on the head may reduce the pain to a mild form, controllable by aspirin. Sleeping or resting quietly in a dark room will also lessen the pain.

The treatment is the same for common migraine.

Prevention: Often before an attack, when the symptoms are a forewarning of oncoming migraine, the headaches can be aborted by simply taking aspirin or ergot. Some women plunge into violent, sustained exercise. Some use snuff, forcing themselves into a paroxysm of sneezing. There are a number of means to upset the oncoming syndrome of headache, nausea, vomiting, and eye pain. The body can be distracted or tricked. Each patient must find a particularly expedient way suited to herself. (See *Part 3, Early warning signals, Migraine* **13b**.)

Outlook: This malady disappears with time, especially after fifty and especially after the menopause.

Cluster headache (histamine headache) 13c

This is a rare form of a vascular headache occurring almost exclusively in men. The most likely sufferer is usually a hard-driving, hard-working, hard-living, aggressive, athletic, rugged middle-aged man.

Cluster headaches are almost as agonizingly painful as classic or common migraine.

The danger: Not fatal or permanently damaging.

Symptoms: The headache comes on abruptly, excruciating and throbbing. It is generally one-sided and can affect that whole side of the face. The eye, if implicated, may become bloodshot and tear, with the pupil contracted. If the nose is involved, it will become stuffy and run; if the mouth, the saliva will be heavy and uncontrollable. Pain may also radiate into the neck. Sweating and pallor are common. The heartbeat may be slowed. In the temple of the related side, the veins as well as the arteries will become prominent and tender.

The attack may last for a few hours to many days.

Oddly enough, cluster headaches may start when the patient has totally let go, when he is most relaxed, especially deep in sleep. When the syndrome of headache has fully developed, they will come in clusters, with only a short period of relief between – often as many as three or four times in a day over a period of weeks. Periods of remission between attacks may vary from weeks to months, even years.

Cluster headaches can be set off by any of the vasodilators (anything that dilates the blood vessels), such as alcohol, wine, nitroglycerine, or histamines (a substance found in all animal and plant tissues). The good news is that in between the headaches, the drinking of any spirits or wines will not set off an attack; during the cluster period, however, a cocktail will precipitate an attack at once.

Treatment: Ergotamine, the basic drug for migraine, is the one most in use.

Prevention: Unknown.

Outlook: Eventual recovery.

Menstrual headache 13d

Menstrual headache is a minor menstrual disorder and is recognized by a characteristic symptom of pelvic discomfort and the usual accompanying malaise and nausea. Treatment is simple: aspirin if necessary and the reassurance that this headache will disappear.

Premenstrual headache 13e

Premenstrual headache may appear as much as seven days before the menstrual period. Characteristics of this headache are irritability and an inability to concentrate. The headache is usually annoying rather than severe but sometimes it can persist until the first moment of the menstrual flow. Aspirin is the most advised treatment.

Contraceptive pill headache 13f

Birth-control pills have been well recognized as a cause of headache in women. The sudden appearance of a headache when a woman has normally been free of them prior to taking the pill demands immediate and total discontinuance. Any one-sided neurological disorder, such as numbness or tingling pain, means that the pill should be stopped immediately. These individuals will probably never be able to take 'the pill', because of the possibility of developing a stroke, particularly young women. Other symptoms of antagonism to the pill may be heaviness and lumps in the breast, skin discoloration, and unusual vaginal bleeding.

The headache is the pressure type, as if the head were tied in a tight band. It may also become migraine or it can manifest itself in a plain but severe ache. There can be accompanying depression, irritability, and insomnia. No woman should try to treat it herself. The services of a doctor are essential here.

Postcoital headache 13g

Immediately after sexual intercourse, a few women (and a few men as well) develop what is usually a minor throbbing headache. Mostly fleeting, but can last about an hour and can affect an eye. This is a variant of the tension headache. The cause is usually anxiety of some form or another. A bottle of aspirin should be kept handy.

The anxious man who is impotent or who ejaculates prematurely will often develop a postcoital headache.

Menopausal headache 13h

Menopausal headaches can vary from quite mild to intense, from being constant to intermittent. When not related to actual change in hormonal balance, menopausal headaches are most likely due to depression. They are precipitated and exacerbated by hot flushes, irregular menses, and other signs of menopausal changes.

The characteristic menopausal symptoms will easily identify the headache. In general, aspirin or stronger analgesics taken early or as soon as the headache has developed will mitigate this symptom. Tension and anxiety will always make it worse. Nausea and vomiting should be treated symptomatically.

Treatment is best accomplished by a gynaecologist for the more basic disorder.

Anyone who has special or chronic headache problems should write to The Migraine Trust, 45 Great Ormond Street, London WC1.

2 The eye

Raphael M. Klapper

'Even in the glasses of thine eyes, I see thy grieved heart,' said Shakespeare – a very perceptive observation of the human eye. This incredible organ of sight not only permits us to see but is most often a barometer of our emotions and our state of health, as well.

The annals of Jewish history include a story of the famed Maimonides, world-renowned physician to the sultan. Between his home and the sultan's palace there was always a line of poor people to whom he would give free medical advice. Merely by looking into a person's eyes he could tell the nature of his ailment.

An impoverished poet, who lived at that time, thought Maimonides was a charla-

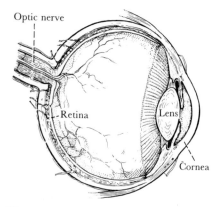

The eye. (*National Eye Institute, National Institutes of Health, USA*)

any other organ. Today we use our eyes far more than our ancestors; we drive cars, watch TV for hours, read books and newspapers and look at movies. Despite this intensive use, our sight seems to meet the demands without undue strain.

The eye is a fantastic, incredible piece of engineering – an instantly self-adjusting camera, with a built-in drainage and repair system. This most delicate instrument looks out at the world from a protected, cushioned socket, requiring only reasonable care from its owner in order to provide good and constant lifetime service.

tan, and knowing himself to be in excellent health, nevertheless stood in line among the ailing poor. Maimonides looked into his eyes for a long time. Then, without a word, he wrote out a prescription and, placing it in an envelope, gave it to the poet. He is a charlatan, thought the poet. Then he opened the envelope to look at the prescription. It said, 'You have the worst disease of all, poverty.' There was some money in the envelope to help alleviate his disease.

The eyes are the greatest clues to diseases elsewhere in the body, more so than

Nearsightedness 14 (myopia)

Myopia is primarily due to the shape of the eyeball, a hereditary factor. The axis of the eyeball is too long, so that near vision (reading and writing) is excellent, but things at a distance are blurred. The condition is easily corrected by glasses. It usually becomes worse, with an ever slowing rate, until age thirty. If after that age stronger glasses are still required, another visit to the ophthalmologist is in order.

Farsightedness 15 (hyperopia)

In farsightedness the axis of the eyeball is too short. Things at a distance or moderate distance are seen clearly, but near vision (reading and writing) is blurred or difficult. The condition, which may cause headaches, is easily corrected by glasses.

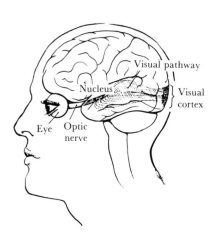

The eye and brain. (*National Eye Institute, National Institutes of Health, USA*)

Astigmatism 16

Astigmatism results from an unequal curvature of different parts of the cornea, which makes it impossible for the images to be focused properly on the retina. A congenital defect, the disorder can usually be corrected by glasses.

Presbyopia 17

A defect in vision resulting from advancing age, usually beyond the age of forty-five, presbyopia is correctable by glasses, most often requiring bifocal lenses.

Dark glasses syndrome 18

The constant use of dark glasses is unnecessary and could be harmful. Only under certain conditions do they have value, such as in glaring snow or on long drives over concrete roads or on sunbright beaches. They are also useful for those suffering from photophobia (intolerance to bright lights), which is common among people suffering from certain eye ailments and is also peculiar to blondes and persons with very light skin.

The normal human eye was designed to take in bright sunlight, and it needs no help from opticians, unless the subject is a celebrity or a hopeful film star in need of seeming to hide from the public. Film stars or not, people who wear dark glasses at night or indoors or on dark days only succeed in becoming more sensitive to light. In fact, older eyes need more light, so that, in general, wearing tinted glasses is not advisable except for persons with cataracts. Before purchasing dark glasses, hold them up to the light and move them slowly, right to left and up and down. If the reflected light beams are irregular, wavy, or if there are bubbles on the lens, they should not be purchased. Another shop may have the proper kind.

Contact lens intolerance 19

Hard lenses

Contact lenses are highly advantageous for the nearsighted, for those who have corneal disorders, for those who have had cataracts removed, and for those who need to be without glasses professionally as well as cosmetically.

The skill and care needed in fitting contact lenses requires an expert. The wearer needs about two weeks to adjust to the lenses.

Contact lenses are unsuitable for those with tremors, severe arthritis, recurrent sties, hay fever, allergies, or any disorder causing excessive watering of the eye and bloodshot eye. All wearers of contact lenses should carry a card with them saying so, in case of an accident or any period of unconsciousness, for lack of blinking can injure the cornea.

Inserting contact lenses and taking them off requires care and proficiency, with particular heed to eye hygiene. Hard contact lenses should never be worn overnight, nor longer at one stretch than the time indicated by the ophthalmologist. Even under the best conditions, the wearer should have frequent check-ups, usually every six months, and should an intolerance develop, he must immediately stop using them and be guided by his doctor. Serious damage can result if the eye's reactions are ignored.

Soft lenses

Easier on the cornea, although the vision may be less sharp than with the hard lenses, soft lenses are well worthwhile, considering the fact that they cause very few pressure problems on the eye. They require a bit more care, a few additional minutes of sterilization every night. And they are more expensive.

Strabismus 20
(cross-eye, walleye, squint)
At birth or very early in childhood

Cross-eye at an early age is due to a lack of eye muscle coordination. The danger is partial loss of vision in one eye, the so-called 'lazy eye'. Early treatment is important, preferably before the age of three. Glasses and drops may help, but often surgery is necessary to set the eye straight. Following surgery, exercises are usually needed to make both eyes function together and remain straight.

In adults

When the eye becomes crossed in adult life the onset may be associated with double vision. This symptom should never be ignored, even if it occurs for only a brief time. Sudden cross-eyedness in adults may be due to pressure on a nerve supplying the eye muscles. An ophthalmologist should be consulted without delay.

Conjunctivitis 21
(pinkeye)

Acute conjunctivitis 21a

An inflammation of the mucous membrane lining the eyelids and the white part of the eye, acute conjunctivitis may be caused by bacteria, by a virus, or by exposure to irritating chemicals.

The danger: Generally, no risk of visual loss is involved. However, conjunctivitis may become chronic. The viral and bacterial types are contagious, and contact with a person afflicted with the disease should be avoided.

Symptoms: The eye tears and becomes red. It may exude a purulent discharge and itch and burn. Eyelids can become swollen. Occasionally the victim may have blurred vision and a feeling that something is in the eye. A form of acute conjunctivitis, the allergic type, is seen during the hay fever and rose fever seasons. This form may also be due to other allergies.

Treatment: Antibiotic drops prescribed by the doctor, sometimes cortisone drops as well, especially in the allergic type of conjunctivitis, give relief. Compresses are sometimes helpful, as are sunglasses. The patient should allow no one else to use his towel and carefully dispose of tissues and handkerchiefs.

Outlook: Good for complete cure.

Chronic conjunctivitis 21b

Chronic conjunctivitis may be caused by the same agents mentioned above, the most common cause in urban areas being air pollution. The symptoms are less severe but just as bothersome. Older people with deficient tear secretions suffer from dry eyes and are much more prone to chronic conjunctivitis.

The danger: Chronic conjunctivitis presents no danger to sight, but the patient may sustain an associated *Blepharitis* **36**, an inflammation of the lid edge that may lead to scarring, cosmetically unsightly redness of the lid edges, and loss of eyelashes. Sometimes the eyelashes grow inward rubbing against the cornea, and this may become painful.

Treatment: When the disease is chronic, the ophthalmologist will generally not want to use antibiotic drops over a long period of time. Treatment in the office with astringents and mild astringent drops used at home are helpful.

Outlook: Good, but generally takes time.

Trachoma 22

A highly contagious viral conjunctivitis affecting both the upper and lower eyelids, trachoma is caused by the trachoma virus. Not customarily found in northern Europe or in the United States, except sporadically in impoverished areas, it is, however, a highly endemic disease everywhere else.

The danger: Of the 400 million people in Asia and Africa affected by this disease, twenty million have been blinded. Untreated cases usually lead to severe eye damage at best and usually blindness. The disease is easily spread by towels, handkerchiefs, and crowded conditions.

Symptoms: The incubation period is about a week. The first symptoms to appear include swelling of the eyelids, bloodshot eye, and photophobia (intolerance for bright lights). The eyelids droop, become painfully inflamed and itch. In a week the upper eyelids become marked with tiny cavities, which in a few more weeks become granular and scarred. The cornea becomes ulcerated and overgrown with wild tissue, which reduces and obstructs vision. Permanent scar tissue forms on the inner eyelids.

Treatment: Local and oral use of sulphonamides, plus antibiotic therapy, can save eyesight. This is a disease of carelessness, filth, and ignorance of hygiene. Generous use of soap and water before and during the disease can counteract infection. Badly deformed eyelids require surgery.

Prevention: Cleanliness.

Outlook: With proper and immediate medical and hygienic care, recovery is practically 100 per cent. Without care blindness will results.

Glaucoma 23

Glaucoma is a serious eye disease that can cause blindness. Essentially it is an increase in pressure inside the eye that, if not controlled, results in irrevocable damage to the optic nerve. It occurs most frequently in people over forty but may occur as a congenital form in children and in younger people. There are dozens of types of glaucoma but the most common are so-called chronic simple glaucoma and acute (angle closure) glaucoma.

Chronic simple glaucoma 23a

Symptoms: The most common form, chronic simple glaucoma has been described as a thief in the night because it steals vision without warning. No symptoms appear early in the disease to warn the patient, and when visual loss is finally noticed, it is already too late to regain lost vision. The only way to detect glaucoma early is by a thorough ophthalmological examination, which should include not only measurement of the pressure but also gonioscopy (an

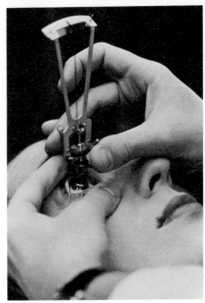

A tonometer is used to measure the pressure within the eye – a test for glaucoma. Procedure is painless and takes only a few seconds. (*National Eye Institute, National Institutes of Health, USA*)

examination to determine if the angle between the iris and the cornea is open for drainage or closed). It is possible to have glaucoma and have normal pressure during the visit to the doctor. Normal pressure alone, therefore, is not a foolproof sign of the absence of the disease. An ophthalmologist may order provocative tests to reveal the disease. One of the more common tests is the use of the tonometer, which measures the tension and pressure inside the eyeball. The finished tonogram looks like an electrocardiogram and helps the doctor to decide whether glaucoma is present.

Later symptoms are seeing halos or rainbows around electric lights, a stony hard eyeball, blind spots, narrowing of the visual field, and seeing poorly at night.

Treatment: Eye drops in the form of miotic drugs, such as pilocarpine and others, are prescribed, which drain fluid from the interior of the eye and thus lower the tension. Close observation is

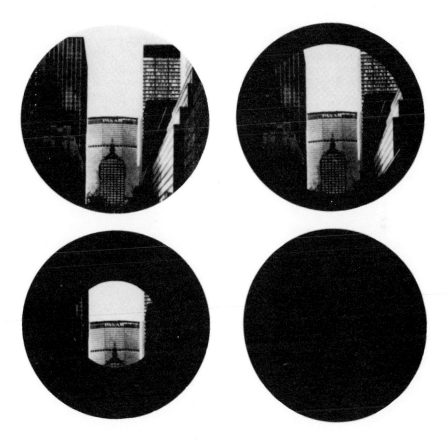

Progress of the disease glaucoma is chronicled in this series of four photographs. *Top left:* The scene is viewed through the eyes of a person with normal vision. He is able to take in the whole panorama. *Top right:* Some loss of side vision due to chronic glaucoma has taken place. Such a loss may not be noticed. *Below left:* Advanced loss of sight – at this stage the patient may still see small print but most of his vision is gone. *Below right:* Final, complete loss of vision is shown in the last illustration. (*National Society for the Prevention of Blindness*)

necessary to determine whether the disease is well controlled. A visual field test should be done at least once a year to ensure that treatment is adequate enough to prevent damage to side vision. When it is impossible to achieve control with medication, surgery is indicated, such as iridectomy, which removes a portion of the iris to deepen the drainage channels. **Prevention:** The best course of action is a periodic ophthalmological check-up

for persons over forty. (See *Part 3, Early warning signals, Glaucoma* **23a** and **23b**.) **Outlook:** Generally good if discovered early.

Acute Glaucoma 23b

The danger: Loss of sight. This is a *Medical Alert.* Every minute counts, since vision might be lost entirely if not treated promptly.

Symptoms: Advance symptoms before an attack are diminished vision, coloured halos around electric lights, some pain in the eye, headache, and dilated pupil. The acute attack is characterized by rapid loss of sight and severe throbbing pain in the eyeball and photophobia (intolerance to light). Headache and vomiting may be so severe that the disease is often mistaken for a gastrointestinal disorder. The eye becomes stony hard, red, and cloudy and the cornea is steamy. After each attack the vision becomes poorer and the visual field narrower.

Treatment: The doctor will immediately attempt to bring down the pressure with medication that will drain fluid from the interior of the eye, thus reducing the tension. No eye drops should be used without specific instruction from an ophthalmologist, since some medication can worsen the condition in susceptible individuals. Surgery is often necessary.

Prevention: Regular check-ups will establish the tendency to such types of glaucoma. Early detection and immediate treatment will limit its development. (See *Part 3, Early warning signals, Glaucoma* **23a** and **23b**.)

Outlook: If surgery is done early, the prognosis is good.

Dacryocystitis 24

When the lacrimal (tear collecting) sac becomes inflamed, the condition is called dacryocystitis. It is usually a result of an obstruction of one of the tear canals that leads into the nose (nasolacrimal duct). The disease occurs in infants and in adults over forty.

The danger: If untreated, dacryocystitis can cause infection of the cornea.

Symptoms: Pain below the eyeball, redness, and swelling below the eye, which may extend to the eyelids, causing conjunctivitis. Profuse tearing with purulent discharge is usual.

Treatment: Frequent application of hot compresses may help but antibiotics are usually necessary. Probing is of no permanent value. The episode may subside but if tearing persists, it becomes necessary to use surgical treatment, that is, opening a new channel into the nose.

Prevention: Contributing nasal and sinus disorders (such as nasal trauma, deviated septum, nasal polyps, and hypertrophic rhinitis) should be treated early, since dacryocystitis may stem from these disorders.

Outlook: The acute symptoms may subside without recurrence. However, if conservative treatment fails or if the tear duct is permanently closed off by scarring, surgery becomes necessary.

Cataract 25

A slowly growing opaqueness in the lens of the eye, cataract results from a number of causes, the far greatest incidence a concomitant of advancing age. It can also occur congenitally, however. In adults, besides the ageing process, diabetes, infection inside the eye, and, very rarely, exposure to chemical or physical poisons can cause cataracts. Cataracts are not peculiar to man; they occur in most mammals. Generally, cataracts are one of the penalties of growing old.

The disorder begins slowly, with an ever-increasing opacity and a corresponding loss of vision, like a window getting frosted by cold until only light can be seen through it. When a cataract reaches this extreme state it is calle 'ripe' or 'mature'.

The danger: Ultimate loss of vision until surgical treatment.

Symptoms: The basic symptom is a gradual and painless loss of sight. The growing opacity in the lens can be seen. There are some dangerous similarities between *Chronic simple glaucoma* **23a** and cataract, because diminishing vision is gradual in both and sometimes glaucoma appears without pain. Whereas vision lost because of cataracts can always be restored, in glaucoma it is lost permanently.

Treatment: Surgical removal of the lens is the only answer for cataract. With the help of glasses or contact lenses, almost full vision is restored. This form of surgery has reached a high level of skill in our times and has become quite safe. Literally it is an eye-opener – from darkness to light.

Usually some postoperative discomfort is felt at first, because after glasses are fitted, the corrections are imperfect. Objects seem bigger than they actually are, but the eye adjusts quickly and soon full eye comfort returns. Contact lenses for those who can abide them bring more normal vision.

Prevention: If the cataract is the result of normal advancing age, nothing can be done to prevent it. If it is due to diabetes or some other disease, particular care and control of the disease can help to slow or at least delay the development of the cataract.

Outlook: Surgical treatment restores sight with a minimum of risk.

Iritis 26

An inflammation of the iris, the coloured part of the eye, iritis has no fully identified causes, although some infections and, rarely, venereal disease have been indicated, as well as some of the fungus and protozoan infections.

The danger: When complications are severe, some form of glaucoma and blindness can set in. Vision can be obscured by degeneration of the cornea and lens. Watchfulness is necessary since this disease has a tendency to recur.

Symptoms: Pain in the eye radiating to the temple, redness, and blurred vision are the cardinal symptoms. A great deal of tearing, and intolerance to light are also present. The iris becomes swollen or muddy looking, and the pupils contract. The cornea and lens may degenerate. The upper eyelid may become swollen. Movement of the eyeball causes pain.

Treatment: Atropine or other medication is used as an ointment or as eye drops. Steroid therapy is employed locally, as well as taken internally. If

there is a suspicious underlying cause, it should be treated concurrently.

Outlook: On its own, one episode usually responds to treatment, but this disease needs constant supervision, since it tends to return.

Choroiditis 27
(uveal disease)

Choroiditis is the inflammation of the middle layer of tissue deep inside the eye, the choroid (a tissue continuous to the iris). The precise cause is always difficult to track down. Syphilis, TB, fungus, and protozoan infections are sometimes responsible.

The danger: Choroiditis is a serious eye disorder that must be attended to promptly, for it can cause retinal damage, and less commonly, a form of glaucoma and cataracts.

Symptoms: The patient experiences such visual disorders as blurring, occasionally black areas in the visual field and also flashes of light. Pain is usually absent unless the iris is involved. The eye to the non-professional observer seems normal, but the ophthalmoscope will disclose a swollen retina. There can be distortion of objects.

Treatment: Steroid therapy is employed for a long period of time. In general, medication cannot be applied directly because the disorder is deep inside the eyeball and cannot be easily reached. However, on occasion, injections of cortisone into the eye may be helpful. If the underlying cause is known, it should be treated promptly. Choroiditis caused by fungus, worms, or amoebic organisms does not generally respond to steroid treatment.

Outlook: Choroiditis is curable but needs determination and very thorough, careful research to discover and treat the underlying ailment.

Retinitis 28

An inflammation or swelling of the retina,

in either one or both eyes, retinitis may be caused by choroiditis, iritis, blood vessel spasm, and injury.

The danger: Retinitis, when secondary to *Choroiditis* **27**, can result in atrophy of the retina, with the most serious visual impairment. Generally, early treatment is effective in preventing scarring.

Symptoms: The characteristics of retinitis include eye discomfort, reduction of visual sharpness, distortion of the form and size of objects, and a narrowing of the visual field. The ophthalmoscope will reveal swelling of the retina.

Treatment: Immediate cortisone treatment will heal the retina. The cause should be determined and, if possible, removed.

Retinitis pigmentosa 29

A chronic progressive degeneration of the retina, causing atrophy of the optic nerve and blindness, retinitis pigmentosa is hereditary. It shows up in childhood, in adulthood, and in later life. Blindness cannot be staved off. Happily, this is not a common disorder.

Side views become narrower and narrower, so that the patient has what is called tunnel vision, as if looking through two tubes. Central vision, however, remains for a long period of time, with some people for a lifetime. Recently, on the theory that excessive light might contribute to this disease, doctors have begun to prescribe a dark contact lens for one eye, thus slowing the process.

Detached retina 30

Detached retina occurs more frequently in nearsighted people. It can be caused by eye injury or diabetes often late in the disease. The separation of the choroid from the retina is partial at first but becomes complete if not treated promptly. The detachment is usually due to a break in the retina through which fluid pours into the space between the retina and the choroid.

The danger: This is a *Medical Emergency.* As long as the retina is attached in most of the eye, blindness can be prevented.

Symptoms: The patient experiences flashes of lights or sparks or stars, followed later by the sensation of a curtain across the eye.

Treatment: If surgery can be performed before total separation of the retina, the detached part of the retina can be re-attached. The eye surgeon conducts a thorough examination to locate all the breaks (there may be many) and maps out the area of detachment. Surgery consists of bringing the retina and choroid together and sealing the breaks with either diathermy or freezing. The use of the laser beam, in which a tiny beam of light of tremendous intensity is used to heal the rupture, is another successful form of surgery.

Pending the arrival of the doctor, the patient should be kept quiet to prevent further separation. The eyes should be bandaged and the patient kept relaxed.

Prevention: The speed in obtaining quick medical attention can mean the difference between sight or blindness in the affected eye.

Outlook: Good. The operation is eighty-five per cent successful.

Keratitis 31

An inflammation of the cornea (the curved transparent part of the eye in front of the iris and the pupil), keratitis is most often caused today by viral or bacterial infections (one of these viruses is the herpes virus, which may also cause blisters on the lips or genital organs). Other less common causes are tuberculosis, syphilis, and other systemic infections (infections affecting the whole body). An important factor in bacterial keratitis may be infection following the embedding of a foreign object in the cornea. This can be very serious and on rare occasions may lead to the loss of an eye.

The danger: Severe loss of vision.
Symptoms: The patient experiences pain in the eyeball and the feeling that something is in the eye with heavy tearing, redness, a sensitivity to light, and blurred vision. The cornea, which is usually clear, becomes cloudy. A coloured dot may appear on the eyeball. This is a *Medical Emergency*. An ophthalmologist should be consulted immediately.
Treatment: The immediate use of antibiotics, sometimes cortisone, is indicated. Also available is an antiviral medication in drop form for viral keratitis.
Prevention: Systemic keratitis can be avoided, of course, by proper treatment of the underlying disease. To prevent the form of keratitis that results from the embedding of a foreign object in the eye, the prompt removal of that object is, of course, imperative. To remove a foreign object from the eye, a person should blink frequently. Sometimes a flow of tears will dislodge the object. If it cannot be dislodged within a short period of time, seeking help from a relative or local pharmacist can be dangerous; only an ophthalmologist can render proper aid.
Outlook: Good, if treated promptly. Otherwise a complete clouding and scarring of the cornea may occur and may be complicated by *Iritis* **26** and *Glaucoma* **23**. When the cornea is opaque and cloudy, a corneal transplant might help.

Optic neuritis 32

An inflammation of the optic nerve, optic neuritis results from syphilis, acute infectious diseases, multiple sclerosis, internal poisoning (such as thallium, wood alcohol, carbon tetrachloride, and lead) and occasionally by extension from meningitis and encephalitis.

The danger: Untreated cases result in impairment of vision or blindness, more likely the latter. Once the optic nerve has atrophied, nothing can save it. This is a *Medical Alert*.
Symptoms: The patient usually experiences a sudden loss of vision (blind spots

and narrowing of the visual field). Movement of the eyeball may cause pain. The adjacent retina may be swollen, and some bleeding into the retina may take place. Spontaneous remission may occur, but the disease can also drag on for months.
Treatment: Immediate and heavy steroid therapy can save the sight of the eye, particularly if the underlying disease can also be treated.
Prevention: Exposure to toxic causes should be avoided; treatment of the underlying disease should be undertaken.

Temporal arteritis 33

An inflammation of the artery that runs along the temple, temporal arteritis can seriously affect the eye. It occurs in people over fifty.

The danger: This is a *Medical Alert*. Temporal arteritis can result in irreversible damage and blindness of the eye.
Symptoms: The patient suffers a headache radiating from the eye into the temple area, a deep aching pain in the temple artery, which becomes prominent, pulseless and often nodular, and a tenderness in the scalp. A sudden loss of vision may occur in one or both eyes. Sometimes double vision is experienced at the beginning.
Treatment: In patients showing early manifestations of this disease systemic steroid therapy is immediately administered.
Prevention: (See *Part 3, Early warning signals, Temporal arteritis* **33**.)
Outlook: Poor unless caught early.

Eye disorders resulting from tobacco and alcohol 34

Alcohol taken in moderation does not generally cause deleterious effects on the eyes. Tobacco from the point of view of the ophthalmologist is generally unsalutary even in small amounts. Both alcohol and tobacco if taken in excess and

227

especially when combined can cause blind spots in central vision and disturbances of colour, especially red and green. Chronic alcholism also causes eye muscle palsies and often involves the nerves that lead to the eye muscles. When a person is both a heavy smoker and alcoholic, the total effect on the eyes is much worse. The outlook is generally good if smoking and drinking is stopped and a proper diet is instituted.

Note: ingestion of methyl alcohol (wood alcohol) is *extremely dangerous* and may lead to optic nerve atrophy and total loss of vision. Symptoms are sudden loss of vision, sometimes double vision at the beginning. Since treatment is difficult, prevention is of the utmost importance. Keep all chemical agents out of reach of children. Have them properly labelled. Never take your medicine in the dark without identifying the label.

Eye disorders resulting from side effects of commonly used drugs 35

Digitalis: One of the most commonly used drugs for heart conditions, digitalis is a marvellous drug, and its discovery has marked a milestone in medicine; it does, however, have some side effects on the eye that should be reported to the treating doctor. Snowflakes may be seen when there is no snow. Vision may become yellow. Rainbows may be seen. These symptoms generally disappear when the dosage is reduced.

Cortisone: Often a lifesaving and sight-saving drug, prolonged use of cortisone may cause cataracts or glaucoma. If the drug is to be used for a long period of time, ophthalmological observation is recommended.

Tranquillizers: These drugs have brought relief to millions of people around the world. Some of the drugs may on occasion cause blurred vision or double vision; some should be used cautiously, as in

cases of glaucoma. The need for treatment will generally outweigh the risk of the eye complications. Any visual disturbances during treatment should be promptly reported to the treating doctor. *Aspirin:* In large doses, aspirin may sometimes cause haemorrhages into the retina.

Important: drugs sometimes used for diarrhoea and gall bladder and stomach disturbances may contain atropine or a belladonna type of ingredient. These may provoke an acute attack of glaucoma. Drugs used against Parkinson's disease and some travel sickness drugs may have a similar effect. When blurred vision occurs during treatment for gout and high blood pressure, it should be reported to the doctor.

According to some opinions, female sex hormones, including contraceptive pills, may cause eye symptoms, such as blind spots, rarely double vision, very rarely a blockage of the retinal artery or vein. Other doctors do not believe that such occurrences are direct results of the 'pill'. It is prudent, however, for any patient on the 'pill' to report visual changes to her doctor.

Blepharitis 36

An inflammation of the eyelid margins, blepharitis is usually due to staphylococcus bacteria.

The danger: In addition to scarring the eyelids and the resulting loss of eyelashes, blepharitis can leave the way open for secondary infections of *Conjunctivitis* **21** and corneal disorders (*Keratitis* **31**). It is also very apt to recur.

Symptoms: The patient experiences a burning, smarting feeling in the eye as well as a swelling and itching of the eyelids, the margins of which become thickened, inflamed, and encrusted with tiny ulcers or blisters. The eyes tear, and the eyelashes fall out. Crusts form, which are tenacious and hard to remove. This is particularly bad upon awakening; the eyelids are glued together and separating them is both difficult and painful. A feeling of something being in the eye is common.

Treatment: This ailment is resistant to treatment and when cured can recur. An antibiotic or sulphonamide ophthalmic ointment is applied directly to the eyelid margins after the crusts have been removed. Antibiotic and steroid drops are used to ward off secondary infections. Continued and prlonged use of steroids requires medical supervision to prevent glaucoma. Home remedies – hot compresses, boric-acid solution – are of mild benefit.

Prevention: Along with the usual hygienic measures – use of individual towels and washcloths – it is very important that mascara brushes, eye cosmetics, applicators, and materials should be kept meticulously clean and not passed from person to person. The disease is contagious.

Outlook: Blepharitis responds well to treatment but tends to recur.

Sty 37
(hordeolum, chalazion cyst)

An acute infection of one of the tiny sebaceous glands of the eyelid, a sty is usually caused by staphylococcus.

Symptoms: The patient experiences a burning, smarting feeling in the eye, a feeling of something being in the eye, tearing, and photophobia. Redness, pain, and swelling in the eyelid occur, along with the appearance of a small, hard, red boil at the base of an eyelash. Tender to the touch, the boil soon ruptures, discharging pus, which usually relieves the pain.

A sty that forms deep inside the eyelid is called a chalazion cyst and is more severe and more painful.

Treatment: Hot compresses over the eye three or four times a day and antibiotic medication applied locally will heal the sty. An eye surgeon will often have to remove the chalazion under local anaesthesia. If a crop of sties keep recurring, a staphylococcal vaccine is sometimes used.

Xanthelasma 38

Xanthelasma, flat or slightly raised yellow nodules of fat on the eyelids, occurs mainly with ageing people. Painless, it may result from excessive amounts of cholesterol in the blood, which may be deposited in the skin or on the inside wall of the arteries. A doctor should be consulted, because proper diet and medication can help. When cosmetically objectionable, lesions may be removed surgically by an ophthalmologist.

Colour blindness 39

This condition occurs mainly in males. Red and green become indistinguishable. In the more severe form of this disorder, all colours are seen as black and white.

Colour blindness is hereditary but can skip a generation – a grandfather can give it to his grandson. There is no treatment and no cure.

Excessive use of alcohol and cigarettes can infrequently cause a temporary state of colour blindness, but cutting out the cause will restore colour sight.

Floating spots 40

Floating spots are specks that float in the vitreous, the semi-solid gelatinous substance that fills the eyeball. They cast black and brown shadows on the retina and are always moving or floating. They can be few or many in numbers and can be annoying as well as alarming. They can occur simultaneously in both eyes.

In a small percentage of cases, they may indicate some more significant eye disorder. An ophthalmologist can answer this question. Generally, floating spots are a result of the ageing process and occur mainly in nearsighted people between the ages of fifty and seventy.

Exophthalmos 41

Not a common disorder, exophthalmos, a protrusion of one or both eyeballs, is caused by a number of varying disorders, such as hyperthyroidism (the most likely cause), tumour in the socket, thrombosis of a vein in the socket, glaucoma, abnormal myopia in one eye, or swelling from infected sinuses.

If the advent of the protrusion is sudden, it is usually due to haemorrhage inside the eyeball socket or an inflamed adjacent sinus. If the protrusion takes several weeks or months to become noticeable, it is usually due to a slow-growing tumour or even a very slowly developing aneurysm, particularly when it is pulsating and affects only one eye.

If both eyes are involved, it is indicative of exophthalmic goitre.

The danger: Concern is directed not so much to the affected eye as to the seriousness of the responsible cause. If the eyeball protrudes too much there is danger of ulceration of the cornea.

Symptoms: The obvious symptom is protrusion of the eyeball with frequent pain in the eye-socket. In exophthalmic goitre there is also lid lag, so that a large amount of the white of the eye is seen and there is an absence of blinking.

Treatment: When the eye itself is affected, measures have to be taken to protect it. Generally, however, the treatment is for the originating disease. In extreme cases, surgical socket decompression is the answer. Steroid medication is often helpful.

When protrusion is caused by hyperthyroidism, the treatment indicated is for thyroid hyperactivity (*Hyperthyroidism* **340**).

Outlook: Protruding eyeball is a symptom rather than a disease. If the causative disease is curable, the protrusion is usually curable as well.

Arcus senilis 42

A result of the ageing process, arcus senilis is the formation of a thin, white,

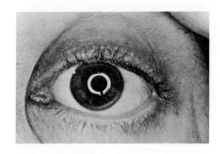

Corneal arcus or arcus senilis appears as white ring around the outer edge of the cornea. (*National Eye Institute, National Institutes of Health, USA*)

opaque ring around the edge of the cornea. Not usually noticeable, except by the subject himself, the disease has no bearing on the health of the eyes or of sight. Mainly, it occurs in people over sixty but has been known to occur in people in their mid-forties. Occasionally, a similar condition may be due to a deposit of fat in the tissues, indicating a problem with the metabolism of certain fats.

Pterygium 43

A triangular, white, opaque growth over the cornea and towards the pupil, pterygium occurs more often in areas where dust, wind, and inclement weather prevail. It is not serious, but if it interferes with sight, it can easily be removed surgically.

Systemic diseases that affect the eye 44

During a complete eye examination the fundus (background of the eye) is examined. This is, in a sense, a miniature physical examination, since this is the only place in the body forming a window, so to speak, through which live veins, arteries, and nerves can be seen. Scores of diseases that originate elsewhere in the body may manifest themselves in the eye. Discovery during an eye examination permits early diagnosis and treatment.

Besides the three major systemic diseases listed below, other ailments that may first manifest themselves in the eye are disturbed function of the thyroid (protruding eyeballs), diseases of the blood, brain tumour or abscess, shingles, kidney diseases (impaired vision, puffiness of eyelids), gout, Hodgkin's disease, meningitis, multiple sclerosis, and others.

Diabetic retinopathy 45
(diabetic retinitis)

Diabetes of many years' duration commonly involves one or more structures of the eye. The blood vessels of the retina may degenerate, causing aneurysms (burst blood vessels that bleed into the vitreous, producing blood spots and blurring). The optic nerve may be damaged and can lead to loss of sight. Diabetes is a common cause of blindness.

In recent years the outlook has become more hopeful with the advent of laser and light coagulating treatment (see *Detached retina* **30**). Many doctors believe that

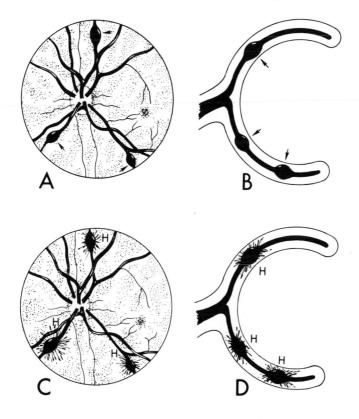

Diabetic retinopathy. A: Damage first occurs in the walls of the retinal capillaries. Arrows point to the capillary walls which balloon out, forming aneurysms. B: Cross-section of the eye also shows aneurysms. C: The walls of the aneurysms are weak; blood can easily flow through them. D: The cross-section shows these haemorrhages contained within the retina. (*Blindness Annual 1969*, American Association of Workers For The Blind).

the diabetic process in the eye can be arrested by means of these treatments. (Also see *Diabetes* **332**.)

Hypertensive retinopathy 46

The ophthalmologist will determine the amount of damage done to the blood vessels in the retina by the high blood pressure. This information, in turn, will help the general practitioner decide how intensive the treatment should be. (Also see *High blood pressure* **138**.)

Arterio-atherosclerotic retinopathy 47

An indication of how far hardening of the arteries has progressed can also be gained by an examination of the fundus. When hardening of the arteries is well advanced, the tiny blood vessels in the retina are damaged as well. The blood vessels either rupture or become blocked, thus depriving the cells of the retina of needed nourishment. Partial blindness can result. (Also see *Arteriosclerosis, Atherosclerosis* **123**.)

3 The ear

Donald R. Weisman

The ear serves the dual purpose of not only hearing but also the vital function of equilibrium.

Although total deafness is comparatively rare, partial deafness is common. People have varying degees of hearing loss, resulting from disease, heredity, and the trauma of exposure to today's noisy environment. Particularly vulnerable are tractor operators, drillers, factory workers, traffic policemen, military and aircraft personnel, and all those who work in very noisy surroundings. The high levels of amplification at which rock music is played are exacting a terrible price in terms of hearing loss in both listeners and performers. Noise pollution is a serious menace. Everyone subject to this destructive influence would be well advised to guard against it.

Here is an oversimplification of how the extraordinary organ of the ear works: Atmospheric sound waves are collected at the ear and strike the eardrum (tympanic membrane), making it vibrate. This, in turn, activates the tiny chain of three bones, or ossicles, in the middle ear, causing them to vibrate and increase the force of the sound waves more than half again.

The sound waves, in turn, through the medium of the clear liquid in the inner ear, transfer the vibrations to very special cells, which convert the mechanical

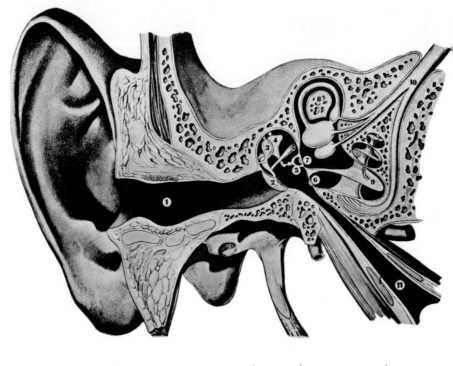

Cross-section of the ear. (*United States National Institutes of Health*)

waves to electrical impulses. The impulses are sent by the acoustic nerve to the brain, where the big computer transforms the electric stimuli into intelligible sound and noises. The mystery is the translation of vibrations into electricity and then into identifiable sounds. It remains incomprehensible and incredibly complex.

Despite the areas of mystery, surgeons are able to reconstruct a disease-damaged or developmentally faulty sound-conduction apparatus and restore most conductive hearing loss. Delicate procedures on the inner ear can restore a sense of balance to one suffering from intractable vertigo. But deafness resulting from de-

terioration of the acoustic nerve is not as yet subject to surgical correction. Active research in this field offers a hope for the future. Acupuncture performed by masters of this ancient Chinese art has been found ineffective in dealing with nerve deafness.

DEAFNESS

There are two basic kinds of hearing loss, conductive and perceptive, or nerve loss. (A third type is the frequently occurring mixture of these two.) Conductive deafness results from obstruction in the transmission of sound through the external ear canal, across the tympanic membrane, and along the chain of ossicles to the inner ear and nerve. Wax in the canal or a collection of water produces an easily remedied form of conductive hearing loss. Otosclerosis is a condition in which the stapes, the stirrup-shaped innermost ossicle, is rigidly attached to the inner wall of the middle ear, thus blocking sound transmission. Surgery performed under the microscope can usually restore hearing. More about this in a moment. As noted above, surgery is not performed for perceptive deafness, but a carefully fitted and engineered hearing aid may provide the acoustically deprived with an awareness of environmental sound.

In addition to the audiometer, which accurately gauges the degree of nerve damage loss, and the tuning fork, which determines whether the hearing loss is conductive or perceptive, the otologist's arsenal now includes newly developed tests and highly sophisticated electronic equipment that can pinpoint with great accuracy the site of small tumours and other lesions.

Conductive hearing loss 48

People who suffer from this form of hearing loss tend to speak in a much lower voice because they hear their own voices at amplified loudness levels by conduction through the bones of the skull.

The doctor can test for conductive hearing loss by using a tuning fork. A vibrating fork is first placed close to the ear. If the ringing sound is heard better on the bone, deafness is of the conductive type. (A home test for hearing loss is described in *Table 7*.)

In addition to wax and water in the ear and to the otosclerotic stapes fixation described above, conductive hearing loss is encountered in such diseases as otitis media, mastoiditis, eustachian tube blockage (usually a concomitant of a cold), and boils and growths in the ear. (See *Part 3, Early warning signals, Deafness in infants and children* **48** and **49**.)

Note on hearing aids: there are two kinds of hearing aids, air conduction and bone conduction. Air conduction aids are worn in the ear, while bone conduction types are worn against the bone behind the ear. Hearing aids can only improve hearing; they do not bring the hearing back to normal.

A hearing aid should be expertly prescribed by an otologist or an audiologist at a speech and hearing centre and dispensed by a reputable dealer. Everyone who is partially deaf has a unique and particular hearing problem that needs special designing and fitting, which can be done only by a specialist. It is the specialist who can devise the best possible improvement in hearing. Buying a hearing aid 'off the counter' is like buying a pair of spectacles from a pushcart. Bargain-priced hearing aids or 'miraculous new invisible wonders' will invariably prove to be a waste of money.

Perceptive hearing loss 49

People who suffer from perceptive hearing loss, or nerve damage, tend to speak quite loudly to compensate for their own voice, which they hear much more faintly.

They cannot hear sounds in the high frequency range. Sounds like *p, k, t*, and hard *g* are also out of their range, although other sounds are heard normally, so that often ordinary speech is unintelligible to them. The word 'tall' is heard as 'all'. 'Sit' may sound like 'fip', that is, if hearing is not so severely impaired that the sounds cannot be heard at all. Such persons hear no better on the telephone, because bone conduction is even more severely impaired than air conduction.

What are the causes of perceptive (nerve) hearing loss?

1. The repeated loud sounds of a noise polluted environment can cause permanent hearing loss, as well as a single, sudden loud blast.

2. Presbycusis, a result of old age,

accounts for sixteen per cent of all hearing loss and cannot be alleviated.

3. A blow to the ear can cause permanent injury of the acoustic nerve.

4. Trauma to the head of sufficient force to cause loss of consciousness (cerebral concussion) can often result in deafness as a result of irreversible brain damage.

5. Certain medications and drugs, such as quinine, may cause deafness (occasionally recovery is possible after discontinuance). Streptomycin and certain other antibiotics, such as the recently available gentamicin, may have effects upon the acoustic nerve, particularly if kidney function is in any way impaired. Overdosage of aspirin and other salicylates on sensitive individuals can cause hearing loss and noises in the ear. Arsenic and mercury are known poisons, which not only affect the body but hearing as well. Over-indulgence in alcohol can often cause permanent hearing loss. Mescaline (peyote) causes distortion of tone and hallucinatory sounds.

6. Arterio-atherosclerosis can cause presbycusis as a result of reduced blood supply to the acoustic nerve.

7. Deafness can be a symptom of Ménière's disease, tumours of the brain, and tumours of the acoustic nerve.

8. Congenital deafness is most often caused by rubella (German measles) during the first three months of pregnancy. The risk of deafness in the newborn is so high that abortion should be performed in all such cases.

9. Other causes of perceptive hearing loss are the use of forceps during delivery, Rh blood incompatibility, and complications from such diseases as syphilis, meningitis, mumps, measles, strep infections, anaemia, and leukaemia. (See *Part 3, Early warning signals, Deafness in infants and children* **48** and **49**.)

Otosclerosis 50

A common ear disorder, otosclerosis is mainly a result of some inherited factor. Although this form of conductive deafness occurs mainly in women from sixteen

to forty, it is far from uncommon in men. The stapes (the smallest bone in the body, smaller than a grace of rice) in the middle ear is fixed and prevented from vibrating because of a new growth of spongy bone around it. This lack or loss of vibration makes it impossible for the nerve to send any message to the brain.

The danger: Progressive conductive deafness and tinnitus (a ringing, buzzing, or hissing sound in the ears), will become chronic unless surgically treated. Perceptive deafness sometimes occurs late in the course of the disease.

Symptoms: First, the patient experiences a slow, stealthy loss of hearing. Then tinnitus sets in, followed by a distortion of sounds, which is noticed more easily by singers and musicians. The low tones are the first to go. This condition is worsened by pregnancy, and an increasingly soft voice may be noticed, although it seems normal to the subject. Pregnancy should be avoided or terminated in a young woman with an established diagnosis of otosclerosis.

Treatment: Surgery has a ninety per cent success record. The operation, a stapedectomy, has been improved with newer developments and a greater incidence of success in recent years. A brilliant new method removes the stapes and replaces it with a vein graft or a plastic device. Within a week, the patient has returned to normalcy, with either significant improvement or total restoration of hearing. The operation poses no danger to life.

Prevention: None known.

Outlook: Favourable with surgery. For those not so inclined, a quality hearing aid is advised.

THE OUTER EAR
Wax in the ear 51
(cerumen)

The most common cause of conductive hearing loss, wax in the ear is often a medium for bacteria, which can cause infections. For that reason, it is better to have a doctor remove the wax. He can see if the eardrum has been perforated or whether there is some form of middle-ear infection, which can cause dizziness. When infection is present, he will not wash out the wax by syringing, which might spread the infection and further contaminate the middle ear, but will remove it by other means, usually a small hand-held instrument called a cerumen curette. For most persons, such treatment once a year may be enough. For others, prolific wax producers, a visit to the ear doctor every three or four months may be necessary. Self-treatment, which includes instillation of so-called wax solvents or olive oil and syringing one's own ear, is fraught with danger.

Boils in the ear canal 52
(furunculosis)

The symptoms of boils in the ear canal include pain and diminished hearing and a feeling of fullness in the ear. Often there is pain along the jaw. The ear canal may be swollen or totally blocked by the boils, which can occur singly or in multiples with consequent blockage of sound. If the condition is mild, insertion of a cotton pledget saturated with easily available Burow's solution or dilute acetic acid can be done by the patient himself. The pledget should be changed ever two or three hours. Aspirin will help to relieve pain. Water should be kept out of the ear. If the condition progresses, an ear specialist should be consulted. He may have to incise the miniature abscess and release the pus, leading to immediate relief.

Furuncles of the ear canal are almost always caused by the staphylococcus, which has gained its unlawful entry through a small crack or fissure in the skin. For this reason one should use great restraint in scratching an itchy ear, particularly avoiding the use of keys, hairpins, and other such implements. A penicillin derivative is extremely effective against many forms of staph and will often be prescribed for a person who is not allergic to penicillin.

External otitis 53
(swimmer's ear)

External otitis is simply an inflammation of the ear canal, usually caused by swimming in less than the purest waters – crowded or excessively chlorinated swimming pools, for example. Pain is usually moderate but can be severe. There may even be some fever. If the fever is mild, self-treatment as indicated under *Boils in the ear canal* **52** will soon correct the condition. If the fever or the pain is more than moderate, a doctor should be called. Antibiotic therapy may be necessary.

Fungus infected ears 54
(otomycosis)

Poor hygiene and swimming in polluted waters may cause a fungus infection in and around the ear canal. Although the patient usually may feel some pain, the infection is mainly characterized by strong itching. There may be grey or black particles (fungi) in the ear. Mild cases may be treated with Burow's solution or dilute acetic acid; severe cases require the services of a doctor. Any effect upon hearing will be temporary.

Misshapen ears 55
(cauliflower ears)

Plastic surgery can do wonders for both congenitally misshapen ears and cauliflower ears, a result of bleeding under the skin from blows or trauma which when untreated become deformed.

237

THE EARDRUM
Perforation of the eardrum 56

The eardrum can be traumatically perforated when toothpicks or hairpins are stuck into the ear, by the careless use of Q-tips to clean the ear canal, or by a blow to the side of the head. A playful slap with an open palm may rupture the drum by implosion.

The position of the eardrum in the ear canal is far nearer the outer ear than anyone would suspect, and perforations are very easily produced. Perforations of infectious origin occur when the pressure of pus in the middle ear bursts through the drum at its weakest point, usually its central portion. This is unfortunate since a central puncture often fails to heal. A small surgical incision called a myringotomy will release the pus and cause it to heal promptly.

The danger: Small perforations of traumatic origin are usually self-healing. Large ones need complicated operative procedures in which a portion of a vein or other donor tissue is placed as a graft to cover the hole.

Symptoms: The pain accompanying traumatic rupture can be agonizing. There is loss of hearing and a hollow reverberation in the head, possibly dizziness, nausea, and vomiting. Blood may appear in the ear canal.

Treatment: Drugs are used to control the pain. A small pledget of clean, *dry* cotton wool should be loosely placed at the orifice of the canal, and a doctor consulted without delay. Even if the perforation is large it may be able to promote spontaneous closure.

Prevention: There is, of course, no way to avoid trauma. Ear infections should be evaluated and treated. Diving, either in sky or sea, should never be undertaken without intensive instruction and training. Persons with small perforations may insert an ear plug, enter the water without diving, and enjoy their swim. Those with large perforations must avoid immersing the head in water.

Outlook: Treatment always effects a cure.

THE MIDDLE EAR
Blockage of the eustachian tube 57
(eustachian salpingitis)

The eustachian tube, which runs from the middle ear to the postnasal air channel (nasopharynx), is a safety outlet for secretions from the middle ear and also serves to equalize the air pressure on both sides of the eardrum. Violent blowing of the nose, without the mouth open, can force infected material into the eustachian tube and contaminate it and possibly the middle ear as well.

The eustachian tube is not normally a wide-open channel. It is closed by muscle and mucous membrane at its lower end behind the nose, opening only as we swallow, yawn, or chew, so that a small amount of air can pass into the middle ear to replace the air that has been absorbed by the mucous lining of the middle ear, and thus maintain an equilibrium with the atmosphere of the surrounding environment. If anything should impair the ventilatory function of the eustachian tube, such as enlarged adenoids, a bad cold or allergy attack, an enlarging tumour mass, or a sudden descent in a poorly pressurized aircraft, the middle ear will be denied the air it needs. The resulting negative pressure, or suction, will cause the drum to be retracted or drawn inward. If the condition progresses without relief, fluid (actually serum) is drawn out of the bloodstream until it fills the middle-ear space, surrounds the ossicles, and severely impairs hearing. Treatment is usually simple, swift, and relatively painless. In an adult, if a short course of steroid treatment fails to clear the ear, the fluid is drawn out by a needle placed through the anaesthetized eardrum. Children must be hospitalized and placed under a general anaesthetic. The fluid is drained from the middle ear by a small suction tube placed through an incision in the eardrum. Sometimes, particularly when the fluid encountered is thick and gummy, the surgeon will insert a Teflon tube through the incision to keep it patent for many weeks. In any case, a child should undergo concomitant adenoidectomy and tonsillectomy, if adenoids or tonsils are the cause.

Symptoms: Impaired hearing, fullness in the ear, cracking noises during swallowing, occasional dizziness, noises in the ear, and a sensation of fluid in the ear.
Treatment: Nose drops or nasal spray during the early phase may alleviate the blockage. If there is no response, professional help should be sought.

Otitis media 58

A potentially major ear disorder, otitis media is always secondary to an infection of the nose and throat. It is very common in childhood, Basically, otitis media is an infection of the middle ear, by either a virus or a bacteria such as strep, staph, or pneumococcus. It can also develop as a complication of scarlet fever, mumps, pneumonia, measles, flu, diphtheria, whooping cough, and tonsillitis.

The danger: In the non-purulent form, the clinical course may be mild, with a slight pinkness of the eardrum as the only positive finding in addition to the cold. Complete recovery is usually spontaneous. Where progression does occur, medical treatment is essential since complications range through mastoiditis to possibly fatal meningitis or brain abscess.
Symptoms: (Listed hereafter)

Acute otitis media 58a

The primary symptom is a severe stabbing earache, which may be constant or intermittent and may radiate over the side of the head. Other indications are fullness in the ear (which changes with a change of position), tinnitus, tender-

ness over the mastoid bone, and a high fever (up to 40·5°C, 105°F).

Chronic purulent otitis media 58b

An earache may be present. The outstanding symptom is a discharge of offensive pus from the ear. There is also a sense of fullness in the ear plus hearing loss. The eardrum is almost always perforated. A constant stream of pus can cause fatty tissue to grow around the eardrum so that skin can grow through the perforation into the middle ear. This dangerous condition is called cholesteatoma.

Chronic secretory otitis media 58c

Once antibiotics are started the earache of acute otitis media will quickly abate, but fullness, a sensation of fluid in the ear and loss of hearing may remain because of congestion in the lining membrane of the eustachian tube. Pus may still be present in the middle ear.

Treatment: Surgical drainage of the middle ear is usually essential in severe or refractory otitis media. No form of swimming is permissible for some time, even after apparent healing. Alert and watchful treatment is especially recommended in purulent otitis media to prevent mastoiditis.

Antibiotics and other medications should be started as early as possible and continued until all symptoms have disappeared completely. The sinuses, nose, and throat are treated simultaneously. Treatment often will require removal of adenoids, since they are the principal cause of otitis media in children. If there is exuding pus, the ear canal must be kept clean.

Chronic purulent otitis media **58b** is difficult to treat because the germ is resistant to antibiotics and because this disease involves the bony margins of the middle ear. Cholesteatoma must be removed surgically to avoid possibly serious consequences. The pus in chronic otitis not complicated by cholesteatoma should be cultured to determine the type of offending micro-organism so that the most effective antibiotic can be employed, perhaps even as an ear drop. X-rays can demonstrate the extent of the disease as well as the presence or absence of erosion of bone such as might be caused by cholesteatoma. Persistent and vigorous local treatment will often succeed in drying up a chronically draining ear without surgery. A foul-smelling discharge from the ear is a danger sign that warrants immediate medical investigation. In the case of *Chronic secretory otitis media* **58c**, if pus is still present in the middle ear after treatment with antibiotics, surgical incision in the eardrum is necessary to effect drainage.

Prevention: Otitis media is often a preventable disease, particularly in a child. If great care is employed when he has a cold, an upper respiratory infection, or any of the infectious diseases of childhood, accompanied by a rash, and he is taught how to blow his nose properly and is also not allowed to resume his normal activities too soon, he can often avoid this most unpleasant ear ailment.

Outlook: Antibiotics, with the help of some minor surgery, have drastically cut down the dangers of this disease. Barring complications, hearing will always return to normal following recovery, and the affected eardrum will assume an entirely normal appearance.

Mastoiditis 59

Mastoiditis, the inflammation of the several small air spaces within the mastoid bone behind the ear, is most often caused by *Chronic purulent otitis media* **58a**. It can also be due to inflammations of the nose and throat, measles, scarlet fever, and diphtheria, although these last diseases are rapidly becoming extinct thanks to modern immunization procedures.

The danger: This is a *Medical Alert* and requires immediate medical attention. A

serious disease, mastoiditis can end in permanent damage to the middle ear (cholesteatoma) and deafness. Since the mastoid bone is close to the brain, complications of mastoid disease are meningitis, brain abscess, and infected clots that block the large blood vessels at the base of the brain.

Symptoms: Beginning as a sore throat, a cold, and a moderate earache, mastoiditis in its acute form will progress to severe pain, high temperatures, a red tenderness behind the ear, and occasionally a stiff neck. Examination will reveal an abnormal eardrum, sometimes a bulge in the roof of the ear canal, and a discharge from the external ear.

Treatment: In most cases vigorous antibiotic treatment, if begun early, will make surgery unnecessary. Occasionally, surgery to remove the diseased parts of the mastoid bone is required.

Prevention: To prevent mastoiditis with its complications, every earache that does not disappear in a day or so must be considered serious, especially if there is pus in the ear.

Outlook: Acute mastoiditis has become relatively rare because of antibiotics and can be kept under control by advanced surgery in nasopharyngeal medicine. If surgery should become necessary, the operation is quite simple, non-mutilating, and yields good results.

THE INNER EAR
Ménière's syndrome 60

A disturbance of the inner ear, or labyrinth, Ménière's syndrome is most common in later life, involving both sexes about equally. Ménière's syndrome, a disease of equilibrium, is caused by tumour, allergy, infections, leukaemia, arterio-atherosclerosis, toxicity from quinine, salicylates, genetic factors, streptomycin, and physical or emotional stress.

The danger: Besides the possibility of accidental physical disability as a result of severe imbalance, Ménière's syndrome may also cause deafness.

Symptoms: This disease usually begins with a mild perceptive deafness in one ear. The most dramatic symptom is loss of balance (vertigo), which is often preceded by a sense of fullness in the ear or an increase in the loudness of the tinnitus, but can also occur without warning.

The attacks often come on abruptly, last from minutes to hours, and are often associated with nausea and vomiting. Attacks are intermittent. The patient may feel fine for months or even years at a time. The degree of deafness often fluctuates.

Treatment: There is no universally accepted medical or surgical treatment. One approach is to reduce fluids in the inner ear by the use of diuretic drugs and abstinence from salt. Tranquillizers and seasickness pills are often used. Antihistamines and blood vessel dilators are additional forms of medicinal therapy. Since many feel that the effect of stress upon a sensitive labyrinth is a contributory factor, psychiatric counsel may help to achieve a more placid emotional response to the pressures of living.

In severe cases where medical treatment has failed to relieve the disabling symptoms (a very small percentage), various surgical procedures are available to destroy all or part of the inner ear. One such operation, called labyrinthectomy, should be performed only on an ear that is already severely or totally deaf, since it will accomplish its goal of relief of symptoms while sacrificing any residual hearing in the operated ear. There are conservative procedures designed to relieve the vertigo while sparing or even improving the hearing. Ultrasonic vibrations applied to the labyrinth through a special probe require a preliminary mastoidectomy. A recently developed operation uses a tube-like shunt to decompress and drain the fluid-filled inner-ear sac.

Prevention: Unknown.

Outlook: Prolonged remissions are not uncommon, and the disease may disappear completely with time.

Motion sickness 61
(seasickness, mal de mer)

Motion sickness is caused by a disturbance in the sensitive nerve receptors of the inner ear as a result of shifting fluids (endolymph) within three semi-circular canals. Why some people become seasick while others do not is poorly understood. Any kind of motion can produce motion sickness, plane, bus, automobile, train, and, of course, boats, large and small. Sometimes riding facing backwards will produce symptoms, while riding forwards will not. This phenomenon is a demonstration of the intimate liaison between the nerve centres of the eye and the ear.

People with a chronic infection of the eustachian tube, the sinuses, or the ears are more prone to this ailment. Small things can trigger the symptoms, such as a hot, stuffy compartment on a train, strange or loud sounds, or seeing the horizon go up and down.

The danger: In itself, seasickness, although a dreadfully disabling experience, is not serious. But unabating symptoms over a prolonged period, as in a sea voyage, can lead to dehydration, acidosis, and profound mental depression. Recovery is usual after a few days on terra firma.

Symptoms: The basic symptoms are, of course, nausea and vomiting, often in recurrent waves. There is also dizziness, a greenish pallor, cold sweat, and difficulty in breathing. The extreme unpleasantness of motion sickness will cause physical and mental prostration.

Treatment: The best treatment is prevention. Once nausea and vomiting have taken hold, cure or even alleviation is poor. The three main drugs are Dramamine, Bonine, and Marezine. The last one does not usually make one sleepy, but its duration is relatively brief, whereas the first two may last all day long but tend to cause drowsiness.

When symptoms appear during travel, one should place oneself in a reclining position and try to keep one's head still.

He should not try to read, look at the passing scenery, or, if on a boat, watch the undulating horizon. Alcoholic drinks, including that old but useless remedy iced champagne, should be avoided, but small amounts of ginger ale, cola drinks, or fruit juice may be tolerated. The sucking of ice is sometimes beneficial. Inhalation of oxygen, if available, will often relieve symptoms.

Prevention: The distress of seasickness can be prevented by taking the indicated drugs in advance of a trip. Anyone convalescing from an illness should delay travel until he is fully well. A good way to prevent seasickness is to take anti-motion sickness pills all during the trip, even when feeling fine. Additionally, the traveller should have plenty of sleep and eat sparingly before departing and while en route.

Outlook: Good, but possibly not until after the trip is over.

Flying and earache 62

Some people are prone to earache while flying, particularly those who have a history of eustachian tube trouble. An infection of the nose and throat may lead to contamination of the middle ear during flight. Any susceptible person with an upper respiratory infection should postpone his trip.

Chewing, swallowing, and yawning during the descent of the plane may prevent problems. Any drug (inhalant or spray) that shrinks the mucous membrane should be employed just before descent.

4 The nose and throat

Donald R. Weisman

THE NOSE

Tradition holds the nose in great esteem, as an indicator of character, a mirror of the ego, and even at times a sexual symbol. For Rostand it was the source of great personal pride and magnetism. Comics have made it the butt of their humour. Who can think of famous personalities without picturing their distinguished nasal profiles: Cleopatra, Caesar, Barbra Streisand, John Barrymore. Although no longer considered an indicator of character, the nose is, nevertheless, an important functioning organ in both health and disease.

The nose is truly a unique and vital structure – a self-cleaner that filters out all particles and some bacteria, thus preventing them from reaching the lungs. In addition, the nasal secretion contains an antibacterial substance called muramidase. The nasal passages also act as an air conditioner – all air breathed in through the nostrils is adjusted to body temperature even though the temperature outside might be far below zero, and humidified by the turbinate bones in the nose. Mouth breathers lose this vital function.

Injuries to the nose

The nose is the most frequently injured bony structure in the body. Its prominent location on the face makes it subject to traumas of various sorts. When subjected to a blunt force such as a fist, a batted ball, or a dashboard, its bony skeleton is easily fractured. Two main questions arise in connection with a fracture of the nose: Is the displacement of

243

the fractured segments sufficient to cause a cosmetic deformity? Is there an impingement of the breathing space with or without a visible external deformity? If the answer to both of these questions is negative, no corrective procedure is necessary. The fracture will heal and the bones will unite within a period of some two or three weeks, and the nose will be as stable and attractive as it was before.

Injuries to the nose are always accompanied by considerable swelling and tenderness, making precise clinical evaluation of the bony alignment or lack of it quite difficult. Fortunately, speed in correcting any resulting deformity is unnecessary. The swelling will subside in several days, following which a careful examination will delineate the extent of injury. This is well within the time period during which a simple corrective realignment procedure can be performed under local anaesthesia, even in a child. X-rays are of little help and will often be negative even in the presence of an obvious clinical fracture.

Initial treatment of an injured nose should consist of nothing more than rest, early application of ice packs to prevent swelling, and control of any bleeding. Once swelling has set in and the eyes have become black and blue no local treatment will be effective. Treatment with certain enzymes or even steroids may hasten the resolution of the oedema (swelling).

Common cold 63
(acute viral rhinitis,
acute coryza)

The organ that most expresses the distresses of the common cold is the nose. It bears the full brunt of this most common ailment afflicting man.

About forty viruses can produce the cold. Many of these viruses can be found in healthy, asymptomatic people (carriers who do not have the disease).

A cold is spread by droplets from a person who has one of the viruses – coughing, talking, sneezing – or by con-

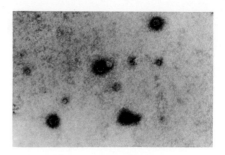

Electron micrograph of a cold virus. Magnification: 175,000 times. (*United States National Institutes of Health*)

tact with objects upon which these droplets have been sprayed. The incubation period is from one to four days.

Good health is not necessarily a barrier to catching a cold, although depression, fatigue, and nervous tension can help bring it on much faster. Experiments in England have shown that chilling is not a major factor.

The danger: By reducing body resistance, particularly in children and the elderly, the common cold can lead to such complications as pneumonia, tracheobronchitis, laryngitis, sinus infections, and ear disorders. Whenever a cold is accompanied by a high fever (more than 38·9°C, 102°F) or pain in the ear, chest, or lungs, a doctor should be called.

Common bacteria normally found in a healthy nose or throat can proliferate, because of the weakened defences of a body struggling with a heavy cold, and cause bronchitis, otitis, and sinusitis, especially in children who have not yet developed toughness or immunity.

Symptoms: A cold usually comes on suddenly, often taking the subject by surprise. The throat is frequently irritated, the nose runs, there is some sneezing, and a feeling of discomfort. In children, there may be some moderate fever.

The ensuing headache is moderate; if it is severe, other diseases or complications should be suspected. Often there is loss of smell or of taste, vague aches in the back or legs, occasionally a cough. Later, the nose becomes obstructed, necessitating constant blowing. The voice may become either weak or husky.

Serious diseases that resemble a cold

Measles **370**, *German measles* **371** and *Chicken pox* **372** can simulate a cold, having similar symptoms except for the telltale sign, a body rash.
Flu **376** begins like a cold but soon the malaise and fever become quite severe, with strong aches in the back and legs.
Diphtheria **358**, after the initial cold symptoms, moves rapidly to unusually deep fatigue and a severe sore and swollen throat. Swallowing becomes very difficult. Childhood immunization procedures have all but eliminated this onetime killer.
Whooping cough (pertussis) **357**, after early cold symptoms, soon develops into a virulent cough, which gets even worse in a few days. Pertussis vaccination prevents this disease.
Meningitis **7** begins with cold symptoms that soon worsen to high fever with a characteristic stiff neck.
Strep throat (pharyngitis) **73** usually begins with a cold and is soon accompanied by severe chills. Parents should be sensitively alert if a sore throat and a high fever follow. Swallowing becomes difficult, the pulse very rapid and irregular. Complication may be serious and may involve distant organs, such as the heart and kidneys. Fortunately the causative organism, the beta haemolytic streptococcus, is easily destroyed by penicillin and other antibiotics.
Acute bronchitis **103** and *Chronic bronchitis* **104** begin with a cold but soon progresses to include a prolonged, pronounced cough accompanied by shortness of breath.

Treatment: No really useful medication is available for the common cold. Antihistamines do not cure; they only mask

or temporarily relieve some of the symptoms.

Nose drops or one of the better nasal sprays are safe if used for only a few days and may relieve the congestion that usually accompanies a cold. They may also prevent sinus and ear complications.

Antibiotics are of no value unless there are bacterial complications. Since a cold is a virus disease, antibiotics, which destroy or prevent the growth and proliferation of bacteria, are ineffective against it. Thus, repeated and unnecessary use of antibiotics creates a tolerance for the drug in the bacteria normally found in the body. Accordingly, when a bacterial infection does occur, the antibiotic may be far less competent.

Vaccines, alkalis, ultraviolet rays have not proven to be of value.

Decongestants may help to relieve symptoms but should be carefully prescribed. Medications obtained over the counter are usually of insufficient strength to be effective and may be unsuited to the illness being treated. Sweating out a cold by hot baths or heavy exercise only weakens the body and makes one more susceptible to secondary infections. Inhalators are at best palliative.

Vitamin C in large doses remains controversial. For some, it can be quite effective, while for others, eating a pound a day won't help. It is worth a try – at least two grams a day.

The best procedure is rest. Bed rest makes sense if the cold is heavy or if there is fever, especially in children. Fatigue always worsens the disease. Drinking great quantities of fluids is helpful.

A doctor cannot cure or shorten the duration of a cold, but he can be helpful in preventing secondary infections and complications.

Prevention: The rules are simple: avoid crowds in winter, maintain a healthy remoteness from coughers and sneezers. Smokers should put away their cigarettes, pipes, and cigars, preferably for all time.
Outlook: If the patient relaxes, does nothing about the cold, makes no effort to fight it or to return to work sooner than he should, the period from incubation to

recovery will usually last from a few days to a week or two. Nostrums peddled in television commercials should be left to those with a need to throw money away.

Chronic rhinitis 64

An inflammation of the mucous membrane of the nose, chronic rhinitis is a recurrent upper respiratory infection caused by any one of a number of diseases – sinusitis, nasal blockage from a deviated septum, polyps – or other factors, such as a bad climate, continuous exposure to dust and other noxious materials, sensitivity to air pollution, and overuse of decongestants. Smoking greatly increases one's proneness to this disease.

The danger: Chronic rhinitis can sometimes weaken body resistance, thus making it more susceptible to other diseases.

Symptoms: The characteristics of the disease include obstructed nasal breathing, constant nasal discharge, postnasal drip, and mouth breathing. Other symptoms that appear occasionally are sore throat (pharyngitis), inflammation of the eyelid (conjunctivitis), some loss of smell and therefore loss of taste and intermittent headaches.

Treatment and outlook: The best treatment is removal of the offending agent if it can be identified. Industrial and atmospheric pollutants pose an admittedly difficult problem. Humidification of environmental air during cold months may help.

The use of nasal sprays or drops is harmful because constant use eventually thickens the nasal mucosa, causing rebound congestion. The spray or drops do give temporary relief, but the payment for this may be a worsened condition later.

Hay fever and allergic rhinitis 65

Hay fever is caused by wind-borne pollen,

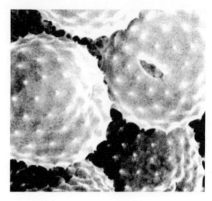

Pollen highly magnified. (*United States National Institutes of Health*)

fungus spores, and moulds. Spring hay fever is due to tree pollen such as oak, maple, and others. Summer hay fever is caused by grass pollen, including wheat and corn, as well as fungus spores.

Perennial allergic rhinitis, however, is not seasonal, as is hay fever, but runs a continuous course throughout the year. Usually the contributing cause is house dust, animal dander and furs, some foods, feathers, industrial fumes, drugs, and polluted air.

Symptoms: Hay fever is characterized by a profuse thin watery nasal discharge, violent sneezing, excessive tearing, and itching of the nose, roof of the mouth, and throat. Often there is photophobia, frontal headache, loss of appetite, insomnia, and exhaustion.

The same symptoms occur in allergic rhinitis, but they are somewhat less severe.

Treatment: The offending allergen must be found in both allergic rhinitis and hay fever. Usually a skin test will reveal the cause. Once this is identified, a specific desensitization programme will usually bring immunity. Antihistamines bring relief in 70–90 per cent of the cases. They are most effective if taken prophylactically, that is, before the attack occurs.

Allergic rhinitis sometimes progresses to sinusitis, nasal polyp formation, or chronic rhinitis.

Prevention: If the causative agent is identified, the elimination of the allergen from the environment can prevent attacks.

Outlook: Most people can be helped if not cured. Allergists have much to offer, and treatment is no longer the endlessly extended process it once was.

Sinusitis: acute and chronic 66

The sinuses are air spaces that empty their secretions into the nasal cavity through narrow ducts. The drainage system is not very efficient, and in some cases the duct is so placed that one would have to stand on one's head for proper drainage. Many feel that the sinuses are a fault of nature, an arrest in the evolutionary process.

The sinuses do have a function, however. They are the resonating chambers for the voice. They also help to heat and moisten the air we breathe and are an integral part of the nasal filtering system. The air within the sinus cavities helps reduce the weight of the skull. When fluid or pus replaces the air, headaches are likely.

Sinuses can become infected from a deviated septum, polyps, nasal allergies, and colds. The infecting micro-organism can range from one of the cold viruses to strep, staph, or pneumococcus germs. Inadequate and poorly placed drainage makes the sinuses ideal feeding grounds for these micro-organisms. Blocked drainage can be caused by polyps, deviated septum, allergies, chronic rhinitis, and dental disorders.

The danger: Untreated sinusitis can progress to more serious complications such as otitis media, acute bronchitis, asthma, pneumonia, and even meningitis. Most cases of sinusitis are mild and of brief duration. When drainage is blocked, however, it can result in severe discomfort.

Symptoms: The basic symptom is headache, which is usually frontal or peri-orbital (around the eye) regardless of which sinuses are affected. The headache may be constant or recurrent. Acute sinusitis may produce chills, fever, mental sluggishness, loss of smell, and occasionally dizziness and vomiting. A serious sign is the development of oedema of an orbit (swelling around the eye).

The degree of blockage determines the degree of the headache and of tenderness over the affected sinuses. The discharge from the nose is thick and yellow, which under a microscope is seen to contain many pus cells and bacteria.

In the chronic form, the mucous lining in the sinus becomes thickened or polypoid, and nasal and postnasal discharges are continuous; the sinuses are laden with pus.

Treatment: Medication for acute sinusitis is not much help, except where the infecting micro-organism is microbial, indicated by the very sick appearance of the patient and a persistent fever. In such cases, antibiotics are quite beneficial, particularly after a culture of the sections has identified the offending organism so that the antibacterial agent most capable of destroying it can be employed.

Vasoconstrictors, in common use, can often do harm because of the greater dilatation that occurs once the effect of the drug has worn off. Basically, the object is to obtain drainage of the infected sinus. This is usually accomplished by the nose and throat specialist, who has many ways of evacuating the pus, most of them both painless and effective. Application of heat over the area is sometimes beneficial. Many specialists use infrared treatments with excellent results.

Convalescence requires about four weeks.

The treatment for chronic sinusitis includes humidifying the patient's room during those periods of the year when steam heat deprives the air of its needed moisture. Forced hot air heat is most unhealthy for chronic sinus sufferers. In general, this disease is frequently difficult to manage. If the cause is an allergy, the allergen must be found and the patient desensitized; if the cause is a nasal growth, it must be surgically removed. The sinuses must be cleaned and irrigated, sometimes repeatedly. The disease-thickened mucosa in the sinus may also have to be surgically removed and effective drainage re-established.

Blowing the nose should be done with care – only one nostril at a time (never violently) with the mouth wide open. This is always helpful in clearing the sinus passages.

Outlook: Usually good with proper treatment. As in other problems involving the upper air passages, smoking in any form should be avoided. Recent studies have shown that a smoking roommate may provide a climate inimical to the patient.

Deviated septum 67

A condition that may be congenital, developmental, or traumatic (blow or fall on the nose), a deviated septum occurs when the long septum, or bony wall, that divides the nose into two breathing passages is twisted or deflected. This condition can lead to obstructed nasal respirations, headaches, postnasal discharge, and even to visible curvature or deformities of the external nose. The remedial process is surgery, in which the nasal contours are aesthetically enhanced.

Postnasal drip 68

Although most of the time postnasal drip is caused by an overactive production of mucus by the glands of the nasal lining membrane, it can also be caused by sinusitis, allergy, and irritation of the mucous membrane of the nose by smoke or dust.

Symptoms: Postnasal drip is characterized by constant hawking in an attempt to clear the throat. Coughing also occurs in some cases, and an occasional choking sensation in others. Bad breath is common in chronic conditions.

Treatment: No specific remedies are available, but some household hints, such as sleeping in a room with a vaporizer during the winter months, sleeping on two or more pillows, and blowing the nose, even if there is no obvious need to do so, may be helpful.

Some people have the bad habit of unconsciously drawing the nasal secretions to the back of the throat, rather than letting them drain out through the nose. This habit should be avoided.

Outlook: Since the causative factors are numerous and variable no statement as to outlook can be uniformly applicable. Generally the condition tends to be chronic.

Nasal polyps 69

Polyps are soft, moist, grape-like growths hanging on a stem in the mucous membrane of the nose. The cause is usually an allergy. Polyps can prevent proper drainage from the sinuses, interfere with breathing, and become a focus of chronic infection. They can occur singly or in huge numbers, completely obstructing the flow of air through the nose. They often arise within the sinus cavities and enter the nose through small drainage openings called ostia. Sometimes the nasal cavity will be entirely free of polyps, but respirations are blocked by one or more polyps hanging by a long pedicle, or stalk, in the space that communicates between the back of the nose and the throat. These are called antrochoanal polyps and are often missed on routine examinations because of their hidden location.

Symptoms: Polyps in the nose may be indicated by a loss of smell, headaches, excessive nasal discharge, and nasal obstruction.

Treatment: Surgical removal of polyps from the nose is performed in hospital or the outpatient department, depending on the extent of the disease, and is a painless procedure under local anaesthesia. A more extensive procedure is required for polyps of sinus origin.

THE THROAT

The throat houses the tonsils and adenoids, the protective fortresses of the body against infections during early childhood. They should not be *routinely* removed, but because their ability to perform their protective function is weakened by repeated acute infections, they may, in turn, become reservoirs of infection, as evidenced by persistent enlargement of the glands of the neck and repeated feverish episodes, as well as altered speech and breathing patterns. In such cases the indication for surgical removal is clear.

Tonsillitis 70

The danger: Severe and untreated tonsillitis can be the source of many serious systemic diseases, such as diphtheria, mastoiditis, septicaemia (blood poisoning), endocarditis, and rheumatic fever.
Symptoms: The onset of acute tonsillitis is generally sudden. Chills and high fever (40·5° or 41°C, 105° or 106°F) are accompanied by extreme pain in the tonsil area. Headache, malaise, pain in the back of the jaw, in the neck, and occasionally a stiff neck also occur. Swallowing is painful and difficult. The congestion results in snoring. The tonsils are clearly enlarged, very red, often ulcerated, and spotted with white streaks. Occasionally there is some coughing.

Chronic tonsillitis is characterized by frequent sore throats throughout the year, a constant nasal discharge, bad breath, frequent colds, loss of strength, fatigue, low energy, frequent low-grade fever, and failure of the child to grow or to gain weight.
Treatment: Antibiotic or sulphonamide therapy relieves the acute form. Anything cold, such as ice cream, is soothing. A tonsillectomy is performed when indicated.
Outlook: Antibiotic therapy is most effective. Mild tonsillitis is a self-limiting disease. Age has nothing to do with the extent of disease. Tonsillitis in adults is quite common and is treated as in children.

Adenoiditis 71

The adenoids are situated in the back of the pharynx, near the nasal passages at the eustachian tube. Like the tonsils, they are guardians against diseases, becoming infected themselves rather than allowing the body to become infected and, like the tonsils, terribly inefficient performers.

The danger: Extreme infection of the adenoids can cause otitis media, fluid collections in the middle ear, and hearing loss.
Symptoms: Mouth breathing is the primary symptom. Other significant signs are snoring, loss of appetite in children resulting from a loss of smell and taste, halitosis, nasal speech, and a very significant symptom, lowered mental ability resulting from chronic air hunger. A dull facial expression, the adenoidal facies, is the clue. If the adenoids are shrunken by medication or removed, the slow child may suddenly become alert, brighter, and leap ahead in learning and intelligence.
Treatment: Antibiotics will relieve mild infections. Drinking or eating anything cold (ice cream) can bring about some relief. Repeated infections may require operation. Gargling is useless.
Outlook: Excellent when medically treated.

Quinsy 72
(peritonsillar abscess)

An abscess between the tonsil and the nearby muscle of the pharynx, quinsy usually occurs on one side of the throat and can be caused by tonsillits.

The danger: The abscess can interfere with breathing, prevent swallowing in some cases, and spread to adjacent soft tissue spaces. This may be a *Medical Emergency.*
Symptoms: Quinsy is indicated by a large swelling on the affected side, often occupying a third of the throat area. Pain is severe at the site and at the back of the jaw. The patient speaks in a nasal

twang and endures the near impossibility of swallowing. Trismus, the inability to open the jaw, is a common occurrence. Even in the more moderate form of the disease, the soft palate and the uvula (the elongated tissue hanging down in the back of the mouth) are swollen and easily noticeable. Pain can radiate into the neck. The lymph nodes on the side of the neck are enlarged. The patient is toxic, very sick, with a high temperature.

Treatment: Occasionally the abscess ruptures on its own, but in most cases a surgeon is obliged to incise the abscess and drain the pus, affording the patient immediate relief. Peritonsillar abscess is an absolute indication for tonsillectomy since it is likely to recur in a more virulent form.

Pharyngitis: acute and chronic 73

(simple sore throat and strep throat)

An inflammation of the throat, ranging from mild to serious, pharyngitis is usually caused by an extension of the common cold, tonsillitis, adenoiditis, or sinusitis.

Viral pharyngitis, by far the more common, is mild and usually uncomplicated, but bacterial infections, such as strep throat, are quite frequent and can be quite serious in children. Diphtheria, at one time a more serious disease causing pharyngitis, rarely occurs today.

The noninfectious forms are due to prolonged irritation of the throat resulting from excessive use of the voice, the swallowing of irritating foods (spicy food, alcohol, red pepper), dusty working conditions, smoking, an overindulgence in alcohol, or the breathing of industrial fumes.

Chronic pharyngitis may in rare instances be due to tuberculosis or late syphilis.

The danger: One of the serious dangers of a sore throat, in the bacterial form, particularly strep throat, is that it can lead to rheumatic fever in children. Another hazard of pharyngitis is the formation of an abscess which must be surgically incised.

Symptoms: In acute pharyngitis the throat feels dry, burning, and often as if there were a lump in it. It is bright red and along with the tonsils is flecked with white spots. Swallowing is painful. Often there is a swelling of the lymph glands on the sides of the neck.

In addition, chills and fever occur, and the patient has difficulty in speaking. If stiffness of the neck also occurs, it may indicate meningitis.

In chronic pharyngitis the tissues in the back of the throat are swollen, and the patient endures a heavy, sticky mucus, which is often difficult to clear away and causes gagging, nausea, and vomiting. There may be a persistent cough.

Treatment: The causative organism should be identified by a swab culture to determine whether the disease is a mild viral form or a virulent bacterial type.

If the infection is viral, gargling might bring some relief, as can many of several mildly anaesthetic proprietary throat sprays.

In chronic pharyngitis identification of the cause of the irritation will determine the appropriate treatment (intranasal medication, tonsillectomy and so on).

Malaise and/or fever above 38·3°C, 101°F indicates the possibility of a more serious condition requiring examination by a doctor. If the sore throat is caused by bacteria, namely streptococcus, the doctor will prescribe antibiotics for a full ten days even though the patient has returned to good health days earlier. This will ensure protection against rheumatic fever.

Prevention: Avoid people with pharyngitis as you would those suffering from a common cold. If the cause is specific, such as overuse of the voice or an overindulgence in whisky or smoking, the answer is apparent.

Outlook: The uncomplicated viral form will disappear in three to six days, with no specific treatment and without medical aid or counsel. The bacterial variety needs medical attention and alert care for complete recovery.

Laryngitis 74

An inflammation of the larynx (voice box), the causes of laryngitis are many – the common cold, pharyngitis, sinusitis, tonsillitis, bronchitis, flu, pneumonia, whooping cough, syphilis, measles, excessive or improper use of the voice, inhaling irritating gases or vapours, and poor ventilation.

Chronic laryngitis is due to the inhalation of industrial dust or noxious materials, overindulgence in whisky and smoking, and a thickening of the vocal cords due to the presence of polyps.

The danger: If hoarseness persists for more than ten days, a check-up for possible serious disease is essential. Although the designated period is three weeks before serious consideration of malignant possibilities, one would be well advised to be on the safe side and consult a doctor as early as possible, even though the likelihood of cancer is remote. The examination of the larynx is simple, quick, and painless.

Symptoms: Laryngitis is characterized by a change of voice, hoarseness, rawness in the throat, loss of certain speech sounds, and a constant urge to clear the throat. When the condition is more serious, fever, pain, difficulty in swallowing, and malaise also occur.

Treatment: Absolute voice rest is essential as determined by the doctor. Also, the 'No Smoking' sign is up. Bed rest in a well-humidified room and quantities of fluids are also indicated. Antibiotics will be prescribed by the physician if the cause is bacterial.

Prevention: Most chronic sufferers know the cause and can prevent it. This means abstaining from smoking, heavy drinking, working in places that fill the lungs with dust or noxious fumes, and avoiding poorly ventilated places.

Outlook: If the laryngitis is not a result of some serious disorder, recovery is almost certain within a week if treatment is followed as described.

Benign growths on the vocal cords 75
Polyps 75a

Varying in size and shape, polyps are usually small, warty growths on the vocal cords or hanging from a stem attached to the cords, causing hoarseness and other changes of voice. They can be easily removed by a surgeon.

Fibrous nodules 75b

Sometimes called 'singer's nodes' or 'screamer's nodes', fibrous nodules occur from misuse or overuse of the voice or from excessive smoking. They are easily observed by direct or indirect laryngoscopy (examination of the larynx by observing its reflection in a mirror). Even very small nodes can affect the voices of singers and have been known to bring about a prompt termination of many careers, both promising and established. They tend to occur on the opposing surfaces of the vocal cords and prevent them from contacting one another cleanly during vocalization. The air that escapes through the defect may produce hoarseness. Surgeons are now using an operating miscroscope to facilitate the precise delineation and excision of these tiny lesions. See also *Cancer of the larynx* **439**.

5 The mouth and tongue

Alfred I. Winkler

Perlèche 76

Perlèche, inflamed ulcerations beginning at the corners of the mouth and continuing from the exterior to the inside of the lips, is caused by an excessive folding of the lips, a result of a collapsed bite (the jaws are closing too deeply from inadequate dentures), smoking, and licking the lips. Some clinicians are considering malnutrition as a predisposing factor. Occasionally perlèche is accompanied by secondary infections of staph and strep bacteria, or fungus (thrush).

Symptoms: The corners of the mouth are an intense red, inflamed, and fissured or ulcerated. The area is tender with a painful burning sensation.

Treatment: Correction of the predisposing factors, such as avoidance of smoking or licking the lips, will help to alleviate the condition. New, well-fitted dentures with a normal vertical dimension will decrease the wrinkles. Application of steroid ointments with neomycin or nystatin is the usual procedure.

Trench mouth 77 (necrotizing ulcerative gingivitis, Vincent's angina)

An inflammatory condition of the gums, trench mouth is characterized by necrosis (death) of the gums between the teeth and occurs most frequently among adolescents and young adults. It may be localized to a few spots or it may envelop the entire mouth. A dirty grey membrane forms over the infected area.

The condition is caused by several types of bacteria but mainly by the fusospirochetal organism. No longer considered highly contagious, trench mouth can be triggered off by a run-down condition, insufficient rest, emotional stress, poor oral hygiene, faulty dental arch, untreated cavities, poor fillings, vitamin C deficiency, malnutrition, and heavy smoking. Lead and bismuth poisoning can induce this disease. Other systemic disease factors are diabetes, blood disorders, and gastrointestinal and endocrine disturbances.

The danger: In some cases trench mouth can loosen all the teeth and cause necrosis of the jaw.

Symptoms: The major symptoms are pain, bleeding gums, excessive salivation, a foul taste and bad breath. The gums, which are red and spongy, will bleed at the slightest touch. The dirty greyish membrane that appears in the mouth can be removed. Swallowing and talking are painful. Sores and ulcers appear on the gums and the inside of the cheeks and on some occasions on the tonsils and the pharynx. Fever and malaise are often present.

Treatment: Although trench mouth responds quickly to penicillin or tetracycline, such measures are often not necessary. In mild cases the disease can be treated at home with appropriate hygienic care of the mouth. Good results are obtained from rinses of such oxidizing agents as hydrogen peroxide solution (to twice that amount of water) or sodium perborate (one teaspoon in a glass of water).

Plenty of rest is indicated, but brushing the teeth is contraindicated until so advised by a dentist. The diet should be soft but nutritious without spicy foods or alcoholic beverages. Smoking should be avoided.

If the patient remains sick with a temperature of more than 37·8°C, 100°F, a doctor should be consulted.

Prevention: Good mouth hygiene, good nutrition, and, where possible, avoidance of stress.

Outlook: At worst, trench mouth is quite manageable with antibiotics and is no longer considered a dangerous disease.

Thrush 78
(moniliasis, candidiasis)

An infection caused by the fungus *Candida albicans*, thrush is much more frequent today because of the intake of a broad spectrum of antibiotics, which kill off bacteria and thus leave the field free for fungus infection. Malnutrition and faulty dentures are often implicated.

The danger: The fungus can spread to the pharynx, larynx, gastrointestinal and respiratory tracts, skin, and vagina.

Symptoms: In general, the mouth is dry. Slightly raised white patches that look like milk curds appear inside the cheeks, lips, and on the gums, tongue, and soft palate. These patches later become shallow ulcers. Removal of these white spots is not easy and can cause bleeding.

Treatment: Home treatment is simple. It consists of swabbing the mouth with a one per cent solution of gentian violet or employing Bradosol lozenges or mouthwashes containing Zephiran. With suporting multivitamins, the condition should clear up in a week. If a doctor is called, he will usually prescribe a specific drug for fungus called nystatin or advise amphotericin B locally.

Aphthous stomatitis 79
(canker sores, aphthous ulcers)

A recurrent disease of unknown origin,

aphthous stomatitis is characterized by painful ulcers of the mucous lining of the mouth. The latest belief in the medical profession regarding these most common mouth lesions is that they are induced by psychosomatic factors – mental or emotional distress, business troubles, sexual difficulties, intense grief, anxieties, and so on. More women contract canker sores than men, and more people in higher rather than lower income brackets. Recurrence ranges from once a year to once a month, prior to or after menstruation.

The danger: None. However, occasionally the sore or sores might be some other more significant ulcer. If the ulcerations do not show signs of healing within a week, a biopsy should be considered.

Symptoms: Hours before the appearance of the ulcers, the mouth becomes oversensitive, or there is a pronounced tingling or burning sensation. Soon blisters appear that have red margins; when they erupt they produce small egg-shaped ulcers – yellow or white centres on red. They are very tender and painful. Speaking, smiling, or frowning becomes difficult. Within a week the ulcers are covered with an opaque yellowish coat, which lasts less than four days. A week or two later the ulcers heal without permanent scars. There is no fever and no underlying symptoms. The ulcers may appear singly or in batches; they may heal in one place and break out in another.

Treatment: No specific treatment is required; anaesthetic cough drops or lozenges may help to relieve the pain. A mouthwash, several times a day, of a ten per cent solution of sodium bicarbonate in warm water is soothing. High potency vitamin B complex has on occasion shortened the duration and prevented recurrence. Corticosteroid medication may be applied topically.

Prevention: High-strung persons should try to tune themselves down.

Outlook: A little suffering, but no permanent or serious damage will be experienced.

Herpetic stomatitis 80

Herpetic stomatitis is somewhat similar to aphthous stomatitis, except that the cause is known, the herpes virus, which is dormant until stimulated by traumatic dental treatment, chapped or broken skin, or sunburn on the lips. Food allergies, menstruation, and anxiety can also bring it on.

The danger: None, although the affliction can give the patient a bad week or two.

Symptoms: The gums are inflamed and painful. White plaques and ulcers appear on the mucous membrane of the mouth, producing a foul taste. Before the lesions appear, the patient is sick with fever. In a child the pain may be so severe as to keep him from taking food. The intense phase of the disease lasts less than a week. Within another week all symptoms will disappear. This is a self-limiting disease.

Treatment: There is no specific treatment, but several general measures are helpful. Mouthwash of ten per cent sodium bicarbonate in warm water is soothing and helps in healing. Anaesthetic cough drops or lozenges may be helpful to relieve the pain. Large doses of high potency vitamin B complex can shorten the duration and often prevent recurrence. If the patient is a child, the parents must be on the alert for dehydration.

Prevention: Avoid sunburned lips and extended anxiety states.

Herpes labialis (cold sores, fever blisters) 80a

In herpes labialis, a milder form of herpetic stomatitis, the blisters appear on and around the lips, preceded by a feeling of itching and burning. The blisters last a few days, then burst. The ensuing sore is hard and crusted and takes about a week or so to heal. The blisters should be kept as dry as possible, since moisture delays healing. Applications of drying lotions – camphor, alcohol, or any cold sore medication – can cut the remedial time in half by inhibiting the blisters from erupting and protecting them against secondary infections.

Gangrenous stomatitis 81

(noma, cancrum oris)

A rapidly spreading gangrene of the inside of the cheek, which strikes mostly at undernourished or weak children and the elderly, gangrenous stomatitis often is a result of complications from measles or whooping cough in children between two and six years old.

The danger: This is a *Medical Emergency*. Gangrenous stomatitis is a very grave ailment and must be treated immediately. The patient's life can be saved only by prompt treatment and surgery.

Symptoms: Gangrenous (dead) tissue, grey or black, appears on the gums or the mucous lining of the cheeks or inside the lips. Externally the cheeks become swollen and red, glazed, then black. There is pain and fever. Halitosis and a foul taste in the mouth are minor but consistent symptoms.

Treatment: Massive doses of antibiotics can control the disease.

Outlook: If caught in time, gangrenous stomatitis can be stopped and cured.

Stomatitis traumatica 82

Stomatitis traumatica is not caused by a germ or virus but by a mechanical injury, such as badly fitting dentures or incompleted dental work that leaves exposed rough or sharp surfaces and jagged teeth. Bad chewing habits and accidental biting of the cheek can also bring it on.

The symptoms can be pain, excessive salivation, and bad breath. Stomatitis traumatica can lead to increased susceptibility to other mouth diseases.

Oral lichen planus 83

Basically a skin disease, which can also manifest itself in the mucous lining of the mouth, the cause of oral lichen planus is unknown. It can occur at any age but mostly in the young adult.

It has been noted that the disease will show up more often after an emotional shock or when the subject is under great mental strain or under physical stress. (See also *Lichen planus* **296**.)

The danger: None. Although many patients torment themselves with believing that the ailment is cancerous or pre-cancerous, this notion is false. Although a chronic disorder, oral lichen planus is not pre-cancerous, as is *Leukoplakia* **84**.

Symptoms: Both the erosive and non-erosive forms of this disease are characterized by bluish-white lacy lesions on the lips and inside the lips. In the simple non-erosive form the bluish-white circular lines appear in the mucosa of the mouth but not on the gums. Although the affected parts of the mouth feel rough and itchy, there is no pain.

The lesions that appear in the erosive form vary in appearance and can be felt with the tongue. There is pain and the gums can be involved. The ulcerations keep recurring. The erosive form is often confused with *Herpetic stomatitis* **80**. Sometimes a biopsy is performed to rule out other more dangerous maladies.

Treatment: Anaesthetic troches, benzocaine, topical steroids, and tranquillizers are administered to lessen the pain.

Outlook: The disease may or may not disappear, but it has very little effect on the general health or life of the patient.

Leukoplakia 84

Whitish growths on the mucous lining of the mouth, usually on the tongue and cheek, leukoplakia occurs mostly in men (about two-thirds) who are middle-aged or elderly.

The suspected causes are derived most often from a combination of local (the mouth) and systemic (the body) conditions. Local conditions, include bad dentures, jagged teeth, faulty dental work, nicotine from cigarette, cigar, or pipe smoking, whisky, hot spices, and the habitual taking of very hot food. Systemic conditions include the secondary stage of syphilis, a vitamin A or B deficiency, of gonadal (ovarian or testicular) deficit.

The danger: Leukoplakia can be precancerous and should be carefully checked. It is insidious, since there is no pain or discomfort until late in the development of this disorder. Lesions on the floor of the mouth are particularly likely to become malignant.

Symptoms: White patches, or yellowy-white patches appear on the inside of the cheeks, on the tongue, or on the floor of the mouth – somewhat leathery or thickened. They can be fissured and become ulcerated. Pain, unfortunately, as mentioned above, is a late symptom.

Treatment and prevention: The mouth should be kept scrupulously clean. Bad or faulty dentures, most especially over one of the lesions, should immediately be corrected or removed. All irritants listed earlier must be avoided. Vitamin A buccal tablets should be sucked two or three times a day.

The lesions are removed surgically if the doctor deems it necessary after a biopsy. **Outlook:** Every patient with leukoplakia should be on the alert. Frequent biopsies, even though the previous biopsy was negative, should be performed until the leukoplakia has disappeared. If the disease lasts too long, removal of the lesions should be considered even though they are not yet cancerous.

Tumours of the mouth 85

Benign tumours of the mouth are usually part of some known mouth disorder or systemic ailment. Wisely, however, one must be forever vigilant of the doubtful tumours, possibly malignant tumours, as follows:

1. A single lesion, with no signs of any known disorder, that is not painful and does not heal within a few days;
2. A painless ulcer that is indurated (hardened) and/or cratered without known cause and does not heal within a few days;
3. An ulcer with a soft underlying mass of tissue that grows slowly and is not painful;
4. A benign polyp or papilloma that is constantly being irritated by a tooth or dentures.

The first three should be subjected to a biopsy. In number 4, the condition that is irritating the benign growth should be corrected. Constant irritation of a benign growth can often make it turn malignant.

In mouth cancer the seriousness of the tumour is out of all proportion to the severity of the symptoms. Early malignancies are not dramatic or painful; the lesion might be small and unimportant looking.

A rule of thumb: any lesion, tumour, ulcer, growth, or thickening of mucosal tissue that does not show signs of healing within five days should be seen by a doctor. The medical rule is that any lesion that does not heal within two weeks should be considered cancerous until proven otherwise. But why wait two weeks? Mouth ulcers are curable if the growth is caught while it is still local and prompt treatment is initiated. The reason most mouth cancers do not have an encouraging rate of cure is that the doctor sees them only after they are far advanced. Early diagnosis and proper care are a must. See also *Cancer of the mouth* **437**.

Tonguetie 86 (ankyloglossia)

Tonguetie occurs when the lingual frenum (the mucous membrane that connects the tongue to the floor of the mouth) is attached very close to the tip of the tongue, thus limiting the mobility of the tongue. A common cause of speech deficiency, the condition may be congenital or hereditary, and is easily remedied by surgical incision of the frenum.

Tongue disorders 87
(glossitis)

Symptomatic conditions of the tongue are often indications of disorders elsewhere in the body. Ulcers, which may be due to cancer, syphilis, an injury from the sharp edge of a decayed tooth, and mouth disorders, may cause heavy salivation and difficulty in swallowing as well as a foul taste and bad breath. A swollen tongue can be caused by a fish bone, accidentally biting the tongue, an irritating substance, aspirin, thyroid disorders, digestive disorders, and mouth diseases. An enlarged, flabby, pale tongue, which may leave indented teeth marks, is most often due to chronic dyspepsia.

The tongue is subjected frequently to injuries from chewing, accidents, or convulsive seizures. Usually injuries self-heal quickly unless the cut is severe, in which case suturing is required.

Glossodynia 87a

Characterized by a painful or burning tongue, glossodynia is usually due to such local origins as rough teeth edges, faulty dental work, and calculus. Quite frequently, however, this condition is of psychosomatic origin, especially in menopausal women. A large number of systemic disorders can also produce this disorder. Treatment includes removing the local irritant or treating the underlying disease. Psychosomatic glossodynia needs psychiatric help.

Scrotal tongue 87b

In scrotal tongue the surface is fissured with deep haphazard grooves starting from the centre. These fissures may trap food and bacteria, inducing a mild glossitis (inflammation of the tongue). This congenital anomaly occurs in as much as ten per cent of the population. If there is no superimposed infection, no treatment is necessary.

Geographical tongue (benign migratory glossitis) 87c

Geographical tongue occurs more in children and young adults and more frequently among females, usually those with an allergic background or those under stress and occasionally during menstrual periods. The lesions begin as irregularly outlined, non-hardened white or pink to red patches or spots on the tongue that are devoid of the normal papillae (the nipple-like protrusions on the tongue). These patches are multiple and constantly changing. They vary widely from day to day, giving the appearance of a geographical map. Occasionally some patients will complain of discomfort when eating heavily seasoned foods, drinking carbonated beverages, or smoking. There is no specific treatment, just reassurance that the disease is not carcinogenic.

Black hairy tongue 87d

The result of a fungus that turns the tongue black and causes the papillae of the tongue to elongate, black hair tongue is generally neither harmful nor painful. The papillae, however, can be very long, so that on occasion they may touch the roof of the mouth, causing a tickling or gagging sensation. The discoloration will disappear on its own.

The disorder occurs most frequently after the topical application of antibiotics or prolonged antibiotic treatment, which kills off bacteria and thus creates an unbalanced oral flora with a predominance of fungi. Treatment consists of brushing the tongue several times daily and employing some antifungal medication such as nystatin or sodium caprylate.

Ranula 88

A ranula is a large retention (closed) cyst

on the underside of the tongue, which can be small or as large as a robin's egg. The veins over it are translucent. Although uncomfortable, the tumour is usually painless unless inflamed. The clear viscous fluid can be needle aspirated to provide temporary relief. Often surgery is necessary to remove the growth. It is neither cancerous nor precancerous.

Mucocoele 88a

A mucocoele is also a retention cyst of the small glands found in the lips, cheeks, and palate. Mucocoeles are small, round, translucent, bluish, and elevated lesions, that frequently rupture and heal. If they have a tendency to recur, they should be surgically excised.

6 The teeth, gums, and jaws

Alfred I. Winkler

TEETH

Of all parts of the human body, the teeth are, perhaps, least able to withstand civilization. They have failed to adapt. For some reason, teeth, which are the hardest part of the body, are also the weakest, unable to bear up against the soft living of contemporary society.

In a lifetime, the teeth are subjected to wear from normal mastication. If the diet contains much raw food with abrasive material, the attrition will be faster. The grinding surfaces of the teeth develop highly polished surfaces with the cusps flattening or disappearing. Nothing much can be done about this wearing down process. Another form of attrition results from periodontal (gum) diseases, which can be helped by the dentist. Gum disorders, the major cause of tooth loss, affect ninety per cent of the population.

During development of the teeth in the foetal or postnatal stage some abnormalities can occur, such as extra teeth crowding the mouth or missing teeth, or teeth not properly formed or badly positioned. These defects are usually indicative of a family trait.

Yellowish-brown teeth in infants are often due to the mother's taking tetracycline during some period of her pregnancy, even if only for a week or two. Mottled enamel in infants and very young children is due to too much fluorine in the drinking water. Light brown or brownish black discoloration of the permanent teeth can develop.

If from childhood to old age one maintains constant communication with a good dentist, the likelihood is that he will have a good set of functioning teeth all

259

his life. In the long run, this is far less expensive than the cost of negligence, which will eventually require a great deal of dental work – and expense – to replace lost teeth.

Dental caries 89

The gradual decay and dissolution of the enamel and dentine (the layer immediately under the enamel), dental caries, if untreated will reach and infect the pulp, the central core of the tooth that houses the blood vessels, connective tissues, and the nerve. Caries causes cavities. The general belief is – although no one is certain – that a number of different kinds of bacteria work on the sticky, gelatinous coating of the tooth to produce an acid that eats away at the tooth.

The danger: If allowed to go too far, the pulp becomes inflamed and later infected, with eventual loss of tooth vitality and abscess at the tip of the root. Simply, the tooth will disintegrate.

Symptoms: The obvious symptom is a cavity in the tooth or general decay of the tooth. If the cavity or decay has been allowed to progress until it hits the pulp, there will be varying degrees of pain and possibly a swelling of the face.

Treatment: The only treatment of a cavity is surgical scouring with a burr and restoration, with various materials such as silver, gold, silicate, or composite.

Prevention: Prevention is the big issue. Caries is as common as the common cold and whereas the common cold is difficult to prevent, caries has a more hopeful outlook.

1. Brushing. A plaque on the teeth is a gummy, sticky, sugar film that is both colourless and transparent. Ordinary tooth-brushing will help but not completely. The dentist will prescribe a 'disclosing tablet', which is chewed. This tablet contains a harmless dye that is swished over all the teeth by the saliva, staining the plaques so that they can be seen and brushed off. It is messy, particularly for children, but it is effective.

Brushing requires a special technique. On the upper teeth the toothbrush (bristle) should be placed above the gum line and worked down; on the lower teeth brushing should be upward from below the gum line. The toothbrush should be replaced often.

Brushing should be done after each meal and especially before going to bed. Bacteria act on the sugar film minutes after sugar has been eaten and reach their highest activity within fifteen minutes. Heavy brushing or brushing too often can rub off the thin tooth enamel.

2. Rinsing. If possible, the mouth should be rinsed after each meal and before bedtime. Commercial mouthwashes mask the odour for a brief time; their germicidal effect lasts only about an hour.

3. Toothpaste. The value of toothpaste increases if it contains fluoride.

4. Fluoride. It has been proven that fluorine combines with the calcium in the tooth, making it a much harder substance and thus slowing down the action of the bacteria. Fluorine works best when it is part of the drinking water, but in some communities this is not available. Fluorine in a toothpaste or in a mouth rinse or taken internally in the form of a pill can be substituted. Fluorine can cut down tooth decay by half, and for children who are prone to caries this chemical is vital; overuse, however, can mottle the teeth.

5. Dental floss. The unwaxed kind is best, easier to get between the teeth where the toothbrush is not effective. Floss should be gently inserted and worked in all directions with care not to irritate the delicate gums.

6. Other inter-dental cleaning agents. Triangular, soft wooden picks to massage the gums and brush away food particles are helpful. Some dentists recommend the water pic, which thrusts streams of water under pressure between the teeth. It should not be turned on too high, for it can harm the gums.

7. Sugar. Avoid sugar as much as possible. Sugar is a prime cause of caries. A good point to remember is that sugar is

added to many processed foods, even foods not considered sweet. It is not so much the amount of sugar consumed but the frequency of putting this substance in the mouth that is significant.

8. Children's teeth. All children should have their teeth examined every six months, for only a dentist can detect the making of a new cavity.

Pulpitis 90

The pulp, the central soft tissue of the tooth which encases the nerve, becomes infected by tooth decay that has eaten through the enamel and the dentine so that the micro-organisms of the saliva invade it. Pulpitis can also be caused by a fracture of the tooth that exposes the pulp or by over-heating the tooth, especially from the new high speed drills, or by trauma (an injury of violence to the tooth) or even by bruxism (grinding the tooth during sleep so that the pulp becomes irritated or inflamed).

There are two types of pulpitis: reversible and irreversible. In reversible pulpitis the nerve and the pulp can yet be saved and brought back to sound condition. Produced by bad contact with the opposing tooth or by a new filling that is irritatingly close to the pulp or by a deep unfilled cavity, reversible pulpitis may degenerate into irreversible pulpitis. When the pulp is abscessed and dying and cannot be resurrected, the pulpitis is irreversible. A painful response is elicited when the tooth is tapped with an instrument or a finger.

The danger: If not treated the tooth will become abscessed and removal might be necessary.

Symptoms: The tooth becomes sensitive to cold, the pain lasting a few minutes and then disappearing. In advanced stages, pain will appear without any cause and last for a much longer time, occurring more frequently when the patient is in a horizontal position. There may be swelling of the face. The tooth will now be sensitive to hot substances

as well. The toothache is sharp, stabbing, or throbbing; the pain is difficult to pinpoint, often manifesting itself in a different place, sometimes even in the opposing jaw.

Treatment: In reversible pulpitis the dentist will apply a suitable germicide and seal off the exposed pulp, thus preventing further invasion from salivary bacteria. In irreversible pulpitis the pulp will be removed and the canals sterilized and filled.

Prevention: Care should be taken that a cavity does not develop too far without treatment. On some occasions an over-enthusiastic dentist might drill too near the pulp, thus destroying it.

Outlook: Removal of the pulp in root canal work does not mean that the tooth is dead; it is still attached to the bone, very much alive, and can do a useful job for a long time, providing that the root canal treatment is well done.

Tooth abscess 91

If the underlying pulpitis has not been treated, an abscess will form at the end of the root. The infecting germ is either staph or strep or some other kind of bacteria or even a fungus.

The danger: Pus from the abscess can leak into the bloodstream, causing swelling in the adjacent area. Staph or strep are no germs to treat casually. This is a *Dental Emergency* and should be treated at once.

Symptoms: A steady, relentless gnawing ache accompanied by a swelling of the face near the tooth characterize tooth abscess. The tooth becomes so tender it cannot occlude with the opposing tooth without excruciating pain. The gum swells. Heat makes it even worse.

Chronic abscess: usually there was a toothache in the recent past or a previous acute abscess followed by a gum boil. As long as the abscess is draining through the gum boil, which acts as a safety valve, the patient is comfortable. Warning: the patient should not swallow pus from the boil if he can help it.

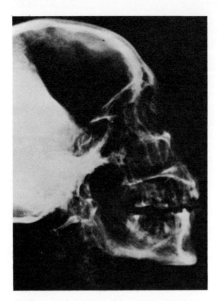

Skull x-ray shows that this man had badly worn teeth with dental abscesses. When he lived good dental care was not available. This man was Ramses II, pharaoh of Egypt 3,300 years ago. (*United States National Institutes of Health*)

Treatment: The tooth is opened for drainage and left open until all the acute symptoms have subsided.

If it is not too late, root canal treatment is undertaken. Otherwise an apicoectomy (cutting a flap in the gum near the root and sewn back after removal of the abscess). If nothing else can be done, extraction becomes necessary as a last resort. Penicillin or other antibiotics are always administered, because of the possibility of serious systemic infection. Saline rinses every half hour which might help rupture the abscess spontaneously are also employed.

Prevention: The fault is usually the patient's for letting the pulpitis go on too long without treatment. All pulpitis should be treated at once.

Outlook: In the hands of a good dentist, the tooth can sometimes be saved.

Tooth abrasion 92

The loss of tooth substance through factors other than mastication or decay is called abrasion. The most frequent causes include a faulty method of tooth brushing (horizontally), holding nails or pins between the teeth, or chewing tobacco or smoking a pipe.

The danger: If abrasion is not treated, the tooth or teeth can crack off, leaving the root behind.

Symptoms: Abrasion is characterized by a loss of tooth substance (hard decay) at the gum margins (especially from horizontal brushing), causing V-shaped notches. Teeth may become sensitive.

Treatment: If the loss of tooth substance is substantial, the erosions should be filled to avoid an accumulation of food there and consequent decay.

Prevention: Proper brushing technique will avoid abrasion.

Malocclusion 93

An imperfect meshing of the upper and lower teeth is called malocclusion. The bite is wrong and contact between the grinding teeth is poor. A dental speciality called orthodontics devotes itself completely to straightening teeth, concentrating mostly on children so that their permanent teeth will grow in straight and strong. If the permanent teeth have already appeared, they are kept in a brace and forced to go straight. This not only ensures attractive teeth but healthy teeth as well. Correcting the bite and straightening the teeth will not only help the patient speak better, but also chew better, and as a consequence help him avoid all forms of gastric disorders from bad chewing and gulping.

One child out of three needs orthodontics.

There are a number of reasons for crooked teeth and malocclusion:

1. Baby teeth that stay in the mouth too long often cause the permanent teeth to come in irregularly.

2. An impacted tooth that will not erupt, thus allowing the whole line of teeth to drift towards the empty space.

3. A tooth that erupts too slowly, causing the normally erupting opposite teeth to grow longer in order to meet it.

4. A prematurely lost baby tooth that causes the other teeth to shift.

5. An unwelcome extra baby tooth that crowds the rest of the teeth.

6. A poorly formed tooth, caused either by insufficient calcium or the inability of the body to utilize calcium properly.

7. A bad siege with measles or scarlet fever, which can interfere with proper bone development.

Orthodontic treatment for children has in the main been highly successful. The orthodontist has a whole series of devices, bands, and braces to fit every possible contingency. This is perhaps one of the most vital forms of dentistry; preventive medicine at its best, orthodontics prevents the ailment before it can begin and thus ensures a longer life for the teeth.

Malocclusion in the adult is corrected by grinding down some teeth and building up new crowns and jackets so that the teeth will mesh properly.

Complications in tooth extraction 94

If the dentist has not taken proper precautions before extracting a tooth to inquire whether the patient has any blood disorders (anaemia), bleeding diseases or rheumatic fever, then the patient himself should advise the dentist so that he can be given an antibiotic injection or other necessary preventive treatment.

Normally, the extraction site heals in a few days if it has not been irritated or over-rinsed and if the patient has followed the dentist's instructions in post-extraction care. Usually the dentist will discourage the patient from .insing the first day, and if that is not completely possible, the patient is advised to rinse only with cold water. The dentist will further recommend that the patient avoid hard foods and advise him to treat the extraction as an operation, which it assuredly is, by refraining from all activity.

Symptoms: Complications arising from extraction include bleeding, swelling, and pain. Early (primary) bleeding, that is, on the first day following the extraction, is due to rinsing that is done too vigorously and too soon. The patient may also be over-conscious of the extraction and engage in constant sucking and spitting. Sometimes bleeding is caused by the failure of the dentist to properly treat the lacerated tissue and injured bone. Secondary bleeding occurs two or three days later, the result of an infected clot.

Prolonged or uncontrolled bleeding, the result of an underlying pre-existing blood disorder or other systemic disease is occasioned by the negligence of the dentist and the patient.

Continuous pain that appears two or three days after the extraction is called dry socket. It becomes worse, remains acute for several days, and then may subside. Often it may go on for weeks in a chronic form. This delayed pain usually signifies an infection prior to the extraction. After the socket is carefully cleaned it will reveal an exposed portion of the alveolar bone.

Treatment: An ice bag a half hour every hour for the first day will reduce swelling. To control bleeding, a small piece of gauze (5 by 5 centimetres, 2 by 2 inches) is folded into a hard pack and placed carefully in the socket and held in place for fifteen minutes by biting down firmly. If the bleeding has stopped, the gauze treatment should be repeated again for forty-five minutes. Sucking or spitting is highly irritating. All activity for the day should be stopped or cut down to keep the blood from circulating too strongly. If the bleeding persists, the dentist will pack the socket with gauze treated with a blood-clotting medication. A cold, wet tea bag can often do the same. If necessary, the dentist will suture the wound.

To alleviate dry socket, the extraction site is gently irrigated with warm water and packed with iodoform gauze treated with eugenol or some other anaesthetic solution. Pain can be reduced by aspirin or some other analgesic. It will take upwards of a week for the body to cover the naked bone with a protective membrane. If the area remains swollen and there is high fever, the dentist will prescribe an appropriate antibiotic. As in bleeding, taking it very easy for a day or so will hasten the healing process.

Broken or chipped tooth 95

If a tooth is chipped or broken, a dentist should be consulted at once. If the pulp is exposed (often not apparent to the patient), it will become infected by salivary bacteria, thus causing pulpitis and abscess. The dentist can frequently patch up the pulp and save the vitality of the tooth. If the injury has destroyed the pulp, immediate root canal work can save the tooth. If the crown of the tooth has been broken off, the dentist can build an artificial crown over the root or stump with a new jacket. Small chips can be smoothed off with an emery board.

Missing tooth and implantation 96

Every tooth that is missing is sorely missed. It should be replaced by an artificial tooth to prevent the nearby teeth from drifting or leaning. Usually the opposing occluding tooth will grow longer, thus compounding the loss. The unsightliness needs no description.

When the missing tooth is one vital to the entire set of teeth, such as one needed an an anchor for a bridge, some of the bolder dentists will do an implantation of an inert metal or plastic, attaching it to the bone below with an artificial tooth above the gum. The success of this procedure is slippery. Although highly commendable, it is not in general practice, either because of a lack of success or of sufficient skill at the present time.

Knocked-out (evulsed) tooth and replantation 97

If a tooth has been knocked out in a fight or accident, the victim should hurry to his dentist with tooth in hand. The sooner he gets to him the better. Within the hour is best. The dentist will immediately clean the tooth, remove the pulp, sterilize it, refill it, and replace it in the gum, splinting it to a nearby tooth for a month or two until the tooth takes hold. Often, if the patient strongly believes the tooth will hold, this emergency measure can be imminently successful. Sometimes, however, the root is absorbed and the tooth eventually gives up and falls out. But since this can take several years, the patient at least has the use of the tooth during that time.

Tooth eruption and impaction of wisdom tooth 98

The twenty deciduous teeth (baby teeth, milk teeth) begin to appear when an infant is six months old and begin to disappear in the sixth year, when the permanent teeth begin to erupt (thirty-two in number). By the fifteenth year all are in except the wisdom teeth (third molars), which show up between seventeen and twenty-five.

Sometimes these third molars do not erupt but stay inside the gum and jawbone. Most of the time they give no trouble and the patient is unaware of their existence unless he has a full-mouth x-ray done. Occasionally, the gum surrounding the impacted wisdom tooth becomes inflammed and irritated, causing pain and swelling. Removing the tooth by cutting open the gum and yanking it out is not a cheery prospect. In addition, the operation can provide the possibility of a deep-seated infection. The dentist will try to avoid extraction if at all possible and employ an alternate line of action. On some occasions the inflammation will disappear on its own.

However, when the impacted wisdom tooth erupts only partially, the dentist will try all sorts of procedures to force it into full eruption. If all efforts fail, extraction is necessary, but it is far less of an ordeal than having to cut away the gum.

Bruxism 99

Many people develop a habit of grinding their teeth (bruxism), usually when asleep. It is bad for the teeth, injuring and irritating the pulp and eventually damaging the pulp to the point of killing the nerve. Grinding the teeth is like rocking a pole that is implanted into the ground until it has become thoroughly loosened.

Dentists have devised an appliance they call a bite plate to be kept in the mouth during sleep. It prevents grinding, is not uncomfortable, and will save teeth and periodontal tissue.

GUMS (PERIODONTAL DISEASES)

The greatest cause of teeth loss after the age of thirty-five is periodontal (peri = around; odont = teeth; located around the teeth) disease, which is preventable. Sound teeth require good oral hygiene (see *Table 6*) and regular visits to the dentist.

Gingivitis 100

Gingivitis is an inflammation of the gums; it can be acute or chronic. The local causes, which are the most common, are mouth infection, plaque, unremoved tartar (calculus) around the teeth, faulty dental work, malocclusion, and even mouth breathing. Records show that good oral hygiene produces a low inci-

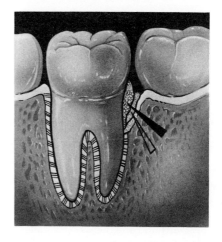

Periodontal disease. The gums at the neck of the tooth have become swollen, bled, and separated from the tooth, causing pockets. (*American Diabetic Association*)

dence of periodontal diseases, while poor oral hygiene produces a high incidence.

Gingivitis may also be the primary sign of some underlying systemic disorder, such as diabetes, leukaemia, scurvy, pellagra, and pregnancy (the early months).

The danger: Gingivitis, if not checked, can develop into periodontitis (pyorrhoea), with loss of bone and teeth.

Symptoms: The gums are inflamed in a band at the neck of the teeth; they are swollen, red or purple, and bleed at the slightest touch. Pockets in the gums (a separation of the gum from the teeth), in which bacteria gather and multiply, are formed from an accumulation of tartar.

- Diabetic gingivitis: severe gum inflammation, abscesses, and the growth of polyps between the teeth.
- Leukaemia gingivitis: a painful and discoloured enlargement of the gums; the entire mouth is inflamed.
- Scurvy gingivitis: blue-black or purplish spots on the gums and mouth.
- Pellagra gingivitis: reddened and cracked lips, a scalded feeling on the tongue, which is bright red and smooth,

and ulcerated lesions on the gums and in the mouth
• Pregnancy gingivitis: enlargement of the gums with tumours, a condition that usually disappears by the second month but on occasion may persist for full term.

Treatment: Local gingivitis is treated by removing the tartar. Gross malocclusion, as well as faulty dental appliances, should be corrected. Rinsing the mouth with an antiseptic solution will help alleviate gum ulceration.

Gingivitis resulting from a systemic underlying disease should be treated at the source.

Prevention: Tartar must never be allowed to accumulate on the margins of the gums and teeth. The pockets formed by an accumulation of tartar can never be remedied. Only regular visits to a dentist can save teeth and gums.

Outlook: Gingivitis can be arrested; but whatever damage has already been done can only be alleviated, not cured. Keeping in close touch with a dentist is essential.

Periodontitis 101
(pyorrhoea, parodontitis)

In periodontitis, a direct result of untreated gingivitis, the gums have recessed, or drawn away from the teeth, thus forming large pockets in which bacteria flourish.

The danger: Loss of bone and teeth and chronic ill health result.

Symptoms: Large gum pockets and a loosening of some or all of the teeth characterize periodontitis. Decaying food and active bacteria enlarge the pockets further. Pus is discharged between the gums and teeth. A constant swallowing of the pus causes dyspepsia (indigestion) and chronic ill health. The eroded gums bleed at the slightest touch. The breath is foul.

Treatment: If pockets have begun to form, the gum that has separated must be removed surgically (gingivectomy).

Gums that have separated can never be made to adhere again. Cutting off slices of gums may seem like a drastic procedure, but it is far better than losing the affected teeth.

Bone loss cannot be replaced, but the dentist can stop the downward process and preserve what is left. He will scrape off the tartar, remove the diseased sections of the gums, correct the bite, and if possible shore up and strengthen the loose teeth. Bone graft is done to stabilize the teeth.

It is most important to obtain the advice and care of a specialist as soon as possible. Most of the teeth can be saved.

Prevention: Pockets in the gums can never be remedied. Therefore, tartar, the cause of pockets, must never be allowed to accumulate. Regular visits to a dentist can save the teeth and gums. Any gum disorder should be treated early.

JAWS
Temporomandibular joint disorder 102

When the sliding hinge that connects the upper and lower jaw on each side of the mouth is lopsided from deviation or dislocation of the lower jaw, the patient is suffering from temporomandibular joint disorder. The disorder is caused by malocclusion, cusped interference, poorly fitted dentures, bruxism, and emotional distress resulting in altered muscular balance. It may also be associated with such systemic conditions as rheumatoid arthritis, septicaemia, scarlet fever, typhoid fever, influenza, and gonorrhoea.

The danger: None, but since the patient has difficulty in speaking, chewing, and swallowing, the disorder is most uncomfortable.

Symptoms: The mouth cannot be opened fully and the affected side of the face is sore; severe pain is experienced by any movement of the jaw, as in speaking, chewing, or swallowing. A clicking sound is often heard when the mouth is opened. Other symptoms are headaches, neck pains, and pains radiating from the jaw. **Treatment:** The acute symptoms will usually subside in less than a week if the jaw is kept inactive and somewhat immobilized. The diet should be soft for two weeks to avoid painful chewing.

Tranquillizers and analgesics are the usual form of treatment. Application of moist heat is relieving. In extreme cases the injection of cortisone or other related steroids directly into the area is frequently employed.

Also, the occlusion of the teeth should be properly adjusted. Faulty dentures should be replaced or repaired. The periodontist or the dentist will advise the patient on special massage and jaw exercises.

Outlook: Always eventually correctable.

7 Respiratory disorders

Walter L. Phillips

The respiratory system consists of air tubes and two lungs, each of which is enclosed in an airtight space called the pleural cavity. The main air tube, the trachea, extends from the larynx and divides into two main tubes (the bronchi), each of which enters a lung where they branch into a multitude of smaller tubes called bronchioles.

Respiratory diseases are becoming more common all over the world, particularly in highly industrialized countries such as the United States and in Europe. Air pollution, cigarette smoking and overcrowded living conditions are important factors. The average human being inhales about 14 cubic metres, 3,000 gallons of air per day, which is contaminated with carbon dioxide, carbon monoxide (a poison), nitrogen dioxide (a lung irritant), hydrogen sulphide (a poison), various hydrocarbons from automobile exhausts (some toxic, some irritant), asbestos, carbon particulates, rubber compounds, and so on.

These pollutants reduce our lifespan. Although somewhat less hazardous, rural areas are actually not much safer, as winds carry industrial pollutants all over the land and perhaps hundreds of miles from their sources of origin. Rubber particles subjected to air pollution undergo changes, becoming brittle; our respiratory tracts become damaged as well from breathing in contaminated air for long periods of time.

The answer to this problem is to reduce environmental pollution at all costs. An individual response would be to leave the heavily polluted atmosphere of a city or town for short periods in order to breathe fresher and cleaner air elsewhere.

THE BRONCHI
Acute bronchitis 103

Inflammation of the bronchial tubes may be caused by viral or bacterial infections. Bronchitis occurs more frequently in winter and more commonly in cold, damp climates. Commencing as a common cold or infection of the throat, nose, or sinuses, the inflammation may spread into the chest. Contributing factors may be those that reduce individual resistance, such as fatigue, severe chilling, overcrowding, inhalation of irritant gases, and exposure to others already suffering from respiratory infections. Excessive cigarette smoking is an important cause of bronchitis.

The danger: This mild disease in otherwise healthy people is short-lived. It may prove dangerous, however, for infants and the elderly. The duration of the disease may become prolonged and lead to chronic bronchitis possibly complicated by pneumonia.

Symptoms: Commencing as a head cold, running nose, malaise, slight fever, and chills, the muscles soon begin to ache and there may be pain in the back. The cough is the outstanding symptom, starting as a tickle in the throat and later becoming more frequent, distressing, and racking. It causes a sensation of soreness behind the breastbone. At first dry, unproductive, and painful, the cough becomes less distressing when phlegm begins to appear. The phlegm is white and mucoid at the start and subsequently becomes yellowish and purulent; it may become tenacious and copious. The cough is usually worse at night. Fever may be high and prolonged during the full-blown stage of the disease.

Treatment: The patient is kept in bed in a warm room in which the atmosphere is humidified with a vaporizer, which tends to lessen the cough. Drinking fluids should be encouraged.

Medication consists in administering aspirin to reduce the fever. A teaspoonful of terpin hydrate will relieve a dry cough by helping to produce sputum. The severe, exhausting cough will be relieved by terpin hydrate with codeine, a cough suppressant, for which a doctor's prescription will be required. Patent expectorants (medicine to loosen phlegm) are of small value.

If the patient is also asthmatic (wheezing and having difficulty with breathing), the doctor will prescribe bronchodilator drugs.

Fever may persist for as long as five days, while the cough may last for weeks. The fever may remain high, and the patient continues to feel ill and to produce purulent sputum. Superadded infection with bacteria is the usual cause, and treatment with antibiotics or sulphonamides is indicated. Care must be taken to determine whether the patient is sensitive to these drugs, and, of course, the patient should be given the appropriate drug for the particular bacteria in the sputum.

Physical rest is very important for complete recovery. Recurrent pulmonary infections complicate incomplete treatment and convalescence.

Prevention: Cold, damp climates should be avoided by those prone to bronchitis. Cigarette smoking is definitely harmful. When possible, the individual should move away from smoggy, overcrowded, polluted communities.

Outlook: The disease is usually self-limiting and the outlook is good.

Chronic bronchitis 104

Chronic bronchitis is a degenerative disease. After repeated attacks of bronchitis, the walls of the bronchial tubes become thickened, inelastic, and narrowed. The mucous membranes of the bronchi are permanently inflamed and the airways become filled with tenacious mucus.

Chronic bronchitis occurs four times more frequently in men than in women, and it occurs more frequently in cities than in rural communities. Cigarette smoking is a major factor, the number of cigarettes smoked being large in most cases. Many more smokers than non-smokers die of chronic bronchitis.

The danger: Chronic bronchitis is one of the causes of chronic obstructive lung disease, which results in interference with breathing and a diminished gaseous exchange in the lung air sacs. Retention of carbon dioxide and reduced oxygen uptake occurs in the blood, resulting in carbon dioxide narcosis (stupor). Pneumonia and heart failure follow and frequently terminate fatally.

Chronic bronchitis is frequently associated with emphysema, which also may develop into chronic obstructive lung disease.

Symptoms: The cough is the main symptom, often occurring in paroxysms. The strain caused by coughing may induce a hernia, cause a rib to fracture, and occasionally cause an eye haemorrhage resulting from a temporary rise in blood pressure. Other symptoms include:
● Breathlessness: known as dyspnoea,

breathlessness is due to a loss of elasticity of lung tissue and also to retention of secretions in the rigid bronchi. The secretions may induce a wheeze resembling an asthmatic attack.
● Phlegm: the amount and colour of sputum varies according to the presence of infecting bacteria. Characteristically, the sputum is sticky and ropy and expectoration may be difficult.
● Cyanosis: blueness (cyanosis) of the lips and fingernail beds is due to diminished oxygen absorption from the lungs.
● Barrel chest: the loss of elasticity of the air tubes and lung tissues causes diminished lung ventilation. The lungs become over-distended and this, in turn, alters the shape of the chest. Air becomes trapped in the lungs.

Treatment: The removal of bronchial irritants is all important. Cigarette smoking should be stopped, and the patient should avoid working in any environment in which irritating substances or noxious fumes are present. It may take a considerable period of time before benefit is seen. Purulent sputum should be analysed to determine the specific organisms involved, and these should be tested for sensitivity to specific antibiotics. Treatment of the patient with the correct antibiotic often results in improvement of the disease.

Carbon dioxide retention and cyanosis may require special oxygen therapy. This can be supplied only in a hospital, for it may be necessary to use special breathing machines. In order to maintain a clear airway, seriously ill patients will require tubing through the trachea and the aspiration of secretions.

Slight to moderate shortness of breath can be assisted by special breathing exercises. The yoga breathing system (*Table 9*) is helpful in many cases.

Postural drainage (*Table 8*) is used to help the patient remove secretions from the bronchial tree. Adoption of the correct position allows secretions to flow out of the lungs. Tapping the chest and coughing help this form of drainage.

Any drug that depresses respiration is absolutely contra-indicated. It is for this reason that cough suppressants should be avoided when shortness of breath and copious secretions are the main symptoms.

Prevention: Chronic bronchitis is usually progressive and treatment should be started as early as possible. All bronchial irritants should be avoided.

Outlook: It is impossible to predict the course of the disease. Preventive treatment is important.

Bronchiectasis 105

Bronchiectasis is an abnormal dilation of the bronchial tubes in which mucoid secretions collect. Infection of these secretions may be superadded, causing inflammatory changes in the bronchial walls. As the inflammation extends more deeply, blood capillaries become eroded, causing the secretions to become not only purulent but also bloodstained. The introduction of antibiotics has diminished the incidence of this lung ailment.

Children and adolescents suffering from measles and whooping cough often develop this disease as a complication, resulting from the retention of secretions. The aspiration of foreign bodies, such as peanuts, into the bronchi and occasionally pulmonary tuberculosis may be complicated by the development of bronchiectasis.

The danger: Originally there was a high mortality rate. The purulent secretions flowed from one lobe into the next and frequently into the opposite lung. Chronic ill health is often due to infected pulmonary secretions. Recurrent attacks of pneumonia are frequent.

Symptoms: The cough is an outstanding feature, occurring with changes in posture; thus the cough starts as the patient arises in the morning and when he retires to bed.

The phlegm is profuse and foetid and the breath is so foul-smelling that the patient may become a social outcast. Bloodstaining of the sputum occurs frequently, but this is not a serious symp-

tom. Shortness of breath (dyspepsia) depends on the amount of sputum that has to be expectorated.

As in all cases of chronic sepsis, malaise, anaemia, and diminished capacity for work is common.

Cough, sputum, haemoptysis (coughing blood), and shortness of breath are also characteristic of *Pulmonary tuberculosis* **112** and *Lung cancer* **411**. Examination of the phlegm may help establish the cause.

Treatment: Removal of bronchial obstructions before additional infection can occur allows the air tubes to return to normal. Once infection has developed and the bronchial secretions have become foetid the condition is irreversible.

Bronchiectatic lung tissue is useless and dangerous. Cure can be obtained only by the removal of the damaged parts of the lung. Occasionally the disease is so extensive that all the affected tissue cannot be removed. Before any surgery, a prolonged period of postural drainage (*Table 8*) is necessary. This helps to bring the patient into as good a condition as possible.

In non-surgical patients (when the disease is too extensive) regular daily postural drainage is necessary. Deep-breathing exercises are helpful. The yoga breathing system (*Table 9*) is helpful. At the same time inhalation therapy should be prescribed by the doctor.

Expectoration of sputum is assisted by coughing; cough suppressants, therefore, should be avoided. The use of the appropriate antibiotic will help to keep the sputum free from added infection. Long-term therapy with tetracycline is often valuable.

Prevention: Prompt treatment of *Atelectasis* **114** (lung collapse) will help avoid the complication of bronchiectasis. Mucus plugs and foreign bodies should be removed by bronchoscopy.

Lung collapse, which may result from aspiration of mucus or pus from infected sinuses, frequently complicates operations and, therefore, should be treated before any lung surgery is contemplated.

Outlook: Bronchiectasis is probably never fully cured but progressive destruction can be halted.

Foreign body in the bronchi 106

A foreign body in the bronchi is a dangerous event that occurs in adults as well as in children. In adults, the breathing in of foreign objects can happen under the influence of alcohol, particularly while eating. Loose dental fillings may be inhaled during sleep, or nails or screws held in the mouth by workmen may also be aspirated.

Breathing in particles of food is most common and the most destructive – kernels of peanuts, seeds, beans, bones, crumbs. Peanuts lead the group by far. Dust or liquids are not in the category of foreign bodies.

The danger: If the foreign object has moved into the bronchi it may ultimately cause bronchiectasis or lung abscess. Removal of foreign objects from the bronchi is always a difficult matter, particularly if it is a food particle. This is a *Medical Emergency* and surgery is essential if the person's life is to be saved.

If the foreign object is lodged in the windpipe, first-aid procedures must be applied immediately. The subject should be made to lie over a bed or table with his head or shoulders hanging down lower than his body. A hard slap or blow between the shoulder blades can dislodge the object. A child should be held upside down by the heels and slapped hard between the shoulder blades.

Symptoms: A large object blocks the trachea and causes asphyxiation. A small object causes choking, gagging, severe shortness of breath, and cyanosis until it passes into the bronchi. Symptoms will then subside, often suggesting that it has either been expelled or swallowed. The symptomless period may last for days or weeks. Non-irritating smooth objects often present no initial symptoms even when in the trachea.

Inevitably, the patient has fever and a cough of varying intensity. Often the doctor, if he has not been informed of the choking incident, might mistake the symptoms for those of *Pneumonia* **109**.

Food particles are the deadliest, because they become a focal point of infection in the bronchi, eventually becoming lodged in the wall, causing toxaemia, high fever, severe shortness of breath, and chills from resulting lung abscess. The sputum will be bloodstained and foul during the heavy coughing bouts.

Between the initial event of choking and gagging and the ultimate obstruction and infection of the bronchi the patient may be symptomless and the cause can be easily overlooked.

Treatment: A foreign body in the bronchi can only occasionally be expelled by coughing. Usually, it must be removed surgically and at once, by aid of a bronchoscope (a long metal tube inserted into the trachea).

The presence of a foreign body in the bronchial tree may cause bronchiectasis or lung abscess. After removal of a foreign body, it is important to determine the presence of bronchiectasis by a special x-ray investigation known as bronchography.

Prevention: Pins and nails should never be kept in the mouth, because of the danger of aspiration. Since loose dental fillings may also be aspirated, proper attention to dental work will prevent this occurrence.

Outlook: The removal of all foreign objects from the trachea or bronchi has become quite safe for the patient.

Laryngotracheo-bronchitis 107
(croup)

Croup is a dangerous disease that most often affects infants and young children but may also occur at any age. Fatalities run very high. The mucous membrane of the larynx, trachea, and bronchi become severely inflamed and swollen, producing a sticky, heavy, choking mucus.

The danger: Life is threatened by respiratory obstruction and the toxic effects of acute inflammation of the airways. The mortality rate is greater than fifty per cent. This is a *Medical Emergency*.

Symptoms: The onset is sudden and usually there are no premonitory symptoms. Fever mounts swiftly, running up to 41·5°C, 106°F. At first, there is a croupy, non-productive cough, but later a thick tenacious phlegm forms in the bronchi and trachea. A major symptom is shortness of breath. The mucus in the laryngotracheobronchial tree is so heavy and clinging that it blocks the airways; breathing becomes a raspy gasp, causing pallor or cyanosis. There is hoarseness when the inflammation involves the larynx.

The swollen, obstructed throat, plus the heavy, sticky mucus, makes this a deadly ailment that will cause death if not relieved. The patient appears anxious and frightened.

Treatment: Hospitalization is advisable, because of the constant risk that respiratory obstruction may require resuscitation measures. The doctor will administer the maximum dosage of appropriate antibiotics and be prepared, if necessary, to perform a quick tracheotomy (an incision in the neck to allow the insertion of a breathing tube) to prevent suffocation. If the patient is kept at home his room should be highly humidified with one or two vaporizers of a steaming kettle. Humidity of ninety per cent is best (the temperature not higher than 24°C, 75°F).

After overcoming the first effects of the disease, sputum should be examined for the causative organism so that the correct antibiotic can be administered.

Prevention: There are no specific preventive measures.

Outlook: If this disease is treated quickly and energetically, full recovery can be expected after some weeks of convalescence. Too often, however, treatment is too slow, too late, or inadequate. Sharp vigilance can save a life.

Asthma 108
(bronchial asthma)

Asthma is Greek for 'panting'. This is a chronic disease characterized by paroxysmal attacks of shortness of breath and difficulty in breathing, accompanied by wheezing caused by a spasm of the bronchial tubes and a swelling of their mucous membranes. Asthma occurs in childhood, in young adulthood, in middle age, among all races, and has no regard for sex. The intervals between attacks can be symptomless, but some attacks (status asthmaticus) can last for hours or days without letup.

The cause: In infancy asthma is usually a reaction to food; from age ten to the late twenties it results from an allergen that is inhaled; over forty the cause is infectious. However, any of the above determinants can happen to anyone in any age in any combination. About a third of those who become asthmatic after age ten develop a severe even life-threatening reaction to aspirin.

The two kinds of asthma are extrinsic, caused by some outside agent such as pollen, feathers, animal dander, dust, insecticides, moulds, and so on, and intrinsic (infective asthma), caused by infection within the respiratory system. Although some authorities once considered that intrinsic asthma might have a psychogenic origin, this idea has been discounted (surgical excisions of the autonomic nerve factors of the bronchi have not been successful). Emotional problems can, however, exacerbate the disease.

Intrinsic asthma, which usually begins later in life, starts off with long periods of remission between attacks, but as the years roll by the intervals become shorter and shorter. If the asthma attacks take place mostly in winter, it is most likely infectious, or intrinsic; if only in summer, it is likely to be allergic, or extrinsic.

The danger: Less than a third of asthmatic children recover spontaneously before they are in their twenties; an equal number not only do not recover but get worse – unless they are under constant care and treatment.

Chronic asthma, if not properly treated, can cause *Emphysema* **113**.

The asthmatic is hypersensitive to many drugs, often including penicillin, in reaction to which they can occasionally suffer fatal anaphylaxis (a hypersensitive state of the body to a foreign protein or drug).

In a severe, prolonged, continuous attack of asthma, status asthmaticus, the mortality rate can be high if the response to many of the drugs including cortisone is negative.

Symptoms: Asthma is a dramatic disease. It will awaken the patient in the middle of the night in a state of near suffocation. He sits up in alarm; his intake of air is quick but his exhalation is agonizing, prolonged, seemingly impossible, noisy, and wheezing. His chest feels tight, constricted, and is conspicuously distended. The veins of his neck stand out. He is sweating. His face is flushed or worse, sometimes pale and cyanotic. His gasping efforts to breathe panic him and terrify his family. It seems as if he will not survive, but he does – fatalities are rare in uncomplicated asthma.

After a half hour or several hours, the patient will go into the final stage – coughing, bringing up copious amounts of very thick, tenacious mucus, which at last brings him relief. The violent cough finally abates; the attack is over, leaving his lower chest muscles aching.

Between attacks he is symptom free.

Some patients suffer a mild chronic state of asthma in which any exertion or activity, such as anger, laughter, or even a sneeze, can bring on an attack.

Treatment: Treatment for asthma is complex, extensive, and constant. It consists of finding the causative allergen and of directing efforts for the relief and general care of the patient.

If the cause is extrinsic, that is, induced by an allergic reaction to some pollen or mould or drug, the outlook is far better. The responsible substance can usually be found and a programme of desensitization undertaken, with partial and possibly total cure.

For the intrinsic form of asthma there is rarely any cure, but the disease can be held in check by constant treatment and medication.

Medication: the new isoproterenol in-

halant is a very potent drug, which needs very careful instruction for the patient. It is entirely safe when used correctly but deadly when overused. Isoproterenol is the most effective bronchodilator. From four to six inhalations a day is the advisable maximum.

In intrinsic cases (infective asthma) the best treatment is with antibiotics, but there are problems. Penicillin is usually the most effective, but asthmatics, being hypersensitive (that is usually what made them asthmatics in the first place), frequently respond badly to penicillin, sometimes fatally.

Bacteria vaccines are in wide use for asthmatics but there is considerable question regarding their value.

Adrenalin (epinephrine) given subcutaneously (under the skin), aminophylline given rectally, or ephedrine taken orally will usually reduce or stop an attack. All these drugs have side effects – aminophylline causes rectal irritation, the other two cause jitteriness, palpitations, and worsened conditions for patients who also suffer from high blood pressure, heart disease, and hyperthyroidism.

Antihistamines are of no value and sometimes can do additional harm.

To loosen phlegm, potassium iodide (0·6 grams) may be taken three times a day after meals.

Cough syrup has value, but its purpose must be better understood. The cough reflex is so strong, the body so anxious to get rid of the dangerous mucus, that it goes far beyond its needs. Cough syrups prevent the body from overdoing it. The drug of choice is a solution of terpin hydrate and codeine (a teaspoonful every 4 hours) or hydrocodone bitartrate (10 mgs, or about a third of an ounce, every 4 hours).

Steam inhalations are also helpful.

During a prolonged asthma attack in which none of the above drugs is working, oxygen administered by mask or tent can make the difference between surviving or not. If the patient has gone into status asthmaticus, he should be hospitalized, where he will be treated with hydrocorti-

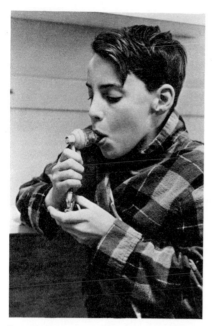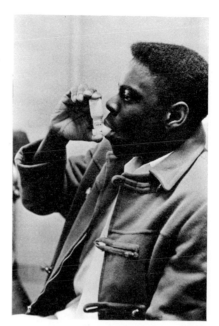

Bronchodilators give relief to asthma suffers (*United States National Asthma Center*)

sone (prednisone) or if the case remains intractable, a tracheostomy will be performed (an incision in the trachea to allow the insertion of a tube to facilitate the passage of air) and the patient will be placed in a respirator. This last desperate measure, accomplished only by a skilled, practised team in a hospital, can often mean the saving of a life.

General measures: general good health practices are absolutely essential for an asthmatic, as are emotional factors. The asthmatic by the very nature of his disease is anxious and fear-ridden. A constant state of anxiety can trigger off more attacks than would ordinarily take place. He must be knowledgeable about his disease and know that the attacks are rarely fatal, so that he can meet them without terror and with some degree of patient calm.

He must know that intense emotional and stressful situations can bring on an attack. Although life is not possible without stress, every effort should be made

on his part to avoid it as much as possible. It is interesting to note that the use of psychotherapy has never been successful with asthmatics.

The asthmatic must make every effort to avoid colds or any other respiratory infections; he must not let himself become too fatigued and must try to avoid overcrowded places. He must also avoid nasal and bronchial irritants, such as smoke, dusty places, wet paint, and if possible heavy air pollution.

Breathing exercises can give him a new lease on life. One of the best is the yoga system of deep breathing (*Table 9*), developed a thousand years ago.

An asthmatic can do much to help himself. He should analyse his last attack. What did *he* do to bring it on? Was he in a new place? Did he eat any new food? What animal was near him? Had he been upset, angry? Was he in a garden or park? Did he get into freshly laundered clothes? Was it a windy day?

He should keep a detailed list. He may

not be able to cure himself, but he can assuredly cut down the number of attacks.

Prevention: There seems to be no known way of preventing asthma. Asthmatics are people born with supersensitive bodies.

Outlook: Asthma, if not outgrown early in life, settles down to become chronic, needing constant medical care. The doctor can help the patient avoid many attacks. Without medical help the attacks might be threefold more. The wise asthmatic makes peace with the disease and his reliance on the medical profession.

In status asthmaticus, relief may not follow any of the approved methods of treatment. The continuous state may eventually cause heart failure. Relief of the spasm, which results in inadequate blood oxygenation, is vital. The cause of continuous spasm of the bronchi is the presence of thick, tenacious secretions. Hospitalization is necessary. Bronchoscopy, performed under local anaesthesia, allows the removal of much of this sticky material. It may be necessary to wash out each main bronchus separately, at the same time providing the patient with oxygen. This washing process may have to be repeated. In most cases the acute bronchospasm can be relieved.

Even a small quantity of thick, tenacious secretions can be responsible for this serious symptom; its removal frequently gives relief.

THE LUNGS
Pneumonia 109
(pneumococcal pneumonia, staphylococcal pneumonia, Klebsiella [Friedländer's] pneumonia)

Pneumonia, an inflammation of the air cells (alveoli) of the lungs, is due to a bacterial, viral, or chemical irritant. There are more than fifty causes, but the most significant and the most common are the bacterial forms – pneumococcal, streptococcal, staphylococcal, and Klebsiella (Friedländer's) pneumonia. By far the most frequent is the pneumococcal variety – the prototype of all pneumonias. There are more than eighty types of this pneumonia, but only nine of them make up three-quarters of all pneumococcal forms. Types II and III are the least common but the most dangerous.

When bacteria enter the lungs, their presence and activity produces fluid in the air sacs, which is exactly what they need to multiply.

The lungs are divided into five lobes. If one or more lobes are infected it is called lobar pneumonia; if both lungs are infected, double pneumonia, and if the infection of the lungs is near the bronchial tubes it is called bronchopneumonia.

The disease is airborne, spread usually by breath; often the carrier may be resistant to the disease yet still spread it around. Contact with the pneumococcal germ does not mean a person will automatically get the disease. The conditions must be right: he must be undernourished, an alcoholic, debilitated, elderly, an infant, or weakened by an attack of flu or other chronic systemic disorder, or his lungs stagnated by his being in bed too long (a long period of bed rest can make one susceptible, as can anaesthesia).

The incubation period is from one to seven days.

There are many who dismiss the disease as no longer important. This is as untrue as it is dangerous. About one out of every five hundred persons gets pneumonia every year, which means that in a lifetime the chance of any individual becoming ill with pneumonia is one out of seven or eight. Once the disease was a major cause of death, but thanks to antibiotics it has plummeted down, but not out.

The danger: Antibiotics have made most pneumonias curable, but some pneumococcals, types II and III, for example, are still not within medical control. Many people die of pneumonia, especially those who are suffering from a chronic disease, particularly meningitis and endocarditis. The elderly often are not helped by antibiotics.

The Klebsiella type is particularly virulent although considerably lessened by antibiotics. An additional and tragic danger with Klebsiella, though an uncommon form of the disease, is that it is sometimes mistaken for pneumococcal by the laboratory. This diagnosis can be fatal because Klebsiella does not respond in the slightest to penicillin, which is the ideal medication for the pneumococcus germ.

The doctor has a great responsibility, together with the laboratory, to identify the causative germ. If he or the laboratory believes the patient has viral pneumonia when he has staphylococcal, the patient might not survive.

Staphylococcal pneumonia, which is resistant to antibiotics, can also leave the patient with a lung abscess; it is also particularly lethal to infants under four months, to the aged, and to the debilitated. (Staph pneumonia usually follows epidemics of flu.) All patients suspected of having staph pneumonia should be hospitalized.

Symptoms: Pneumonia either begins as or is preceded by an upper respiratory infection like a cold. The only difference is that the secretions are unusually heavy, more than any cold produces.

Then the disease hits dramatically, beginning with sudden, paroxysmal, shaking chills, often so violent that the bed trembles and the teeth chatter. This may go on for several minutes to a half hour. The oncoming fever is high; the patient is prostrated; his face is flushed; he looks and feels quite ill; his skin is hot and moist; beads of sweat appear on his forehead and face. Cold sores may break out around the corners of his lips; his tongue can be furred. He appears apprehensive.

The basic symptoms are severe chills, pain in the chest, a painful cough, and rusty brown or blood-streaked sputum. Pneumonia is not hard to identify.

The patient will try to suppress the cough because of the exacerbating pain in the chest. Rusty phlegm is brought up.

Breathing is painful and rapid, from 25 to 45 times a minute, the pain often causing an odd expiratory grunt.

The pulse rate can run from 100 to 130 per minute.

The crisis (turning point of the disease), which formerly appeared in five to ten days, now appears within one day because of antibiotic therapy.

The doctor will listen with his stethoscope for rales (sounds of air passing through bronchi that contain phlegm). He will also listen for pleural friction rub to identify pleurisy.

The symptoms are much the same for all bacterial pneumonias. Occasionally there might be a clue to the causative germ. Staph pneumonia will often start with great prostration, the fever being remittent. If there is cyanosis with a peculiar reddish-blue colour, it is usually a serious sign of a very grave form of the disease. If pus forms in the pharynx or tonsils it might suggest strep pneumonia. Klebsiella pneumonia also begins with early severe prostration; the sputum is bloody and gelatinous.

Treatment: The patient should be isolated with few or no visitors. Masks should be worn if possible.

Complete bed rest is in order, plus plenty of liquids and a soft diet high in proteins and lots of salt, because of salt loss (except when the patient has congestive heart failure). The patient should be allowed all the liquids he wants, which will be considerable.

When breathing is difficult, oxygen should be administered (especially if there is cyanosis) through a nasal catheter or the use of a tent; a mask is unsuitable because of the continuous cough.

A tight chest binder is most helpful for the patient to cough against.

Antibiotics should be started at once, the earlier the better, even before identification of the causative germ. While the sample of phlegm or smear is being sent to the laboratory, therapy should begin. Penicillin, totally effective against the pneumococcus – none have been known to survive this drug – should be administered. Once the germ is identified, the doctor may change the antibiotic to a more specialized type.

If penicillin does not work, the following reasons should be considered:

1. The germ is either a staphylococcus (a resistant strain) or Klebsiella, which is immune to penicillin, but very susceptible to gentamicin.

2. The patient is also suffering from empyaema, endocarditis, or meningitis.

3. The patient responds badly to penicillin.

4. If the pneumonia has been curbed but not cured and the disease is still holding on, the pneumonia has been caused by other bacteria. The pneumococcus has been knocked out, but the others are still there. A change of antibiotics will usually do the trick.

Antibiotics must be continued for several days after the patient is free of fever; a relapse can occur if the antibiotic is discontinued too soon. The patient may get out of bed two days after all signs of fever are gone. A follow-up x-ray of the lungs should be taken three to four weeks after recovery.

If there is shock, it should be treated in the normal way for shock. If the neck is rigid, it could be a serious complication, pneumococcal meningitis.

Prevention: Anyone who allows himself to get run-down, leaves himself more vulnerable to pneumonia. In areas where, or during periods when pneumonia is prevalent, immunization with pneumococcus polysaccharide might be advisable. This is also suggested for those in the high risk bracket, the old and those suffering from chronic ailments.

Outlook: About ninety-five per cent of those who contract any form of pneumonia survive. Best results are from those who receive antibiotic treatment within the first few days. The prognosis for those under fifty is always excellent, providing they have no complicating chronic diseases. Untreated cases (without antibiotics) have between a 20 per cent and 40 per cent fatality rate. The factors that militate against recovery are old age, infancy, late treatment, involvement of more than one lung, heart disease, cirrhosis of the liver, complications resulting from shock, meningitis, bacteraemia, pregnancy (last three months), and last but hardly least, type II and type III pneumococcal pneumonia and Klebsiella pneumonia.

Klebsiella, if untreated, has an 80 per cent fatality rate; if treated, 40 per cent; if treated at once less than 30 per cent. Happily it is not common, less than 5 per cent of all cases. The lung abscess that it produces can persist for months.

Atypical pneumonia 110
(virus pneumonia)

Atypical pneumonia is a pulmonary virus disease with symptoms resembling those of pneumonia. Frequently called virus pneumonia, it is most often caused by organisms of the genus *Mycoplasma*. The characteristic signs are similar to those of true pneumonia, and like all other pneumonias, the alveoli (air spaces) of the lungs are infected. This form is spread from person to person by nose and mouth discharges – coughing, sneezing, spitting – but, unlike the common cold, casual contact will not transmit the disease. The receiver has to be very receptive – by being run-down and debilitated, or by suffering from flu or other systemic diseases. In general, what holds true for pneumococcal pneumonia is also true for atypical pneumonia. It affects all ages, but more often younger age groups.

The danger: The mortality rate is low, less than one per cent. Even in severe cases full recovery is usual.

Symptoms: The onset is gradual as compared to the pneumococcal variety. Often the patient might not appear or feel ill. Atypical pneumonia is frequently referred to as 'walking pneumonia'. The respiration rate and pulse are often normal even if fever is present. The chills are mild, but the cough can be incessant and paroxysmal, bringing up much phlegm, but rarely rusty or bloody.

In the average, moderate case the temperature usually remains elevated for about ten days and then gradually returns to normal. However, convalescence is lengthy, leaving the patient fatigued for a long time.

Complications are relatively rare.

Treatment: This form of pneumonia is not easy to identify. If the causative germ is Mycoplasma bacteria, the disease will respond well to tetracycline. Nevertheless, the disease is self-limiting, even without medication.

Treatment should include codeine for the characteristic constant cough. Inhalation of steam is useful. If the disease is quite severe, oxygen therapy should be employed.

The patient must be kept in bed for several days after the fever has dropped to normal. Early return to daily duties will leave the patient feeling fatigued and weak for a long time afterwards.

Outlook: Excellent. Even those who appear critically ill recover fully.

Aspiration and lipoid pneumonias 111

Pneumonias caused by foreign matter that gets into the lungs, such as regurgitated material that is breathed in, are called aspiration and lipoid pneumonias. They can also be induced by insufficient care in inserting and removing a stomach tube. Other causes are eating while under the influence of whisky, the administering of cod liver oil to infants; and the taking of mineral oil or oily substances, such as nose drops, especially before bedtime, by elderly patients whose gag reflex is impaired.

If a sufficient amount of foreign material has been taken into the lungs, there will be fever, chest pains, shortness of breath, and cough.

Various forms of antibiotics are indicated for this form of pneumonia, in which there may be a mixed infection.

The administration of oily nose drops to children should be done with utmost care. While being treated, the child or patient should be placed on his back with his head tilted far back and turned to the side or he may lie on his side with no pillow.

Pulmonary tuberculosis 112
(TB, consumption)

Tuberculosis is a worldwide bacterial (tubercle) infection of the lungs that causes the growth of fibrous tissue, calcification, abscess, necrosis (death) of lung tissue, and cavities in the lung. The two types of tuberculosis that affect man are the human and the bovine. The pasteurization of milk has eliminated the bovine variety.

The danger: The tuberculosis germ is one of the fiercest, most persistent enemies of man; it will attack with equal virulence every part of the body (these ailments will be described in the appropriate sections), but about ninety per cent of all tubercular diseases is tuberculosis of the lungs.

By the age of fifty, practically everyone has some TB scars on the lungs. Many have been infected with the germ but do not have the disease – one out of twenty will show active signs of tuberculosis. The death rate is about five per 100,000 (a decline from 200 at the turn of the century), or out of every 250 people who have active TB, only one will die of it, a great testimony to medical advancement. But this should not lull anyone into believing that this ancient enemy has been beaten. Unfortunately, in recent years, a slight but significant rise in the incidence of this disease has occurred in the Western World, indicating the growing resistance of the tubercle bacillus to current drugs.

Tuberculosis is the most pervasive communicable disease in the world. Men have it twice as often as women, and non-Caucasians seem more susceptible, probably because of their greater poverty, poorer nutrition, and over-crowded living conditions.

Who is susceptible to the disease? Children who have been weakened by other pulmonary ailments, such as whooping cough, diphtheria, or measles, or other debilitating diseases. The same tendency is shown by people in occupations that jeopardize the lungs – miners, steel grinders, cement workers, and so on. Although tuberculosis is no respecter of wealth, it nevertheless strikes far more frequently at the poor. Heredity has not been proven, but some families have less resistance to the germ than others.

Contagion: The disease is spread from tubercularly diseased persons, particularly those with open cavities in their lungs, by coughing, sneezing, or spitting or the careless disposal of tissue. Unpasteurized milk is always a potential danger.

The tubercle bacteria invade the lung and are immediately attacked by the white blood corpuscles, which ingest them, imprisoning them. Scar tissue then forms around the germ (causing fibrous lung tissue); the germ is further encased in lime salts (calcification). But this microbe cannot be killed; it has formed a protective waxy coat around itself, lying dormant, quiescent, waiting for an opportunity to get free – which unfortunately does happen often. An infection with the tubercle bacteria means a life-long infection; but the germ can be kept inactive for the rest of one's life.

Test for tuberculosis: when the body is infected with the tubercle bacillus, it becomes allergic to the germ, and its presence can be ascertained by a skin test (Mantoux test). A prepared amount of t. berculin (a sterile liquid substance prepared from the bacteria) is injected into the skin. The body will react allergically if it's already infected. Within two or three days a redness, swelling, and hardening will occur at the area of injection. If the hardened area measures about half an inch the test is positive. This is only one of many tests but the most reliable.

The chest x-ray: a positive tuberculin test indicates that a chest x-ray should be taken at once. Although the x-ray is far from infallible, it will show signs of tuberculosis by shadows on the lungs, before any active symptoms show up. The earliest signs can be seen in the apexes of the lungs. However, the benefits of early diagnosis of tuberculosis must be judged against the harmful effects of radiation exposure.

Symptoms: Cough, bloody sputum, severe fatigue, loss of appetite and consequent loss of weight, and a drenching night sweat are some of the classic easily recognizable symptoms, but they vary considerably in types and degree of intensity.

Tuberculosis of the lungs has two forms, primary and progressive.

The primary form is not always recognized because it often does not have the obvious symptoms of the progressive type. But more children are affected by this form. There may be mild fever, some weight loss. Even x-ray may not show signs of lung damage. The early phase in children can seem like mild flu, but the fever might last for weeks. The child is abnormally tired and his appetite is poor. Even though the child may be alert, a sharp-eyed parent will know he is off his norm. There may be no cough, no pain in the chest, and no shortness of breath. But sooner or later the x-ray will begin to show patches on the lungs. Although the symptoms may be minor, the lung involvement can be serious and advanced.

In the adult, early signs of primary tuberculosis are the slow sapping of his strength and developing shortness of breath, especially on effort. On slight exercise his pulse will accelerate rapidly and be slow in returning to normal. There is always a weight loss early in the disease.

Progressive pulmonary tuberculosis in the adult can occur insidiously with a slow loss of weight and a gradual insidious fatigue and then explode in what was often chillingly called 'galloping consumption'. In a short time the patient becomes emaciated, his skin turns greyish, he develops a cough with bloody sputum, and almost every night he drenches his bed with sweat. Before the advent of new drugs, 'galloping consumption' would kill in a matter of weeks.

Blood in sputum: when the blood loss is severe – profuse, bright red, and frothy – leaving a strong salty taste, the patient is faced with a life-threatening situation – this is a *Medical Emergency.*

Cough: at first the cough will appear only in the morning, but it soon grows worse in severity and frequency. The pus-filled sputum is green, then becomes yellow, but is always blood. *Pleurisy* **118** is a common finding, causing pain in the chest or side. Often this pain (always aggravated by breathing) is a primary symptom.

In the early stages of tuberculosis, there may be no sign at all of breathing insufficiency, but as the disease progresses there is a marked loss in vital capacity.

Note of warning: there may be a seeming period of remission in which the symptoms appear to have abated – coughing, pain, fatigue, sweating, become greatly reduced. Although this often signifies that the tuberculosis has been arrested, it sometimes turns out to be a false 'cure' and the disease may actually be getting worse. The cavities in the lungs may be getting even larger, especially if the patient should elect to stop treatment.

Treatment: Modern treatment employs several drugs to combat the disease. Although each drug, on its own, is powerful enough to contain tuberculosis, a single drug is never used separately, because the tubercle germ, one of the most resilient, tenacious bacteria that afflict man, rapidly develops resistance to a medication. Using three drugs divides the germ's ability to resist by three. It must be remembered that there are side effects to the use of these drugs. Originally the number one medication was isoniazid (also called INH); number two was streptomycin; and the adjunct to the primary drugs was number three, aminosalicylic acid (PAS). Now, however, there are many other effective drugs, the safest being rifampicin, which is given by mouth.

These drugs must be taken for a minimum of eighteen months to two years. Interrupted drug treatment is hazardous, for it gives the tubercle germ a chance to develop more resistance. What is astonishing is that in a recent survey a major problem in treatment indicated that patients were too often remiss in taking their medication, even though the new drugs could mean the difference between life or death or a life of invalidism.

There are cases where these drugs are not effective, where the tubercle bacteria have developed total resistance. There are also patients who develop an intolerance for the drugs or pulmonary bleeding. In such situations some of the older therapy is used, such as artificial pneumothorax (collapsing a lung) or resection (cutting out diseased tissue). These patients require hospitalization and constant observation.

Response to chemical therapy is poor in people suffering from malnutrition, anaemia, and diabetes. The underlying disease must be treated simultaneously.

Hypersensitivity to the drugs develops early in the therapy and should be closely watched. Even two or three days of adverse reaction can endanger a patient's life. Late hypersensitivity, after the patient has been on the drugs for four or five months, is rare.

Relapse and re-treatment poses serious problems. Premature cessation of treatment can also be deadly when treatment is resumed. The second time around the germ is usually far more resistant. Often it becomes necessary to try the other drugs. The bacilli may have become so drug resistant that in spite of drug therapy the sputum remains bacilli positive. In such cases the question of surgical intervention requires special consideration.

Once a major part of the treatment, strict bed rest is no longer advised, although rest is still highly advisable. Nor does climate seem to have any significance in convalescence and treatment.

Isolation is no longer required, but the rules of proper hygiene must be stringent indeed. Patients under treatment should be schooled in taking essential precautions against spreading the disease – covering the mouth with disposable tissues, then burning them; separation of soap, towels, and dishes; not spitting in the wash basin, and other good sense rules.

Children should not live in the same household where a tuberculous patient with an active disease (open cavities in the lungs) is also residing. In fact, older people with chronic lung disease should be examined medically if they are living in a home where children are running about.

After the tubercle germ has disappeared from the sputum, after the lung cavity has closed and the symptoms of cough, fatigue have stopped, the patient can return to normal life – but with strings attached. He must remember he has not been cured; tuberculosis has only been brought to quiescence. He must remember he has no reserve – overwork, overdoing anything, or loss of sleep can reactivate the disease.

Precautionary treatment: when an infant or a very young child shows a positive reaction in the tuberculin skin test, and even though there are no other signs of tuberculosis, the wise and practised procedure is to administer special therapy (usually isoniazid) in sufficient dosage and of sufficient duration to prevent not only pulmonary and general body tuberculosis but tuberculous meningitis.

Note: women who have tuberculosis should consult a doctor regarding pregnancy. Each case requires individual consideration.

Prevention: TB is preventable. By avoiding overcrowded living conditions, by paying attention to nutrition, by considering all coughs as suspicious, by staying away from people who have the active form of the disease and from people who have undiagnosed chronic bronchitis, by considering loss of weight and drenching sweats sufficient reason to see a doctor, and by maintaining good health, resistance to the tubercle bacillus can be achieved.

Everyone in the medical profession and close relatives of someone who has tuberculosis should be considered for BCG vaccination against the disease. Children living in the same house with a tuberculous patient should be given the vaccine plus protective treatment with isoniazid. (Note: Many authorities now deny the efficacy of BCG vaccine.) (See *Part 3, Early warning signals, Pulmonary tuberculosis* **112**.)

Outlook: Some major battles against TB have been won, but the war is still going on. As it stands now, TB is controllable but not yet curable. Thanks to the new chemotherapy, most patients who would previously have died now survive. But the disease is still rampant in less prosperous countries. Eradication of tuberculosis must mean eradication everywhere.

Emphysema 113

In emphysema the lungs lose their elasticity, causing them to be continuously overdistended. As a result, not enough air is moving in and out of the lungs. The patient can breathe in, but breathing out is difficult and inefficient. The lungs are in a constant state of inflation. As a result of advancing age, heavy smoking, or familial weakness, emphysema usually is part of bronchitis or bronchitis is part of emphysema.

The danger: The seriousness of the disease varies widely. Some persons never reach a stage of incapacity and go through life with relatively little inconvenience, while in others the disease worsens progressively until final degeneration of the ability to breathe. Life is shortened by this incurable disease. A usual complication is right heart failure (failure due to venous and capillary engorgement).

Symptoms: The cardinal symptom of emphysema is shortness of breath on exertion. There is a hard cough, which is very tiring and haphazard in occurrence and is usually brought on by talking, shouting, laughter – or any effort. The phlegm that is brought up is minimal but thick and heavy.

Exhaling can become arduous; the chest, as a result, takes on a barrel-like appearance. Cyanosis appears frequently in more advanced cases as a result of insufficient oxygen. Between exhaling and inhaling the patient often takes a moment's pause. The vital capacity is significantly decreased.

Treatment: Although emphysema is irreversible (the lung tissue can never regain its former elasticity), the patient can be helped to feel considerable relief and his lungs can be made more efficient.

The use of bronchodilator aerosols (atomizers) is most effective for many sufferers. The patient deeply inhales the fine mist, holds his breath, then exhales. A half dozen such deep inhalations will give relief. It is better to employ the aerosol method regularly at fixed times every day rather than when the symptoms appear.

In severe cases the patient should be hospitalized and given oxygen or Intermittent Positive Pressure Breathing in which the patient breathes through a mask connected to a device that produces intermittent air pressure. When pressure is increased the lungs are inflated, when pressure is released the patient exhales.

The patient is usually not confined to bed but kept active within the limits of his capacity, never to such effort, however, that will cause him shortness of breath.

Several drugs are employed to loosen and thin the bronchial phlegm, which interferes with his breathing: Potassium iodid solution 30mg (5 to 10 drops in water 3 times a day) or ammonium chloride (1 gram every 4 hours). There are a number of other drugs that are helpful in dissipating bronchial phlegm. Cough remedies are not used because coughing is essential to clearing the passageways.

Respiratory infections that can aggravate emphysema are treated with antibiotic therapy.

An abdominal belt is often advised for those with breathing problems.

The abdominal breathing exercises described in Modified Yoga Breathing (*Table 9*) are highly recommended.

Prevention: Cigarette smoking should be avoided, and when possible, one should live in a clean, dry environment.

Outlook: With medical care the patient suffering from emphysema can prolong his life.

Atelectasis 114

Atelectasis is due to the collapse or airless condition of a lung or portion of it. It is caused by obstruction of a foreign body, a tenacious mucus plug, heavy bronchial secretions, enlarged lymph nodes, pressure from a tumour, and postoperative complications. Atelectasis may also be the first sign of a lung tumour.

If the collapse is massive (a full lung) and developing rapidly, there will be severe shortness of breath, pain on that side, cyanosis, a drop in blood pressure, rapid heartbeat, and shock. The heart might even be displaced. In slowly developing atelectasis, the signs are severe shortness of breath and weakness.

The postoperative patient should be compelled to early ambulation; he should not be allowed to lie in one position for as long as two hours; narcotics should be used sparingly because they depress the cough reflex. To be on the safe side an Intermittent Positive Pressure Breathing machine should be employed for five minutes every hour or so for three or four hours after surgery.

A patient suffering from atelectasis should be treated with aerosol bronchodilator drugs, in which he can quickly breathe in the spray. He should be made to cough; if necessary, a cough-inducing machine is used. Since collapsed lungs tend to get infected, antibiotics are administered.

If the obstruction is removed, there are usually no aftereffects.

Lung abscess 115
(pulmonary abscess, gangrene of the lung)

A lung abscess forms in localized areas of the lung in which there is pus formation and necrosis of tissue surrounded by inflammation. The causes can be pulmonary embolism, staph or Klebsiella pneumonia, lesions from bronchiectasis, or any bronchial obstruction with infection.

The abscess can bring about a cavity in the lungs, as in tuberculosis, but the germs in the abscess are more easily destroyed. Eventually the abscess ruptures into a bronchial tube and is coughed up – a very foul-smelling, purulent matter.

The danger: This is a serious disease that can be controlled with antibiotics and surgery, but for those already weakened by chronic disease, the abscess itself can become chronic with the risk of complications that are occasionally fatal.

Symptoms: Lung abscess is quite similar to pneumonia – severe chills, high fever, painful cough, drenching night sweats, and great malaise. The difference between the two diseases is that in lung abscess the chills are repeated whereas in pneumonia they occur usually only at the inception.

Another distinguishing feature is that when the abscess ruptures, perforating a bronchial tube, the sputum coughed up is extremely foul, purulent, bloodstained, and contains bits of gangrenous lung tissue. The rupture can cause a severe worsening of the condition and even shock.

Additional symptoms are often weight loss, weakness, shortness of breath on exertion, anxiety, pallor or cyanosis, and considerable prostration.

Treatment: Penicillin should be instituted as soon as the sputum tests have been made. Since abscess almost always is a result of several different types of bacteria, more than one antibiotic is employed. Penicillin is dramatically effective except when one of the bacteria is Klebsiella pneumococcus, against which penicillin is ineffective.

The cough should not be curbed unless it becomes too harassing.

Creosote carbonate in milk (5 drops after meals 3 times a day) will help deodorize the foul odour. However, the antibiotics work so quickly that this is not always necessary.

Surgical drainage is essayed only if the bacteria resist antibiotics (not very common).

If the cavities in the lungs persist after considerable antibiotic therapy, further treatment consists of excision of the diseased parts of the lungs.

This is a very serious disease, requiring complete bed rest and the employment of postural drainage (*Table 8*). Nutrition is important; the diet should be high in proteins and vitamins.

Outlook: The full healing of a lung abscess depends on the adequate drainage of the bronchial tubes into which it has ruptured. Without proper drainage the cavity will not heal and the abscess will become chronic. With good drainage and antibiotics, 85 per cent of the patients recover completely. The other 15 per cent can be helped by surgery.

Oedema of the lungs 116
(pulmonary oedema, 'wet lungs')

An accumulation of tissue fluids in the lungs, oedema of the lungs is most often caused by left heart failure (engorgement of the blood vessels of the lungs). Other causes include lung infection from pneumonia and chemical injury from irritants, most of which are industrial, such as chlorine, ammonia, bromine, and others. The disease can also be excited by some noxious gases, such as sulphur dioxide and nitrogen oxide, which pollute the atmosphere.

A unique cause is depression of the cough reflex – people who don't cough often or well and thus allow fluids to accumulate in the windpipe. Morphine, which is given to patients suffering from asthma, emphysema, and chronic bronchitis, depresses the cough mechanism. These patients are often overdosed, causing an accumulation of phlegm. Overdosage of barbiturates will also interfere with normal coughing.

The danger: This is a *Medical Emergency.* A disease with a high level of fatalities, oedema of the lung often requires heroic efforts on the part of the doctor. When there is a combination of circulatory failure and poor tracheobronchial drainage, the condition is often terminal.

Symptoms: The primary symptom is extremely difficult respiration, in which breathing is rapid and laboured; the cough is often asthmatic and wheezing, occasionally producing bloody phlegm. Insufficient oxygen causes cyanosis; the extremities are cold, the veins in the neck protrude. The doctor can hear moist rales in the chest. The patient has a sense of oppression in his chest; he appears pale, apprehensive, and sweats profusely. Hypertensive patients are particularly anxious; their breathing is deep and especially laboured.

Treatment: If an attack of breathing difficulty has occurred, tourniquets are placed on all four limbs, one at a time. This measure, to obtain better circulation of the blood, keeps the fluid from gathering in the lungs. The tourniquet should be kept on each limb no longer than fifteen minutes, with enough pressure to block the venous return but not enough to impede the arterial flow to the limbs.

A high concentration of oxygen (50 to 100 per cent quality) should be administered immediately along with an atomized spray of epinephrine, which should reduce the patient's anxiety and restlessness. If the patient is struggling and anguished it might be necessary to give him a hypodermic injection of morphine.

Other treatment consists of intravenous injection of aminophylline and diuretic therapy.

Bed rest is imperative.

Prevention: The answer is crystal clear, as the air in the lungs should be, untainted with fumes. Normal coughing should not be suppressed; the body is simply acting automatically to rid itself of harmful phlegm.

Outlook: In mild attacks the prognosis is generally good. In serious attacks the outlook is much dimmer because oedema of the lungs is usually a very late symptom of some serious pulmonary or cardiac disease.

High altitude lung oedema 116a

Caused by an excessively rapid descent plus heavy exertion, the symptoms of high altitude lung oedema appear within thirty-six hours and often in as little as six: shortness of breath, malaise, cough worsening to bloody cough, noisy breathing, cyanosis. Unless oxygen is given at once and the patient brought down to a lower altitude, he will die.

Pneumoconiosis 117 (dusty lungs)

An occupational disorder, pneumoconiosis is caused by the inhalation of dust particles. The several varieties include:

Silicosis 117a

Produced by the inhalation of silica dust, silicosis is the most widespread and important of all industrial, man-created lung diseases; it is a forerunner of tuberculosis. The disease is wide-ranging among miners of lead, coal, copper, silver, gold, talc, mica, and bauxite (aluminium) as well as stonecutters, sandblasters, metal grinders, and others.

Anthracosis (black lung) 117b

Produced by the inhalation of coal dust, anthracosis causes miners' lungs to turn dark or even black.

Siderosis 117c

This disorder is produced by the inhalation of iron particles. It is a benign disease and no treatment is necessary.

Asbestosis 117d

Produced by the inhalation of asbestos fibres, asbestosis was previously confined to those working in asbestos factories, but the use of asbestos in the manufacture of automobile brakes has allowed it to be spread in the air in congested areas of the world. It is a worrisome and unknown factor in many lung disorders, especially since asbestos fibres remain and accumulate in the lungs (the white blood corpuscles are unable to ingest and dispose of asbestos fibres as they do with most foreign bodies and all germs). In addition, asbestos is the cause of a special type of carcinoma of the lungs, in which asbestos particles are found in the sputum.

The danger and symptoms: All the above, in varying degrees of virulence, eventually cause shortness of breath, which sometimes develops slowly and at other times more rapidly, particularly on exertion. Later symptoms are fibrosis of the lungs, wheezing, coughing without phlegm (if serious, there will be phlegm and bloody phlegm), all of which can eventually lead to pneumonia, tuberculosis, and lung cancer.

Treatment and prevention: All forms of pneumoconiosis are generally irreversible. Treatment is palliative. Bronchodilators in the atomizing spray form can bring some relief. Continuing to smoke adds a serious hazard. One of the best palliatives is getting out of the occupation. Economically this may not be easy, but it is financially superior to lying in a hospital. Young people with sensitive lungs must change their jobs before it is too late.

It is essential for both labour and management to devise better methods of dust suppression and better safety measures for the workers.

Outlook: If a victim removes himself from this hazardous employment, he can at least prevent the disease from progressing further. If he elects to stay on the job, he may be faced with the problem of how to survive with both lungs damaged.

THE PLEURA
Pleurisy 118

Inflammation of the pleura, the double membrane that covers the lung, pleurisy is caused by any disease that also inflames the lung, such as pneumonia, tuberculosis, or tumour. Pleurisy also can be brought on by flu, show up after a severe cold or during kidney diseases, acute rheumatism, rheumatic fever, or bronchitis – and, then again, it often appears for no reason at all. There are two varieties, dry and wet.

The danger: Generally pleurisy is a disorder that will disappear with treatment. Often, however, it is a forerunner of tuberculosis or empyaema, or a symptom of an underlying disease, occasionally carcinoma of the lungs.

Symptoms: In dry pleurisy the comparatively dry surfaces of the double membrane rub against each other. The pain is sharp, knifelike. The friction rub is heard by the doctor when listening with a stethoscope. Pain is always worsened by breathing or coughing. The pain is often displaced to the shoulder, abdomen, or neck. There is considerable shortness of breath.

The pain of pleurisy can simulate a heart attack, the difference being that in a true heart attack there is no differentiation in pain when breathing, while in pleurisy pain is always worsened on inhalation or exhalation.

Wet pleurisy is usually a continuation of dry pleurisy. Now, additionally, tissue fluid gets in between the membranes. Breathing is rapid and shallow; temperature may run up to 38·3°C, 101°F. There is, of course, pain on breathing, on bending and twisting. If the tissue fluid is excessive, some vital capacity will be lost because of the reduction of lung volume. Usually there is a cough.

Treatment: Fever or not, the patient should be confined to bed. Absolute rest is essential, with lots of fresh air and sunlight if possible and no exertion of any kind until the convalescence stage is reached.

Pain can be relieved by analgesics. The affected side is often strapped to help immobilize the chest and reduce the pain. Opiates are sometimes necessary to keep the patient from becoming too agonized and depressed. A cheerful outlook can hasten recovery by a week.

Deep, slow careful breathing can help prevent pleural adhesions. The lung can be expanded and vital capacity improved by making the patient blow up balloons.

In wet pleurisy it is often necessary to remove the fluid by needle aspiration. This is without danger and is performed with local anaesthesia. The diet should be high in proteins and vitamins.

Prevention and outlook: Pleurisy is often due to the neglect of some underlying lung ailment, but just as often it can appear without reason. If there is no causative disorder the prognosis is complete recovery.

Empyema 119
(putrid empyema)

Once feared, the ravages of empyema have been greatly reduced by the use of antibiotics. Acute or chronic, empyema is characterized by the collection of pus in the pleural sac. The chronic form often results from inadequate treatment of the acute form. The cause is usually pneumonia or tuberculosis, but it can also be incited by scarlet fever, kidney abscess, or liver or abdomen abscesses. The infecting agents are always bacterial, never viral.

The disease usually begins with wet pleurisy which becomes suppurated.

When pneumonia does not respond satisfactorily, that is, when the temperature does not return to normal as expected, the likelihood is that the patient has developed empyema. The fever becomes capricious – intermittent. When the pus is aspirated from the pleural cavity by needle, it is usually without odour; whereas, when the causal organisms are intestinal bacteria, the pus is foul smelling.

The danger: The disease can cause, if not promptly treated, pericarditis, endocarditis, meningitis, and brain abscess, thus creating an unholy triangle, because empyema is secondary to such other odious diseases as pneumonia or tuberculosis. An unlucky or uncareful patient can go from pneumonia to empyema to meningitis.

Symptoms: A sharp pain in the chest and frequently a short dry cough are characteristic. Additionally there are usually chills, fever, sweating, flushed cheeks with the rest of the face and body pale or grey, strong malaise, foul breath, loss of appetite, and emaciation. Clubbing of fingers is common.

Treatment: Antibiotic treatment is important. It is usually necessary to remove the pus-filled pleural fluid by needle aspiration or by surgical drainage (cutting through the chest wall).

In uncomplicated empyema the patient should be encouraged to get out of bed and move about as soon as his temperature has dropped to normal and the pus has been removed from the chest.

Diet should consist of a high concentration of all vitamins.

Breathing exercises should be part of the convalescent period – exhaling against self-enforced resistance. Deep breathing done with care can be of great value.

Outlook: The outlook is always dependent on the underlying disease. Empyema by itself is quite curable.

Pneumothorax 120

Pneumothorax, collapse of the lung, occurs when air gets into the airless space between the pleural membranes, which are normally flat against each other. Except for artificial pneumothorax (performed by a doctor as a therapeutic measure in combating tuberculosis), this disorder has three forms: traumatic, spontaneous, and that produced by tension.

Traumatic: This form of pneumothorax results from an injury, a bullet wound, a car accident, in which the pleural sac is penetrated, thus allowing an invasion of air.

Spontaneous: spontaneous pneumothorax occurs for no special reason in the majority of cases. Occasionally, however, it is caused by a blister on the pleural membrane that ruptures and allows air into the pleural sac. This blister is a result of either a scar from some infection or a congenital defect. A sudden strain, such as a cough or sneeze, could burst the blister. Or it could burst on its own while the patient is asleep when the blister has reached its point of ripeness. This form occurs five times more often in young men than in young women. Beyond age forty spontaneous pneumothorax is a result of an existing lung disorder.

Tension: in pneumothorax produced by tension a tear occurs in the pleural membrane, allowing air to get in but not escape, something on the order of a tyre valve. When the pleural cavity is filled with air, it collapses a part of the lung and also displaces the heart and other nearby organs.

The danger: The only dangerous form is tension pneumothorax. As the pleural sac fills with air that cannot escape, breathing becomes quite difficult and·the patient becomes quite anxious. This is a *Medical Emergency*; the air must be removed with a catheter and pump. Often it becomes necessary to give needed oxygen by mask.

Symptoms: The onset of spontaneous pneumothorax is sudden, with severe, sharp chest pain, difficulty in breathing, shortness of breath, and a slight cough but no sputum. Pain is usually on the affected side and worsened by inhalation. Pain may go to the shoulder, but does not radiate down the arm, which differentiates it from a heart attack. When an x-ray picture is taken the pneumothorax will be seen clearly.

In tension pneumothorax, as indicated above, breathing becomes difficult, pain is severe, and the patient is anxious. The symptoms are the same as in spontaneous pneumothorax, only more intense.

Treatment: Some cases of spontaneous pneumothorax are self-limiting, requiring only rest until the ruptured pleura heals and the lung expands back to normal (from two to four weeks). When necessary, as in tension pneumothorax, treatment is usually carried out by inserting a catheter into the pleural cavity and sucking out the air, thus allowing the lung to re-expand.

Outlook: In spontaneous pneumothorax the outlook is always benign.

Hyperventilation 121
(respiratory neurosis)

An increase in the rate and depth of respiration and a consequent diminution of the normal carbon dioxide content, hyperventilation can be deliberate, as in the case of swimmers who mistakenly believe they can swim longer under water if they first take a series of deep breaths, or unwitting, as in those suffering from acute neurotic anxiety.

The danger: In the case of swimmers, hyperventilation will cause blackout and drowning. There are a number of such cases every year in which college and high school swimmers are fished out of the water drowned or half drowned.

Symptoms: In the underwater swimmer the symptoms are insidious – the swimmer simply fades into unconsciousness before he comes up for air.

In respiratory neurosis there is a feeling of panic, a tightening in the chest, and suffocation. Oppression occurs in the heart area, along with a fast heartbeat and a sense of unreality. The blood pressure falls and the person (most often a woman) faints, with residual numbness or coldness of the extremities. Sometimes this can occur several times a day.

Treatment: The patient is made to breathe into a paper bag for several minutes to restore the carbon dioxide in the lungs and blood. Overbreathing can be dramatically curtailed by demonstrating to the patient what is actually happening. The patient is deliberately asked to breathe in deeply for a few minutes. As soon as the symptoms return, the patient breathes into a paper bag. Thus reassured that the disease is not fatal, the patient is now conscious of overbreathing and rarely does it again.

Hypoxia 122

Hypoxia occurs when the body tissues are under-oxygenated. Under-oxygenation of the tissues may be due to such drugs as morphine, alcohol, barbiturates, almost all anaesthetic agents, or electric shock or respiratory muscle paralysis – but more often to high altitude.

The danger: Severe hypoxia can affect the brain, causing mental deficiency, and produce blindness if not properly and promptly treated.

Mountain sickness 122a (acute hypoxia, high altitude sickness, Monge's disease)

Occurring in unacclimatized persons within a few hours after exposure to high altitudes, the vulnerability of each individual to mountain sickness is unpredictable, depending much on his physical condition, his rate of ascent, and the amount of energy he is exerting.

Symptoms: Respiratory difficulties may begin at 2,000 metres, 7,000 feet. Indi-

vidual tolerance varies greatly; some persons begin to show symptoms at 1,500 metres, 5,000 feet, others not before 4,000 metres, 14,000 feet. In either case, the signs are shortness of breath on exertion, headache, giddiness, restlessness, difficulty in concentration, palpitation, cyanosis of the lips, and nausea.

Above 4,000 metres, 14,000 feet there are stronger and varied reactions: some persons will feel indifferent, show lassitude, while others may become euphoric. Judgement is poor – a real hazard to mountain climbers. There is loss of peripheral vision, a dimness of vision, and muscular incoordination above 5,000 metres, 17,000 feet.

Above 5,500 metres, 18,000 feet the mountaineer begins to lose consciousness. Without oxygen or rapid descent, death will overtake him.

The symptoms can be mild to severe headache, impairment of judgement and concentration, cyanosis of the lips, shortness of breath on exertion, rapid heartbeat, malaise, weakness, nausea, restlessness, and sometimes even euphoria or delirium.

Treatment: Usually mountain sickness will subside gradually in a few days. Occasionally, however, the symptoms do not abate. The patient will then need oxygen and descent to a lower level.

Prevention: Any form of shortness of breath is a contra-indication to mountain climbing.

Outlook: Sudden hypoxia can occur to anyone without climbing high mountains. Jet planes fly in the 9,000-metre, 30,000-foot to 12,000-metre, 40,000-foot range. When an accidental loss of cabin pressure occurs, breathing in oxygen from a mask can be a lifesaver. Seconds count.

8 The heart and circulatory system

Abner J. Delman

Many people are burdened with misinformation regarding overtaxing the heart. They feel that the more energetic they are, the sooner their hearts will wear out. Nothing could be further from the truth. The heart does not need rest in the conventional sense. Indeed, it rests two-thirds of the time. Between one beat and the next, one-third of the time is work, two-thirds is rest.

The heart, like any other muscle, needs exercise. It would be most unusual for a healthy, well-conditioned heart to be jeopardized by an extended period of heavy physical exertion, because it is, by far, the most powerful muscle of the body – all other muscles will give out before it will. In running, for example, the feet will tire before the heart will; but if the heart has been weakened by defective or diseased blood vessels, of course, any sudden exercise can knock it out and often seriously damage it further.

Basically, appropriate exercise is vital for good functioning of the heart; although it has not been completely proved, it is suggested that the more the heart is exercised, the longer it will last, and appropriate exercise will improve the entire cardiovascular system.

A regimen of exercise must begin mildly if the person is middle-aged and has not been exercising regularly. He must slowly build up to a sustained vigorous daily stint. The faults of our age are psychic stress and physical indolence perhaps even more than diet, although diet is indeed most important. (Diet must be individualized in each case.) If one exercises vigorously every day, diet becomes less significant. An interesting proof is the research conducted by London University. Two sets of people were used to test the value of exercise, the bus drivers and the conductors of the London transport system. The driver sits at the wheel all day long, while the conductor constantly runs up and down the double-decker bus collecting fares several hundred times a day. The results of the investigations were astounding. From three to four times as many bus drivers had coronary attacks as did the conductors and those conductors who did eventually have coronaries survived them far better.

Coronary thrombosis is by far the greatest cause of death than all the other heart ailments put together. Under the age of forty, it is a male disease. Above fifty, when most women have reached the menopause, the attack rate is equal.

Prosperous countries or communities have a higher incidence of coronary thrombosis, because they can afford to exercise less and eat richer foods, usually high in cholesterol and saturated fats. (*Tables 2, 3,* and *4* deal with cholesterol and saturated foods.)

Susceptibility: who is susceptible? Who is more prone to coronary attacks? Can this group of diseases be prevented or beaten back? Many authorities have been struck by the familial cycle of these diseases, and some of the more despondent ones have come to the conclusion that not much can be done for those who have an inherited tendency. But this is patently untrue. If the inherited tendency is real, a great deal can be done to alter it – by medication, by changing diet and living habits, and by altering metabolism.

The 'inherited tendency' might be only the acquisition of some bad family habits, such as overeating, eating foods high in cholesterol, an aversion for physical exercise, and a wrong attitude towards stress. These habits can be changed. Heart disease can be pushed back to where it belongs – a disease of old age. We all have to go sometime, but getting it in the forties or fifties or even early sixties is really punishment for our sins against our bodies, sins of omission and commission.

A note about stress: many doctors still believe that stress is a major cause of heart trouble. Stress is part of living, for all of us, no matter what age or society we live in. In fact, the human body is magnificently built to stand up to it; all sorts of glands are provided to take care of stress impact. Even primitive man, trying to bring down a mammoth for his home and family, was under tremendous tension. But having said all that, we must still identify the factor that can induce heart disease. Primitive man was under great stress in killing game, but it was over in a short time; modern man, however, undergoes sustained psychic tension – a relentless pressure that can go on for years. No set of glands can stand up to it without some harm.

Heart disease is nature's way of saying we're doing it all wrong.

Arteriosclerosis, atherosclerosis 123

Actually, arterio- and athero- are different sides of the same coin. Arteriosclerosis is a hardening of the arterial tubes, a loss of suppleness. The doctor taking the pulse can sometimes judge their tonicity (elasticity) by the springiness of the radial

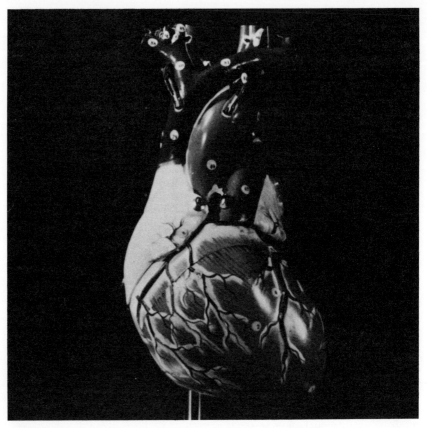

Life-size model of a normal heart. (*United States National Institutes of Health*)

artery in the wrist. Atherosclerosis occurs when the inner lining of the arteries has been layered with hardened cholesterol or other fats so that the passageway has been narrowed.

Requiring scores of years to develop, the disease often starts in childhood, where patterns of eating and sedentariness are determined. It strikes men in not inconsiderable numbers in their thirties and forties. It is the number one killer of both sexes in their fifties, sixties, and seventies. This disease will kill more people in any given year than all the other diseases of man put together.

The basic disease, atherosclerosis of the coronary arteries, is the prime cause of angina pectoris, coronary thrombosis, and coronary insufficiency.

Arterio-atherosclerosis, a silent disease that produces no symptoms until it is far advanced, causes the serious heart and vascular disorders listed below. However, a thorough medical examination including an electrocardiograph can usually determine the presence of this disease.

A very simplified physical-fitness heart test (*Table 5*) can be administered by the subject himself. The results are not a specific judgement but a general evaluation of the person's condition.

Here is a list of nine determinants that

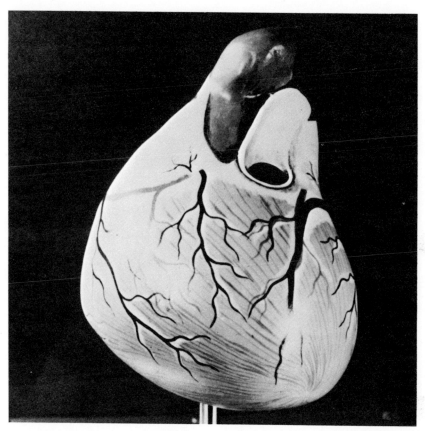

Model of the sick human heart. The heart responds to many heart and circulatory ills by enlarging up to four times its normal size, a condition common in atrial fibrillation and long-standing high blood pressure. (*United States National Institutes of Health*)

may advance the arterio-atherosclerotic configuration:

1. *Exercise*. The lack of sufficient, vigorous, appropriate, daily activity may advance early arterial damage. The heart and blood vessels, as well as the body, need regular exercise to keep fit. The heart, like all other muscles, can become flabby and weak if not exercised. Many people think of the body as a machine. Nothing could be more incorrect. A machine wears out with use – the more it is used the quicker it wears out. Not so the human body – the more it's used, the stronger it becomes, the *longer it lasts*! Experiments with animals have shown

that exercise also widens the very small arteries around the heart – collateral circulation that can take over and resupply needed blood if the coronary artery is blocked.

Daily cardiovascular exercise, whether in the form of jogging, swimming, or bicycling, should be done with complete relaxation. The mind should be free of business or personal problems and be concerned only with the activity at hand. Tensing up with impatience to get through the discipline as quickly as possible can only undo the good of the effort.

Besides regular exercise, those who work at a desk must find ways and means to

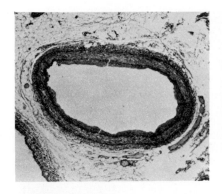
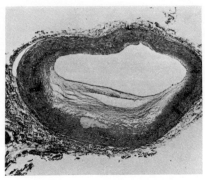
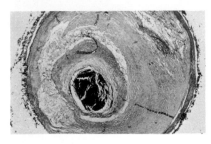

Above left: Normal artery – cross-section.
Above right: Atherosclerotic deposits formed in inner lining of an artery.
Left: The narrowed channel is blocked by a blood clot. (*American Heart Association*)

keep active, such as getting up from the desk frequently, walking instead of driving, taking the stairs instead of the lift. Those who keep moving are less of a target for heart disease.

2. *Overweight*. See *Table 13, Standard table of desirable weight for men and women*. Anyone who is 20 to 30 per cent above his proper weight according to sex, body structure, and height is two to three times more prone to a coronary attack.

3. *Cholesterol and triglycerides*. Levels of these fatty substances in the blood are age-dependent. Under forty, 260mg of cholesterol and 140mg of triglyceride is the maximum for normal readings. Over the age of forty, the maximum is 280–300mg for cholesterol and 180–200 for triglycerides. The separation between normal and abnormal readings remains far from clear-cut. Many doctors feel that any triglyceride reading above 140 or any cholesterol above 220 is abnormal and increases the risk of a heart attack. A high level (above 300) will increase susceptibility to heart disease by three to one. Keeping these levels down can be accomplished by diet, exercise, and, if necessary, by appropriate medication.

Note: cholesterol and triglycerides are not baneful substances; they are vital for various body functions. If the body does not receive enough cholesterol and triglycerides it will manufacture them in the liver. They only become harmful when the metabolic system does not handle them properly, or can't cope with them when too much of these fatty substances are ingested. Then cholesterol and triglycerides are deposited on the inside of the arteries in hardened plaques, thus hardening and narrowing the arteries.

4. *High blood pressure*. It is generally agreed by most cardiologists that 140 over 90 is the maximum for normal pressure. Determination of blood pressure require

a number of readings to evaluate the actual condition. Blood pressure fluctuates in everyone depending upon emotional and nervous stress, physical activity and fatigue. It is only when the figure remains consistently high after many readings that it is diagnostic.

High blood pressure for a long sustained period increases susceptibility to arterio-atherosclerosis and coronary thrombosis by a factor of four to one. Keeping the elevated pressure down by keeping the weight down, by diet and medication, is essential.

5. *Cigarettes*. Smoke, particularly tobacco smoke, constricts the arteries. Ten cigarettes a day can double the chance of getting a coronary; a full pack will quadruple the probability. Women who smoke run an even greater risk than men who smoke.

6. *Metabolic diseases. Diabetes* **332**, *Gout* **334**, *Hyperlipidaemia* **335** (excessive amounts of fat in the blood), or *Hypo-thyroidism* **339** can all lead to coronary artery disease. With proper medical care they can be treated and kept under control.

7. *Low vital capacity*. This is the relationship between the lung capacity and the amount of air that can be expelled. When the vital capacity is low, it will affect the heart. Many lung diseases will lower vital capacity. Exercise in most cases will improve the status.

8. *The muscular man*. Statistics show that a man who puts on weight after twenty-five is far more prone to arterial disease than the smaller boned, less robust-looking man. The muscular type should try to maintain the same weight as at twenty-five for the rest of his life.

9. *The family history*. The incidence of early arterio-atherosclerosis is usually inherited as a result of an innate metabolic abnormality. But this family phenomenon may only be the acquisition of bad habits, such as eating foods high in cholesterol or shunning exercise. Even if there is such an inherited tendency, it can often be counteracted.

Notes on prevention: sedentarianism is an evil that should be overcome.

Weight should be reduced to several pounds below the standard weight.

Restriction of saturated fats is always advisable, but restriction of all fats should be individualized under the care of a doctor. Some blood fat abnormalities may be due to sugar as well as fat intake.

Note: those who drink skim milk to avoid cholesterol should read the label on the cartons, particularly those of fortified skimmed milk. Presumably it is fortified with vitamins, which is good, but it may also be fortified with monoglycerides and diglycerides, forms of saturated fat. In other words, the butter containing cholesterol is removed and supplanted by another saturated fat. One might as well be drinking regular milk.

Metabolic diseases, even the low-level varieties, are particularly significant in young men – they can increase susceptibility to arterio-atherosclerosis.

Huge or even heavy meals should be avoided.

A middle-aged man who has been sedentary all his life should not attempt sudden, vigorous exercise or activity, especially in extreme cold or hot weather. He can induce a heart attack. This is in no way a contradiction to the need for exercise. All exercise programmes for the sedentary man must begin mildly and gradually with the counsel of a doctor and should be preceded by an appropriately monitored electrocardiograph exercise test.

Those who have a known arterial disease should avoid extremely emotional scenes; they can bring on an attack.

Since arterio-atherosclerosis is a degenerative disease, which has taken decades to develop, cure is not common, but considerable reversion can take place, and at least further advancement of the disease can be arrested so that the patient can live out his life almost to the fullest.

Unfortunately, people who are young give little heed to diseases they may be subjected to several decades later. This does not mean one should develop a lifelong preoccupation with heart disease but rather a lifestyle that is consonant with good health in terms of appropriate daily exercise and proper diet.

Inevitably, we all must die, but we can stave off this event to old age, where it belongs. (See *Part 3, Early warning signals, Heart disease* **123**)

Angina pectoris 124

A chronic condition of pain in the chest, angina pectoris, also known simply as angina, is usually brought on by exertion, emotion, a heavy meal, or sudden exposure to extreme cold. A few minutes' rest and the pain usually disappears. Its most common cause is coronary artery disease. The typical pattern is sudden exertion, pain, rest, relief.

The danger: Angina is usually a forerunner of coronary thrombosis.

Symptoms: The outstanding symptom is pain or pressure in the centre of the chest behind the sternum (the flat bone in the centre of the chest), usually brought on by effort. The pain can radiate to the left shoulder and down to the elbow or wrist, or occasionally to the right arm and/or the jaw. The pain is not really so sharp as it is a squeezing, gripping, constricting feeling ranging from mild discomfort to severe distress. Typically, it lasts only a few minutes. Other symptoms are often shortness of breath, palpitations, and dizziness. If it lasts for a half hour or longer, it is most likely *Coronary thrombosis* **125**. In the most severe form, there is a fear of death, ashen face, and cold sweat.

A very early symptom is mild pain on the first exertion of the day that disappears quickly.

Treatment: Much depends on the condition of the blood vessels of the patient. Some cardiologists are doubtful of exercise; others believe it's one of the answers. With proper care, proper diet, and appropriate exercises, the collateral circulation around the heart can develop to the point of partially taking over for the narrowed coronary artery. If the collateral circulation develops satisfactorily, a dramatic reversal can be seen – the symptoms will disappear; the progression towards coronary artery disease halted.

It can go either way, into coronary thrombosis or remission.

Nitroglycerin and amyl nitrite can relieve pain instantly. If the distress does not abate at once with these drugs, the attack is most likely coronary thrombosis. Propranolol (Inderal) is a newer drug that slows the heart rate and force of contraction. Other drugs are hypertensive medications, digitalis and diuretics. Anticoagulating drugs are no longer recommended for angina.

Prevention: All doctors agree that reducing overweight, cutting out foods high in cholesterol, avoiding extremes of fatigue, stress, emotion, and temperature are essential. Smoking is completely forbidden. Appropriate exercises should be taken under proper supervision. (See *Part 3, Early warning signals, Heart disease* **124**)

Outlook: The average life expectancy is about ten years, but many patients master the disease by a determined attitude and sensible care and go on to live out their lives to the full. Those who are stoical, fatalistic, and proceed as before do not have the better odds of those who will not give up and do not give their consent to die.

Most patients with angina pectoris remain fairly stable under treatment. However, those who develop an acceleration of their symptoms, manifested by more prolonged attacks and decreased exercise tolerance, may be potential heart attack victims. In this group, coronary angiograms are performed to determine the feasibility and necessity of bypass surgery. In most cases this surgery will be effective in relieving the symptoms and the patient will be able to return to active life.

Coronary thrombosis 125
(heart attack, coronary occlusion)

This is the great killer. The coronary artery has become so narrowed from arterio-atherosclerosis that a clot forms

WHAT IS A HEART ATTACK?

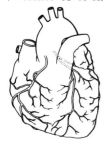

The heart, hardest-working muscle of the body, requires a large and constant supply of blood to do its work. This is supplied through the coronary arter-ies which completely encircle and penetrate the heart muscle, as shown in the drawing. A heart attack occurs when the blood flow through the coronaries is impeded – for example, by formation of a clot.

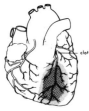

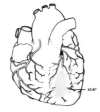

The clot blocking a main coronary branch has deprived the shadowed area of blood. At this early stage of a heart attack, the patient must remain quiet to speed healing.

Some weeks later, the body's repair system has reduced the extent of the injury. A scar has formed and the patient may begin to resume activities under the doctor's supervision.

(*American Heart Association*)

(thrombosis), cutting off the vital blood supply to the heart itself and causing death to a part of the heart muscle (myocardial infarction). (See illustrations under *Arteriosclerosis, atherosclerosis* **123**)

The danger: About eighty-five per cent of those who get to a hospital survive the first attack. Unfortunately, a large number of patients die before they get there. Survival often depends on how soon the victim can get professional help, especially in the prevention of *Ventricular fibrillation* **133** and other complications.

Symptoms: A coronary is usually preceded by a history of *Angina* **124**, but often it will appear suddenly, without warning, without previous symptoms. Any sudden exertion such as running up the stairs, by a man who has led a life of physical indolence, an emotional outburst, a heavy meal – can trigger an attack. Such an incident is only the tip

of the iceberg – the degenerative condition of the patient was already poised on the brink of disaster. Quite often an attack comes without evident cause, during sleep.

The pain is far more intense and longer lasting than in angina; instead of minutes, it often persists for hours or even days. The constrictive, vice-like grip in the chest is usually so profound that the patient lies quite still, not restlessly tossing and turning. The patient often describes the pain by clenching his fist.

The second important symptom is shortness of breath. Additional signs are frequently pallor, cold sweat, a fear of impending death, fast pulse, palpitations, and occasionally nausea and vomiting. A true sign is that nitroglycerin will not relieve the pain as it does in angina.

Treatment: Either a doctor must be called at once or the victim must be sent to a coronary care unit – these are being set up at most hospitals. Speed counts – delay can cost a life. Even if all the symptoms abate, immediate help is still vital. Often, too often, the attack will be repeated within the hour.

The amount of bed rest is determined by the doctor in order to give the damaged heart a chance to recuperate. Hospitalization is usually best because of the immediate availability of emergency measures, such as oxygen, powerful drugs, defibrillating machines, and, of course, the instant availability of a doctor.

Further treatment is then up to the patient himself. If he seriously wants to help himself, he must reorganize his life, not just for a few weeks but for good. With the help of his doctor, he must begin a programme of very mild but increasingly vigorous exercises as well as proper dieting and carefully observe the warnings described in the arterio-atherosclerosis configuration on pp291–6. He may not work himself up to running the marathon, but he will be able to jog as much as a mile a day after a while. Sexual intercourse is rarely forbidden after recovery.

Clinical tests will show how much damage to the heart has taken place. On some occasions a coronary by-pass operation (the substitution of a vein from the leg or a plastic tube for the diseased coronary artery) will be advised.

Prevention: Every home should have a series of emergency numbers handy: the family doctor, the number of the nearest hospital, especially the coronary care unit, and ambulance service.

The belief that coronary thrombosis is the inevitable result of living in our western civilized society has some merit. But one does not have to submit to our society's very serious failings. One can go against the stream – become active instead of sedentary, keep well exercised, avoid saturated fats, avoid smoking, avoid watching TV for long hours every night. We all know the health rules. Practising these rules can mean dying at the right age when it is not a major family tragedy. (See *Part 3, Early warning signals, Heart disease* **125**)

Note: there have been a considerable number of articles and some investigations regarding the value of vitamin E and the sub B groups of choline and inositol in heart disease. Choline is essential in the metabolism of fat, but the other two vitamins have not been proven to be essential in human nutrition – not yet. No one can say positively that they are either worthwhile or worthless. At any rate none of them can do harm.

Outlook: Generally, average life expectancy with medical treatment is seven years. With additional help from the patient, life expectancy may run to decades.

The patient must achieve a positive attitude towards full recovery. He must take over responsibility for his recovery in terms of willpower, cheerfulness, and knowledge. He must know the limits and the extent of things he can possibly do for himself. He must not be influenced by the histories of those among his peers who have had heart attacks. The variety of recovery is too great. One man succumbs, another lives on for decades.

The patient undergoes several phases of adjustment during his hospital stay and later. Usually he goes through a period of anxiety, then depression, and then he emerges with a new appreciation of life, wanting to enjoy it to the fullest. He can do so, if he has learned not to chase after buses or money.

Heart failure 126
(congestive heart failure)

Heart failure results when a weakened heart is unable to adequately do its job of pumping blood to the lungs and the rest of the body. Usually the causes are arterio-atherosclerosis, high blood pressure, or rheumatic heart disease. Any damage to the heart, whether it be in the muscles or valves, can progress to heart failure, especially when the heart is further strained by obesity, anaemia, or some infectious disease.

The two lower chambers of the heart, the ventricles, pump blood into the arteries. The right ventricle forces the blood into the pulmonary (lung) artery; the left ventricle into the aorta, the main trunk of the arterial system of the body.

Right heart failure is failure of the right ventricle to fully do its work, so that the blood backs up into the veins and results in oedema (tissues filling with liquid) and liver enlargement. Left heart failure is a failure of the left ventricle, usually from hypertension or rheumatic fever (a leaking or narrowing of the valves, causing fluid in the lungs, making it difficult to breathe).

The danger: Heart failure does not have to be the end of the line. If the cause can be removed and if the precepts of good health indicated on pp 291–6 are followed, there can be reversion. With proper treatment, one can survive with comfort for years.

Symptoms: The common early symptom of heart failure is a gradual loss of energy over months or even years.

The basic symptom of left heart failure is shortness of breath (dyspnoea) on exertion. This can come on gradually or suddenly. Often this symptom is accompanied by wheezing and coughing that

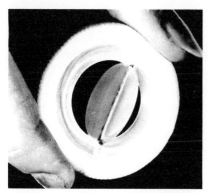

An artificial heart valve employing airfoil design and jewelled bearings is now undergoing experimental trials. (*United States National Institutes of Health*)

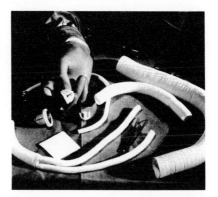

Heart and blood vessel surgery. These spare parts, consisting of synthetic valves, blood vessels, and patches, have enabled surgeons to save the lives of many patients. (*United States National Institutes of Health, Jerry Hecht photo*)

does not produce anything from the bronchial tube or lungs. As the disease progresses, shortness of breath worsens and occurs even at rest, and the subject may awaken from sleep gasping for breath. He will always feel better sitting up than lying down. Left heart failure occurs three to four times as often as right. There may also be palpitation, sweating, and fainting. A severe attack of breathlessness can last as long as half an hour.

The basic symptom of right heart failure is oedema of the ankles and/or legs, which may come and go. Cyanosis is common. There is often tenderness around the stomach because of liver enlargement, loss of appetite, and indigestion. The jugular and other veins in the neck become more pronounced. The urinary output is scanty.

In advanced cases of left or right heart failure there is some loss of mental vigour, judgement becomes impaired, the memory begins to lapse. Breathing becomes laboured with alternating periods of rapid and slow respiration.

Treatment: Proper attention must be given first to the primary causes, such as arterio-atherosclerosis or high blood pressure and wherever possible alleviation of rheumatic heart damage. Physical activity must be maintained, short of shortness of breath. Relaxation is the key word,

whether by vacation, taking an extra day off a week, a nap in the afternoon, or all of them.

The state of mind is vital. Anxiety will do the man with heart failure no good at all, but telling a man to stop being anxious is like telling a man who is panting to stop panting. However, keeping busy and usefully active and doing something constructive for one's health can do marvellous things to lessen anxiety and depression.

Medication such as digitalis and diuretics, which increase urinary output, are valuable. Avoidance of salt and other salt- or sodium-containing foods (even milk has sodium) may be important (*Table 1*). But total abstention from sodium can be harmful. The diet should be under the supervision of a doctor.

In some cases other procedures are helpful, such as aspirating the chest or abdomen to remove excess fluid or surgery to correct valvular defects. For severe cases of breathlessness, oxygen is one of the best forms of treatment.

Prevention: (See *Part 3, Early warning signals, Heart disease* **126**)

Outlook: Variable. So much depends on the condition of the heart, the age of the patient, and his attitude. Not infrequently some people recover almost completely.

Rheumatic heart disease 127

(rheumatic fever)

Of all the diseases that occur in childhood, rheumatic fever is by far the most dangerous and the most frequently contracted of the dangerous diseases. It can be insidious, sometimes difficult to recognize, and often masquerades as so mild as to be ignored or worse, often hard to know when it has subsided because it can lie dormant and at that time do great damage to the heart.

The period of active infection may go on for months. During this active phase inflammation of the heart is at its worst. A mild version of the infection can still commit serious harm. Thus anyone with rheumatic fever must be kept in bed. Penicillin, by reducing streptococcal infections, has cut the hazards down by a factor of five. The children most affected, and most vulnerable, are between seven and fifteen years of age.

Causes: The disease begins with tonsillitis, or pharyngitis – usually a streptococcal infection. In this stage it is infectious, as is any respiratory disease, but when it develops into rheumatic fever it is no longer contagious. Rheumatic fever is a very personal susceptibility. Why some children go on to develop rheumatic fever and others just recover from a sore throat remains a mystery. This disease shows up more often in low income families, and more commonly among those children whose parent or parents have had this ailment. A child from a well-to-do home, neither of whose parents have had it, can still contract the disease; the likelihood is only somewhat lessened.

The danger: The big danger, of course, is permanent damage to the heart, varying from leaking valves to muscular scarring. It can be a crippler of children and too often a killer. Alert parents can prevent *almost* but not all recurrences.

Symptoms: The disease can appear suddenly, dramatically, or it can arise insidiously. Rheumatic fever begins to develop when a child is recovering from a streptococcal throat or other respiratory ailment. Fresh fever appears, plus migratory arthritis. Large joints are affected first, then the smaller ones. Ankles, knees, wrists become red, swollen, hot, and range from tender to painful. Other characteristic symptoms are anaemia, rapid heartbeat, sweating, malaise, loss of appetite, pallor, and failure to gain weight.

Rashes are common. Nodules are found around bony places and purple or round red spots may arise on the skin.

Occasionally there are nosebleeds.

Abdominal complaint is very common, but in the absence of more specific symptoms this is usually not a sign of rheumatic fever.

The most serious symptom is carditis, or inflammation of the heart, and *Atrial fibrillation* **132**. In severe cases there is also cough, pain in the chest, and shortness of breath.

Low-grade rheumatic fever of the smouldering type, is dangerous, because it can be overlooked. It is seen mainly in younger children. Most of the obvious signs are missing *except* an unusually rapid pulse. Also, the child will fatigue easily and his weight gain and growth are far less than normal.

Treatment: Immediate bed rest is essential. Medication (antibiotics) is imperative. Drugs like cortisone and aspirin only minimize the pain, and their overuse can cause nausea, vomiting, and ringing in the ears. The child is usually kept in bed for two weeks *after* all symptoms have subsided and remain absent *without the use of aspirin* (which can mask the symptoms) and the pulse rate is normal.

Improvement will usually be manifested by increased weight and improved appetite. Nutrition is important; the diet should be well-balanced. If the child's appetite is small, his food should be supplemented with vitamins and cod liver oil. Obesity should be avoided. In general, treatment requires practicality and wisdom. Rheumatic fever is not like other diseases. It runs its course, subsides, or seems to subside, but can return again and again. Recurrence is characteristic, generally within three years of the first attack. Everything possible must be done to prevent the recurrence, since every bout may further injure the heart.

In many cases open-heart surgery to repair the valves has effected startling improvements and even cures.

Every effort must be made to avoid inducing invalidism in the child. As soon as he is over the active stage of the disease, he must be helped to return to normal life. The doctor can determine what his capacity is for normal play and exercise. Some will allow the child to govern the amount of activity he can safely tolerate. Over-eager children must be confined and under-eager ones encouraged.

During the long convalescence the child should be kept busy, useful, but not pushed to exhaustion. Particular attention should be paid to his mood and frame of mind. The parent must avoid looking concerned or apprehensive or falsely lighthearted. An imaginative child will need special handling. He must be helped to talk freely about how he feels about his sickness. What he really believes can often come as a stunning surprise.

Cheerfulness is a must in attitude and environment. He will need constant reassurances and above all should be kept in good spirits. No one has yet been able to measure the incredible ability of the human spirit to effect its own therapy.

Lifestyle for a child who has had rheumatic fever
• Nine to ten hours of sleep.
• Outdoor activity whenever possible.
• Lots of fresh air and sunshine.
• A short rest every afternoon.
• Good health must be maintained – with more than ordinary attention to teeth, minor infections, and colds.
• Diet should include plenty of vegetables, fruit, cereals, fish. Coffee, tea, and processed foods are contraindicated. Because of his limited activity the child may become overweight. This can often be worse than not gaining weight normally.
• Aspirin or any salicylate must be administered with care – too much will

produce side effects that can interfere with improvement.
• He should be made to believe in himself and in his ability to get well.

Prevention: Rheumatic fever can almost always be prevented by alert and prompt action! All patients with fever, sore throat, pus in the throat, and enlarged neck glands should be seen by a doctor. If the infection is streptococcal, he will probably prescribe antibiotics. This is also true for tonsillitis or pharyngitis, when accompanied by fever. All upper respiratory infections in children should be treated with concern.

Proper treatment can prevent rheumatic heart disease or mitigate its severity if already contracted.

Prevention of recurrence: The outlook is extremely good, usually without heart damage, if the disease can be limited to one attack.

1. The child should have medical supervision from the time he first contracts the disease.

2. If, after a period of remission, the child tires easily, appears paler than usual, or is slow in gaining weight, he may be going into a recurrence. This is a particularly dangerous time in reference to heart damage.

3. After his first attack, everything possible must be done to keep him from being exposed to colds or respiratory infections. For parents, it means walking a tightrope between being over apprehensive and sensibly firm in keeping him from overcrowded places where respiratory germs abound.

4. An ache in the joints or a slight rise in temperature is a warning of another attack.

5. Antibiotic treatment is usually continued without interruption for eight to ten years after the attack.

Outlook: Dependent upon the number of repeated attacks and the amount of valve damage, with the continuous use of antibiotics, the outlook for this disease has made extraordinary improvement and concomitantly an enormous decline of recurrence has been observed. With penicillin, heart damage has been reduced tenfold. Nevertheless, it remains a serious, widespread affliction – the greatest contribution to childhood heart ailments and a significant cause of heart disease in adults.

When rheumatic heart disease is at the chronic stage, many years after an attack of rheumatic fever, there is usually deformity of one or more valves of the heart. This abnormality will ultimately end in heart failure, fainting spells, and sudden death. The most effective treatment is open-heart surgery, to repair the defective valve or replace it with an artificial one. The degree of heart and valve damage can be determined by cardiac catheterization (slipping a tube through a blood vessel into the heart chamber and recording blood flow pressures).

In spite of the fact that most patients are quite ill, heart surgery will usually be successful, remarkably improving the condition and prolonging life.

The outlook is getting better. With improvement in treatment and advancing knowledge of the basic cause, there is real hope for eliminating this disease.

thalidomide to the offspring of the mothers who took this medication are well known. Pregnant women should avoid every drug that is not absolutely essential, including aspirin, tranquillizers, antihistamines, and even antibiotics. It is advisable to read the small print on all packaged foods, for the amount of chemicals in these foods is astonishing. Short of an emergency, pregnant women should try to live without chemicals, drugs, or medication.

Pregnant women must particularly avoid contracting *German measles* **244**, which can result in cardiac damage to the unborn child.

During the first three months of pregnancy, living at high altitudes where the oxygen level is low (which can result in *Hypoxia* **122**) or even flying very long distances is not advisable.

Outlook: More and more is being learned about how to protect the pregnant woman from the dangers of chemicals and disease that might affect the foetus. New operative skills are being developed to help repair a congenitally damaged heart.

Congenital heart disorders 128

Congenital heart disorders begin before birth. Some are so serious that the infant does not survive, but all of them put together do not add up to a really significant percentage of disorders of the heart.

Symptoms: In some congenital defects the infant has a blue appearance, fails to grow properly, fatigues easily, and often suffers from breathlessness.

Congenital heart disorders often escape detection, because the symptoms do not develop before the teens. Sometimes not until adulthood.

Treatment: The basic procedure is surgery. With the great advances that have been made in congenital heart operations, the surgeon can repair some of nature's mistakes.

Prevention: The big factor in this disease is prevention. The tragic consequences of

Heartbeat disorders 129
(cardiac arrhythmias)

Ranging from harmless to deadly, heartbeat disorders often exist unknown to the patient until the beat becomes violent or very rapid and prompts him to consult his doctor. Since palpitation is not a disease but a symptom, it is not included in this section.

Slow heartbeat 130
(bradycardia, brachycardia)

A heartbeat of less than fifty beats per minute is generally a sign of good health, characteristic of athletes and people who keep themselves in top condition. A regular, daily, vigorous regimen of activity or exercise increases the beat but slows the rate when at rest.

However, there are a few heart disorders, as well as diabetes, some infectious diseases, and jaundice, that will on occasion cause the heart to beat slowly. A very slow heartbeat can cause fainting. Other factors can be opium, convalescence, and anaesthesia (particularly the inhalant type such as ether or chloroform).

Rapid heartbeat (*sinus tachycardia, paroxysmal tachycardia*) *130a*

Frequently, a rapid heartbeat (more than one hundred times a minute) is benign, caused by exertion or excitement, or resulting from menstruation, pregnancy, or the menopause. Often, however, it can be due to such diseases as hyperthyroidism, Addison's disease, heart failure, coronary occlusion, hypoglycaemia, most infectious diseases, and all the anaemias. Many drugs can induce tachycardia, such as adrenalin, the amphetamines, and belladonna. Over-indulgence in coffee and alcohol can also speed up the heart.

There is a form of rapid heartbeat called paroxysmal tachycardia, which can appear abruptly, often for no known cause. The heartbeat may be around 180 but can reach 250 times a minute and persist for hours or even days. It can stop as abruptly as it came but can recur later. Usually there is no other abnormality.

Symptoms: If the heartbeat is very rapid it can produce nausea, weakness, pallor, fainting, and sometimes even shock.

Treatment: There are a number of ways to stop an attack of paroxysmal tachycardia:

1. Closing the voice box and attempting to breathe out against it.
2. Lying down with the feet higher than the head.
3. Bending forward from the waist, as far over as possible.
4. Applying pressure on both eyeballs.

5. Inducing vomiting, using warm bicarbonate of soda.
6. Applying pressure against the carotid artery in the neck. The area around the pulse in the neck is gently massaged while the patient is lying down. Pressure and massage should be very gentle and very gradual, for it can induce cardiac arrest in the elderly.

If these procedures fail, there are several effective drugs.

Extra heartbeat 131
(extrasystole, premature beat, skipped beat)

This extra beat is generally not serious *in the absence of any demonstrable heart trouble or hyperthyroidism*. It can be brought on by fatigue, tension, a cold, caffeine (tea or coffee), chocolate, tobacco, and any unusual medication. In the absence of any heart disease it has no damaging effect upon the heart.

Symptom: A flutter or jump in the chest, quite alarming at first; a feeling of a skipped beat or an extra heartbeat but no pain.

Treatment: If there is no known major disorder, treatment consists of a mild sedative and reassurance. Should it persist, a variety of drugs are available, which a doctor can administer with good results. In the presence of heart disease it is important to treat and eliminate these beats. In a healthy heart, exercise can often make the extrasystole disappear.

Outlook: If without known cause, the prospects are always good.

Atrial fibrillation 132
(auricular fibrillation)

A rapid, continuous but irregular, fluttering heartbeat, this form of fibrillation occurs with all forms of heart disease and with hyperthyroidism. Rarely, it can also appear in apparently normal hearts. Further investigation will indicate if this form of fibrillation is innocuous.

The danger: Atrial fibrillation if prolonged can contribute to heart failure and may also increase the likelihood of an embolism.

Symptoms: A continuous but irregular, fluttering heartbeat, an eerie feeling in the chest, a twitching rather than a beat. The pulse is irregular in changing from a heavy to a light heartbeat. There is also pallor and weakness.

Treatment: In severe cases the patient must rest in bed until told otherwise by his doctor. Methods of treatment include various drugs. In selected instances, direct current electroconversion (direct electric stimulation of the heart) is employed. In the presence of valvular heart disease the doctor might find it advisable to administer anticoagulants.

Outlook: Determined by the degree of the underlying heart disease, the outlook is usually good with effective treatment.

Ventricular fibrillation 132a

A totally disorganized heart pulsation, in ventricular fibrillation the heartbeat is no longer a beat but a flutter, the heart twitches, rapidly and weakly. Although the heart is still in action, it is so completely out of order that it cannot pump blood into the arteries. Ventricular fibrillation can be brought on by a coronary attack, an overdose of drugs, anaesthesia, or by a strong electric shock. It may be seen in the late stages of severe heart disease.

The danger: This is a *Medical Emergency*. Blood pressure falls to zero and sudden death occurs.

Symptoms: Total collapse, no pulse, pallor.

Treatment: Treatment is always on an emergency level. Most hospitals have a defibrillator, an electrical device that shocks the heart through electrodes placed directly on the chest wall. (See *Table 22* for emergency treatment before the arrival of help.)

Prevention: Exclusive of heart attacks, prevention is in the hands of the doctor

in terms of watchfulness during operations, during the administration of anaesthesia, and in the use of cardiac drugs.

Shock 133

One of the most mysterious and most dangerous of emergent conditions is shock (not to be mistaken for electric shock or electric shock therapy). Shock is best described as a collapse of the circulation of the blood – the flow of blood back to the heart is inadequate to keep the body functioning. The larger vessels dilate, 'pooling' the blood and diminishing the amount of circulating blood.

Shock can result from trauma, such as severe wounds, broken bones, massive bleeding, extensive burns; dehydration (loss of body fluids from extensive vomiting, intense diarrhoea, or profuse sweating); an allergic reaction to an insect sting; an overwhelming infection; a heart attack; poisoning (there are 200 well-known drugs and medications that will cause shock); a reaction to major surgery (usually anticipated by the surgeon).

The danger: Shock is always a *Medical Emergency*. Death can ensue even if the precipitating cause itself is not fatal. Immediate medical treatment is essential.

Symptoms: Great pallor, very dry mouth, cold and clammy skin, and lips, nails, earlobes, and fingertips are cyanotic. The patient may feel faint and chilled; his pulse is fast and weak; he experiences shortness of breath and rapid, shallow breathing; his eyes can become sunken or staring and his pupils may be dilated. At first the patient is anxious, then apathetic and disinterested in his surroundings. If not treated, he may become comatose and in danger of dying. The blood pressure keeps dropping and finally is unmeasurable.

Shock can be extremely deceptive. Often the symptoms may appear mild and not very serious, but the victim can take a sudden, disastrous turn for the worse.

Treatment: The best case for survival is in a hospital. While waiting for an ambulance the patient should be kept relaxed, reassured, and calmed – this is quite important. His body should be kept prone with his head lower than the rest of his body by placing a pillow, clothing, anything under his buttocks and legs. The patient must be kept warm with blankets (no electric blankets). No food should be given; he may be very thirsty but offering him a drink should be done with extreme caution – he may vomit and breathe it all in. If there is bleeding, control is essential. If he has stopped breathing, artificial respiration (*Table 22*) should begin immediately.

At the hospital he will be given narcotics to stop the pain and blood transfusions if he has lost too much blood (if proper blood is not available the fluid volume of the blood will be restored by artificial substances to maintain plasma levels). Various drugs (similar to adrenalin) will be administered to raise the blood pressure. Oxygen is often valuable.

Outlook: Most cases of treated shock survive. The prognosis for untreated cases is poor.

Heart block 134

In heart block the impulse that governs the beat has been deranged, like a blocked electric wire. As a result, the ventricles, the main chambers of the heart, beat at a slow rate, usually less than fifty beats a minute. Heart block may occur in any form of chronic heart disease. It may be a consequence of an overdose of digitalis, quinidine, or other cardiac drugs.

The danger: Potential heart failure, cardiac arrest, and fainting spells. For emergency treatment, see *Table 22*.

Symptoms: After a number of regular beats, one will miss. Palpitation and a fluttering feeling in the chest are common but dizziness and fainting are the significant signs. The patient with heart block may keel over when he abruptly changes position, such as jumping out of bed, standing up suddenly, or bending over too rapidly.

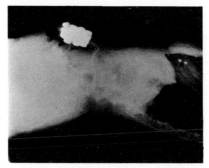

X-ray of heart patient with the newest in artificial pacemakers. A miniature *internal* pacemaker, stitched inside her body, keeps her heartbeat regular and she can go about her house without fear of fainting or falling unconscious. Small long-life batteries in pacemaker provide direct and repetitive electric stimuli to the injured heart. (*United States National Institutes of Health*)

Treatment: The patient with heart block should avoid sudden movements or abrupt changes in position. The only effective procedure is the surgical implantation of a pacemaker, which is a small battery-powered gadget implanted in the body that controls the heartbeat by a series of electrical impulses. It initiates a rhythm, called the pacemaker rhythm, that can generate a suitable rate of ventricular beating. Many thousands of people are alive because of this electrical device and are leading fairly active, useful lives – who otherwise would be invalids. Every year or so the skin is reopened and new batteries are inserted.

Outlook: With a pacemaker, a patient can survive heart block and lead a normal and useful life.

Endocarditis 135

A bacterial infection, usually either streptococcal or staphylococcal, of the protective inner linings of the heart chambers, mostly in the heart valves, endocarditis may be precipitated by a tooth extraction or any surgery of the mouth or of the urinary tract. The basic cause is septicaemia (blood poisoning). Under normal conditions, the linings of the heart do not get easily infected. Patients with rheumatic fever or congenital heart disease are more disposed to this ailment.

The subacute (near chronic) form occurs more often with those who have damaged heart valves (usually from rheumatic heart disease). Undamaged hearts usually develop the acute form. All unexplained fevers should be treated with suspicion.

The danger: If the disease persists, it can develop into congestive heart failure, intense anaemia, cerebral or pulmonary embolism, or kidney failure – all of which can be fatal.

Symptoms: The subacute form is not easy to identify; it creeps up deceptively, without early signs of cardiac trouble. People between the ages of twenty and forty are more likely to be affected. When a fever can't be explained, endocarditis should be suspected. Later there is pain in the chest and irregular heartbeat. The fever is intermittent but usually reaches a daily peak of 39·4°C, 103°F. Chills, pain in the joints, and a worsening anaemia exacerbates fatigue and loss of appetite. Small red or purplish spots break out all over the body. Thin red lines show up under fingernails and toenails; and palms and soles have large discoloured blotches. Clubbing or swelling of the fingertips is usual. The spleen becomes enlarged and painful; bleeding from the nose or blood in the urine is frequent. Some form of blood poisoning is always present.

Treatment: *Bed rest is absolutely essential* with no activity during the acute stage. Food intake must be kept up. Transfusion is indicated if the anaemia is severe. The proper antibiotic, determined by the infecting organism and its sensitivity, is life-saving and medication should be continued for a month or longer. Without antibiotic therapy the disease is fatal.

Prevention: For those who have damaged heart valves or have had rheumatic fever, all surgery should be performed with extreme caution, and a prophylactic antibiotic given in advance.

The disease can recur. Patients should be medically supervised for some months after recovery. Relapses are all too common.

Outlook: Prior to penicillin this disease had a mortality rate of 99 per cent. Now it is down to 15 per cent. In untreated cases the outlook is always poor.

Pericarditis 136

An inflammation of the pericardium (the double-membrane sac that encloses the heart and allows it to work without friction), pericarditis is caused by a direct viral or bacterial infection or is a disease secondary to coronary thrombosis, rheumatic fever, TB, or uraemia. In a wide number of cases the cause is totally unknown.

The danger: Some forms of pericarditis are associated with severe failure of cardiac function and compression of the heart.

Symptoms: The chest is tender to the touch, and the pain, which may be intense, sharp, and penetrating, is increased by breathing and lying down and decreased by sitting up and leaning forward. Fever is moderate.

If significant fluid accumulates in the pericardium, with distension of the neck veins, low blood pressure, and a rapid, weak, irregular pulse may develop. In a small number of patients this may later develop into chronic constrictive pericarditis. In advanced cases there is shortness of breath.

Treatment: *Bed rest is absolutely essential.* During the acute phase, if the cause is bacterial, the proper procedure is antibiotic therapy, plus drugs to relieve the pain. In other form, salicylates or steroid therapy is valuable.

If fluid has accumulated in the pericardium, the recourse is drainage by aspiration (withdrawing the fluid through a needle by suction). In chronic constrictive pericarditis, surgical removal of a piece of the pericardium can sometimes lead to a total cure.

Prevention: A close watch should be kept on all patients who have recovered from this disease to prevent its recurrence, which unfortunately is common.

Outlook: With proper treatment, the mild form usually subsides in a few days, and the patient almost always recovers. In constrictive pericarditis or where it is secondary to another ailment, such as tuberculosis, rheumatic fever, histoplasmosis, the outlook is dependent on the primary disease.

Peripheral vascular disease 137
(Buerger's disease)

In peripheral vascular disease the arteries and veins are obstructed by clots usually caused by arterio-atherosclerosis. The legs are most often affected. Smoking may be a major contributor to this condition, and diabetes mellitus is another factor. The disease is seen more often in men than in women.

The danger: Gangrene of the foot and consequent amputation. Coronary thrombosis is also a lurking danger.

Symptoms: The most common indication is intermittent claudication (a cramping pain in the leg on physical exertion with relief immediately obtained upon resting). Intermittent claudication occurs almost twice as often among cigarette smokers as among those who don't smoke at all. The heavier the smoker, the greater his risk. An additional symptom is associated numbness and coolness of the leg or foot, which may be highly sensitive to cold. When lowered the foot and/or toes become reddened; when raised they turn white. When pain in the foot or leg appears while resting, the disease is more serious. Persistent pain heralds the onset of gangrene.

Treatment: No treatment is effective without total renunciation of tobacco. In the milder form, or before the acute stage, exercising and peripheral vasodilators may be beneficial. When the disease has progressed, surgery is the best procedure,

either to remove or by-pass the obstruction.

The patient must be especially careful about foot care. Minor infections (even getting the foot wet) can be serious; the danger of gangrene is considerable. If the patient develops athlete's foot, a badly growing toenail (from being improperly cut), a corn or a bunion, a nick or bruise on the leg, or gets himself chilled (cold further constricts the blood vessels), he should go to bed and call a doctor. This might seem to be hypochondriacal behaviour, but it is most advisable.

Walking should be stopped at once if pain is felt, and a doctor should be consulted. When sleeping or resting in bed, the feet should be lower than the heart.

One bit of good news – an occasional drink of wine or whisky can be beneficial.

Prevention: Proper treatment of diabetes mellitus if present will do much to prevent this disease. Early diagnosis and treatment will, of course, minimize its extent. Since smoking may be a major cause, giving up tobacco seems like a good way to begin.

Outlook: If the patient cuts out smoking and gets sufficient exercise, the prognosis is quite hopeful. Surgery will frequently alleviate the symptoms.

Heavy blood pressure 138
(hypertension)

Blood pressure is the force of the blood against the arterial walls, a measure of the force of the heart pumping blood so that it can circulate throughout the body. Without it, the blood would not move. Blood pressure varies in all of us not only from day to day but from hour to hour, upon the ceaseless demands of our bodies and minds. It rises when we are physically active or emotional and drops when we're at rest or asleep. There are normal ups and downs. When it goes up and stays up, however, this condition becomes hypertension or high blood pressure. What is most affected are the arterial walls, which are muscular and elastic so that they can absorb the ups and downs of pressure. Too much pressure over an extended period of time can injure them.

The actual physical cause of hypertension is in the arterioles, the tiny arteries that lead into the capillaries, where the blood delivers oxygen and nutrients to every cell and removes the waste into the veins. When these arterioles (too small to be seen by the naked eye) contract, clamp up for whatever reason, the heart must pump harder to force the blood through.

Twice as many women have high blood pressure as men, but the disease is more deadly to the male. Black people under fifty have the disease seven times more frequently than white people under fifty. Above fifty, the percentage tends to even out. Those who have hypertension and are treated have far fewer strokes.

The danger: Hypertension in itself is not fatal, but it is the greatest contributor to premature death. It is a major cause of heart ailments; it weakens and destroys the arteries; it is a prime cause of kidney failure and is the single most significant cause of cerebrovascular disorders that end in stroke.

Uncontrolled hypertension is the most consequential shortener of life of our times. In recent years, the death rate from this disease has declined as a result of an increased public awareness of its dangers and the availability of more effectual treatment.

The causes: Only about ten per cent of the causes are known, such as kidney diseases or adrenal gland tumours. The great majority of cases are of unknown origin. This is called essential hypertension. Essential is an absurd word in this context. It does not mean necessary as the word indicates, but obscure. Why some people suddenly develop this major form of the disease is not known, but what can make it worse is known:

Sodium (salt): see *Table 1* for low-sodium diet. Sodium lurks unsuspected in many common foods. Milk, for example, contains sodium.

Birth-control pills: women who take them should be examined regularly. If there is a rise in blood pressure, the pills should be discontinued and other devices used.

Pregnancy: one of the dangers of the latter stage of pregnancy is toxaemia (*Pre-eclampsia or eclampsia* **246**), which is always accompanied by a rise in blood pressure. Pregnant women should have their blood pressure regularly checked.

Consistent, prolonged emotional stress.

Drugs: benzedrine, cortisone, epinephrine, Privine, all of these are common drugs. Some of them are useful in treating other ailments, but they do raise blood pressure.

Obesity.

Lack of sufficient exercise.

Symptoms: Half of all hypertensives are not aware that they have the condition. In the early stages of hypertension, there are no signs or symptoms, because the arteries have not yet been damaged; in fact, there is every likelihood that the patient is feeling fit and even vigorous (a result of the incitement of the abnormal blood pressure). A doctor, however, can detect hypertension by the pressure reading and also by examining the retina of the eye.

Typically, the patient discovers he has hypertension after medical examination for some other reason. He may be put on a regimen of powerful anti-hypertensive drugs whose side effects are apt to make him feel poorly compared with his earlier robustness.

What often happens is that he gives up the drugs and goes back to the drugless life of feeling vigorous. Unfortunately, this cannot last long, for time is running out. The hypertensive has been constantly drawing money from a bank account with a limited deposit. Eventually the disease catches up with him, but by the time he goes back to his doctor with symptoms, his arteries have been damaged, often beyond repair.

In the middle and later stages of the condition there are some highly distinctive symptoms. The most characteristic is the throbbing headache – usually described as rhythmic pulsation at the top or back of the head, occasionally running to the upper part of the neck and worsened by bending over. These headaches are more common in the morning before getting out of bed, oddly enough when the pressure is lower. The intensity of the pain is not a reliable guide to the degree of the blood pressure. The pulse is usually more rapid than it would be normally.

Dizziness is common; spots before the eyes are a frequent but unreliable sign. Fatigue is more significant, especially if it seems to get worse. Unexplained nosebleed often appears as the ailment progresses. A sudden bloodshot eye, or an unusually excessive menstruation are other signs. None of these symptoms, however, can be attributed routinely to hypertension. Shortness of breath appears later and is more related to the underlying heart or arterial impairment. Only a doctor, by frequent tests on a sphygmomanometer (blood pressure machine) or observation of the arterioles in the retina, can tell whether the subject is hypertensive. The subject cannot rely on how he feels; he can feel in the pink of health and still have creeping hypertension.

Treatment: A part of the treatment must be in the form of reassurance and counsel concerning the need for relaxation, the need to keep from being overweight, and the need to change from a sedentary lifestyle to a more active one. In general, the patient must be made aware of all the things that can intensify his hypertension, and he must act on them.

Besides the low sodium diet, the basic medical treatment is the administration of anti-hypertensive drugs. A large array of these drugs have been discovered recently which are literally lifesavers. They can keep the pressure down for long sustained periods. To name a few, these are hydrochlorothiazide, reserpine, hydralazine, methyl dopa, and guanethidine. Appropriate use of these medications has dramatically lowered the blood pressures of literally millions of people.

The longevity of patients treated with these drugs is five times greater than that of untreated subjects. Heart failure deaths resulting from hypertension have dropped from one out of three to one out of thirty-six.

Prevention: A healthy, active way of life can do much to cut down the incidence of this disease. Early treatment of any contributing cause, such as kidney trouble or obesity, can mean the difference between a normal, reasonable longevity or a short and ailing life.

Outlook: From the onset of the disease, the average life expectancy is about twenty years. The untreated subject rarely gets into his fifties. The malignant rapid form, if untreated, rarely allows the subject more than two years.

Strokes, heart failure, and uraemia can be avoided by an alert doctor and an even more alert patient. The outlook for the patient who is willing to take control of his high blood pressure problem is encouraging.

Stroke 139
(apoplexy, cerebral haemorrhage, cerebrovascular accident)

When a rupture, spasm, blockage, or hardening of the arteries cuts off the blood supply to the brain, a stroke occurs. The nerve cells die in that part of the brain affected, and the part of the body controlled by those nerve cells can no longer function, thus producing a numbness or paralysis or a loss of speech, comprehension, or vision. The effects range from severe and permanent to mild and transitory. Stroke is largely a disease of older people but can occur among the young.

A stroke occurs when a clot formed elsewhere in the bloodstream lands in the brain or may be caused by a clot (thrombosis from arterio-atherosclerosis) formed locally in one of the cerebral arteries; or by a rupture from an arteriosclerotic blood vessel; or by an aneurysm (the rupture of a blood vessel weakened by high blood pressure) in the head. Thus a stroke can be due to blockage of a blood vessel in the brain or from a bleeding rupture.

More than eighty per cent of those suffering from a cerebrovascular accident have a previous history of high blood pressure. More than half have some form of heart disease; ten per cent of these have already suffered a heart attack. Characteristic findings of those who have suffered a stroke are high cholesterol levels, diabetes mellitus (including the mild form), and obesity. They are often heavy smokers.

The danger: Stroke results in paralysis of the body or mind and often ends in death. Fatalities usually occur from a few days to a month after the stroke. Decline of the death rate in strokes has been largely due to curbing the underlying causes, such as coronary disease, rheumatic heart ailments, and high blood pressure.

A temporary paralysis of a muscle if not attended to at once can mean a shrinkage and wasting away of the muscle beyond recall.

Symptoms: The basic symptom is paralysis, sometimes affecting the whole side of the body, but more often just the legs or arms. Often the patient is unconscious with stertorous breathing (snoring), or if conscious, he may have lost his speech or memory; his physical movements are impaired and uncoordinated with a loss of equilibrium. He has spells of confusion, vertigo, and emotional instability. His eyeballs may be paralysed. In many cases his valued personal habits may deteriorate. Vomiting is a characteristic symptom.

Headaches are common before and after a stroke. If they are at the temples, the carotid arteries are affected; if any of the blood vessels have ruptured (aneurysm), the pain can be excruciating. The pain is usually localized at the back of the head and at the base of the skull.

Disturbances of vision are likely, either as blind spots, actual blindness in one eye, or temporary loss of total vision.

To determine susceptibility to stroke, the doctor employs a number of tests. The same tests can be applied to those who have already had a stroke to evaluate the nature and seriousness of the attack. One of these is x-ray examination of the blood vessels to determine their condition.

Symptoms of a more serious, perhaps fatal, stroke are continuous or recurrent coma, continuous high temperature, high pulse and rapid breathing, lasting for days.

Treatment: Immediate treatment is crucial. Rehabilitation should begin the same day, if possible. The right exercises can often bring about recovery in many situations, and a good physiotherapist can be of inestimable value. Information regarding rehabilitation can be obtained from the British Heart Foundation, 57 Gloucester Place, London W1.

Various surgical techniques can often bring about recovery, including thrombectomy, the removal of a clot from an artery, and arterial by-pass, the reconstruction of an impaired artery by substituting one of the patient's own veins or using a plastic material. Such surgery can often head off an incipient major stroke. When performed by an experienced and competent surgeon, these operations have minimal risks and very few fatalities. Recovery is rapid and the patient is back at work within weeks.

Prevention: (See *Part 3, Early warning signals, Stroke* **139**)

Outlook: Death at the time of the stroke is not common. However, extensive haemorrhage can be fatal.

In less severe cases a slow and gradual degree of recovery, sometimes requiring weeks or months, occurs. Usually there is some permanent damage, such as impairment in walking or some residual defects in speech. All recovery reaches a maximal point of improvement within six months.

The doctor can reduce oedema (swelling), he can help stave off other attacks with artery-relaxing drugs, anti-hypertensive medication, and a large array of other life-saving medicines. A good doctor can not only prolong a patient's life, but can enable him to make a quicker and more complete recovery.

Pulmonary embolism 140
(pulmonary infarction)

A clot in the major artery in the lungs that destroys part of the tissue of that organ, pulmonary embolism is caused by a thrombosis (clotting) in one of the deep veins in the leg (*Phlebitis* **141**) or pelvis that travels to the lungs. This is more likely to occur in patients with congestive heart failure, rheumatic heart disease, in the elderly whose physical activity is progressively curtailed, in patients subjected to prolonged bed rest, and in those who have undergone extensive orthopaedic operations of the lower extremities. Varicose veins and the use of contraceptive pills may be predisposing factors for some people.

The danger: A large embolus can cause death in a few minutes or hours. Susceptible people should take precautions on long automobile or plane trips by getting up, stretching and moving around as much as possible.
Symptoms: Initially there is pain in the leg. Later there may be a sudden onset of pain in the lungs, followed by shortness of breath, coughing, and bloody sputum, the symptoms are often similar to coronary thrombosis, pneumonia, or pleurisy. Sometimes the symptoms take a less dramatic form, such as fever and a rapid, irregular heartbeat, but always involve rapid breathing. A large embolism will cause shock, acute shortness of breath, and cyanosis (blueness).
Treatment: The administration of anticoagulant medication remains the most vital form of treatment. Surgical ligation (tying off) of the superficial femoral vein in the leg has fallen into disuse because of too many failures. However, the heart-lung by-pass machine allows the surgeon immediate access to the blocked vessel often with lifesaving results.
Prevention: Many lives can be saved by the early diagnosis of phlebitis (venous thrombosis) and the prompt administration of anticoagulants.
Outlook: Very much depends on the general health of the patient, the size of the clot, the condition of his heart and his treatment. If he survives the first day, his chances are good.

Phlebitis 141
(venous thrombosis, thrombophlebitis, milk leg, white leg)

Often called milk leg or white leg, phlebitis is a clot in the outer veins of the thigh or leg. The basic cause is not well-known. Too much bed rest can bring it about. Other factors are obesity, heart failure, varicose veins, and infections. The incidence is not very high.

The danger: A clot in the vein can end up in the pulmonary artery and cause that too often fatal disease, *Pulmonary*

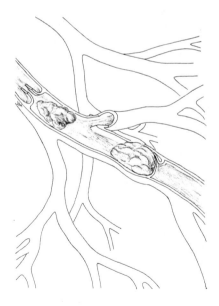

Venous thrombosis. Clots in a vein in the leg. (*Julian A. Miller*)

embolism **140**. It is, in fact, the prime cause of embolism in the lung.

Symptoms: The leg is unusually white. The swelling may range from mild to very pronounced; generally it is quite noticeable. Pain is always present and may be severe. The leg feels heavy, weighted, and sensitive to the touch. Often there is pain in the joints. Surface veins become clearly prominent and the area affected may become discoloured. A low-grade fever is continuous; the pulse is always rapid.

Phlebitis is often brought on by surgery or childbirth. The post-operative early warning signs are an unexplained fever and unexplained rapid pulse.

Treatment: Feet should be raised in bed. A hot water bottle over the affected area can relieve pain and discomfort. Analgesics are helpful, as is whisky in moderation. The doctor will decide on the necessity for anticoagulant therapy.

Occasionally surgery is employed to tie the impaired blood vessel.

Prevention: People with poor circulation and those who are bed-ridden must take particular pains to keep their legs fairly well exercised. An early warning sign is pain in the calf when the toes are moved towards the sole of the foot. In general, long periods of inactivity should be avoided.

Outlook: When the disease is confined to the leg or thigh the outlook is good, especially with prompt treatment. Under good control, most people recover.

Aneurysm 142

When a weakened or diseased artery balloons out, it is called an aneurysm. Aneurysms can occur anywhere in the circulatory system, but the aorta, the largest artery in the body, is most often affected. An aneurysm in the chest section of the aorta is somewhat less serious than one in the lower abdominal section.

When aneurysm is a late complication of syphilis the danger of total rupture is very great. Hypertension and arterio-atherosclerosis are two other most com-mon causes. Far more men than women acquire this disease and people under forty are usually not prone to it.

The danger: Rupture of the blood vessel. Without immediate surgery internal bleeding will inevitably result and end fatally.

Symptoms: Often there are no symptoms in the earlier stages of the disease. Later, there is a high pulse rate and rapidly falling blood pressure, especially when bleeding is already occurring.

The most hazardous area is the abdominal aorta, where throbbing can be felt because of the distension. If the distension is pressing on the vertebrae there will be excruciating pain in the back or abdomen.

Aneurysm in the chest may produce constant or paroxysmal pain radiating to both shoulders, to the back, and to the neck. Additional symptoms are shortness of breath, a husky voice, and a metallic cough. Swallowing becomes difficult.

Aneurysm in the thigh produces a rounded swelling, which can be seen and felt, expanding and contracting with each heartbeat.

Because of the calcium deposits in the artery, an x-ray will clearly define the aneurysm.

Treatment: Aneurysm caused by syphilis should be treated as if the old infection were still active, by penicillin.

The major and perhaps only real treatment is surgery. The diseased section of the artery is cut out and replaced by by-pass grafts. This operation is generally successful and by now a fairly common procedure. There are some hazards for the patient, but they are far less hazardous than allowing the disease to take its inevitable course.

Prevention: Those who contract syphilis and do not seek immediate medical help are prone to this disease later in life. Syphilitic aneurysm is a disease of neglect.

An aneurysm is one of the penalties of high blood pressure. Since high blood pressure is controllable, prevention of this disease is in large measure up to the patient himself.

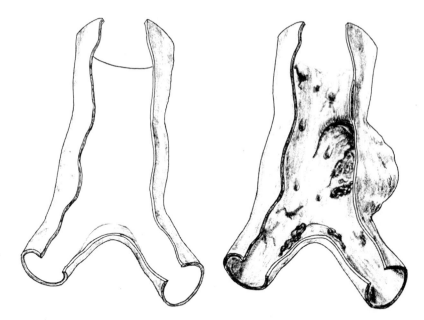

Left: Normal aorta (bifurcated). *Right:* Arteriosclerotic aneurysm of the aorta. (*Julian A. Miller*)

Outlook: Extremely variable, depending on the stamina of the patient and the condition of the disease. The sooner the patient knows he has this disease and the sooner he seeks medical help, the better are his chances. Prompt surgery before bleeding has started or soon after can give the patient reasonable hope of survival.

Varicose veins 143

Varicosity occurs mainly in the legs. The veins are prominent, bluish, enlarged, twisted, and lumpy. More women have this than men. When the valves in the vein are faulty and unable to keep the blood from flowing backwards, the blood stagnates in these vessels and varicosity results.

This is often a familial trait. Contrary to popular belief, those who stand or walk a great deal do not develop varicose veins but the activity can exacerbate a pre-existing condition.

Pregnancy can produce this ailment, particularly in the early months. If this happens, the patient must be carefully watched because of the danger of phlebitis. Usually the varicosity diminishes after childbirth.

Obesity is another cause, as is prolonged weight-bearing, occupational hazards for such workers as porters and movers. Sometimes an abdominal tumour will bring it about.

The danger: A slight injury at the area can cause serious bleeding. Phlebitis is always a danger, especially when the varicosity is not hereditary.

Symptoms: Mostly none. In some cases there is soreness and increased leg fatigue. When there is swelling it will disappear after a rest or a night's sleep. Occasionally the area might become discoloured. In severe cases, ulcers will appear at the vein sites.

Treatment: If the leg becomes troublesome, the patient should avoid standing, and attempt to keep off his feet for a while. The leg should be elevated and rested. Tight clothing is harmful; obesity can worsen the condition.

If bleeding develops from injury or spontaneously, the leg should be elevated and gentle pressure applied over the wound. The patient should avoid walking for a while. This is not true for the non-bleeding varicosity.

The use of an elastic bandage or stocking, which forces stagnant blood into more viable veins, has proved helpful.

Surgery is a common form of treatment, which removes the affected veins and ties up the ends. The result is not only of cosmetic value but also a benefit to health by increasing the circulation. There is very little danger of phlebitis from this operation. Ninety-five per cent of these surgical procedures are successful.

Treating varicose ulcers consists of bed rest and elevation of the leg so that the knee is higher than the heart and the heel higher than the knee. Antibiotics are effective.

In general, after surgery it is important to keep the leg from being immobile for any length of time. Very shortly after surgery the patient is requested to walk for a few minutes every hour.

Prevention: If varicose veins are not a legacy from one's grandparents, then much can be done to keep the condition mild and untroublesome, by not being obese, by avoiding any employment that places a strain on the legs, and by exercise such as cycling.

Cardiac neurosis 144
(functional heart trouble, soldier's heart)

Cardiac neurosis, of course, is not a physical disease, but a mental condition in which pseudo-heart attack occurs. The causes are stress, both conscious and sub-conscious, often brought on by fear of heart attack, by hearing about a friend or relative who succumbed to the disease, or by being in battle or in any dramatic or life-endangering situation.

The danger: The psychological damage can be enormous.

Symptoms: The symptoms are plentiful – too plentiful: palpitations (but the pulse is regular), vague non-radiating pain in the chest, shortness of breath, giddiness as opposed to dizziness, headaches, sighing, flushing, cold extremities, mental and physical fatigue, apprehensiveness, restlessness, anxiety.

Some immediate tests can rule out actual organic disease: exertion or exercise will not worsen the condition or intensify the pain (in true heart attack, exertion always worsens the pain or distress); very often the doctor can distract the subject even during an 'attack'.

Treatment: The doctor or a friend or relative should treat the underlying anxiety with consideration, for that is a real trauma and should be properly evaluated. The patient must never be derided or reproached. Some method should be found to allay his anxieties.

Prevention: The sufferer is usually a high-strung individual who needs special attention. His mental distress and physical symptomology can be mitigated by a sensitive, understanding family. His doctor will never minimize his distress or dismiss him but will treat cardiac neurosis as a real disease.

9 The digestive system

Max A. Teslar

With the exception of the common cold, digestive ailments have the distinction of being the most frequent disorder of man, causing more workdays lost than any other class of disease.

Advances in this field have been extraordinary. New instrumentation has made diagnosis easier, more revealing, and less dangerous. Fibreoptic instruments, for example – thin, pliable glass or plastic tubes through which light can be transmitted – allow doctors to examine without danger almost every part of the alimentary system without resorting to surgery. Liver biopsy is now a routine and easy procedure. The cause of coeliac disease (intestinal malabsorption) is known, and a cure has been found. Many cases of diarrhoea are due to toxins from virus and bacteria, and, as such, can now be cured. What causes gallstones is known and a method of dissolving them without surgery is being developed. Whipple's disease, once fatal, is now known to be due to bacteria and, as such, is easily restrained by antibiotics. Significant progress has been made in controlling internal haemorrhage, and the disasters of obstruction and perforation can be managed far better; a great advance in knowledge is that some tumours secrete harmful hormones; and a vaccine for hepatitis is being developed. The war has not been won, but victory has been achieved in countless battles.

Malignancies of any part of the digestive system are described in *Chapter 23, Cancer.*

THE OESOPHAGUS (THE GULLET)

The oesophagus is the passageway for food from the mouth to the stomach. It is ten inches long and lies between the windpipe and the spine, flanked on either side by great blood vessels and the vagus nerve (the most widespread of cranial nerves, servicing the heart, lungs, stomach, pharynx, and larynx). In the chest, the oesophagus lies behind the heart. Oesophageal trouble in this region is easily mistaken for heart disease.

The muscles along the gullet are exquisitely complex, working in marvellous synchronization to help the food go down. (Gravity alone does not do it.) The wave-like action of these muscles is called peristalsis, best described as a kind of automatic milking machine. Considering the highly intricate structure of this tube it has amazingly few disorders.

Right upper quadrant | Left upper quadrant

Right lower quadrant | Left lower quadrant

The four regions of the abdomen.
(*Julian A. Miller*)

Zenker's diverticulum of the oesophagus 145

An unnatural pocket or pouch (diverticulum) that develops somewhere along the walls of the oesophagus, usually in the section in the neck, Zenker's diverticulum affects mainly older people, men four times more frequently than women.

The danger: The spillover of food collecting in the pocket may cause a variety of lung infections.
Symptoms: The chief complaint is difficulty in swallowing. The first few swallows of food are made in relative comfort, but as soon as the pouch fills with food it begins to cause distress by obstructing the oesophagus. Further swallowing is difficult, then impossible. During eating or drinking a peculiar gurgling noise comes from the pouch. Regurgitation is usual; cough is characteristic and occurs most frequently at night.

Eventually there is loss of weight. Sometimes the pouch can be felt in the left side of the neck.
Treatment: A small diverticulum requires little or no treatment. When the pocket is larger, the patient can be helped if he leans towards the side as he eats, as the pouch always grows downward. In this way gravity keeps the pouch from being filled up – the food slides past it.

When difficulty in swallowing is extreme and weight loss is significant or if chest infections are frequent, surgical correction is essential.
Outlook: Zenker's diverticulum is an annoying ailment, but it is not fatal and can be completely cured.

Achalasia of the oesophagus 146
(cardiospasm)

When the peristaltic action fails at the juncture of the oesophagus and the stomach, causing food to stick at this point and inducing a progressively increasing dilatation of the oesophagus above it, the patient is suffering from achalasia (failure of the muscles to relax) of the oesophagus. The cause of this neuro-muscular disturbance remains unclear.

The danger: This is a *Medical Alert*. The frequent night vomiting characteristic of this disorder can cause aspiration of food into the lungs with possible asphyxiation. Aspiration pneumonia is a serious complication. Malnutrition is another dangerous possibility.
Symptoms: After making great effort to swallow a mouthful of food, the patient often regurgitates it. Pain is at first intermittent, but as the disease becomes worse, the pain becomes continuous (usually behind the breastbone) and can be felt over the entire abdominal area, radiating, in some cases, to the jaw, neck, and back; it can mimic the pain of heart attack.

Although the disease usually becomes progressively worse, there are some temporary remissions.
Treatment: The dilatation found at the time of treatment is irreversible. Cutting the oesophagogastric sphincter is desperate surgery but has a good degree of success. General treatment is to avoid emotional upsets. Mealtime should be pleasant, neither hurried nor stressful. Food should not be too spicy, too hot, or too cold (iced drinks are particularly harmful). Food must be thoroughly masticated. The use of a sedative before eating is effective.

Among other forms of medical treatment is the dilatation of the oesophagus by means of a graduated series of bougies (olive-shaped dilators). Dilatation should only be handled by a skilled specialist, since a rupture of the oesophagus can have fatal results.
Outlook: The disorder can be arrested. Without treatment, it becomes progressively worse.

Ulcer of the oesophagus 147

An ulcer of the oesophagus resembles a stomach or duodenal ulcer. The cause, as in the other forms, remains obscure but is usually related to the presence of a *Hiatus hernia* **149**.

The danger: Unlike peptic ulcers of the stomach and duodenum, the oesophageal form rarely ruptures. However, the disease can become chronic and lead to strictures of the oesophagus unless vigorously and properly treated.

Symptoms: Oesophageal ulcer is characterized by very severe pain that occurs soon after eating, originating underneath the breastbone and radiating to the back. Heartburn, belching of acid or water, loss of weight and appetite, and excessive salivation may occur.

Treatment: If hiatus hernia is present, that, of course, should be treated. Otherwise, treatment is similar to that for *Peptic ulcer* **157**: very bland diet, plus antacids; food should be eaten slowly and milk taken every hour or two. A local oral painkiller can be very helpful. Lying down after meals should be avoided to prevent the flowing back of gastric juices.

Outlook: With proper care and treatment this disease is curable.

Oesophagitis 148

An inflammation of the lining of the oesophagus, oesophagitis can be acute or chronic. Any number of disparate conditions, such as eating irritating food, the residue of an infectious disease, irritation from various drugs, excessive vomiting, reaction to a gastric tube after surgery, or cigarette smoking, may cause the acute variety. The chronic condition is more often associated with hiatus hernia and acid reflux from the stomach.

Symptoms: A severe burning pain behind the breastbone and difficulty in swallowing are the major symptoms, usually accompanied by heartburn. A fear of eating, resulting from the intense pain produced by swallowing, causes a corresponding loss of weight. The pain is often mistaken for a heart attack.

Treatment: As in ulcer of the oesophagus, treatment includes a bland diet, slow and careful eating, antacids every hour or two, and the avoidance of lying down after meals.

Outlook: Quite curable with proper care.

Hiatus hernia 149
(hernia of the diaphragm)

The protrusion (hernia) of a small part of the stomach through an opening (hiatus) in the diaphragmatic muscle at the juncture of the oesophagus and the stomach, hiatus hernia is seen more frequently in the obese and in women who have borne children. Its incidence increases with advancing age.

The danger: Repeated inflammation of the oesophagus can lead to strictures or hidden but continuous minute bleeding, resulting in iron deficiency anaemia. This type of bleeding is one of the most frequent causes of blood loss in older people.

Symptoms: Five out of six cases produce no symptoms; neither is there any relationship between the intensity of the symptoms and the size of the hernia.

Pain ranging from mild heartburn to a deep-seated ache is located behind the breastbone at its lower end and may be associated with belching. Often it may radiate to the left shoulder and arm, simulating a heart attack. It does not worsen with effort, which should help to rule out coronary thrombosis. The onset of pain occurs immediately after meals, especially when lying or bending down. A sneeze, cough, and straining at stools may aggravate it. Sleep may be interrupted by the pain, obliging the patient to get out of bed and walk around fretfully.

Bleeding, which can vary greatly, is seen in vomit and in the stools. Bleeding may also be minute, but steady – so minute that on occasion it does not alter or discolour the stools. This form of hidden bleeding is dangerous, causing severe anaemia that is often unnoticeable except for pallor.

If a stricture develops later in the disease there may be difficulty in swallowing, particularly solid foods.

Treatment: The patient should eat six times a day, with the last meal scheduled two hours before bedtime. Aerophagia (swallowing air) can exacerbate the symptoms (see *Table 12: How to avoid swallowing air*). The following are contra-indicated: carbonated drinks, constrictive clothing, citrus fruit, tobacco, coffee, tea, and overeating. All bending should be done at the knee, not at the waist, to avoid increasing intra-abdominal pressure.

In mild cases, standing up and drinking liquids after meals is beneficial. Most importantly, the head of the bed should be elevated 15–20cm, 6–8in.

Antacids should be taken in the periods between eating. Surgery is recommended only as a last resort for the relatively few in whom symptoms of oesophagitis persist despite several months of intensive medical therapy.

Prevention: The incidence of hiatus hernia can be reduced considerably by avoiding obesity and learning the proper way of lifting weights (*Table 15*).

Outlook: Most people are helped by following the indicated regimen. Repairing the affected weak muscle by surgery is occasionally necessary.

Benign tumour of the oesophagus 150

The size of the tumour varies from a pea to a mothball – it rarely grows larger.

Symptoms: Difficulty in swallowing is the major symptom, accompanied by a feeling of pressure in the oesophagus; the larger the tumour, the greater the pressure or fullness.

Treatment: Diagnosis can be made only by x-ray or oesophagoscopy (using an optical device for looking into the oesophagus). Surgery is indicated.

Outlook: Good.

Varices of the oesophagus 151

Varicose veins of the oesophagus, oesophageal varices are almost always caused by *Cirrhosis of the liver* **191**. The swollen veins in the gullet may rupture and bleed.

The danger: This is a *Medical Alert.* Massive vomiting of blood produces anaemia, shock, and in severe cases even death.

Symptoms: The basic symptom is the vomiting of bright red blood.

Treatment: After x-ray and/or oesophagoscopy has determined the disease and the site of the bleeding varicose veins, therapy, a stopgap measure, utilizes a special tube with a series of balloons that is inserted into the oesophagus. When in the proper position and inflated, the balloons press the veins flat and stop the bleeding. It is a painless procedure and may be lifesaving. However, often the only permanent solution is surgery (ligation of the bleeding vein), directed at decreasing the pressure in the liver blood supply.

Prevention: Since this disorder is caused by cirrhosis of the liver, most often a result of heavy, lifelong alcoholic intake, its prevention, obviously, can be achieved by moderation.

Outlook: Guarded.

Globus hystericus 152
(hysterical dysphagia, lump in the throat)

A psychiatric disorder in which the subject feels a lump in the throat, globus hystericus occurs most often in middle-aged married women and occasionally in men. It usually occurs after an emotional upset or when under intense nervous strain.

Symptoms: Both liquid and solid foods are swallowed with difficulty and the patient is distressed by a constant feeling of a lump in the throat.

Treatment: After the x-ray reveals no abnormality, and all other organic diseases of the oesophagus and nearby organs have been ruled out, the patient should be calmed and reassured by his doctor, friends, and relatives. If that does not help, a qualified psychiatrist should be consulted.

Rupture and/or foreign body in oesophagus 153

Perforation, or rupture, of the oesophagus can be caused by swallowing a foreign object, such as fish or chicken bone, by severe vomiting, or by a severe crushing injury to the chest; infrequently the rupture can be caused by a medical or dental instrument during an examination.

This is a *Medical Emergency.* Symptoms are severe chest pains, breathlessness, and sometimes shock. X-ray will indicate the presence of air and fluids in the chest cavity. The perforation must be closed immediately by surgery. Antibiotics are administered to prevent fatal infections.

The swallowing of foreign objects is not confined to children – adults have swallowed their dentures, chicken bones, and so on. If the gullet is merely blocked and not perforated, a skilled specialist can usually remove the object with special forceps after an x-ray and oesophagoscopic examination. Sometimes open surgical removal is necessary.

THE STOMACH
Indigestion 154
(dyspepsia)

Indigestion is not really a specific ailment, it is a generalized class of symptoms that can be due to gastrointestinal disorders or various other often unrelated diseases. Most often it's the body's outcry against an inclement lifestyle. Various expressions that have crept into our language – 'sick with worry', 'I've had a bellyful!' 'I've no guts for that', 'he's off his head', 'a dyspeptic old man' – deal heavily with the digestive tract and particularly with indigestion.

The causes of indigestion are so indicative of tension and anxiety, and the disorder is so widespread, that it must reflect on our whole highly geared society or, to put it more precisely, our neurotic age.

Here are some of the peculiar behaviours of Western Man that produce dyspepsia:
- Overeating – a compulsion, never a real need.
- Eating too fast – a sign of anxiety and tension or stress of disappointment.
- Swallowing air (aerophagia) – a major cause of indigestion that is characteristic of nervous people.
- Improper chewing – caused by improper attention to teeth and dentures.
- Improperly cooked food.
- Too much fat in the diet.
- Constipation – usually a result of a long history of physical indolence.

The danger: Losing the joy of living.
Symptoms: Heartburn – what is it really? So many people complain of heartburn, but each has his own personal interpretation of it. Heartburn has two forms: 1. a burning, boring pain behind the lower end of the breastbone that appears an hour or so after meals. The distress may come on slowly or suddenly and lasts from a half hour to an hour or more; 2 an acute, painful attack around the heart; the patient cannot breathe deeply; characteristically, forced to breathe shallowly, he will put his hand on the chest. The attack will last a minute or so but may occur again minutes or hours later. Usually there is palpitation. The patient is always sure he is having a heart attack, which this pain mimics so well. In both cases antacids relieve the distress.

Nausea: a sick feeling, a feeling of wanting to vomit, nausea is frequently associated with such other symptoms as dizziness, weakness, headache, sweating.

Flatulence: an undue amount of gas or air in the stomach or intestines, the discomfort of flatulence in the stomach is relieved by belching, in the intestines by the passage of flatus, or passing wind. One of the principal causes of flatulence is aerophagia (the swallowing of air), which is practised unconsciously by tense or nervous people. Swallowing air can produce very alarming symptoms – chest distress that simulates cardiac pain and shortness of breath. When the subject tries to relieve the air pressure by belching, he oddly enough swallows more air. Drinking too much carbonated beverage (soda pop or beer) will also add unwanted air to the stomach. (*Table 12* describes how to avoid aerophagia.)

Treatment, prevention, outlook: Eating a meal should always be leisurely – food must never be gobbled nor eaten at stand-up counters. Nor should food be water logged, that is, drinking water should be confined to before or after meals. The atmosphere during a meal should not be marred by airing problems and conflicts. Quarrels should never be started until an hour, at least, after eating. Smoking is bad before, during, and after meals. A cocktail before dinner is a good custom.

The correction of constipation needs a regimen of exercise, taking a long, brisk walk, running a mile, bicycling, swimming, or digging a hole – anything that will keep the body physically active for at least a half hour a day. Eating cooked fruit twice a day will help, as will drinking more than a quart of water daily.

Any of the antiemetic (anti-vomiting) agents can help subdue nausea.

Positive note: the dyspeptic sufferer is, in a way, quite fortunate. Everyone finds some way to release his frustrations. Some do so in the form of high blood pressure, ulcers, or asthma – all of which can be fatal. No one dies of dyspepsia.

Acute gastritis 155

An inflammation of the mucous lining of the stomach, acute gastritis is usually sudden and violent but of short duration. There are three important forms:

Acute simple gastritis: most often caused by too much alcohol or the excessive intake of such drugs as aspirin, coal-tar products, and ammonium chloride (a diuretic and phlegm loosener), as well as iodides, bromides, and quinine. Also, spicy foods may precipitate gastritis.

Acute erosive gastritis: caused by the intake of strong alkalis or other poisons.

Acute infectious toxic gastritis: caused by flu, diphtheria, pneumonia, scarlet fever, or any intestinal fever.

The danger: Erosive gastritis is a *Medical Emergency*. The degree of danger is dependent on the type and reaction of the corrosive material ingested.

Symptoms: Acute simple gastritis usually occurs eight to twenty-four hours after a bout of heavy drinking or the excessive ingesting of the offending drug. There may be a severe burning pain or pressure at the pit of the stomach, loss of appetite, malaise, nausea, vomiting, and coated tongue. Occasionally headache and vertigo occur. The symptoms usually subside in two days.

In acute erosive gastritis the patient suffers from severe stomach pain, collapse, very fast pulse, cyanosis, difficulty in swallowing, excessive thirst, possibly the vomiting of blood and blood in the stools. The skin is cold and moist; the stomach may be rigid and tender.

Acute infectious toxic gastritis is characterized by a loss of appetite, vomiting, and a feeling of fullness in the stomach.

Treatment: Acute simple gastritis: bed rest, no solid food or half-solid foods. The food at first should be strictly bland. If the patient cannot tolerate even that, he should be fed dextrose sugar in a saline solution intravenously. After the third day, the patient should begin a bland diet. The doctor may administer antiemetic (anti-vomiting) medication.

Acute erosive gastritis: immediate hospitalization, for the patient will need prompt and vigorous treatment in the form of antidote and gastric lavage (stomach pump). The lavage must be handled with extreme care, for the acid of alkali might have so damaged the lining of the oesophagus or stomach that the insertion of the tube might perforate the organ. Until the danger is past, usually several days, the patient must be fed intravenously.

Acute infectious toxic gastritis: along with treatment of the underlying disease, antiemetics are employed. A bland diet, if tolerated, is indicated.

Outlook: Recovery is generally the rule.

Chronic gastritis 156

Occurring in about three per cent of the population, chronic gastritis is a disease that persists for months, even years, and is often the sequel to the acute form as a result of continuously insulting the stomach by habitual alcoholic or excessive drug intake or overindulgence in coffee.

The danger: Some forms of this disease, such as chronic atrophic gastritis, can lead to cancer of the stomach.

Symptoms: Usually there is mild nausea, a loss of appetite, heartburn and flatulence, constipation, a sense of distension and fullness in the stomach even after eating a small meal, a bad taste in the mouth, a furred tongue that is red at the tip and edges, and a foul breath. Pain in the stomach is mild to acute. There may be vomiting with blood, blood in the stools. If the disease has been around for a long time, the complexion becomes sallow and the patient is irritable and depressed. However, often there are no symptoms.

Treatment: Antispasmodics, antacids, and sedatives may help. Plain but varied food is recommended, while spicy fried or rich foods are to be avoided. Intake should be small to moderate, and meals should be eaten at regular times, the last one at least two to three hours before bedtime. In severe cases a bland diet is advised, similar to the one suggested in *Peptic ulcer* **157**. Medication is confined to any tonic that will promote appetite. Occasionally gastric lavage is indicated for chronic atrophic gastritis.

Outlook: With proper attention to the diet, much of the discomfort can be relieved.

Peptic ulcer 157
(gastric ulcer, duodenal ulcer)

If indigestion is the body's outcry against our stressful, anxious age, then peptic ulcer is open, flaming rebellion. Peptic ulcer is man's response to his own self-punishment. The major cause seems to be psychogenic. Peptic ulcer afflicts those persons who respond more painfully to frustrations and anxieties, including the obsessive personality, the phobic, and the perfectionist. Peptic ulcer is a disease of unfulfilled aggressiveness, in which the mucosal lining of the stomach or duodenum gives way under the strain and pressure of the follies of our age. It occurs more frequently among professionals and administrative people, where competition is usually high. Ten per cent of all men will have a duodenal ulcer at some time in their lives.

A peptic ulcer is a sore on the stomach or the duodenum (the first section of the small intestine) which, if allowed to continue, could eat its way through the wall of the organ. A significant factor is an over-secretion of hydrochloric acid in the gastric juice.

The ulcer, which varies from 3 to 19mm, an eighth to three-quarters of an inch, is seen in all age groups, especially from twenty-five to fifty-five, with the highest incidence between forty-five and fifty-five. People with type O blood have a much higher incidence of the disease than those who are type A, B, or AB, and it is common among those suffering from arterio-atherosclerosis, coronary thrombosis, chronic pulmonary diseases, and those who are under extensive steroid therapy.

The danger: Of the many serious complications of peptic ulcer, two are *Medical Emergencies*: massive haemorrhage and perforation.

Symptoms: Steady rather than intermittent pain in the abdomen is the most common symptom. It is usually absent in the morning before breakfast, but often appears at night between 1 and 3 a.m. Occasionally the pain may be only a vague distress and heartburn, but more often it is a burning, boring feeling or constant cramp in the abdomen between the end of the breastbone and the navel. The pain is caused by an oversecretion

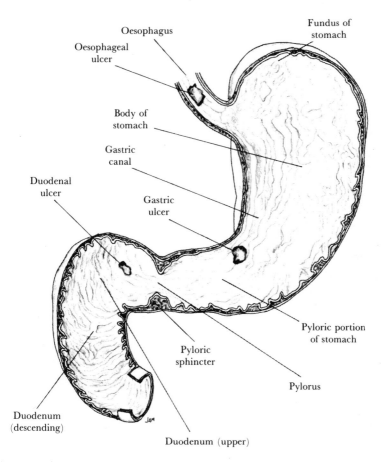

Oesophagus

Oesophageal
ulcer

Fundus of
stomach

Body of
stomach

Gastric
canal

Duodenal
ulcer

Gastric
ulcer

Pyloric portion
of stomach

Pyloric
sphincter

Pylorus

Duodenum
(descending)

Duodenum (upper)

The stomach and duodenum, showing an oesophageal ulcer, gastric ulcer, and duodenal ulcer. (*Julian A. Miller*)

of hydrochloric acid, which reaches a peak one to one and a half hours after eating. Relief is almost invariably obtained by eating, antacids, and rest. Pain can be exacerbated by not following the indicated diet or by allowing oneself to become emotionally upset, overexcited, overly fatigued, or by resuming smoking.

Vomiting is the second symptom. It can also relieve the pain, particularly in gastric ulcer. If there is blood in the vomit it will have the typical coffee-grounds appearance (the gastric juices acting on the blood darken it).

Another symptom is blood in the stools – not bright red, but appearing black and tarry.

The belief that peptic stomach ulcer can induce carcinoma (cancer) of the stomach is no longer popular. As one doctor said: 'Once a peptic ulcer, always a peptic ulcer.'

Distinguishing symptoms between peptic ulcer and carcinoma of the stomach:

• Average age of patients with peptic ulcer is forty, while for carcinoma it is fifty-five.

• In peptic ulcer duration of the disease

is long; in carcinoma the history is short.

● Loss of appetite is not characteristic of peptic ulcer; it is decidedly so in carcinoma.

● Good response to treatment is rapid in peptic ulcer, slow in carcinoma.

● Feeling full upon eating happens normally in peptic ulcer, but the full feeling is encountered long before the meal is over in carcinoma (it is one of the early symptoms).

● In peptic ulcer, traces of blood in the stools soon disappear with treatment; this very rarely occurs in carcinoma.

● Peptic ulcer usually heals within a reasonable time (four to six weeks), except for debilitated elderly people. In carcinoma, if it heals at all, it will take a far longer time. Any ulcer that does not improve within the indicated time should be suspected of being cancerous.

Note: those who have been cured of peptic ulcer should be re-examined to be positive that it was not a hidden cancer (*Stomach cancer* **430**).

Treatment: The average healing time is 40 days, with a range of 13 to 230 days. Basically, healing means controlling the secretions of acidity in the gastric juice.

A bland diet is the treatment of choice, though eating regularly is far more important than what is eaten. The emphasis is on *when* rather than what to eat. Some foods, however, should be avoided, such as heavy fibrous vegetables and very hot or very cold foods. Meals should be small and frequent. Eschew all substances that stimulate gastric acid secretion, such as spices, coffee, tea, and alcohol (including beer and wine).

Some drugs are ulcerogenic (causing or aggravating ulcers): steroids, salicylates, rauwolfia (for high blood pressure), and the arthritic medications Indocin and butazolidin.

A variety of antacids are available, such as aluminium hydroxide combined with magnesium trisilicate and calcium carbonate in the liquid form (usually more effective than the tablet), one or two tablespoonsful an hour after meals when acid secretion is at its peak. Anticholinergics or belladonna may be pre-scribed by the doctor though they have side effects (drying of the mouth, blurred vision). Phenobarbitol or other suitable tranquillizers are given to the particularly highly-strung patient.

Surgery is a lifesaver for those who develop such complications as perforation, obstruction, or a massive haemorrhage that is not helped by transfusion.

Lifetime directions for patients with peptic ulcer

● Allow plenty of time for meals; make mealtime a friendly, pleasant interlude and not a time to air your social or financial problems.

● Eat slowly and chew thoroughly.

● Never go more than three hours without eating.

● If you're in a hurry and are compelled to rush through your meal, cut the food intake in half; just assuage your hunger, not your appetite.

● A cold or any respiratory infection can set you back. Take especially good care of yourself if you feel a cold coming on. Get into bed and stay there for a day or so and drink plenty of milk.

● Cut out all smoking and cut down on drinking.

● If your symptoms return, it usually means you have not had enough sleep, not enough rest, been eating the wrong foods, getting too upset, worrying too much. When this happens, go on a two-hour feeding schedule, with plenty of appropriate antacids.

Prevention: Those individuals prone to ulcers must choose a career in which the work is suitable for the stomach. Changing one's character is, of course, very difficult but avoiding the pitfalls only needs wisdom. Such an individual must learn to take out his aggression externally, never internally. Hitting a punching bag, taking up karate, running a mile or so every day are simple, excellent means of avoiding that ulcer.

Recurrence: About 25 to 50 per cent of peptic ulcer patients have a recurrence within a two-year period. In some measure, this can be avoided by keeping off ulcerogenic foods and drugs. A regimen of care and constant alertness to the threat of recurrence can do much to ward it off.

Outlook: Peptic ulcer remains a distracting disease that can be cured but recurs again and again if the hypersecretion of hydrochloric acid is not permanently contained. Generally, the outlook isn't bad, providing there are no complications (15 to 20 per cent develop complications). The disease is not always progressive and the recurrences are often conspicuous by their absence.

Obstruction in peptic ulcer 158
(stenosis, pyloric obstruction)

The most frequent complication of peptic ulcer is a narrowing of the pyloric channel (the opening between the stomach and small intestines) either by a swelling of the inflamed tissues or by actual scar formation, an obstruction that blocks the passage of food.

The danger: Actual scar formation is not usual. When it does occur, however, surgery is indicated. This condition is a *Medical Alert.*

Symptoms: Vomiting, most often bloody, rather than pain is the major symptom. There is considerable distension of the stomach after eating, loss of appetite and weight, foul belching, and dehydration.

Treatment: The retained food is pumped out through stomach lavage. Nourishment should be given intravenously to correct the dehydration and loss of protein in the blood. After two or three days, liquid protein may be given. In this way the inflamed tissue can return to normal, thus relieving the obstruction and avoiding removal of inflamed or scar tissue by surgery.

Outlook: The obstruction is usually helped by prompt treatment. This disorder is usually transient.

Massive haemorrhage in peptic ulcer 159

About fifteen per cent of all peptic ulcers develop the complication of haemorrhage in varying degrees. This can be due to nervous tension, emotional upset, not sticking to the prescribed diet, or, rarely, performing some strong physical exertion – or no reason at all.

The danger: This is a *Medical Emergency.* Severe cases, if not immediately and vigorously treated, can result in bleeding to death.

Symptoms: In mild haemorrhaging some weakness occurs, along with sweating, black, tarry (bloody) stools, and vomiting small amounts of blood.

In severe cases, blood in the vomit is profuse. There is persistent blood in the stools (black, tarry stools and red blood). The sharp drop in blood pressure is manifested by physical collapse, shortness of breath, a rapid, thready pulse, cold, moist skin, fainting, severe weakness, dizziness, thirst, and profuse perspiration. The patient is very pale, restless, and shows all the symptoms of shock. The pain usually disappears when the haemorrhage begins. If the pain persists, the situation is grave.

Treatment: If the loss of blood is twenty-five per cent or more, a blood transfusion must be started at once, as well as treatment for shock. Frequent milk feed may be continued despite the bleeding. Most ulcers respond to conservative treatment. If moderate episodes of bleeding occur more than twice, or if bleeding continues after a transfusion, surgery becomes imperative.

Outlook: Surgery in patients under fifty has a mortality rate of less than one per cent. Over fifty, the rate can rise to as high as fifteen per cent.

Perforation in peptic ulcer 160

Although a perforation in the peritoneal cavity usually occurs to peptic ulcer patients when symptoms are at their worst, it is just as likely to occur at any time for no apparent reason and without any warning at all.

The danger: The direct result of perforation is peritonitis, which has a very high rate of fatalities. This is a *Medical Emergency.*

Symptoms: Sudden, agonizing, writhing pain in the abdomen is the prime symptom. The abdomen is rigid and tender. The pulse and temperature rise, blood pressure falls. The patient is ashen grey. Vomiting blood may occur shortly after onset and increases with peritonitis. If it is a gastric ulcer, pain in the shoulder tip is present, more often in the left shoulder; if it is duodenal, the right shoulder is affected.

Peritonitis sets in rapidly. Characteristically, the patient lies motionless, panting for breath, his hands on his stomach to protect it from the slightest motion.

Treatment: The tear in the stomach or duodenal wall must be closed; the sooner this surgery is performed the better the chance of survival. A delay of as little as eight hours after perforation can mean a drastic change in outlook. Shock prevention treatment should be instituted at once. A stomach tube is employed to empty the stomach continuously. Treatment for *Peritonitis* **179** should begin as soon after the operative procedure as possible.

Outlook: If caught in time, the outcome is usually good. If surgery is performed within the first eight hours, the mortality rate is less than 10 per cent. With the lapse of twenty-four hours, it has risen to more than 50 per cent.

Postgastrectomy syndrome 161

Postgastrectomy syndrome is the development of the same or new symptoms after the surgical removal of all or part of the stomach (gastrectomy). Subtotal gastrectomy, the removal of part but not all of the stomach, has a mortality rate of 1 to 5

per cent. Although a major surgical procedure, the serious, disabling postoperative symptoms are usually temporary. However, in about one out of five cases of peptic ulcer surgery postgastrectomy syndrome develops. The syndrome has two forms: (1) a new ulcer forms accompanied by the same symptoms experienced with the original ulcer (about eight per cent of the cases) and (2) new symptoms or tumours appear, sometimes as serious as the original disease, even though the surgery was successful.

Symptoms: The new symptoms fall into a pattern, most evident after meals – fullness in the stomach, nausea, and pain in the upper abdomen, which often worsens unless relieved by vomiting. The patient cannot eat a normal-sized meal.

The basic characteristic is the 'dumping' syndrome, the too rapid emptying of the gastric contents of the stomach into the intestines. About a quarter of an hour after eating the patient will break out in a sweat, have heart palpitations, feel light-headed (often to the point of fainting), and become prostrate. His pulse and blood pressure will go up, and he'll suffer abdominal cramps but not real pain. A major indication will be explosive diarrhoea with the passage of considerable foul-smelling stools. In long-standing cases, inevitable weight loss occurs, as well as anaemia and weakness. About half the patients who have had half or more of their stomach removed will show signs of this symptom to some degree (more common in women, particularly the highly emotional).

Weight loss is the dominant feature of postgastrectomy syndrome because of both the inability to take full meals and the malabsorption of fats, proteins, and carbohydrates as well as vitamins. Patients often prefer voluntary starvation rather than undergo the agonies of eating.

Treatment: The patient is advised to eat in a recumbent or semi-recumbent position. If that is not possible, he should lie down immediately after meals. Little or no liquids should be drunk during and immediately after meals. Appropriate sedatives and antispasmodics to delay dumping should be taken before meals. Dining time must always be a relaxed time – for the rest of his life. Harsh foods, hot spices, alcohol, and smoking can only irritate the gastrointestinal system.

The same factors that produced or aggravated the ulcer – emotional stress, psychological conflicts – can exacerbate the intestinal tract in postgastrectomy. Nervous tension is perhaps a more important determinant in this conditon than the food that is eaten.

Outlook: Most patients who suffer from postgastrectomy syndrome eventually settle down to a way of life that will minimize flare-ups, but they will need constant medical attention.

Acute gastroenteritis 162

An inflammation of the lining of the stomach and of the intestines, acute gastroenteritis is caused by food poisoning, overindulgence in alcohol, intestinal flu, virus, and allergies to certain foods. It can also be precipitated by such drugs as cinchophen (commonly used in analgesics and fever-reducing drugs) colchicine (an antirheumatic, antineuralgic medication), salicylates, cocaine, stilbostrol, and nicotine. Other causes are chemical poisons such as cadmium, mercury, lead, and all the heavy metals. There are more than 250 drugs and chemicals, running from aconite to zinc, that can induce varying degrees of this disease. Gastroenteritis also occurs in many infections, most especially in typhoid, dysentery, and cholera.

The danger: Even though fatalities are rare, except for the elderly and the very young, gastroenteritis is always a *Medical Alert.*

Symptoms: The disease co:..es on suddenly, with nausea, vomiting, stomach cramps, rumblings in the bowels, and diarrhoea. Depending on the intensity of the disorder, there are varying degrees of prostration. The abdomen is distended;

tenderness is more likely in the lower quadrants than in the upper. If vomiting and diarrhoea are persistent, severe dehydration will occur. Other symptoms are rapid pulse, cold skin, dryness of the mucous membrane, weakness, and shock.

Treatment: Bed rest is essential. No food or drink should be given as long as vomiting and nausea persist; afterwards, light tea, strained light soup with some added salt, and thin cereal gruel.

If vomiting continues, the doctor may administer an intravenous injection of salt or potassium to ward off dehydration, urinary suppression, and acid-base imbalance. When shock is impending, blood plasma therapy is indicated. Vomiting can usually be held in control with proper sedative medication.

Outlook: If the offending cause is removed, recovery is usual.

Infected food gastroenteritis 163

Infected food gastroenteritis is usually due to eating food that is infected by salmonella bacteria.

The danger: Rarely fatal, except occasionally among the elderly and infants, this disorder is, nevertheless, a *Medical Alert.*

Symptoms: The onset is usually twelve to forty-eight hours after eating the infected food. The basic symptoms are nausea, cramps, vomiting, and diarrhoea. There can also be headache and chills and fever. Severe cases develop dehydration, kidney failure with urinary suppression, and shock. The disease can be so mild as to allow the patient to continue his normal activities with only minor discomfort, or it can cause death (a rare contingency). Infected food gastroenteritis can be easily identified when other diners become ill as well.

Treatment: The treatment is the same as in *Acute gastroenteritis* **162**. In severe cases, the doctor will occasionally prescribe streptomycin, although some authorities feel this is of no real value.

Prevention: Doubtful food, particularly when served in doubtful places, should be avoided. If any food from any place, home included, tastes even slightly off, it should not be eaten.

The greatest source of salmonella infection is poultry, which includes all fowl and their eggs, from chicken to turkey. The incidence in fresh eggs is low, but frozen and powdered eggs have a large rate of contamination, most especially in prepared food mixes made with powdered eggs. Pork, beef, and lamb also harbour the germ. Actually, salmonella is found everywhere in varying degrees, in almost all foods we eat.

Persons who have had major gastric surgery have a greater predisposition for the disease. Individual resistance can make the difference between a serious attack and no symptoms at all.

Since the faeces of patients even after recovery contain large numbers of the salmonella germs for weeks, months, and even years, food handlers who have had the disease should be barred from their work until they are clinically free of the germ.

Another good rule is that everyone acutely ill or convalescing from this disease should be kept isolated.

Outlook: Symptoms subside in two to five days. Recovery is normal and uneventful.

Staphylococcal gastroenteritis 164

The most common form of food poisoning, staphylococcal gastroenteritis is caused by the toxins (poisons) produced by the staphylococcal germs in food. The food becomes infected from a diseased food handler through nasal discharge or even a skin infection. The bacteria multiply in the food and produce a toxin. The toxins, rather than the bacteria, are the cause of this disorder. Such foods as custards, cream pies, processed meats, cheeses, ice cream, mayonnaise and hollandaise sauce, potato and chicken salads are highly appreciated by the staphylococcal germ as an excellent place to raise a large family. It takes only four hours at temperatures above 27°C, 80°F for the infected food to produce enough toxins to make the food poisonous. Unfortunately, such contaminated foods have a normal appearance, odour, and taste. Boiling or cooking kills only the germs; the toxin remains unaltered.

The danger: Most people simply suffer an extremely uncomfortable twenty-four hours, but the elderly and infants can often succumb. This is a *Medical Alert*.

Symptoms: Incubation from the time of eating to the first symptom runs from two to four hours. Onset is abrupt, with the usual gastroenteritis symptoms – nausea, vomiting, pain, diarrhoea, and occasionally, excessive salivation and sweating. In severe cases there is prostration, shock, and blood and mucus in the stools.

The attack is short, usually from three to eight hours, rarely ever more than twenty-four. Fatalities are rare, individual resistance and susceptibility are as much determining factors as the amount of toxin ingested.

Treatment: The treatment is the same as in *Acute gastroenteritis* **162**. In a majority of cases, no specific therapy is needed, nor is any antibiotic or other antimicrobial medication.

Prevention: Food can become contaminated by careless food handlers who fail to take normal hygienic precautions, and through the improper storage of food. Legislation preventing food handlers from working until they are free of staph infection should be enacted and handlers should be required to have regular medical check-ups. All perishable food should be refrigerated at 5°C, 42°F or below to prevent the growth of toxins. It should never be exposed to room temperature for any length of time.

Outlook: Almost always good.

Botulism 165

A highly fatal type of food poisoning,

botulism results from eating food containing the toxins (poisons) produced by the *Clostridium botulinum* bacteria. This toxin is probably the most poisonous substance known to man – one drop evenly divided could kill 50,000 people. The spores of this bacteria are found everywhere in the world. Improperly preserved food can initiate botulism. Home-tinned food is an example. Less frequently, it occurs in such commercially prepared foods as tinned olives, corn, spinach, string beans, beets, asparagus, seafood, pork products, beef, and in improperly smoked or canned fish. This does not mean these tinned products are dangerous, only that contamination occurs more frequently in these foods.

Ten minutes of boiling or a half hour of heating food at about 63°C, 176°F will destroy the toxin.

The danger: This is a *Medical Emergency*. Botulism has a 10 to 70 per cent mortality rate, depending on which type of botulism is involved. There are six distinct varieties.

Symptoms: The disease strikes eighteen to thirty-six hours after eating the contaminated food. The earlier the symptoms appear the more extreme the disease will be. Since the poison attacks the nervous rather than the digestive system, most of the symptoms are not characteristic of gastrointestinal tract disorders.

The first signs are fatigue and dizziness, followed quickly by blurred sight and double vision. The mouth becomes extremely dry; swallowing and speaking, very difficult. The muscles of the extremities and the trunk are weakened, creating serious breathing problems. In some forms of botulism nausea and vomiting are extreme. Cramps and diarrhoea are other distinctive signs. The pupils become dilated and fixed. Death results from airway obstruction, respiratory and cardiac paralysis.

Some forms of botulism are often confused with polio, encephalitis, stroke, central nervous system syphilis, myasthenia gravis, and poisoning from atropine and belladonna.

Treatment: Stomach lavage should be initiated within a few hours of swallowing the infected food. Fatal respiratory blockage, which can come on suddenly, requires the quick availability of a respirator; tracheotomy can be a life-saver.

If the victim can be kept alive for ten days or longer, he will survive without permanent damage. An enema is helpful in clearing away the unabsorbed toxins in the colon. The doctor will first test the patient for sensitivity to serum; if negative, he will administer antitoxin intravenously. The antitoxin should also be given to those who ate the same food but have not yet shown signs of the disease.

The patient must be kept in bed in a darkened room, no visitors. Chloral hydrate is the indicated drug to relieve anxiety (morphine is not used since it has a depressing effect on the already weakened respiration). Feeding and medication must be administered with extreme care because of the difficulty in swallowing. Rectal or tube feeding (water, dextrose, salt, vitamins B complex and C) might be necessary.

Prevention: Choose fresh vegetables rather than canned. Doubtful foods should be boiled. Home canners must be sure they know exactly what they are doing.

Outlook: Vigorous medical management can substantially reduce the death toll. If a patient survives the paralytic phase of the disease, recovery will be full, rapid, and complete.

THE PANCREAS

A rather large glandular organ that lies behind the stomach in a horizontal position, the pancreas produces both an external and internal secretion. The external pancreatic juice is a thick, saliva-like fluid containing the enzymes that break down starches, fats, and proteins. The internal secretions are hormones, among which is insulin. If the output of insulin is insufficient, diabetes results.

329

Acute pancreatitis 166

An inflammation of the pancreas, running from mild to extremely grave, acute pancreatitis is divided into three types: oedematous, haemorrhagic, and necrotic. Of the three types, haemorrhagic and necrotic are quite serious. The majority of cases occur in people with biliary tract disease or those who are heavy indulgers in alcohol. Such infectious diseases as mumps, scarlet fever, typhoid, viral hepatitis, mononucleosis, and uraemia can also induce the disease, as can pregnancy. The majority of cases occur in women in their early fifties.

An attack can be precipitated by a drinking spree or by overgorging on food or, less likely, be set off by steroid therapy or as a reaction to chlorothiazide (a diuretic used to lower high blood pressure).

The danger: Acute pancreatitis is often hard to distinguish from gallbladder disease or perforation of a peptic ulcer (both of which require immediate surgery). An unnecessary operation can be forestalled by a careful laboratory test of the blood, which will show a high amylase (pancreatic enzyme) content. This is a *Medical Emergency*, for in severe cases the disease can worsen dramatically and end in death in a few hours.

The diseased pancreas discharges some of its enzymes directly into the peritoneum causing peritonitis, a very grave disorder. Insulin failure can add diabetes to the deadly list.

In the haemorrhagic and necrotic forms of pancreatitis the mortality rate ranges around fifty per cent.

Symptoms: Sudden, relentless, writhing pain high in the abdomen, often radiating to the back, can be so intense that even opiates will not relieve it. There is a tenderness over the pit of the stomach. In the two pernicious types, haemorrhagic and necrotic, there is severe vomiting and shock; the skin is blue, cold, and clammy; the pulse is rapid and feeble and the blood pressure is low. Outstanding symptoms are pain and shock. If the bile ducts or gallbladder are involved, jaundice will appear.

In the milder form, oedematous pancreatitis, in addition to pain there are metabolic disturbances.

One of the difficulties the doctor faces in this disease is its similarity to other acute disorders, such as heart attack, peptic ulcer perforation, appendicitis, and inflammation of the gallbladder.

Inflammation of the gallbladder: pain in pancreatitis is high in the abdomen, while in the gallbladder, the pain is confined to the upper right quadrant. The patient appears quite sick in pancreatitis, while in gallbladder attacks the patient does not seem very ill.

Perforated peptic ulcer: while board-like rigidity of the abdomen is found in perforated ulcer, only some slight rigidity is found in pancreatitis.

The amylase enzyme rises in the blood in pancreatitis. This is the only sure way to differentiate the disease and often prevent unnecessary surgery.

Treatment: Strict bed rest and absolutely no food is allowed; the stomach must be kept empty by gastroduodenal suction. The suppression of pancreatic fluids is essential; hence, no food is given that will stimulate the pancreas to action. The doctor will prescribe atropine to reduce pancreatic secretions and propantheline to reduce gastric secretions.

Fluids are given intravenously. Broad spectrum antibiotics are prescribed against potential peritonitis. If the attack is severe, calcium replacement is indicated.

Pain is relieved by meperidine rather than morphine or codeine, since the latter two can cause spasms of the outlet of the common bile duct. *Shock* **133** must be treated at once.

Between attacks, the diet should be high in carbohydrates and low in fats and proteins. Heavy meals, as well as alcohol, should be avoided.

Surgery has value only if the underlying cause is gallstones; operative procedures must wait until the attack has subsided.

Prevention: Basically, prevention should be geared to avoiding future attacks, which, unfortunately, are a dangerous and common occurrence. However, by maintaining a low-fat diet, eating small, frequent meals, and avoiding alcohol, overeating, and obesity, attacks can be minimized. Any drinking spree can precipitate a new attack. Some drugs can be a predisposing factor.

Outlook: Mild cases of oedematous pancreatitis are self-limiting and recovery is usual. Haemorrhagic and necrotic pancreatitis need vigorous medical attention for survival.

Chronic relapsing pancreatitis 167

Although the causes are the same as in *Acute pancreatitis* **166**, chronic relapsing pancreatitis is not due to the acute form; actually, they are not the same disease. In the chronic form repeated attacks injure the pancreas, making it fibrous, scarred, and calcified. Seventy-five per cent of the sufferers are chronic alcoholics, almost 15 per cent have diabetes, and 10 per cent have cirrhosis of the liver. The majority are men in their late thirties; the disease can also occur, however, in childhood and old age.

The danger: This is a *Medical Alert*. Chronic pancreatitis has a poor longevity, and diabetes is a constant complication.
Symptoms: The main symptom is pain, sometimes mild but more likely severe, which can be continuous, intermittent, or fluctuating. Pain may persist for days or weeks and often leads to an addiction to opiates. The periods between attacks can be symptomless, but the periods between get shorter.

Additional characteristic signs are nausea, vomiting, jaundice, chills, and tachycardia (rapid heartbeat). Weight loss can be considerable. The stools are fatty, foul-smelling, and frothy.
Treatment: Chronic pancreatitis is always difficult to treat. The replacement of pancreatic enzymes is the standard procedure. The alleviation of pain requires strong drugs. Bed rest is essential. A high

carbohydrate diet is prescribed; food should be easily digestible and minimally stimulating to the pancreatic secretions.

Oral intake of fluids must be cut down and the fluid balance maintained intravenously. Nasogastric suction (stomach pump through the nose) to keep the stomach dry of secretions that might trigger off the pancreas to greater inflammation, is essential from time to time.

Benefits have been derived from surgery to re-establish some form of drainage, but the greatest surgical successes involve the removal of stones from the bile or pancreatic ducts or the gallbladder. The desperate measure of excising all or part of the pancreas has occasionally been effective. Replacement therapy is then necessary to resupply the body with insulin and other enzymes.
Prevention: The chronic form can be prevented by employing the same procedures described in *Acute pancreatitis* **166**.
Outlook: Hopeful; no reasonably dependable therapy has as yet been found, but neither does the medical profession consider this disease one of its failures. There are a number of specific medications and various surgical procedures that can help the patient, although perhaps even more important is his own determination to be cured, especially if alcoholism is a causative factor.

THE INTESTINES
Regional enteritis 168
(Crohn's disease, ileitis)

A non-bacterial inflammation of the small bowels causing a heavy thickening of the intestinal wall and a hardening and narrowing of the passageway, regional enteritis can occur in one place or simultaneously in several places along the lower half of the small intestine (ileum). Striking men and women of all races equally, half the cases occur between the ages of twenty and thirty.

Until recently the cause had been declared unknown. Lately, however, evidence indicates that the roots of this disease lie, as in peptic ulcer, in nervous tension, worry, and emotional conflict. It is a disease of persons who cannot sustain the pressures and emotional conflicts of a competitive society.

The danger: Although it produces a sense of deep illness in the patient, mortality is low. However, the disease can lead to malnutrition and invalidism. A peculiar danger of regional enteritis is the difficulty in differentiating it from appendicitis. To be on the safe side, many doctors perform appendectomies rather than risk the ensuing peritonitis from a diseased appendix. It is always advisable to call in one or more consultants to avoid diagnosis through surgery. If time will permit, which is unhappily not often the case, the doctor can differentiate the disease from appendicitis by the barium x-ray technique (barium helps visualize the internal organs). If there is narrowing of some parts of the small intestine, as indicated by the x-ray, the diagnosis is regional enteritis, not appendicitis.

Symptoms: The early symptoms include anaemia, malnutrition, transient changing arthritis (migratory), and weight loss, producing a wasting effect. Mid-abdominal cramps and diarrhoea complete the picture. Loose stools occur four or five times a day. Another characteristic symptom is a sausage-shaped, palpable mass in the lower right quadrant of the abdomen. Later, pain occurs in the lower right quadrant, and the patient suffers from nausea and vomiting.

Another characteristic symptom is the formation of fistulas, ulcerated or scarred tube-like passageways going from one cavity to another or to a free surface. Fistulas appear in the late stage of the disease; they carry the diseased contents of the intestines into the rectum with the inevitable infections.

Fever is mild. Because of the rapid intestinal transit time, there is a loss of essential nutrients in food and a poor absorption of vitamins, which can cause the skin, as in pellagra, to appear dry, scaly, and shrunken.

As the disease progresses, the all too common complication of partial obstruction of the bowels occurs.

Treatment: Bed rest is essential for the patient with fever, diarrhoea, and weight loss. Vitamins help to offset malnutrition and medication can relax cramping muscle spasms. The diet should be bland but highly caloric with large amounts of protein. Every effort should be made to improve the appetite. However, no milk products should be offered, as they are not well tolerated by patients with regional enteritis.

Surgery has produced very poor results and should be performed only under life-threatening conditions such as obstruction.

There are differences of opinion regarding antibiotics. Secondary infections can be prevented by this medication, but many doctors feel that it's not worth further irritation of a delicate intestine. Steroids are employed in severe cases.

The most overlooked and probably the best therapy is psychiatric. Emotional and psychological problems are an important instigating factor of the ailment. If possible, the patient should take a six-month vacation to give himself plenty of time to examine his attitudes, his values, and his way of life. A change of scenery and a new sense of values might help put him on the road to recuperation and health.

Prevention: Every effort should be made to prevent recurrence; surgery should be avoided if possible – it will neither cure the disease nor prevent its recurrence. The patient must find some way to externalize his problems; change his living patterns, his habits, his way of life; and cut down emotional conflicts. Getting that trophy while writhing in pain in a hospital bed makes him a losing winner. (See *Part 3, Early warning signals, Regional enteritis* **168**)

Outlook: In ten per cent of the cases there is full recovery, more from spontaneous remission than from medical help. In this disease, the patient is probably the only source of cure. Regional enteritis is certainly partially a psychiatric disorder and should be treated as such.

Hypertrophic pyloric stenosis 169

Although primarily a disease of infancy, hypertrophic pyloric stenosis is occasionally seen in children and adults. In infants, it develops between the second and fourth week after birth. It is considered a familial disease, although there is uncertainty regarding its genetic character. Pyloric stenosis occurs in one out of two hundred live births, more frequently in males than in females; neither breast-fed nor bottle babies are immune.

Pyloric stenosis is marked by a narrowing and thickening of the pylorus, a sphincter muscle connecting the stomach with the small bowel (the duodenal section) that permits food to pass through. The narrowing of this orifice causes obstruction.

The danger: If not treated, the patient will suffer a long period of malnutrition, resulting in weight loss and stunted growth. There is always the possibility of fatal obstruction of the intestines.

Symptoms: Although symptoms usually appear between the second and fourth week, they may be delayed until the third or fourth month. Newborn infants normally lose weight for a while after birth but they soon begin to gain; in pyloric stenosis the loss is continuous. Projectile vomiting (sometimes containing blood), constipation, loss of weight, and dehydration occur. Vomiting, however, does not seem to interfere with appetite, as the infant may continue to feed immediately thereafter.

In some cases the pylorus – a hard lump about the size of a small hazelnut – can be felt in the baby's abdomen. X-ray will confirm the diagnosis, although in most cases x-rays are not needed.

Treatment: The doctor will consider conservative treatment first: an antispasmodic plus a mild sedative administered a few minutes before a feed; in between

regular feeds, small feeds of breast milk and cereal. Water can be restored by giving fluids intravenously.

Once diagnosis is definite, surgery is advised after the infant is in better condition. Surgical mortality in expert hands runs from 1 to 5 per cent. Permanent cure is the rule.

Older children and adults: treatment is the same as for *Peptic ulcer* **157**. If obstruction is not relieved in four to six weeks, surgery is advised.

Outlook: Always excellent after surgery.

Intestinal obstruction 170 (ileus)

An intestinal obstruction will block or severely curb the passage of intestinal contents. The causes are many:

Inguinal hernia **255**: Half of all obstructions are due to inguinal hernia (a hernia in the region of the groin), in which a loop of the small intestines is caught in a muscle opening.

Adhesions: an abnormal sticking together of adjacent tissues, adhesions are usually a result of previous abdominal operations.

Volvulus: a twisting, kinking of the small bowels, volvulus will cause block-

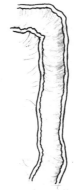 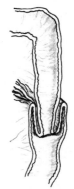

Normal   Colic intussusception

(*Julian A. Miller*)

age in the same way the kinking of a water hose will stop the flow.

Intussusception: when a section of the small intestines telescopes on itself, intussusception occurs, more often where there are tumours or polyps. Also common in infants.

Cancer: a significant percentage of cases are due to this condition.

Impacted foreign objects, gallstones, pressure from adjacent tumours: not common.

Paralytic ileus: peristaltic failure of the intestines (failure of the intestines to move their contents), paralytic ileus is due to peritonitis, abdominal surgery, or a severe injury in the bowels.

Vascular blockage: a situation similar to a heart attack, which occurs when the coronary artery is blocked, in intestinal obstruction this blockage of a blood vessel (embolism or thrombosis) occurs in the abdomen.

The danger: If total blockage is unrelieved in the small intestines, it can cause death within three to six days.

Symptoms: The cardinal symptoms of intestinal obstruction are cramping abdominal pain, vomiting, constipation, and abdominal distension. All of us, on some occasions, have suffered from these symptoms. Relief is usually obtained by antacids or allowing time to pass. However, if the symptoms do not go away or if they worsen, the condition is not one of the transient ills of the body but a serious ailment that demands immediate medical attention.

Pain: cramping, intermittent, mid-abdominal pain, lasting from a few seconds to a few minutes, with the free periods becoming less frequent.

Vomiting: an early symptom, first just the stomach contents, which are greyish, are ejected. Later, if the condition worsens, the contents become brownish, indicating bits of faecal matter, a very serious manifestation.

Constipation: always prevalent in intestinal obstruction.

Abdominal distension: if the blockage is high in the small intestines, distension is minimal; if low, distension is extensive.

The other indications are the usual nausea, belching, and heartburn. A later sign is a diminished output of urine.

If, in addition to the above, there is also bleeding from the rectum, the cause may be an intussusception. If the obstruction persists, strangulation of the intestine is probably taking place, along with shock, dehydration, a fast pulse, and low blood pressure. Outward signs are cold hands and feet, cold sweat, and anxious sunken features. The patient will go into collapse, with constant vomiting, thirst, high fever, and a total suppression of urine.

In volvulus, if the kink is sharp and completely twisted, circulation will be cut off, causing necrosis (gangrene of the local tissue). Immediate surgery is required.

In colon obstruction, the symptoms develop slowly and are less immediate. Pain is less severe and constipation may alternate with diarrhoea.

In paralytic ileus, the patient appears extremely ill, abdominal distension is severe, and gas fills the entire bowels.

Treatment: The doctor will try to determine the precise cause of the obstruction so that he can treat it properly. He will also keep a sharp watch on the pulse rate, temperature, and white blood cell count; if these indicators increase and if the patient's condition worsens (an indication that total strangulation of the bowels has taken place), he will advise immediate exploratory surgery.

The basic objectives of treatment are to reopen the passageway as soon as possible, either by decompression (preferred) or surgery, to replace fluid and nutrient losses intravenously (requires extreme care and expertise; a mistake can do great harm), and to relieve the pain.

Decompression is accomplished by means of suction. A long tube is inserted into the intestine, and through suction, the obstruction is often relieved.

If total obstruction lasts more than twenty-four hours and conservative (nonsurgical) therapy is not successful, surgery is essential. Immediate surgery is always indicated when the doctor is convinced that total strangulation, or infarction (blockage of the blood vessel in the area, causing death of local tissue), has occurred.

In intussusception, the patient is often given a barium enema for x-ray. If this is done early, before the disease has progressed too far, the enema itself can often undo the partial obstruction. If the enema is given too late, just the opposite can occur – from partial blockage it can induce total strangulation.

In paralytic ileus, a result of previous abdominal surgery or some other exterior derivation, an attempt is made to stimulate bowel motility (peristalsis) by locally applied heat (hot damp towels or electric pad) or certain drugs. It often does the trick.

Prevention: Some of the sources of obstruction are avoidable, such as developing a hernia from improper lifting (*Table 15* describes the proper way to lift), obesity, the impatient habit of straining at stools, and a slack, unexercised body.

Outlook: Very much dependent on the degree of blockage, vigorous, proper, decisive treatment, and the patient's physical condition, intestinal obstruction is generally a controllable and curable disease.

Ulcerative colitis 171

An inflammation of the mucosa of the colon, ulcerative colitis is a nonspecific (not caused by any organism), noncontagious, worldwide disorder.

A form of chronic diarrhoea, it is more common to nervous people between ages twenty and forty, but can start at any age, with peak incidence in the thirties.

The fact that milk and milk products have exacerbated this disease has suggested to many doctors that ulcerative colitis is an allergic disorder. Other authorities, however, insist that it is basically a psychogenic ailment. They believe the colon is a target organ for neuroses, bearing the brunt of emotional instability, frustration, dissatisfactions, inability to cope, self-hate, and maladjustment to society and to life. In turn, this theory is countered by the argument that ulcerative colitis victims are made nervous and anxious by the nature of the disease. Still another theory is that it is an autoimmune disorder, that the body is creating antibodies to attack its own harmless mucosa.

Ulcerative colitis is an incapacitating, disheartening, grim affliction very resistant to cure: it causes swelling of the mucosa of the colon, abscesses, haemorrhages, and ulcerations. The colon loses its elasticity, becomes fibrous, and extremely susceptible to secondary infections.

The danger: The first attack can be sudden and severe with massive haemorrhaging, perforation, and toxaemia, which can end fatally. Usually, however, it is a longstanding disease of attrition that wears down the patient, often to the point of invalidism.

Symptoms: The chief symptom is severe, sometimes bloody diarrhoea, with ten to twenty bowel movements daily; the patient is forced to live in the bathroom.

The disease can start suddenly, explosively, or it can come on insidiously with an ever-increasing need to move the bowels and mild lower abdominal cramps. The stools soon become full of mucus and blood. The cramps can become severe with the additional development of rectal tenesmus (urgent need to defecate without results).

The inevitable attendant ills are loss of appetite, nausea, vomiting, anaemia, malnutrition, weight loss, and a fluctuating moderate to high fever.

The sudden, explosive form is characterized by violent diarrhoea, extreme abdominal cramps, abdominal distension, high fever, profound toxaemia, faeces that are watery, foul-smelling, full of mucus and red blood, and a tenderness in the lower abdomen. Occasionally perforation of the colon occurs, followed by peritonitis. The victim can die of peritonitis or toxaemia before the disease is even diagnosed.

The proctoscope (an instrument for inspecting the rectum) and x-ray, in which the colon appears ulcerated and scarred, will always verify the diagnosis.

Additional difficulties include annoying rectal and anal haemorrhoids, fissures, fistulas, and abscesses. The more serious complications include perforation and the consequent deadly peritonitis, acute haemorrhage, and colonic cancer (5 to 10 per cent of patients who have had ulcerative colitis for ten years or more develop this malignancy). Other developing symptoms are nutritional deficiencies, and in children, growth retardation and sexual immaturity.

After a few years, the lower colon becomes shortened, rigid, and thickened, preventing proper bowel functioning.

Treatment: During an attack bed rest is advised. The bowels should be kept as inactive as possible. Supportive nutrition should be taken to make up for the losses resulting from diarrhoea. The body must be resupplied with proper nutrients so that it can combat the disease. The body is its best source of help, since medical aid can only be of limited value.

Intake of fluids is unrestricted. A daily intake of 2,500 calories, high in protein, is advised. Only natural foods should be taken; all concentrates, processed foods (especially those loaded with additives), iced drinks, and coarse, fibred foods should be shunned. Fruit juices and most uncooked foods are also on the proscribed list.

If the patient is unable to eat or drink, water including salts, acid bases, vitamins, and other nutrients, is given intravenously or intramuscularly.

If the patient has developed severe anaemia, a blood transfusion is advised.

The drugs that can be helpful are belladonna, morphine, propantheline, and promazine. A form of sulfa drug can also be used with good results.

Patients severely ill with peritonitis resulting from perforation who are toxaemic and running a high fever are usually given a broad spectrum antibiotic but with caution, because this medication can further irritate the colon if given orally.

Steroid therapy can be dramatically remedial (not a permanent cure). The drug can bring about a temporary remission in 60 to 85 per cent of those so treated. It has, however, two disadvantages: It can reactivate an old peptic ulcer or create a new one, and it can make the disease worse as soon as it is withdrawn. Steroid therapy is always employed when the disease has worsened and threatens life. Recently, the instillation of a steroid retention enema has added to our therapeutic armamentarium.

Psychotherapy: direct treatment by a psychiatrist has often proven to be highly beneficial, occasionally with brilliant results. Even without psychiatric help everyone must be aware of the patient's emotional and psychological problems, which must be allayed, since if they are not the direct cause, they are surely the basis of exacerbation. The doctor, family, friends, must all be alerted to give the patient moral support and encouragement. The patient himself must be urged to fight the disease with every power within him. In this case he can be his own best therapist.

Surgery is required in twenty-five per cent of all ulcerative colitis patients. It is performed when an obstruction develops, when perforation is imminent, when massive haemorrhaging occurs, when the disease is going downhill despite intensive treatment and medication, when carcinoma is real or potential, and when the patient is inevitably on his way to invalidism.

Surgery is radical – either all or a significant part of the colon is removed (colectomy). If only the diseased part of the colon is excised, the two sections are sewn together, making the colon shorter. Usually, however, the entire colon is removed, and the ileum (the lower end of the small intestine) is shunted to an artificial opening in the abdominal wall and projected about an inch (an ileostomy) into a watertight rubber bag that fits snugly to the skin. The bag is efficient, replaceable, and can practically eliminate odour and soiling if proper care is taken. When only the rectum is removed, the colon is shunted to an artificial opening in the abdominal wall (a colostomy).

This artificial way of moving the bowels is not quite as bad as it seems, especially considering the alternatives of invalidism or death. A modern unnoticeable apparatus has been devised that permits the bag to be emptied with a minimum of discomfort. The operation requires a hospital stay of under two weeks, and after a convalescence of four to six weeks, the patient can resume a normal business and social life.

Prevention: If this disorder is diagnosed early, better control of the disease and less virulence can be achieved. Milder cases seem to respond with good results to medical care.

A highly-strung or anxious person would be well advised to analyse why he's giving himself a hard time. Being 'up-tight' often means loose stools. Perhaps there's more to cry about than sing about in today's world, but it's more fun singing, and in addition, there's the not inconsiderable advantage of a longer, healthier life.

Outlook: Ulcerative colitis is a disease of remission and exacerbation. One out of four patients recovers completely after a single attack. Fewer patients are as severely afflicted now because of new medications, more understanding of the disease, and new surgical skills. However, there is still a long way to go. The best hope remains the patient himself; he is the only one at this moment who can effect a cure.

Irritable colon 172
(spastic constipation, mucus colitis)

Also called intestinal neurosis and nervous indigestion, irritable colon, although not well-defined, is responsible for more than half of all disorders of the digestive system. Except for the common cold, it is the most common disorder of man.

Strangely enough, this ailment is hardly known, although everyone, at some time or another, has been indisposed by it, often to the point of requiring medical help. Basically, irritable colon is a nervous disease that attacks the anxiety-ridden people of the world. The varied symptoms imitate every digestive disease known. Usually the disorder is set off by some stimuli, an emotional flare-up due to divorce, trouble at work, illness of a loved one. Emotionally overwrought, the victim becomes lax in his lifestyle – hasty gobbling of food, holding off defecating until a convenient time, often waiting half a day, overuse of laxatives, overuse of enemas – result: irritable colon.

Irritable colon can start at any age, but it is particularly prevalent in early adulthood and even in adolescence. This disease is the intestinal equivalent of weeping. The psychological role of the intestines has crept into our vocabulary. In slang, 'guts' stands for courage and stamina.

The danger: This ailment can mimic many serious diseases to such an extent as to be the major cause of unnecessary surgery in suspected appendicitis. Also, it mimics kidney stones and angina pectoris.

Symptoms: The patient has usually a long history of seeing many doctors with a whole series of gastrointestinal investigations. The single and most characteristic symptom of irritable colon is that the flare-ups coincide with emotional traumas. Onset and recurrence run parallel with the major stresses of life.

The basic symptoms include:

Chronic constipation: small, hard, dry stools covered with mucus. Sometimes only mucus is passed. Most often, diarrhoea is interspersed with constipation. The diarrhoeic patient usually has watery stools several times in the morning and no stools for the rest of the day. If there is blood or pus in the stools, the disease is not irritable colon (except when the blood is from bleeding haemorrhoids).

Pain: in varying degrees, pain is usually prevalent in the upper left quadrant of the abdomen. It can be relieved by manual pressure and passage of faeces or gas. Wearing tight clothing will worsen it.

Distension or bloating: an accumulation of gas is responsible for this symptom.

Other symptoms of importance are headache (common), vomiting (occasional), insomnia (frequent), loss of appetite (but rarely loss of weight), fatigue, and anaemia.

Treatment: The treatment of choice is psychological, for that is where the disease originated. The doctor will try to reassure the patient that the disease is not serious. If the patient has developed the habit of taking laxatives or an enema daily or frequently, it will have to be broken. This may not be easy, since removal of these so-called aids will worsen the condition at first.

The patient with only constipation will profit from reassurance and therapeutic conversations, but if he suffers from diarrhoea as well, help will be more difficult to obtain. He will require, if not direct psychiatric help, then considerable effort from his spouse, a friend, or doctor. Drawing up a chart of his physical flare-ups to show how they coincide with his emotional stresses can be beneficial. For all patients it is advisable to sublimate anxieties in exercise, sports, and hobbies. Long conversations regarding the patient's relationships with his parents, marital partner, children, or about his employment can be of great value.

Diet should be moderately bland with some fruit and some roughage. Bowels should be moved at the same time daily, taking time to perform the act.

Occasionally, the doctor will prescribe sedatives or tranquillizers; antispasmodics and nerve-blocking drugs can be used but with great care. Gas is not a cause but a symptom and is relieved with proper drugs.

Abdominal aches or pains are reduced by the application of heat to the abdomen – not during a period of distress but at regular intervals. Initially, some patients will require a week or so of bed rest.

Prevention: The patient must learn how to employ his excess energy, not in being anxious or tense, but in constructive exercises, hobbies, activities. An excess of neurotic energy can be turned from a fault into an advantage by releasing it in activity and exercise that will keep him physically fit and his cardiovascular system in sound condition.

Outlook: The constipatory patient can be helped enormously by his understanding of the disease and by solicitude from the people around him. The diarrhoeic sufferer is more difficult. Although cure is uncommon, his symptoms can be reduced and the time between attacks lengthened.

Diverticulitis 173

Diverticulitis is a disease secondary to diverticulosis. In the latter, small pockets about a centimetre, half inch in diameter and usually appearing in clusters occur in weakened areas of the wall of the colon. Diagnosis can be made only by x-ray, since in itself the disease is symptomless. About thirty per cent of the people over forty-five have diverticulosis, but only a fifth of them go on to develop diverticulitis.

Diverticulitis is an inflammation of the pockets, obstructed by swelling or impaction of faecal matter. The resulting bacterial infection may die down in a day or so or may go on to abscess, spasm, or obstruction of the colon. The packed diverticula may perforate and lead to peritonitis.

Diverticulitis is often difficult to differentiate from appendicitis and carcinoma of the colon.

The danger: Diverticulitis can become serious if the infected pockets develop complications of perforation or obstruction. If the condition persists beyond the end of the second day, it becomes a *Medical Alert*, which may require immediate surgery.

Symptoms: At the initial onset the patient suffers abdominal distress, which soon resolves into constant pain in the lower left quadrant. The entire abdominal area becomes tender. Other symptoms are distension of the abdomen, nausea, and occasional vomiting. If the

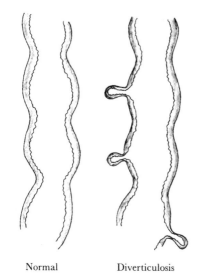

Normal   Diverticulosis
colon

(*Julian A. Miller*)

attack is severe, chills, fever and malaise are added to the list. Often a mass will be palpable in the lower left side of the abdomen.

In the chronic form, constipation alternates with diarrhoea.

Treatment: Most of the time conservative treatment will do the trick – bed rest, liquid diet, antibiotics. In the more severe form food is not taken by mouth but given intravenously. The disease usually abates in a day or so.

Pain is relieved by the appropriate drugs. If the intestines continue overactive, that is, causing frequent bowel movements and cramping pain, relief can be obtained by taking, before meals, such antispasmodic agents as tincture of belladonna (7 to 12 drops in a glass of water) or 15mg of propantheline, and a teaspoonful of psyllium (Metamucil) in water (the only recommended laxative in this disease because it is non-irritating and bulk producing).

However, when the attacks are repeated and severe, or when the disease cannot be significantly differentiated from cancer of the colon, or when perforation, obstruction or heavy bleeding occurs, surgery is clearly indicated.

Prevention: There is some indication that obesity in advancing age can lead to diverticulosis, making one susceptible to diverticulitis. Recent investigations have shown that people who live on a high residue diet – rough vegetables, fruit, whole grain breads and cereals – rarely seem to get diverticulosis.

Outlook: The prognosis is quite good, *if* there are no complications.

Meckel's diverticulum 174

A congenital anomaly, Meckel's diverticulum afflicts about 1 to 2 per cent of the population. A fairly large, blind tunnel attached to the small intestine, the diverticulum (sac) is normally present in the embryo but usually disappears a month after birth. If it elects to remain, it takes the shape of a hollow tube with the usual intestinal mucous membrane. It has no function or value but can be troublesome, like the appendix, by becoming impacted with some intestinal substance and then becoming infected, thus often causing obstruction.

Meckel's diverticulum follows a course exactly like *Appendicitis* **178**.

The only cure is surgical removal.

Megacolon 175
(Hirschsprung's disease)

Megacolon, an abnormally large colon which can be congenital or acquired in childhood or during the teen years, results in severe constipation. The congenital form becomes noticeable within the first year.

In the congenital form, which occurs once in every 2,000 births, most often in male children, the absence of certain nerve cells prevents peristalsis in a section of the colon, thus causing a stoppage of movement. The abdomen is distended with faecal impaction, often grotesquely; nutrition is poor; growth is retarded.

Acquired megacolon is due mostly to

severe emotional stress, in which the child refuses to allow himself normal bowel movements. The rectum is distended and full of faeces, and a characteristic sign is soiled underclothing. Acquired megacolon calls for psychiatric treatment. In addition, stool softeners and mild oil retention enemas can be administered. If this fails, surgical removal of the accumulated faeces is essential to preclude progressive enlargement of the colon.

Constipation 176
(lazy colon, atonic constipation)

Afflicting the old, the bedridden, and the invalided, as well as the highly intestinal neurotic, constipation of physical origin is the result of insufficient physical activity. When children are affected, the cause is usually an overanxious mother exacerbating an imagined condition. Constipation can also be induced by those who habitually ignore the urge to defecate, while those with a long dependence on laxatives and enemas, often starting in childhood, continue that dependence. Also, those who suffer from haemorrhoids and anal fissures and fistulas tend to avoid painful bowel movements and thus develop constipation. Nervous factors, too, are a major cause, for the colon frequently responds negatively to agitation, to continuous haste, to fear and anxiety. Even mild excitement can block up the colon, such as going on a trip or changing jobs.

A considerable difference of opinion exists regarding the actual meaning of constipation. Generally, the accepted medical definition is at least three days between bowel movements and the passage of very dry stools.

The danger: None, unless it is worried into another intestinal disease. Excessive straining at stools among the elderly can sometimes precipitate a heart attack or stroke.

Symptoms: The only serious symptom is constipation, without discomfort or pain, except for the mental anguish of the intestinal neurotic.

Treatment: Constipation can often be overcome by eating naturally laxative foods, such as fruits, plenty of vegetables, particularly rough ones, high bulkage foods (bran), and consuming eight glasses of water and/or a glass of prune juice daily. An attempt should be made to regulate bowel movement for the same time everyday.

In younger, healthier patients a retraining of bowel movements (and a regime of exercise) is in order (see *How to avoid constipation, Table 11*).

If constipation is due to dehydration from a long feverish illness, the patient should drink lots of fluids.

Occasionally a barium enema or swallowing barium will cause faecal impaction, with corresponding stomach pain and unfruitful straining at stools. The treatment is usually a warm enema (50 to 100gm, 2 to 4oz of 100-degree olive oil). If that is not sufficient, a more irritating commercial enema should be employed.

Prevention: Keeping well-exercised, avoiding invalidism, never ignoring the first urge to go to stools, and making every effort not to be an overanxious mother can do much to avoid constipation. If the bowels don't move today there's every chance they'll move tomorrow or the following day.

Outlook: Following the advice of a good doctor or following one's own good sense almost always mitigates constipation and restores evacuation.

Imaginary constipation 177

Some people are deeply disappointed with their entire alimentary canal, most notably the colon and the rectum. They are nettled by a lack of proper frequency of their bowel movements and vexed at the colour and consistency. To improve their status in the world of healthy intestinal people, they bombard their digestive system with all sorts of laxatives, cathartics, purgatives, enemas, and suppositories, like an ageing woman dousing herself with rouge, powders, and perfumes. For them, happiness means a bowel movement every day of the right colour and right consistency.

The study and examination of stools might be commendable in the concerned doctor, but it is a useless, fruitless waste of nervous energy in the nonprofessional.

Daily bowel movements are not essential for good health; the use of laxatives and enemas by persons who are capable of physical activity, who are not invalided or bedridden, is distinctly a wicked act against the body. People who are rectally and anally preoccupied can better serve their needs by transmuting this scatological concern to a concern of greater importance, such as money, sex, love, life.

Appendicitis 178

The vermiform appendix is a small, worm-like, dead-end tube attached to the caecum of the colon (the part that is attached to the small intestines). It serves no purpose and appears to be left over from the early ancestors of man. When it becomes infected, appendicitis results. If the appendix is not removed, it becomes swollen, gangrenous, and soon ruptures (perforates), resulting in peritonitis.

Appendicitis occurs generally in the young, rarely before the fifth year and not often beyond the thirtieth, with a predominance in males. The one per cent mortality rate is always due to complications and late treatment.

The danger: The medical profession has practically total control over appendicitis. However, neglect and delay can cause rupture and consequent peritonitis, a deadly disease that accounts for the one per cent mortality rate. This is a *Medical Alert.*

Symptoms: The anatomical location of the appendix is usually (about seventy-five per cent of the time) in the lower right

quadrant of the abdomen. However, there is no rule that says it must be there. Sometimes it is elsewhere in the abdominal area.

The disease begins with a vague discomfort in the umbilical region, but within a few hours it shifts to the lower right quadrant where it settles down to a dull, more often severe, constant pain. The telltale symptom is tenderness and rigidity in the centre of the lower right quadrant.

There is nausea, often with vomiting, a loss of appetite, indigestion, a fever between 37° and 37·8°C, 99° and 101°F, a pulse rate of about a hundred a minute, and a white blood cell count that rises sharply (from 10,000 to 16,000).

If the fever has risen and the pain has become very severe, lasting beyond forty-eight hours or more, the chances are that rupture is imminent.

Differentiation from other diseases: it is often not easy to differentiate appendicitis from other digestive disorders. The doctor is always in a dilemma when the distinguishing symptoms are not clearly indicated. But delay of surgical removal can endanger the life of the patient; it is often better to perform the operation when in doubt than make the mistake of not doing so and risking peritonitis. Some similar diseases and their distinguishing characteristics are:

● Inflammation of the gallbladder (cholecystitis). The pain of gallbladder radiates, the temperature is higher, and there may be jaundice.

● Gastroenteritis. Vomiting and diarrhoea precede pain, which is not true of appendicitis.

● Kidney infections. Urinanalysis will show excessive pus cells; the lower right quadrant will not be tender or rigid.

● Ovulation. The white blood cell count does not rise.

● Other diseases not so easily differentiated include diverticulitis, pancreatitis, and regional enteritis.

Treatment: Early surgery, the earlier the better, within the first day after the onset of pain; maximum time is forty-eight hours. If done within twenty-four hours mortality drops to half of one per cent. If an abscess has formed, the abscess cavity must be drained before surgery is performed. If the disease is moving towards perforation and peritonitis, large doses of antibiotics are given by injection.

No food, no liquids should be given the patient until the doctor has seen him. The administration of laxatives or enemas can lead swiftly to peritonitis and death. Do not apply heat to the affected area.

As soon as the anaesthesia wears off the patient is put on his feet. His hospital stay is usually less than a week, and within two weeks he is back at work. As long as he lives he'll never miss the appendix.

In the elderly the classic picture of appendicitis is fuzzy. The white blood cell count may not be high and there is no fever. The patient has often administered to himself some laxative or enema, which may contribute to the 10 to 15 per cent mortality in this group.

There is no such disorder as chronic appendicitis. What is called chronic appendicitis is probably a manifestation of other diseases.

Prevention: It's a matter of being lucky. (See *Part 3, Early warning signals, Appendicitis* **178**)

Outlook: Excellent. A dangerous disease has been rendered harmless by the application of modern medicine.

Peritonitis 179

All the vital organs of the body are covered by a thin but strong protective membrane. The peritoneum is the membrane that covers the abdominal organs; it is also richly supplied with nerve endings. When the peritoneal sac is infiltrated by toxins, bacteria, or other substances, such as bile, blood, or urine, it creates a serious disease called peritonitis. This airtight, closely sealed sac can be infiltrated only by the rupture of an organ it contains, such as a ruptured appendix or diverticulitis or a rupture of the other gastrointestinal organs, the pancreas, gallbladder, bladder, or colon.

Additionally, the peritoneum can be infected or intruded upon by blood from an abnormal pregnancy, an infection of the female genital tract (ovaries, the uterus, or fallopian tubes), or from a faulty abortion.

Other causes include the failure of a surgeon to provide sufficient aseptic techniques and, of course, trauma, such as a knife or bullet wound, in the abdomen.

The danger: About ten per cent of those suffering from peritonitis die – from toxaemia, dehydration, and shock. Abscesses are difficult to handle and require surgical drainage. This is a *Medical Emergency.*

Symptoms: The severe, prostrating pain is often intense enough to cause shock. Since movement intensifies pain, the patient is usually motionless, his thighs drawn up, and breathing is shallow. The abdominal area is distended with acute nausea; the abdominal wall is rigid. Pain can often refer to the shoulder. Vomiting is persistent; occasionally there is diarrhoea and hiccups; urine output is low (dehydration). Other signs include rapid heartbeat, fever, progressive toxaemia, low blood pressure, and thirst. The white blood cell count is high, running from 10,000 to 50,000. The patient appears gravely ill with Hippocratic appearance (sunken eyes, hollow cheeks, leaden complexion, relaxed lips). Anxiety is etched on his face. The disappearance of pain does not necessarily mean improvement.

Treatment: The initial cause of this catastrophe must be surgically repaired. Intense antibiotic treatment is prescribed, along with bed rest and opiate injection to control the pain. No food or drink by mouth is permitted, suction by gastric or intestinal tube is constantly maintained, and solutions of saline, glucose, and plasma are given intravenously.

If there is an abscess it must be properly drained, that is if the condition of the patient permits operation. But often in generalized peritonitis supportive measures and intense antibiotic therapy must precede even vital surgery.

Prevention: Somewhere along the line

either the doctor or the patient delayed too long in attacking the underlying disease. An operation that comes a day late, after perforation has already taken place, causes five times as much difficulty.

Outlook: Peritonitis has a ten per cent mortality rate. Under the age of forty-five a patient's chances are better. Over sixty his chances are less than ninety per cent, but then his chances on every disease are less.

THE SMALL INTESTINE – THE MALABSORPTION SYNDROME

Several disorders of the small intestine are characterized by the impaired ability or complete failure of the intestine to absorb nutrients from food. The two most important ailments are sprue and coeliac disease. In addition, the malabsorption syndrome is found in regional enteritis, tuberculosis, and malignancies. When half or more of the small intestine has been removed or the small intestine has received massive exposure to x-ray, or when mineral oil has been used constantly as a laxative (mineral oil absorbs all the fat-soluble vitamins, such as vitamins A, D, and K), the malabsorption syndrome is also present.

Sprue 180
(adult nontropical coeliac disease)

A serious malfunction of the body of unknown origin, occurring mostly in the thirty to sixty age bracket, sprue is a chronic disease causing impairment in the absorption of fats, including fat-soluble vitamins A, D, and K. In addition, vitamin B_{12} and folic acid are also badly absorbed, causing anaemia. Of the victims, twenty-five per cent have a child-

hood history of diarrhoea or a family history of the disease.

The danger: Although treatment is far from satisfactory, without it the patient would just waste away or become a semi-invalid.

Symptoms: The onset is slow and stealthy, taking quite a while before the victim realizes he is ill. The first sign is gas in the colon, expelled through the rectum. Although this, in itself, is hardly significant, other symptoms soon begin to appear: loss of appetite, increasing weakness, loss of weight, brown pigmentation of the skin on the trunk and extremities, very pale skin resulting from oncoming anaemia, and low blood pressure.

The most characteristic indication is, however, diarrhoea three or four times daily, usually in the morning – frothy, bulky, light-coloured, with a very offensive odour, and, particularly, containing large quantities of fat.

The tongue is very red and sore (a vitamin deficiency sign). In acute sprue there is loss or significant diminishment of the sense of taste. The physical picture is of a man whose stomach is badly distended while the rest of his body is emaciated. The patient is usually apathetic, listless, and depressed; he is also suffering from anaemia with small capillary bleeding under the skin (a sign of vitamin K deficiency).

In children the symptoms are retarded growth, failure to attain adult characteristics in mind and body, deformities as in rickets, spontaneous fractures, and all the deficiency signs of insufficient fat-soluble vitamins A, D, and K.

Treatment: Treatment is mostly dietary. The elimination of certain foods, such as gluten, a substance found in wheat, oats, and rye, which for some reason makes the disease worse, can be impressively helpful. Supplementation of lost vitamins A, D, and K are essential, plus a daily intake of calcium and potassium.

Anaemia is most significantly relieved by taking folic acid (5 mg three times a day). This will also relieve the glossitis (sore red tongue).

A daily dose of vitamin B complex has proved quite valuable, while the elimination of milk fats and many carbohydrates is also indicated. Bananas are helpful.

Prevention: Fighting this disease early before it has had a chance to become chronic can do a great deal in terms of remission and cure (see *Part 3, Early warning signals, Sprue* **180**)

Outlook: With appropriate treatment, weight and appetite are usually regained and diarrhoea checked if not stopped. Anaemia can be controlled, but improvement of the ability of the intestine to absorb nutrients proceeds quite slowly, and relapses are frequent. Most patients, however, can be restored to a reasonably normal existence.

Coeliac disease 181
(childhood nontropical sprue)

The childhood form of nontropical sprue, coeliac disease is a chronic intestinal disorder of recurrent nature affecting infants and children up to the age of six. The disease is characterized by a malabsorption of nutrients by the small intestine, causing physical retardation. Various vitamin deficiency signs mark this disorder. The cause remains unknown.

The danger: There is no real danger *if* the disease is kept uncomplicated.

Symptoms: The first sign might be irritability, followed by persistent diarrhoea, usually touched off by some upper respiratory infection. The connection between the two disorders remains unknown.

The stools are bulky, foul-smelling, loose, and upon laboratory examination will show large amounts of undigested fats and starches. The appetite is small, and there is weight loss, general weakening, and a protuberant abdomen with a thin body. The child is cranky and fretful, suffering from malnutrition and vitamin deficiencies.

In time, the diarrhoea subsides and the child rebounds, gaining weight and strength; he is again struck down with

a recurrence of the ailment, most often set off by another respiratory infection.

The attacks keep repeating but with lesser frequency and virulence until they disappear altogether.

Treatment: The attacks can be reduced by eliminating foods containing gluten (wheat, rye, oats). The diet should contain easily digested sugars, such as those found in honey, corn syrup, and bananas, and be well fortified with proteins (lean meat, cheese, and the whites of eggs) plus fruit and vegetables. If the child is still an infant he should be fed raw ground apples and pureed vegetables. The diet must be supplemented with large doses of vitamins A, D, B complex, folic acid, and B_{12}. Considerable vitamin C is also in order.

The cure will take a year or two of alert treatment.

In severe cases of diarrhoea, and consequent dehydration, the child may have to be hospitalized so that he can be properly fed intravenously.

Prevention: No one knows why this disease occurs and prevention remains equally unknown.

Outlook: This disease tends to disappear as the child grows older; its disappearance is hastened and its virulence considerably diminished by proper treatment. Ultimately, the outlook is quite good.

THE RECTUM AND ANUS (ANORECTAL DISORDERS)

Daily bowel evacuation is an age-old as well as current belief but medical facts do not sustain this notion. Normal defecation can vary from twice daily to once every three days. A cardinal rule about this is that *in the absence of any other symptom* bowel movements should be left alone for the body's own determination. The constant use of laxatives and enemas weakens and

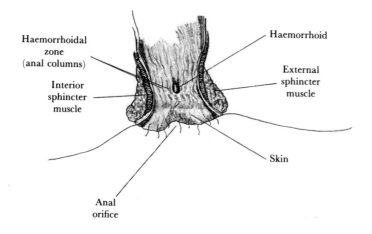

Haemorrhoidal
zone
(anal columns)

Haemorrhoid

Interior
sphincter
muscle

External
sphincter
muscle

Skin

Anal
orifice

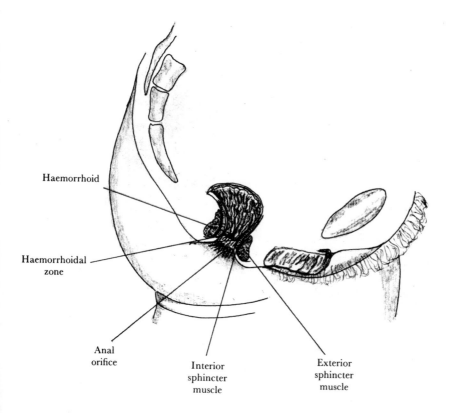

Haemorrhoid

Haemorrhoidal
zone

Anal
orifice

Interior
sphincter
muscle

Exterior
sphincter
muscle

(*Julian A. Miller*)

worsens this normal body function. The best laxative is exercise.

Haemorrhoids 182
(piles)

Probably the most common of all digestive tract disorders, haemorrhoids occur when the veins outside around the anus or just inside the rectum become varicosed. These delicate veins are easily affected by any intra-abdominal pressure, such as obesity, pregnancy, but most frequently by straining at stools and spending too much time at this body function, which causes rupture of the blood vessels or the formation of blood clots as well as scarring and infection of the covering tissues.

External haemorrhoids are easily visible as little folds of brownish skin protruding from the anus; internal haemorrhoids require medical examination to determine the extent and degree of the disorder.

There may be a family tendency for this condition, but it can also be induced by too sedentary a life or an excessive use of laxatives. Highly-strung individuals who have developed constipation and stool-straining habits are the most likely sufferers.

The danger: There is no danger to life, although excess bleeding can produce anaemia.

Symptoms: External haemorrhoids generally occasion only a mild itching with some constriction during defecation. Internal haemorrhoids, however, which are constantly being irritated by the passage of stools, can become quite painful with considerable clotting and bleeding. Frequently the haemorrhoidal mass, the swollen vein and tissue, prolapses (falls) and extends beyond the anus, often having to be pushed back inside.

Treatment: Self-treatment can be dangerous. Commercial ointment only eases the pain, it does not cure; more importantly, it can hide or obscure a more significant cause.

Medical treatment consists of treating the contributing disorders – obesity, chronic cough, sedentariness, cirrhosis of the liver, and others – wherever feasible. (Haemorrhoids that appear during pregnancy usually disappear after birth.) Straining at stools should be stopped, which means not defecating unless there is a real urge that does not require great effort, even if several days go by. The doctor will recommend ways to alleviate the symptoms without resorting to surgery, such as changing bowel evacuation habit patterns, temporary dietary restrictions, removing all rough and irritating foods, sitz baths, application of hot wet packs, and the proper use of local medication, ointment or suppository.

When necessary, he will advise surgery. Unfortunately, this operative procedure has earned a false reputation of being extremely painful. This is not true at all. The results are most gratifying, requiring a stay of, at most, three days in a hospital with total recovery within a fortnight. Seventy-five per cent are completely cured; twenty-five per cent are so improved that only care and conservative treatment are necessary. This is not a dangerous operation.

Prevention: For those who are pregnant, the key word is patience; those who habitually strain anxiously at stool should be less worried. Being sedentary is not salutary.

Outlook: Always good if the underlying cause can be treated. At worst, relief and minimalization of the disorder can be obtained.

Anal Fissures 183

A minor crack or tear either in the mucous membrane of the rectum or in the skin around the anus, anal fissures result from the passage of something hard or sharp in the stools or the passage of an unusually large stool.

An anal fissure will not heal if left alone because each defecation reopens the crack. Repeated defecations build up scar tissue as the body tries to heal the injury.

The cracks are small but very painful.

The pain upon defecation is sharp, knife-like, often so severe that the patient will refrain from defecating, thus causing delay and larger, more abrasive stools.

Treatment consists of scrupulous local cleanliness with the use of cotton wool in preference to toilet paper. Proprietary ointments and suppositories can be helpful. The diet should be low residue and contain fluid to reduce the bulkiness of the stools. Metamucil, or a similar preparation, is excellent as a stool softener.

Physical activities should be cut down and as little time spent at stools as possible. A sitz bath after defecation will nip the pain in the bud. Laxatives are inadvisable because they induce a greater number of bowel movements.

If nothing helps, which is not unusual, the fissure should be completely excised surgically.

Proctitis 184

An inflammation or irritation of the rectum and anus, proctitis has a number of varied sources: colitis, venereal diseases, haemorrhoids, anal fissures, strong laxatives, hard, dry, irritating stools, radiation, allergy, and drugs (in particular, broad spectrum antibiotics).

The basic symptom is tenesmus (straining but inability to pass faeces). The desire to defecate is constant, but the results are mostly mucus and gas. Often the pain is so severe in sitting or standing or walking that the patient is obliged to take to bed.

The mucous membrane of the rectum can range from red and swollen to pinpoint abscesses and tiny ulcerations. A search is required for the underlying cause, but at the same time a direct attempt is made to alleviate the symptoms. An opiate is usually given by mouth or rectum to reduce the tenesmus. Less powerful suppositories can also do the job. Sitz bath, bed rest, and the local application of moist heat can do much to alleviate the discomfort of the patient. Cure can come only from treating the underlying cause or causes.

Anal fistula 185

A fistula is an abnormal tube or opening from a cavity to an opening in the skin or to another cavity. An anal fistula goes from the rectum to an opening in the skin near the anus, serving as another anus without the benefit of a sphincter.

Anal fistulas usually derive from abscesses around the anus. They also occur in *Regional enteritis* **168** and *Ulcerative colitis* **171**.

The fistula discharges intermittently, causing soilage of clothing and a constant unpleasant odour from the faecal substance. The rectum is usually sore rather than painful.

Treatment is always surgical – the fistula is either opened or completely removed. Fistulas never heal by themselves.

Anal pruritis 186
(itching anus)

Anal pruritus is a severe and chronic itch in the anal area. Specific causes should be sought, such as intestinal pinworms, fistulas, haemorrhoids, an allergy to broad spectrum antibiotics (which may also be due to a fungus overgrowth), highly spiced foods, and anxiety. Much of the time there is no known cause. Most patients, however, have an excess of mucus that seeps through the anal canal, keeping the area moist and irritated.

Treatment consists of keeping the area clean and dry. Use of oily medication only worsens the conditions. A dusting powder should be used, preferably a mild antifungal preparation. A low anxiety threshold is perhaps the best therapy of all.

10 The liver and gallbladder

Charles E. Cherubin

The largest (about four pounds) and most metabolically diversified organ of the body, the liver performs more functions than any other organ. It manufactures the blood-clotting agents, prothrombin and fibrinogen, without which we would all bleed to death at the slightest wound. It produces and stores glycogen, a source of glucose needed by the brain and by the muscles for energy. The liver manufactures bile, basic to the digestion of fats, and it aids in the metabolism of proteins, carbohydrates, and minerals. The liver is the body's detoxifier, rendering harmless many noxious drugs and chemicals that find their way into the body. The liver stores vitamins A, B, D, K, and E, and it has yet other functions that have not been fully analysed.

No man-made laboratory could possibly equal what this four-pound human organ can do. It is situated in the upper abdo-

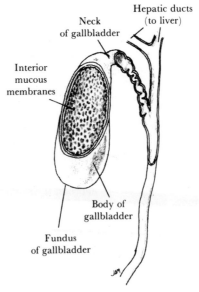

The gallbladder. (*Julian A. Miller*)

Hepatic ducts (to liver)

Neck of gallbladder

Interior mucous membranes

Body of gallbladder

Fundus of gallbladder

men, mostly on the right side, just beneath the diaphragm. Life cannot exist for long with a seriously impaired liver.

The 8cm, 3in gallbladder stores and intensifies the bile made by the liver and, when needed, delivers the digestive juice to the duodenum of the small intestine. The straw-coloured bile from the liver is changed in the gallbladder to a dark green or yellowish-brown. In addition to its digestive properties, bile is also an antiseptic and a purgative.

Acute infectious hepatitis 187
(hepatitis A)

Ranging from a mild infection without symptoms to one that is incapacitating, acute infectious hepatitis crops up both in epidemics and sporadically. Only recently has the elusive virus of hepatitis A, the cause of this disease, been identified. This form of infectious hepatitis is spread by person-to-person contact and through food and water faecally contaminated by poor sewage disposal and insanitary toilet facilities, especially at summer camps, army barracks, schools, and so on. Seafood from contaminated water may be dangerous.

Hepatitis A affects mostly the young, but any age group may be susceptible. Patients with a very mild form of the disease may be unaware of their infection and may pass it on to another person who will develop severe illness. Incubation period is about twenty-five to thirty-five days.

The danger: There are virtually no permanent consequences, once the disease has passed. The death rate is almost non-calculable.

Symptoms: The onset may be sudden or insidious. During the first part of the illness, the symptoms may suggest a viral illness, flu, or gastroenteritis. There may be a fever of up to 38·9°C, 102°F, severe headache, and aching muscles. Loss of appetite is most common (the patient is usually nauseated at the sight of food).

General weakness is usual. The symptoms are very similar to flu except for a tender, aching, and palpable liver and deep pain or pressure just below the ribs of the right side, dark urine, and a loss of taste for cigarettes. This phase lasts about four days to a week when jaundice is usually noted along with an increase in nausea and vomiting, general body itching, the appearance of light-coloured stools, dark urine, and occasionally diarrhoea. This phase persists for about one to two weeks or more. Even after all symptoms have disappeared, convalescence may be slow, running from weeks to months; for a long time the patient may tire very easily.

Although jaundice is the important diagnosing symptom, on some occasions it may not occur. If it does appear, however, other diseases must also be considered, such as medication-induced hepatitis, obstruction of the bile duct by a gallstone, infectious mononucleosis, and many others. The presence of bilirubin (the yellow or orange dye in bile) in the blood provides positive identification.

A specific test to distinguish between mild hepatitis A and the more severe hepatitis B is the hepatitis B antigen (HBAg) test. A positive test indicates hepatitis B, which has a longer convalescence and may produce chronic liver disease. On the other hand, since the test does not pick up more than half or two-thirds of the cases of hepatitis B, a negative test may not indicate hepatitis A. Better, more sensitive tests are being developed, but they are too complex to receive widespread use.

Treatment: No medical treatment is available. General treatment consists of bed rest until the severe symptoms have disappeared, usually a minimum of one to three weeks. Most of the time this is not a problem, for the patient is too sick or fatigued to do anything else. The disease begins to abate within ten days, but the patient can remain in a state of exhaustion for a long time afterwards. Convalescence may take weeks, sometimes months. Most doctors doubt the value of long, continued bed rest, and those patients who are encouraged to be active after the first few weeks seem to get better as quickly as those kept on complete bed rest. The diet should be well-balanced and high calorically to prevent malnutrition.

Most patients usually cease to be infectious two weeks after onset of the disease. However, absolute sanitation is important; hand scrubbing after using the toilet is a must.

Relapses do occur in about five per cent of the cases (this does not mean that the disease is advancing into deadlier liver diseases). Relapses are often due to weakening by other infections (cold, flu, and so on) and to drinking.

Prevention: All those exposed to the patient or those who have swallowed suspected contaminated food or water should be given gamma globulin injections, which will suppress the disease, for a period of about two months. Anyone planning to spend time in a country where hepatitis is common should receive a globulin injection.

In general, alertness regarding sanitation facilities and an avoidance of doubtful waters (for bathing or drinking) can help to avoid this disease. Even clams from waters tainted with sewage can produce outbreaks of hepatitis.

Outlook: Most patients suffering from acute hepatitis recover without incident and generally are immune to this disease, though not to hepatitis B.

Serum hepatitis 188
(hepatitis B)

Similar to hepatitis A except for its greater severity and means of transmission, hepatitis B is often contracted from unsterile hypodermic needles. The drug addict, of course, who is seldom concerned with antiseptic conditions and shares needles with friends, is a prime victim. The virus of serum hepatitis is extraordinarily tough and can survive most ordinary forms of sterilization; it actually takes about thirty minutes of boiling or live steam in an autoclave to kill this virus. A major contributor to the incidence of

hepatitis B is the transfusion of blood, because it is not possible to screen out all donors who carry the virus in their blood. Most often the carrier does not know he has it. A hopeful note is that the hepatitis B antigen (HBAg) test is being used to detect and eliminate some of the infectious blood. (See *Acute infectious hepatitis* **187**)

The infection can also be passed from one person to another by close or intimate contact; kissing and sexual intercourse are suspected means of passage.

The incubation period runs from two to six months (compared with infectious hepatitis which runs from twenty-five to thirty-five days). This form of hepatitis hits adults mainly over twenty; its virulence and mortality rate is far higher than hepatitis A.

Symptoms and treatment: Generally, the symptoms are the same as in hepatitis A, although a distinctive early symptom is the breaking out in hives (itching red wheals). There may also be a brief episode of arthritis (one in five cases) before jaundice appears. The treatment is the same as in hepatitis A. However, because hepatitis B has a greater chance of developing into fulminating hepatitis or cirrhosis of the liver than heptatitis A, it is a far more dangerous disorder.

Outlook: Ninety per cent of the patients suffer no long-term consequences, once the acute phase of the disease has passed. The remaining ten per cent have evidence of liver involvement for months or years. Some of these (very few) develop chronic hepatitis and cirrhosis. The mortality rate for hospitalized patients is low, about 1 to 2 per cent.

Most hospital staffs are quite vigilant about the risks of insufficiently sterilized needles, so that this danger has been considerably lessened. The problem of blood transfusion promises to be solved within the immediate future.

Toxic hepatitis 189

An inflammation of the liver, toxic hepatitis is induced by a large variety of drugs or chemicals, which are either eaten, drunk, inhaled, or injected. While small amounts of milder drugs and chemicals are tolerated and detoxified, a larger dose or continued use may injure the liver and result in jaundice.

Alcoholism and malnutrition greatly increase the susceptibility of the liver to noxious chemicals and drugs. Some of the more important poisons are:

Carbon tetrachloride – a common household dry cleaner, found in spot removers, now banned in most localities.

Cinchophen – an ingredient in many old-fashioned analgesics. Very hazardous for the liver.

Iproniazid – once in common use for mental depression, iproniazid has a particularly nasty side effect on the liver, causing fulminating hepatitis.

Halothane – a widely used anaesthetic, on rare occasions produces a fulminant hepatitic disease leading to death. It is said to happen once in every million patients. The risk increases if there is repeated re-exposure to the anaesthetic as during several successive operations.

Sex hormones – male hormones (methyltestosterone) can cause jaundice but no permanent liver injury; the same applies to female hormones (as in birth-control pills), but this is much rarer.

Other liver-dangerous drugs – phosphorus, all the arsenic compounds, and to a somewhat lesser degree, alcohol, bromates, chloral hydrates, chloroform, naphthol nitrobenzene, Lysol, iodoform, antituberculosis drugs, phenothiazine tranquillizers, sulfonamides, and some of the antibiotics. The risk of liver injury in the last four drugs depends on whether the individual has an idiosyncrasy to them.

The danger: Toxic hepatitis is a serious, frequently fatal medical problem.

Symptoms: The basic symptoms are nausea and vomiting, collapse, and diarrhoea, almost always followed by jaundice and hepatic (liver) failure (apathy, stupor, coma) and often accompanied by generalized itching.

Treatment: The causative agent (the poison) must be removed. Alcohol is strongly contra-indicated. The diet should be heavy in protein and carbohydrates with some restriction in fats. Those who have gone into stupor or hepatic coma must be fed intravenously and require close medical supervision; for them, the outlook is grave.

Outlook: Varies with the degree of poisoning. Some cases end fatally, some patients sustain permanent injuries and some recover.

Gilbert's disease 190
(constitutional hepatic dysfunction)

Although not common, Gilbert's disease occurs often enough to be misdiagnosed. Characterized by an intermittent low-grade jaundice, usually the only symptom, the disease is benign, affecting mostly young adults. All liver function tests are normal. The disease is self-limiting. No treatment is necessary or effective.

To the diagnostician, jaundice is usually a serious sign, but in the absence of other significance symptoms, is often Gilbert's disease, which if recognized avoids unnecessary medical expense and treatment.

Cirrhosis of the liver 191
(portal cirrhosis, Laennec's cirrhosis, alcoholic cirrhosis)

In cirrhosis, a chronic disease, the liver becomes knobby, congested, distorted, and scarred with resulting serious malfunction. Its usual victims are middle-aged men, but not always. A major cause is alcoholism; occasionally hepatitis B virus infection is the agent, and probably other as yet unknown agents are also involved.

The danger: The complications of cirrhosis are quite grave. They include *Oesophageal varices* **151** in which the blood vessels can rupture, causing bleeding and death; hepatic coma, which often ends fatally; the collection of ascites (fluid) in the abdomen because of increased pressure in the veins connecting the intestines to the liver; tumour of the liver; and bleeding from a duodenal ulcer.

Symptoms: Mild cirrhosis of the liver can be asymptomatic. The severe form comes on gradually with nausea, vomiting, flatulence, and loss of weight. Later, jaundice develops, along with emaciation, enlargement (and then contraction) of the liver, which may be felt under the rib cage on the right, rough and hard. The breath becomes foetid in comatose patients. Another late sign is the massive collection of fluid (ascites) in the abdominal cavity, causing great swelling from ribs to groin. Spider angiomas – enlarged blood vessels in the form of red dots from which fine red lines spread out, spider-like – appear on the skin over the chest and shoulders. Reddened areas appear on the palms and puffiness in the feet and legs.

In men, cirrhosis often produces such feminine characteristics as enlarged breasts, along with atrophy of the testicles. Also, there may be loss of pubic hair and impotence. (The liver in this disease is unable to inactivate the female hormones that all men have in small degree.)

Other significant symptoms are large veins around the abdomen and bleeding in various places – nosebleeds, haemorrhoids, vomiting of blood, blood in the faeces in the form of black, tarry stools.

Treatment: Total alcoholic abstinence is absolutely essential. The diet should be rich in protein. If ascites develops, salt must be restricted. In severe cases or in complications, diuretics and steroid therapy are employed.

Prevention: People with early cirrhosis resulting from alcohol can avoid the outcome of this grim disease by abstaining from alcohol.

Outlook: If the patient follows the doctor's order and stops alcoholic intake at once and if no complication develops within the next year and a half, his longevity will be normal. Cessation of alcohol means the difference between survival or death. Unfortunately, this advice is not always taken – and death is then inevitable.

Fatty liver 192

Fat people, persons suffering from protein malnutrition, uncontrolled diabetics, and heavy drinkers usually have fatty livers. An innocuous disease, it is manifested by an enlarged, tender liver with none of the other liver disease signs. In alcoholics, fatty liver precedes cirrhosis.

There is no specific treatment except weight loss in the obese, control of diabetes, or cessation of alcohol intake. If there is malnutrition, a nutritious diet high in protein and low in fats is indicated, supplemented with vitamins. Carbon tetrachloride and phosphorus poisoning may also cause this condition.

Acute yellow atrophy 193
(acute necrosis)

Acute yellow atrophy is the sudden and extensive necrosis (death) of liver cells with a rapid loss of liver function. Alcohol and malnutrition may be predisposing factors. Occasionally pregnancy can provoke the disease. Yellow fever and serum hepatitis can bring it on as well as any notorious liver poisons such as carbon tetrachloride.

The danger: this is a *Medical Emergency.* Acute yellow atrophy is usually fatal; death occurs within two weeks of its onset.

Symptoms: First, the acute symptoms of jaundice – high fever, weakness, and enlargement of the liver, with severe abdominal pain – appear. As the jaundice deepens, the liver shrinks in size and there is black vomiting, often of blood, severe headache, mental torpor and confusion, haemorrhage beneath the skin, bleeding from the mouth, dilated pupils, foul breath, scanty urine, which may contain blood, rapid and feeble pulse, and finally, death.

Treatment: Vigorous action must be taken against shock, dehydration, and acidosis. Comatose patients are fed intravenously. Blood transfusions are initiated at once in severe anaemia. Medication consists of steroid therapy and antibiotics.

Outlook: Occasionally patients with heroic treatment survive; sometimes there is residual liver damage. Fortunately, this disease is not common.

Gallstones 194
(cholelithiasis)

Stones in the gallbladder, or gallstones, as well as stones in the common bile duct, occur four times as often in women as in men. The four Fs designate the type of person prone to it: fat, forty, female, and fair (Caucasian). The causes of the disorder are not clear; the disease is probably metabolic and is probably related to diet and obesity.

The danger: Many of the victims also develop inflammation of the gallbladder (*Cholecystitis* **195**). When the bile duct becomes infected in addition to being obstructed by a stone (*Cholangitis* **196**), the patient may develop gangrene of the gallbladder and peritonitis, as well as jaundice and liver damage from the obstruction.

Symptoms: In some people the presence of gallstones produces no symptoms at all. Common symptoms that suggest their presence are considerable flatulence, belching, acid indigestion, mild jaundice, a fast pulse, and discomfort after meals. However, when a gallbladder attack or biliary colic resulting from a stone in the bile duct occurs, the symptoms are agonizingly painful, with excruciating pain radiating from the upper abdomen to the back or right shoulder.

Treatment: Fried or greasy foods, pastries, and gas-forming vegetables (cabbage, Brussels sprouts, turnips, broccoli, cauliflower, and radishes) are forbidden. Raw fruit and vegetables should be tested for tolerance.

A primary acid of human bile, chenodesoxycholic acid, when taken by mouth

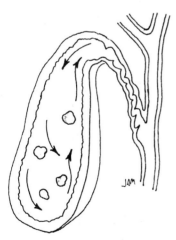

Gallstones may remain in the gallbladder for years without interfering with the bile flow, and often without producing any symptoms of gallbladder disease. (*Julian A. Miller*)

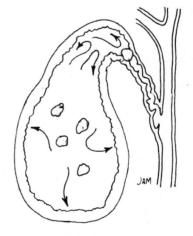

When one of the gallstones becomes lodged in the neck of the gallbladder, pressure builds up causing acute pain. There may be progressive infection of the liver and gallbladder. (*Julian A. Miller*)

for a long period of time, can cause the disappearance of gallstones.

Surgery, however, remains the only standard treatment. The mortality rate is low, around one per cent.

When definitely diagnosed as gallstones, surgery is indicated. However, there is controversy concerning those individuals with 'silent stones'.

Outlook: Surgical treatment is excellent.

Cholecystitis: acute and chronic 195

When inflammation of the gallbladder also affects the bile ducts, cholecystitis results. Commonly seen in women in their fifties or sixties, cholecystitis is most often caused by stones in the gallbladder that obstruct the cystic duct (the tube that leads from the gallbladder to the bile duct), thus damming up the bile. The stone may also be in the common duct, causing retention of bile and jaundice. Other derivations of the disease are infections of nearby organs and pressure from tumours or adhesions.

The danger: This is a *Medical Alert*. The complications – necrosis, gangrene, and perforation of the gallbladder, peritonitis, and occasionally abscess of the liver and pancreas – are serious and require immediate medical care.

Symptoms: The chronic symptoms are those described as *Gallstones* **194**.

In acute cholecystitis, pain may appear abruptly an hour or more after a meal, particularly a heavy meal rich in fats. The pain is likened to labour pains – agonizing, and deep-seated, coming in waves, starting in the mid-upper abdomen, then shifting to the right side, radiating to the back and towards the shoulder. It can also radiate to either the right or left upper pelvis and is usually accompanied by profuse sweating.

Variable jaundice (yellowing of the eyeballs and skin), nausea and vomiting, rapid heartbeat, and temperatures up to 39·4°C, 103°F are seen. The pain can last from a few minutes to several hours,

until the stone or stones have fallen back into the gallbladder or been passed on.

Cholecystitis can often be mistaken for other diseases:

Peptic ulcer: pain is in the mid-stomach, not on the right, and is relieved by food. In cholecystitis food intensifies the pain.

Acute hepatitis: blood tests will usually distinguish it from gallbladder attack.

Heart attack: jaundice is not a symptom in coronary heart disease; an electrocardiogram is helpful here.

Pneumonia and pleurisy: both these diseases are attended by cough, which is absent in gallbladder disorder; an x-ray will distinguish the two diseases.

Cholecystitis will often subside spontaneously.

Treatment: Conservative treatment means bed rest, antispasmodic drugs, and continuous gastric suctioning. Nutrition and fluid balance is maintained intravenously. Narcotics may be necessary for extreme pain, but there is danger in this because it can mask gangrene and perforation.

Surgery is the best procedure and should be done when the patient is symptom-free. However, if his temperature is rising and his pulse becoming faster, surgery should be performed at once, as the dangers of peritonitis and gangrene are high.

Outlook: If the cause is gallstones, removal will effect a cure; if the determinants are other than gallstones, the underlying disorder must be identified and treated. Surgery, cholecystectomy (removal of the gallbladder) and cholecystostomy (opening the gallbladder for drainage), has produced good results. The latter is used in acute situations, with removal of the entire gallbladder left for a future time.

Cholangitis 196

When a stone in the bile ducts blocks the free flow of bile into the small intestine, thus allowing bacteria to flourish, an inflammation of the bile ducts, cholangitis, occurs.

The danger: This disease can lead to serious infection of the liver itself.

Symptoms: The basic symptoms are jaundice, high fever, severe chills, pain in the upper right abdomen, clay-coloured stools and dark urine. As the disease progresses, the liver becomes further damaged.

Treatment: Surgery is usually considered mandatory along with antibiotic therapy. Nutrition and fluids are usually given intravenously. Additional vitamins should be administered such as vitamins B, C, and K.

A stone in the duct – if that is the cause – must be surgically removed. If there is a stricture in the duct, it should be reconstructed surgically. Nutrition, by whatever means, should be continued postoperatively, as well as antibiotic therapy. Diet should be high in proteins and carbohydrates with a modest amount of fats.

Prevention: Concentration should be on vigorous early treatment of the disease to avoid liver damage.

Outlook: Surgical procedures are characteristically favourable.

11 The kidneys and the urinary system

Gordon D. Oppenheimer
with
John G. Keuhnelian

They purify over a ton of blood daily. An awesome pair of decision-making master chemists, the kidneys constantly diagnose and determine which of the myriad substances of the body to excrete and which to retain. The body's needs change from hour to hour; it is the function of the kidneys to anticipate these needs. They eliminate the right amount of urea, ammonia, phosphates, oxalates, urine (three to four pints daily), and other chemicals; they retain the precise amount of sodium, potassium, and other needed substances.

The kidneys also regulate the fluid balance of the body, maintaining the proper amount of water in the blood and in the body at every given moment. They produce hormones and enzymes which interact with similar compounds produced in

other parts of the body in maintenance of blood pressure. In addition, they are responsible for the balance between acidity and alkalinity, for a marked swing in either direction would make life impossible. They have many other functions only guessed at and but dimly understood.

Two bean-shaped forms, each about the size of a clenched fist, the kidneys are situated near the lower ribs in the back on either side of the spine. They are protected by a layer of fat and a glove of connective tissue that also holds them in position. Each kidney contains a million nephrons, each about the size of a grain of sand. The head of a nephron, in turn, consists of a compact mass of capillaries, called the glomerulus, that filters the blood.

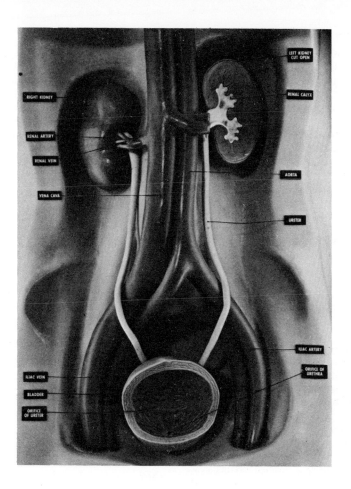

Kidney structure. *Cleveland Health Museum*

From the kidney a tube (ureter) leads to the bladder, a sac for the temporary storage of urine. Normally the bladder can hold a pint of urine. The urethral tube extends from the bladder to the exterior orifice.

Acute nephritis 197
(Bright's disease, acute glomerulonephritis)

Nephritis is a non-bacterial inflammation of the kidneys, particularly of the glomeruli (capillaries) and other renal blood vesseis, induced by a streptococcus infection of the upper respiratory tract. As in rheumatic fever, the streptococcus germ triggers off the disease but is not itself the virulent agent (that is, bacteria are not found in the kidneys). The suspicion is that it is some type of allergic reaction to a substance thrown off by the germ that sets off the kidneys to over-reaction and self-injury.

Nephritis occurs more frequently in children and adolescents than in adults.

The danger: Nephritis is a *Medical Alert.* Although 85 per cent recover, 10 per cent develop the chronic form, and 5 per cent succumb to uraemia and heart failure. Vigorous, prompt treatment will save lives.

Symptoms: Acute nephritis begins as a sudden, severe disease just as the patient is recovering from a streptococcal respiratory infection such as pharyngitis or tonsillitis (usually about one to three weeks later). General symptoms include headache, sharp loss of appetite, nausea and vomiting. The specific symptoms are blood and albumin in the urine (an invariable finding). The urine is scanty and if not frankly bloody, at least smoky. Albumin is a form of body protein, which the diseased kidneys cannot properly retain. Blood pressure rises. A significant sign is oedema (swelling of the body). The face becomes so puffy that the eyes are nearly closed. Ankles swell up. Occasionally some children will have convulsions. Other signs are a mild ache in the kidneys and a furred tongue.

Treatment: Strict bed rest is prescribed, along with limitation of protein in the diet. Basically, the underlying upper respiratory infection should be treated promptly by large doses of antibiotics, tapering off to continued smaller doses. Bowels should be kept open to help the kidneys in their job of removing waste from the body. The following are contra-indicated: diuretic drugs, despite the collection of fluids in the tissues, for they are useless and can be harmful, x-ray treatment, steroid medication, diathermy, or surgical removal of the sheath that surrounds the kidneys.

Fluids (more than a pint above the quantity lost in urination) should be administered. Salt must be decreased to lower hypertension and to cut down on the collection of fluid in the tissues.

Extreme or fulminating cases should be treated in a hospital because the character and the intensity of nephritis can change from day to day.

After treatment, symptoms will subside in a few days to a few weeks. Occasionally blood will continue to appear in the urine for a year or so after recovery.

Prevention: A vigorous handling of the underlying respiratory infection is the best form of prevention. The quick administration of antibiotics will either prevent nephritis or weaken its attack. Any streptococcal infection calls for a urine test. After recovery, every three months for at least a half year, the urine, blood pressure, and body swelling should be checked to make sure the disease is not lingering and developing into chronic nephritis.

Outlook: After a month or so in bed, the majority of patients recover. About ten per cent go on to the chronic form.

Nephritis following a streptococcal infection has a much better outcome than the furtive variety that is only discovered on a routine examination. In such cases the symptoms are vague, the only signs being albumin and blood in the urine. This form needs special attention.

Chronic nephritis 198
(Bright's disease, chronic glomerulonephritis)

About ten per cent of the patients with acute nephritis go on to develop the chronic form. Often the acute form was so mild that it passed unnoticed, but the continued assault on the kidneys eventually produces fibrosis and degeneration with progressive kidney failure. The causes remain more in shadow than in light, and when there is no background of streptococcal infection, the reason is unknown.

The danger: This is a *Medical Alert.* Chronic nephritis is a dangerous disease with fatalities occurring from ensuing hypertension, cardiac failure, cerebral haemorrhage, and uraemia.

Symptoms: In the early, non-symptomatic period, a routine examination, not necessarily looking for nephritis, will discover albumin and blood in the urine. The blood may not even be visible to the naked eye.

As the disease develops, more significant and debilitating symptoms begin to appear such as fluid in the tissues (manifested by puffiness of the face, eyelids, and ankles), distension of the abdomen, a significant rise in blood pressure, and breathlessness on slight exertion. The patient is faced with growing anaemia (caused by the destruction of the red blood cells), poor vision (resulting from tiny optic blood vessels that burst and bleed into the retina, a characteristic of hypertension), signs of heart failure (shortness of breath, swelling of abdomen), and nocturia (excessive urination at night, awakening the patient from sleep).

This advance to full-blown chronic nephritis may take several months or several years, when the patient's apparent good health suddenly gives way to renal (kidney) or cardiac failure. The final blow is *Uraemia* **207**, in which the kidneys are no longer able to remove wastes from the blood and the patient is slowly poisoned to death.

Treatment: In the early stage, when symptoms are absent, fatigue should be avoided. Great care should be taken against all upper respiratory infection. If the latter does occur, prompt, extensive antibiotic therapy is indicated with continued lesser dosage for months or years.

When there is an increase of blood in the urine and swelling appears in the face, abdomen, and ankles to a considerable degree, the patient should stay in bed until the acuteness of the symptoms subsides. If the swelling is pronounced and hypertension is high, salt must be restricted. The ensuing headache, insomia, and irritability are indications of elevated blood pressure and should be controlled with proper medications and sedatives.

Anaemia is a difficult problem and very resistant to treatment in chronic nephritis. All forms of iron compound medication should be tried, but very often the only effective procedure is transfusion. At least nine hours of sleep is advised with rest periods during the day whenever there is feeling of fatigue. The patient should avail himself of the whole spectrum of vitamins unstintingly.

Prevention: All susceptible people who develop any streptococcal infection should immediately combat the disease with appropriate antibiotics before nephritis has a chance to take hold.

Outlook: Chronic nephritis was once a death sentence; today survival is a good possibility, if haemodialysis, in which the blood is circulated through an artificial kidney machine that 'washes' the blood clean of wastes and poisons, is available in a renal unit. For information regarding home dialysis contact the British Kidney Patients Association, Okehanger Place, Borden, Hampshire.

In the past, kidney transplants were not successful – 'The operation was a success but the patient died' – because of the body's rejection of a foreign organ, rejecting it as it would invading bacteria. Today, however, kidney transplants are meeting with growing success because of more care in selecting a kidney to suit the host, and new medication to subdue the body's rejective mechanism. The success rate may be around seventy-five per cent now but there is a constant shortage of donors.

Nephrosis 199

Although nephrosis usually affects children from one to six, no one is actually immune. An unpredictable disease that can run a course from months to years, nephrosis occurs when the tubes of the kidney malfunction, rather than the blood vessels as in nephritis.

The danger: This is a *Medical Alert*. The fatality rate is somewhere just under forty per cent. A good percentage of these deaths result when the nephrotic child is unable to fight off other infections, often succumbing to some respiratory infection that a healthy child could quite easily shake off.

Symptoms: The basic symptom, swelling of the body, in various places, dropsy or oedema, results from the collection of fluid in the tissue that the kidneys have been unable to remove. The face, for example, can become so puffy that the eyes are nearly closed. The abdomen is distended to twice its size. Ankles and feet are other sites for dropsy. Another characteristic symptom is anaemia. The patient is usually pale, weak, and suffering from malaise.

Treatment: Nephrosis requires expert care. A high protein, low sodium (no salt) diet is prescribed. Since nephrosis does not usually respond to medication, blood transfusion is the usual course of therapy. In some cases cortisone, ACTH, or some form of steroid therapy can bring about cures. Often the patient develops a spontaneous diuresis (excreting large amounts of urine), thus reducing the swelling. This remission can last for days or weeks and occasionally permanently.

Prevention: A nephrotic child or adult must be guarded strongly against any secondary infection, which can be deadly to him, until he has recovered from the disease.

Outlook: Half the patients will recover spontaneously in two to five years. Some will die from kidney failure or another disease. About a third will recover from dropsy (oedema) but go on slowly to progressive kidney failure. A patient who can be kept in comparatively good condition during the virulent period of the disease may survive without permanent damage.

Acute kidney infection 200
(acute pyelonephritis, acute pyelitis)

A bacterial infection of the kidneys, pyelonephritis and pyelitis are spread through the blood or lymph system. A multitude of wide-ranging diseases that can precipitate bacterial kidney infection include diabetes, tuberculosis (a not uncommon contributor), kidney stones, and many others. In addition, any remote disorder, such as tonsillitis, a carbuncle, or a boil, can also infect the kidneys.

Young women are particularly susceptible to kidney infections, especially in any gynaecological disorder and in pregnancy. Older men are prone to this ailment when the prostate becomes enlarged, thus inhibiting the bladder and the ureter and causing stagnation of urine and consequent infection.

The danger: Kidney infection is curable. Without treatment, it can be terminal. A severe infection can block urination, causing uraemia and death.

Symptoms: The patient is quite sick – chills, intermittent fever up to 39·4°C, 103°F, headache, and nausea and vomiting.

Specifically, there is a dull to acute nagging pain in the kidneys that can radiate to the lower abdomen and groin. Urination is frequent, urgent, burningly painful, producing urine that is scanty, and cloudy with pus. The odour is of decaying matter. In severe cases, there can be total suppression of urine, making it a *Medical Emergency*. The white blood cell count is high. The kidneys may be enlarged and tender.

Treatment: A kidney infection requires a full urinary tract examination. The underlying infection should be identified and treated.

Antibiotics and urinary tract antiseptics are some of the medications used to combat pyelonephritis. A particular bactericide may suddenly lose effectiveness and require a quick substitution.

In the acute stage, bed rest is the rule with appropriate sedation. The fluid balance of the body is maintained and the urinary output increased. Treatment includes clearing up any obstruction and, if necessary, draining the bladder by tube (catheter).

Prevention: Women should be particularly attentive to genitourinary hygiene. Kidney infection requires medical follow-up examinations to prevent the disorder from becoming chronic.

Outlook: Cure may take weeks or months, but it can be accomplished if pyelonephritis is vigorously treated and the dangers of hypertension, a common companion of kidney infections, are appreciated.

Chronic kidney infection 201

(chronic pyelonephritis, chronic pyelitis)

Chronic pyelonephritis is usually a continuation of the acute from, an infection that has not been successfully treated or that has defied treatment. As in the acute variety, the chronic form affects more women than men, about three times as many.

The danger: Chronic kidney infection can so damage the kidney that it often must be removed surgically. A bad infection of both kidneys can lead to uraemia and death.

Symptoms: Chronic kidney infections can run a course of many years with repeated attacks. Symptoms are similar to the acute form: fever, pain in the kidneys, cloudy, purulent urine with pain on urination, which is urgent and frequent. Nocturia (excessive nightly urination with forced awakening from sleep) is characteristic. Hypertension is a sinister development with many cardiovascular complications. *Uraemia* **207** is another serious complication.

Treatment: Antibiotics and other bactericidals are the indicated medication. Spices and alcohol are contra-indicated, as is any drug that might irritate the kidneys (more than 120 drugs and chemicals, including such mild drugs as aspirin, zinc chloride, and vitamin D, can affect the kidney adversely; medication should be minimal). Often a badly diseased kidney is removed. The underlying cause must be treated simultaneously with pyelonephritis.

Prevention: Every bacterial infection, major or minor, must be thoroughly eradicated. Most cases of chronic kidney infection result from insufficient care of a prior disorder.

Outlook: Although each individual case is different, all treatment is protracted before good results can be seen. Hypertension is one of the dangers that must be kept under control.

Kidney stones 202

The development of stones is one of the most common kidney disorders; it is a disease of middle age and occurs more frequently in men. The stones can range in size from a grain of sand to that of a Ping-Pong ball or larger. Varying widely in composition, from calcium compounds to uric acid compounds, they can be multiple, in one or both kidneys. (One single stone is uncommon.) Some are hard and sharp, others soft and smooth. Almost all of them are insoluble, making the process of dissolving them difficult.

Kidney stones must be either passed through the kidneys, ureter, bladder, and out through the urethra or surgically removed.

Why stones form in some people and not in others is not known. However, some possible factors linked to this disorder are: urine stagnation resulting from a blockage that gives the chemicals in the kidneys a chance to solidify, disordered uric acid metabolism, like gout; abnormal function of the parathyroid gland; poor calcium metabolism; excess drinking of milk and cream (particularly in special diets); overdosage with vitamin D; and long immobilization of bedridden patients or those in a cast. One factor that does not contribute to the formation of kidney stones is the hardness of water.

The danger: This is a *Medical Alert* that can turn into a *Medical Emergency*. A stone may block the ureter, causing *Hydronephrosis* **204**, infection, and uraemia. Lack of treatment can result in total urine suppression, which, if not relieved, will cause death.

Symptoms: Much depends on the size and location of the stones. Small smooth stones can often be passed without incident. Large stones, on occasion, remain 'silent', without symptoms. But generally larger stones obstruct the ureter (the tube connecting the kidney to the bladder), precipitating an excruciating, spasmodic pain in the small of the back that can radiate from the kidney across the abdomen into the groin and genitalia. It can be one of the worst agonies that afflict man. The attack can go on for hours, accompanied by nausea and vomiting, sweating, chills, and shock.

The stone usually scratches the tissues of the kidney, causing blood to appear in the urine.

During an attack, a stone will sometimes pass through the ureter into the bladder, continue through the urethra and be expelled with urine – occasionally without additional pain, but often making itself agonizingly felt every inch of the way.

The passage of one stone does not mean the trouble is over. There is every likelihood that if one stone has formed, the tendency exists and other stones will form as well.

Treatment: Small stones without complications should be treated conservatively by trying to induce the stone to pass into the urine and out. The patient is given large amounts of fluid, three or more quarts daily, antispasmodic medication, and morphine to control the pain.

When the stone is too large to pass and begins to provoke complications – infection, severe bleeding, hydronephrosis, and blockage of the ureter – surgical removal may be necessary.

The complications must be treated simultaneously; infections controlled; and immobilized patients kept in some form of physical movement and on a diet instituted to avoid further enlargement and development of stones.

Prevention: After the first stone has been passed or removed the patient must realize that other stones may form. Most stones are a form of calcium compounds, either oxalates (two-thirds) or uric acid crystals (a small percentage). The patient must cut down but not cut out foods high in calcium, particularly milk and milk products, vitamin D and vitamin D-fortified foods (indicated on the food package), and even calcium antacids.

Stones of the calcium oxalate variety require a diet that includes daily intake of pyridoxine (vitamin B complex) and excludes such high oxalate foods as cocoa, chocolate, celery, cabbage, spinach, tomatoes, and rhubarb.

When stones are formed of uric acid crystals, the patient is advised to lower his protein intake, especially such foods as liver, kidneys, sardines, and sweetbreads, but increase the amounts of high alkaline ash, which is found in most fruits and vegetables (except cranberries and plums). Added alkalines will also be needed. Certain drugs (xanthine-oxidase inhibitors) may be used to decrease the excretion of uric acid in the urine.

Patients immobilized for an extensive period of time must make every effort to maintain some physical movement regularly.

Stones in the bladder 203

Occasionally a stone will either form in or pass into the bladder and remain. The symptoms are urinary frequency, blood, pus, and albumin in the urine in varying quantities, and painful urination. Eventually most stones pass into the urethra and out of the body, but in stubborn cases an instrument is introduced through the urethra into the bladder, to remove the stone. Stones originating in the bladder are usually secondary to prostatic obstruction.

Hydronephrosis 204

Usually secondary to some other urinary tract disease, hydronephrosis occurs when an obstruction within the urinary system cause a back up of urine into the kidneys, overdistending and damaging them, most often permanently. If hydronephrosis is allowed to linger, it will eventually destroy the kidneys.

The several conditions that can provoke hydronephrosis include: infection of the urinary tract, which can produce a narrowing or stricture of the ureter or urethra, causing a back flow of the urine into the kidneys; a stone in the bladder or ureter, making the urine flow back; any tumour (usually malignant) along the urinary system that blocks the free passage of urine; a weakness in the structure of the ureter; an enlarged prostrate pressing against the bladder and obstructing it.

The danger: This is a *Medical Alert.* If the obstruction is bilateral (both kidneys) and considerable destruction of the kidneys has taken place, curing the infection would be like locking the stable doors after the horse has been stolen. Uraemia in this disease is a constant threat.

Symptoms: The basic symptoms are recurring pain, ranging from dull and nagging to spasmodic and colicky, pus in the urine (also blood in ten per cent of the cases), fever, and tenderness in the kidneys. Dyspepsia is also a frequent symptom.

Treatment: If there is doubt in the diagnosis, an intravenous pyelogram can be made, in which the kidneys and bladder are x-rayed after an injection of a dye that shows up on the x-ray as a white shadow. If the function of the kidney is too badly impaired to visualize by this technique, other methods such as cystoscopy, sonar studies (through sound), and others will be used at the discretion of the urologist. Naturally, if a kidney or ureter is dilated this will appear on the film. The iodide is later excreted.

The infection must be cleared up rapidly with an appropriate antibacterial agent before damage is done. Drainage of the kidneys and urinary tract is essential. The surgical goal is relief and correction of the blockage. Fluid intake should be high. Prolonged therapy is needed to suppress or hopefully eradicate the infection.

Prevention: *Any* urinary infection must be treated with dispatch. Even a minor but long-lasting infection can do irreparable harm to the kidneys.

Outlook: If the obstruction has not persisted for too long, if the kidney has not been too badly damaged, if only one kidney is affected, prognosis is good – many ifs but not uncommon. A basic rule is to consider the kidneys as vital as the heart; any disorder should be seen immediately by a doctor – the sooner the better.

Cystitis 205

Cystitis, an inflammation of the bladder, may be secondary to either infection of the kidney, the urethra, or to the retention of an enlarged prostate. It can develop in descending order, from the kidney down to the bladder, or ascending, from the urethra up to the bladder (from a contactual disease like gonorrhoea). Bladder infections are common in women of childbearing age, particuarly those who are pregnant. Normally the bladder is highly resistant to infections, but a constant assault from infected urine or blockage by a stone or tumour or an enlarged prostate can make it susceptible. People who are run-down are especially vulnerable.

The danger: Neglect or inadequate or incomplete treatment will result in a chronic form of cystitis, which is far more difficult to correct.

Symptoms: The characteristic indication is urgent, painful urination. The need to urinate is frequent but with scanty output; it may awaken the patient many times during a night. The urine might appear normal to the patient, but a test will reveal considerable amounts of dead white blood cells (pyuria).

In several cases there is malaise and blood in the urine.

Treatment: Antimicrobial drugs, sulpha, or antibiotic (excluding penicillin, which does not have much effect on cystitis) will clear up the disorder. Some doctors employ an additional medication to ease the pain during urination, aniline dyes, which colour the urine a bright reddish-orange or green.

Immediate subsidence of symptoms does not mean total cure; drugs should be continued for the full time designated by the doctor to avoid the chronic and very resistant form.

The patient should be encouraged to drink fluids – more than a litre, two quarts daily. With prompt treatment, symptoms will disappear within a week and the patient will be back to normal within two weeks.

The underlying cause must be identified and treated to effect a permanent cure.

Outlook: Cystitis is totally amenable to treatment. Acute cystitis will abate within a week, and within two weeks the cure will usually be complete – if properly treated. The chronic variety needs a far greater effort for a far longer period of time.

Benign tumours of the kidneys and bladder 206

Most non-malignant tumours of the kidneys are small, three centimetres, an inch and a half at most; however, large benign tumours do occur, which are difficult to differentiate from cancerous growths (far more numerous). Discovery of a tumour is a *Medical Alert*. All large growths must be excised.

The bladder, on the other hand, has a greater prevalence of benign tumours, papillomas, or polyps. However, they can become malignant and need thorough medical care.

Symptoms for both kidney and bladder tumours are similar to malignant growths. Any show of blood in the urine calls for immediate investigation by a doctor. Since kidney tumours, both benign and malignant, grow slowly, surgery has a great degree of success because many of them are caught early. *Chapter 23, Cancer,* describes malignant tumours of these organs.

Uraemia: acute and chronic 207

Uraemia is a toxic state of the body resulting from poorly functioning kidneys, a condition that occurs when the poisonous waste material normally excreted by the kidneys is retained in the bloodstream.

The causes of kidney malfunction or failure are many: nephritis, urinary obstruction, stones, enlarged prostate, bacterial infection of the kidneys, mismatching in blood transfusion, bad reaction to blood transfusions, severe shock, extensive burns, kidney injury, alkalosis, and overdosage of vitamin D. Systemic diseases that can produce uraemia include lupus, diabetes, and congestive heart failure. Poisons, however, are a major cause; carbon tetrachloride, any mercury compound, cantharides (Spanish fly), bismuth, wood alcohol, Lysol, and occasionally the very useful sulpha drugs such as sulphapyridine and sulphathiazole.

The danger: This is a *Medical Alert*. Uraemia is a frequent cause of kidney deaths. The fatal complications include potassium intoxication, pulmonary oedema (distressed breathing and cyanosis), severe high blood pressure, and gastrointestinal haemorrhage.

Symptoms: The sudden and acute form is marked by an abrupt drop in urine output, 200ml, a third of a pint or less daily (the normal minimum is a half a litre). Severe headache is usually an early symptom. Convulsion may appear without warning. Other signs can be drowsiness, muscular twitching, a transient impairment of vision, double vision with contraction of the pupils, which can herald a coma, a urinous odour of the breath, and urea frost (a powdery rime over the body from the sweat glands, a result of the body's desperate attempt to eliminate the urea that the kidneys have failed to eliminate). Nausea, vomiting, and diarrhoea are common. In children there is swelling and puffiness of the face.

Treatment: The kidney disorder that initiated the uraemia must be controlled or corrected. Contributing aggravating factors, such as heart failure, hypertension, or dehydration, must be treated.

The patient should take in enough fluids to produce 3 litres, two and a half quarts of urine daily. In chronic uraemia, blood transfusions will improve strength and resistance. Restlessness, insomnia, depression, and anxiety can be checked with proper medication.

If the uraemia is due to a correctible, controllable disorder, the artificial kidney machine can save the patient's life, keep

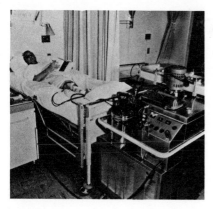

Artificial kidney machine. (*National Kidney Foundation*)

him alive until his own kidneys are well enough to do their job. In chronic uraemia the kidney machine is rarely used.

Kidney transplants (for badly damaged kidneys) have a varying degree of success, depending upon the body's acceptance of the organ.

Potassium must be kept out of the diet, since potassium intoxication is an important cause of fatalities in uraemia. Excessive sedation will produce respiratory difficulties and reduce the rate of breathing. Magnesium antacids can cause serious magnesium intoxication.

Prevention: Besides avoiding lupus, diabetes and heart failure, the subject can often do something about the overdosage of vitamin D and keeping far away from the poisons listed earlier. (See *Part 3, Early warning signals, Uraemia* **207**)

Outlook: Uraemia has a fair to good prognosis if the patient can survive the acute phase. In the chronic form a reasonable extension of life can be anticipated if the blood pressure is maintained at a normal level and the infection is eliminated.

Acute kidney failure 208

(acute renal failure)

Reduction of kidney function is a dangerous condition. The causes are similar to those listed in *Uraemia* **207**, in particular the drugs and chemicals, and in septicaemia (blood poisoning from infection), toxaemia of pregnancy (eclampsia), obstetric accidents, and septic abortion.

The danger: This is a *Medical Alert*. Death can result from sepsis (blood poisoning usually from substances manufactured by micro-organisms), haemorrhage, pulmonary oedema, and potassium intoxication.

Symptoms: In the early stage the first and major sign is failure to urinate or very scanty output. Whatever urine is passed has large amounts of albumin and tiny bits of particles. Later there is persistent nausea, vomiting, lethargy, drowsiness, breathing disturbances, diarrhoea, a dry skin and mucous membrane, convulsions and twitching. The breath smells of urine.

Treatment: An artificial kidney machine can often keep the patient alive until his kidneys have had a chance to recover. There are a number of weapons, such as alkalinization and parathyroid hormones. More than a pint of liquid above and beyond that lost in urine and sweating should be administered to the patient. Complete rest is essential. Potassium must be eliminated from all foods (potassium deaths are common in kidney failure). Diuretic drugs in kidney failure have proved harmful.

Prevention: All accidents involving the kidneys and most other traumas, including severe shock, extensive burns, poisoning, and other disasters, must be treated quickly and energetically to prevent dangerous kidney failure.

Outlook: Prognosis can only be guarded, depending very much on the nature and intensity of the kidney failure and the condition of the patient.

12 Venereal diseases

Gordon D. Oppenheimer
with
John G. Keuhnelian

Early syphilis: primary and secondary 209

Although considerably less prevalent than gonorrhoea, syphilis is a graver and far more serious ailment of man – one of his deadliest enemies. Syphilis is both acute and chronic. In its early forms, primary and secondary, it is a mild to moderate disease; if not cured at that stage, however, it will lie dormant without sign or symptom for years, often a decade or more, and then suddenly emerge into the tertiary or late stage as a terrifying killer.

In its late stage syphilis affects and destroys the heart, aorta, brain, eyes, the central nervous system, the spine, bones, skin, testes, liver, stomach, larynx, trachea – no vital organ is immune.

The tragedy of this disease is that shame, ignorance, and carelessness have pre-served it as a major ailment of our time, when it is so easily cured in its early phases, often by a single injection of penicillin.

Treponema pallidum, the germ that causes syphilis, is spiral in form and very active. The disease is acquired by direct or quasi-direct sexual contact. The number of people suffering from this malady is on a sharp rise, mostly among teenagers from fourteen to eighteen, a large proportion of whom do not seek medical aid, either from ignorance or fear of parental wrath. Parental wrath in such a case is far more evil than the presumed evilness of un-wittingly acquiring the disease.

A good many infectious cases, especially in women, are never seen, diagnosed, or treated, despite the discreet and confidential manner employed by local health departments to locate the original contact so that he or she can also be treated.

Incubation: usually 10 to 30 days after contact, although delays of as much as 3 months have been noted. Secondary symptoms usually appear within 6 weeks of contact.

The danger: If not treated, the disease can develop into a late stage of tertiary syphilis, which can cause cardiac death, moronic premature senility, blindness, deafness, deformities, locomotor ataxia, and various forms of invalidism.

Symptoms: The first indication is a hard chancre (ulcer), which begins as a raised, red, hard spot at the site of infection, usually on the genitalia (penis or vulva) but occasionally also around the lips, pharynx and anus. The chancre, which is hard and painless to the touch or even pressure, soon ulcerates. It has a clear exudate and seems superficial, although it often penetrates deep into the tissues. The germ is spread through the blood and lymph, and lymph nodes become prominent around the groin.

Occasionally primary syphilis is present without a chancre or the chancre is so small as to be dismissed as a pimple. This is more likely to happen to women than men. Any lesion on the genitalia or around the mouth is suspect and must be tested for *Treponema pallidum*.

The chancre, which affects only the genitalia or the mouth, will heal on its own in three to four weeks if not treated. That the patient is cured is a delusion, for the disease is now most likely proceeding to the secondary stage with new and more serious symptoms affecting the whole body.

More than a third of the cases of syphilis go into the secondary stage, which shows up one to six months (occasionally as long as nine months) after the chancre. The secondary form appears as a non-itching body rash, beginning as reddened splotches but soon changing and simulating a large number of various skin ailments (one of the reasons why syphilis is called the 'great imitator'). The skin eruptions are infectious. In the mucous membrane they become ulcerated and covered with a whitish or greyish exudate.

The lymph nodes become enlarged all over the body. Other lesions appear in the bone, liver, kidneys, and central nervous system. Additional symptoms are severe headache, especially at night, pain in the bones and joints, and severe pharyngitis. In addition secondary syphilis may cause baldness, iritis, conjunctivitis hepatitis, kidney disorders, and meningitis.

The secondary stage is actually a desperate attempt by the body to rid itself of the disease once and for all; it succeeds much less than a third of the time. In the majority of cases the germ survives, becomes dormant for a number of years, so that the patient thinks he is well, and then erupts into the deadly late, or tertiary, stage in which it does its greatest harm.

As in the primary stage, all secondary signs are self-limiting and heal without apparent residue. In both the primary and secondary stages the patient is infectious and can transmit the disease to a sexual partner.

Treatment: A massive injection of penicillin, usually delivered into each buttock, can wipe out the disease. Other antibiotics, such as erythromycin or tetracycline, are also employed in large doses for a two-week period, particularly in the case of patients allergic to penicillin. Suspected contacts should be given the same prophylactic treatment as those known to have the disease even in the absence of symptoms.

Several tests have been developed to determine the presence of the germ: darkfield microscopic examination, blood tests (Wassermann and Kahn tests), and spinal fluid tests (mostly used to test for the presence of the disease after treatment).

Prevention: The spiral bacteria of syphilis (deadlier but nowhere near as hardy as the gonococcus germ) are easily killed. Able to survive in only warm, moist surroundings, the spirochaetes die in minutes when exposed to open air.

Syphilis cannot be acquired from a toilet seat unless sexual intercourse is practised upon it. If the genital area is thoroughly washed with soap and water within five minutes after sexual contact with a doubtful partner, the spirochaete in all likelihood will be eradicated. Everyone who acquires this disease must report it, and the person who infected him (or her), to the public health authorities to prevent further spread. The public health authorities are always aware of the sensitivity of the situation and never make public disclosure.

Outlook: Syphilis can be considered cured when repeated blood or spinal fluid tests remain negative for a period of two years. Most relapses occur within the first year. In the primary and secondary stage, the disease is comparatively easy to cure. Immediate treatment as soon as syphilis is recognized will almost surely guarantee a cure if the treatment is adequate and thorough. The longer the delay the worse it is to treat. When it reaches the tertiary stage, therapy is difficult and the harm already done can never be undone.

Syphilis is one of the diseases most capable of medical control. Determination on the part of the patient to be cured and to help cure the partner who transmitted the disease is all that is required.

Late syphilis 210
(tertiary syphilis)

Tertiary syphilis is the final form, the deadly form. Every organ of the body can be attacked by the now deeply entrenched germ. Late syphilis makes itself apparent five to fifteen years after apparent cure of the secondary form, a period that is symptom free and noninfectious. No longer centred in the genitalia but systemically, the disease now involves the brain, spinal cord, heart, aorta, eyes, and will produce tumours in most organs and over the skin. At this stage of the disease it is named specifically, depending upon where it strikes.

The danger: Various forms of invalidism, insanity, death.

Symptoms:

Cardiovascular syphilis: the effect upon the heart and the aorta can be very grave (*Aneurysm* **142** and *Congestive heart failure* **126**).

Paresis (general paralysis): an organic mental disease, paresis begins with damage to the cranial nerves that control facial expression. An early symptom is severe headache, followed by personality changes, growing slovenliness, and tremors of the lips and tongue. Euphoria with delusions of grandeur develops. The patient's memory fails, his mind degenerates, and he lapses into moronic premature senility and finally death.

Tabes dorsalis (locomotive ataxia): tabes dorsalis is characterized by loss of sense of position and balance – when the patient's eyes are closed he is unable to touch his nose or any other point of his body nor can he stand with his feet together without swaying or falling – which becomes increasingly worse. Additionally he is subjected to 'lightning pains', episodes in which the patient feels as if needles are being injected into his skin at various parts of his body, particularly where the bones come near the surface (ankles, knees, wrists). He also suffers from 'crises', severe pain and spasms in the throat, stomach, or elsewhere. A regimen of special exercises, Frenkel's movements, can keep him from becoming a shuffling wreck.

Blindness: visual loss develops from the effect of tertiary syphilis on the optic nerve, causing atrophy (*Optic neuritis* **32**).

Gummas: soft tumours that ulcerate, single or multiple, varying from pinhead to tennis-ball size, gummas, which are slow to heal, occur most often in the liver but are also found in the brain, testes, stomach, and skin. Gummas on the tongue become cancerous.

Treatment: The disorders of tertiary syphilis require very large doses of penicillin or other designated antiobiotics such as erythromycin or tetracycline, which can often stave off the downward plunge of the disease.

Prevention and outlook: As indicated in *Early syphilis* **209**, prompt treatment at the onset can prevent secondary and late syphilis. The outlook for late syphilis is uncertain, depending upon how much destruction of the organ affected has taken place.

Congenital syphilis 211

Without medical control, a pregnant woman suffering from syphilis will deliver a stillborn baby or more likely a baby who is deformed, blind, or deaf.

General procedure for all expectant mothers includes a routine blood test for syphilis, most particularly in the early months of pregnancy, for early discovery will save the mother from anguish and the baby from the ravages of the disease.

The majority of babies born of untreated syphilitic mothers are asymptomatic at birth, but around the third or fourth week they begin to sniffle, blisters appear on the face, buttocks, palms, and soles, and meningitis and sabre shins (curved shin bones) develop. Later destruction of the cartilage of the nose occurs, causing a flattened saddleback shape. The disease can also cause deformed peglike teeth and loss of vision.

Treatment consits of penicillin therapy and a judicious use of steroids. Most doctors usually discover the disease in the mother quite early in the pregnancy. Much and often all the damage to the infant can be avoided.

Gonorrhoea 212
(clap, dose)

Despite the advent of antibiotics and sulpha drugs, both powerful and thoroughly curative medications, the rise of gonorrhoea has made it one of the greatest health problems today. The incidence of gonorrhoea is now of epidemic proportions, the highest in history. The several obvious reasons for the increase of gonorrhoea include the loosening of sexual restrictions that characterizes contemporary society; a comparative increase in homosexuality; the decline in the use of male prophylactic devices (condoms), a result, no doubt, of the reliance on the 'pill'; the gonococcal germ's increasing resistance to antibiotics; the prevalence of a large number of asymptomatic carriers; and last but most importantly, the failure to follow up and treat the partners of the infected patient.

Gonorrhoea strikes in every walk of life but is seen more frequently in the lower income groups. More than half the total number of cases occur between the ages of fifteen and twenty-five. Three times as many men report the disease; women are usually without symptoms.

The disease is most often relayed through sexual intercourse. However, heavy petting among teenagers can be just as infective. The juxtaposition of genitalia without actual intercourse is no safety at all and is no less contagious.

Curing a bout of gonorrhoea unfortunately does not confer immunity – the patient can become reinfected on the very next exposure. The disease is self-limiting, the gonococcal bacteria disappearing within six months. Serious complications can linger on if untreated, however.

Incubation: from contact to symptoms, 2 to 7 days, but on occasion as long as a month.

The danger: Complications of gonorrhoea can cause sterility in both men and women. An inflammation of the fallopian tubes or ovaries can produce infertility, while in men, untreated cases can lead to urethral stricture, and prostatic and epididymal infection. In addition, arthritis, septicaemia, meningitis, and endocarditis are not infrequent consequences of neglect. If gonococcal discharge gets into the eye, blindness can result (to prevent blindness, newborn babies are automatically treated with eye drops of silver nitrate or penicillin against the possibility that the mother may have asymptomatic gonorrhoea).

Warning: syphilis and gonorrhoea are often contracted at the same time. Since symptoms of gonorrhoea appear much earlier, treatment with penicillin, which is usually immediately instituted to kill off the gonorrhoeal germs, may suppress and mask the presence of syphilis.

Symptoms: The major symptoms (when they do appear) include a heavy discharge of whitish or yellowish pus from the vagina and from the urethra of both sexes, which will cloud the urine; a major telltale sign is the staining of the underwear. Urination for both sexes is frequent, urgent, and burningly painful. The meatus (opening) in the penis is red and irritated. About 25 per cent of the women show a vaginal discharge: 10 per cent of the men have no symptoms. Most women are asymptomatic (only 20 per cent show any signs of the disease), and the duration of the disease is much longer in women than in men. Among homosexuals there may be an anal itching where the infecting germ has proliferated. Besides the urethra, vagina, and anus, the pharynx is another site for the infection.

All suspected women should have a culture made of a vaginal and urethral smear.

Treatment: Gonorrhoea responds successfully to early medication, less successfully when treatment is late. Patients respond quickly (ninety-five per cent) to the appropriate antibiotic, usually a large dosage (twice as much for women) of penicillin delivered initially and directly into the muscle. As time passes between onset and treatment, the dosage must be increased. If the reaction to penicillin is negative, other effective antibiotics, such as tetracycline, are available. When the germ is drug resistant, an artificial raising of the temperature to 39·4°C, 103°F is resorted to (*resorted to* are the precise words, since this procedure can be risky).

Failure of treatment is due to various factors: misdiagnoses – the patient may have not gonorrhoea but a *Nonspecific Urethritis* **213**, or *Trichomoniasis* **214**; reinfection; improper dosage of antibiotics (usually a result of a particularly resistant strain of germ).

Differential symptoms between gonorrhoea and nonspecific urethritis or trichomoniasis: All three diseases are spread through sexual intercourse and are also characterized by exudation of pus. However, gonorrhoeal discharge is more pro-

fuse and purulent. To avoid misdiagnosis, discharges should be identified by laboratory tests.

Sexual intercourse should be avoided until treatment is completed. Prostatic massage or the use of urethral instruments is strongly contra-indicated. The elimination of symptoms does not mean the disease has been cured – the germ may still be dormant. Determination can only be made by the proper smear or culture test.

Prevention: With proper concern by the public and doctors, this infection can become a rarity. Every case in which the patient is reluctant to name his or her partner must be reported. The doctor, as keeper of the public health, is obliged to ferret out and treat the partner of every patient.

Washing the genital area with soap and warm water within minutes after sexual intercourse can help reduce the incidence of syphilis and gonorrhoea (especially syphilis; the gonococcus germ is far hardier). Vigorous cleanliness is valuable but in no way guarantees safety.

Even though the ratio of syphilis to gonorrhoea is one to a hundred, the diseases nevertheless often appear simultaneously; patients with gonorrhoea, therefore, should also have themselves checked for syphilis.

Outlook: Gonorrhoea is totally curable – the earlier the treatment the better. Although larger and larger amounts of antibiotics are necessary as the germ grows more and more resistant, the disease can still be thoroughly eradicated in each patient.

Herpes simplex virus 2 212a (HSV-2)

A new, tough ailment that has made a sudden appearance and is increasing with such epidemic rapidity that it has become the second most common venereal disease. Herpes simplex virus 2, HSV-2, is caused by the same virus that produces fever blisters on the lips, herpes simplex. This new ailment is the only significant venereal disease caused by a virus.

The danger: One out of every four children born of a mother who has the active disease will either die at birth or be born with some deformity. Women who have cervical (of the uterus) infection of herpes simplex are eight times more prone to cervical cancer than others.

Symptoms: HSV-2 is transmitted by sexual contact. A series of mostly painful blisters appear on the penis and inside the vagina and/or cervix. They may also appear on the pubic region of women and on the thighs and buttocks of both sexes. Other possible symptoms are enlarged lymph nodes in the groin and fever.

The blisters dry up and vanish within a week or so, even without medical attention, but unfortunately that is not the end of it. Months, sometimes years, later HSV-2 will recur, striking with the same virulence as before. Relapses are usually triggered by physical or emotional stress.

Treatment: A pregnant woman who has HSV-2 should have a delivery induced as soon as possible to prevent further damage to the child.

There are various antiherpetic medications and a variety of therapies, many of them successful, *except* they all may trigger a cancerous response. One successful form of treatment that was abandoned because of its cancerous potential involved painting the blisters with a dye (normally harmless) and then exposing them to light.

Outlook: There is every reason to believe that this disease can be contained and possibly cured by many of the developing vaccines in the near future.

Nonspecific urethritis 213 (NSU)

Nonspecific (simple) urethritis includes the various venereal diseases, other than gonorrhoea, that cause inflammation of the urethra. Sexual intercourse is the primary means of transmission, and those most susceptible are often the sexually highly active and the heavy drinker. It is practically a male disease since women show symptoms very infrequently.

The symptoms include pain in the glans (the rounded head of the penis), the urethra (causing difficulty in urination), and the testicles. Pain is also felt in the perineum (the area between the scrotum and the anus) and in the groin. There may be burning during urination (this is far more common in gonorrhoea), but itching in the urethra is most frequent. The discharge from the urethra varies from heavy pus to thin watery exudate.

Various antibiotics are employed; tetracycline is most in use. If the infecting organism cannot be determined, trial and error of different antibiotics is essayed.

Women are mostly asymptomatic, but should, nevertheless, undergo treatment.

The cause is often psychosomatic. A large number of people still have guilt feelings about sexual intercourse, which can often produce symptoms.

Trichomoniasis 214 (trichomonas vaginalis)

Usually classified under gynaecological disorders, trichomoniasis rightfully belongs in the venereal disease section since its major form of transmission is by sexual intercourse.

Trichomoniasis is caused by a parasitic protozoan called *Trichomonas vaginalis.* Most women have it at some time or another; it is particularly prevalent during pregnancy and during and after menstruation, or on any occasion when the acidity of the vagina is lowered, giving the organism a chance to flourish. The disease is often found in the prostate of men, but it is basically a female disease, transmitted to men through sexual intercourse. A man can harbour the germ and reinfect a woman.

Symptoms: In women there is a greenish or yellowish discharge, an itching in the vulva, painful urination, and an offensive odour in the vagina. In men there is urethral itching and a discharge that ranges from thin to creamy and from scanty to profuse. Often there is urgency in urination and a burning sensation. Frequently, however, there is no symptom at all even though he harbours the organism.

Treatment: Metronidazole (Flagyl) is the drug in use, a very effective medication. Both partners, regardless of the presence of symptoms, should be given identical treatment.

Prevention: The male partner should use a condom to prevent reinfection until both partners are cleared of the disease. Although the parasite exists in the rectum, where it does no harm, the structure of the female genitalia is such that carelessness after bowel movements will contaminate the vaginal area.

Outlook: A very common but minor disease; treatment eventually brings success.

Chancroid 215
(soft chancre)

A common, acute localized venereal disease caused by bacteria that produce ulcers in the genital area, chancroid is spread mostly through sexual intercourse, although infections do occur on the fingers of hospital workers who touch or handle chancroid ulcers.

The incubation period ranges from two to five days but can take as long as ten. The lesions appear as blisters and small, raised, red pimples that soon form into dirty appearing, tender, painful ulcers (differentiating the disease from syphilis whose ulcers are painless and hard) that bleed easily.

The ulcers, between 1·3 and 1·9cm, a half and three-quarter inch in size, vary from superficial erosions, which heal quickly, to sloughing sores (dead tissue separating itself from the live tissue below), which spread rapidly and deeply. If such an ulcer appears on the shaft of the penis it will often penetrate into the

urethra. Another type spreads in one direction while it heals in another.

Untreated, the chancroid lesions will last for months. The highest incidence of this disease occurs in men with long foreskins who do not practice good hygiene. Phimosis (constriction of the penis by the tightening of the foreskin, making erection difficult and painful) can occur during the healing period. When the disease abates, circumcision is advised in cases of phimosis.

The treatment of choice is appropriate sulpha drug medication; antibiotics are also employed (tetracycline is best, penicillin is not successful). Antibiotics are not used until syphilis has been ruled out, since their immediate use would mask the presence of syphilis. Continuous cleaning with soap and water will hasten recovery. Monthly blood tests should be taken for three months to determine that the disease has been eradicated.

Granuloma inguinale 216

A mildly contagious, slow-growing venereal disease of the skin and sometimes of the lymph, granuloma inguinale is usually localized in the genital or anal areas.

It occurs eight times more frequently in the black population than among whites.

Incubation: From 8 to 12 weeks (sometimes shorter), which makes it difficult to trace the original contact.

The danger: The disease often paves the way for secondary infection, which can cause deep ulceration and tissue destruction. The infected lesions can become large and foul smelling, painful and resistant to therapy. Neglected cases give rise to an extensive area of granulated tissue, and lesions of the entire genital region, lower abdomen, buttocks, and thigh. Severe phimosis (constriction of the penis from a tightening of the foreskin) can cause dangerous urinary restriction.

Symptoms: First appearance are pimples, blisters, or nodules, turning into beefy red ulcers with a slight purulent discharge. Small button-like raised spots or a fine granular covering with occasional nodules bulging the surface appear around the genital area. The granulation tissue bleeds easily but is not painful. The ulceration may become stationary for years. The lesions will scar on one side and progress on the other. In time the ulcers are characterized by a sour and pungent odour.

Treatment: Treatment should be postponed until the disease is identified to avoid confusing it with other venereal disorders, particularly syphilis. The cure of this persistent malady can be accomplished by energetic treatment with effective antibiotics.

Prevention: Strong soap and hot water after sexual contact is very successful in reducing the incidence of granuloma inguinale.

Outlook: Always good with treatment.

Lymphogranuloma venereum 217 (LGV)

In lymphogranuloma venereum, a world-wide contagious venereal disease caused by a large virus, a small blister or pimple appears in the genital area, and although it heals quickly, the lymph nodes in the groin later swell up (called buboes). The incubation period is three days to three weeks.

Systemic symptoms are fever, chills, headache, some abdominal pain, nausea and vomiting, aches in the joints, loss of appetite, rashes on the skin, and often haemorrhoids.

In the severe form the penis or vulva become greatly enlarged. Tumours on a stem appear in the labia and clitoris, and growths occur around the anus in both sexes. Inflammation of the anus (*Proctitis* **184**) with a narrowing of the rectum (rectal stricture) occurs mostly in women later in the disease.

There is no specific treatment. Sulpha drugs have been used with some good effects. The more stubborn cases require suitable antiobiotics. In severe proctitis, tetracycline is prescribed for at least a month.

A blood test should be taken every month for three months to determine that the disease has been eradicated.

An excellent preventive measure is the vigorous use of soap and water after sexual contact.

13 The female reproductive system

Divina Gracia Rualo-Pasigan

Far more complex than the male reproductive system, the female genitalia include more organs and, consequently, more potential for disorder. In addition, the female organs are mainly internal, while the male organs are external. It is

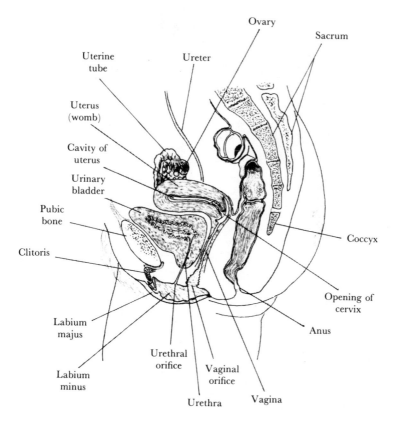

Female reproductive system. (*Julian A. Miller*)

not surprising, therefore, that female disorders outnumber male disorders by four to one.

The interior female reproductive system begins with two ovaries deep inside the pelvis, which produce a single ovum (egg) each month. The egg travels down the fallopian tube to the uterus (womb) and during this travel may meet and be fertilized by a sperm. The fertilized egg then becomes imbedded in the lining of the uterus to develop into another human being. If it is not fertilized, the body discards the egg by the monthly flow of blood (menstruation).

The exterior female genitalia, the vulva, includes the small clitoris, the topmost part, where a great amount of sexual sensation is experienced. Underneath is the urethra and the mouth of the vagina, which is encompassed like double parentheses by the lips of the labia minora and the labia majora.

MENSTRUATION
Absence of menstruation 218
(amenorrhoea)

The absence of menstruation is normal when it occurs before puberty, during

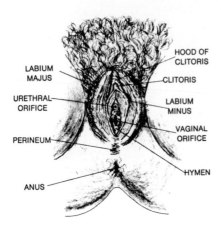

Female genitalia, exterior. (*Julian A. Miller*)

pregnancy, or after the menopause. Menstruation can also be prevented by a congenital defect, such as a deformed or missing uterus or the absence of an aperture in the hymen (the membrane that encloses the vaginal opening).

Amenorrhoea is actually only a symptom resulting from a glandular malfunction, a chronic disease, a metabolic disorder such as diabetes, obesity, malnutrition, and tumours, or more importantly, a neurosis precipitated by emotional distress (unhappy love affair, divorce, and so on). The absence of menstruation can also be the instigator of or result from frigidity. In addition drugs can induce the disorder, such as morphine, nitroglycerin, and thallium (a depilatory agent). A change of environment or travel may also be a factor.

Menstruation usually begins between the ages of twelve to fourteen. If a girl has reached sixteen and has not yet had her menarche (first menstruation), she should be seen by a gynaecologist.

Treatment of amenorrhoea can be effective only if the underlying cause is known.

The danger: If this symptom is not corrected, reproduction may be hindered. It may also mean the neglect of a serious tumour, with all its consequences.

Symptoms: Failure to menstruate at monthly intervals. Some women go through all the motions characteristic of menstruation without bleeding.

Treatment: A complete physical and pelvic examination should be done to identify the cause. This is usually accomplished by various tests – urine, thyroid function, basal metabolism, Pap smear, and maturation index. Sterility is checked by basal body temperature charts and a study is made of ovarian activity. If there is obesity or superfluous hair, adrenal disease is suspected.

In cases of imperforate hymen (absence of an aperture in the hymen) a partial excision is performed.

Hormonal treatment is most frequently employed when the possibility of tumour has been eliminated. Neurotic disorders may require psychiatric help, but even in this circumstance, oestrogen hormones can be very helpful. Hormone therapy can do much to correct amenorrhoea caused by infantile feminism (undeveloped sexual organs as represented by a lack of pubic hair or a neuter sexuality or unusual signs of male characteristics).

Outlook: Variable. Much depends on the underlying trouble; some cases can be completely cured, for others medical help is limited.

Warning: Self-administered hormones can be exceedingly dangerous. Only a competent doctor is qualified to prescribe the proper treatment.

Premenstrual tension 219

Premenstrual tension occurs a week to ten days prior to menstruation and ends a few hours after the commencement of flow. The cause is not fully understood, although *Dyspareunia* **231** (painful sexual intercourse) either contributes to or results from it.

The significant signs are irritability, nervousness, mild to severe headaches, emotional changes, occasionally pain in the breasts and puffiness of the body, more often around the abdomen but elsewhere as well. This symptom has some connection with the salt in the body causing a retention of water in the tissues.

If there are no other symptoms, this is a minor disorder. Treatment is intelligent neglect or aspirin or some sedative. For severe cases, salt should be excluded for several days before the expected onset of the menstrual flow, plus taking of a mild diuretic. If there is bleeding between menstrual periods, a doctor could be consulted.

Painful menstruation 220
(dysmenorrhoea: primary and secondary)

Primary dysmenorrhoea occurs shortly after puberty, affecting half the female population up to the age of twenty-five. Pain begins on the first day of menstruation and lasts about twelve hours.

Secondary dysmenorrhoea can be due to an infection but more often results from long-standing anxiety, sexual pressures, a sedentary existence, constipation, and lack of exercise.

Symptoms: The symptoms include mild to severe cramps, usually in the lower abdomen, sometimes running down the legs and thighs, and a low backache. In some women the flow of blood is copious, while in others it is scanty. Many feel quite sick, their appearance pale and sweating.

Treatment: Organic causes (infectious) should, of course, be treated by a gynaecologist. Otherwise, improvement of pelvic muscles by stretching and exercising them will also improve pelvic circulation. Daily exercise is beneficial. Taking pain-relieving drugs may be necessary. Constipation should be anticipated and correc-

ted without the use of strong purgatives. Avoidance of situations that bring on nervous tension or unusual fatigue is excellent foresight. A hot water bottle can be very immediately effective. Another measure is the relief of pressure from the rectum and/or the bladder by the administration of analgesics.

Outlook: Painful menstruation is most often a manifestation of an unhappy or unrewarding lifestyle or love life expressing itself through the genitalia. For those who can, a change of living patterns is clearly indicated.

Menopause 221
(change of life)

Menopause, the cessation of menstruation, results in a loss of most female hormones and obliges the body to adjust to minimum supplies. Ovulation (the passage of the egg) may cease before the menopause or may continue for a few months after the menopause, which occurs naturally around the age of forty-seven but can occur anywhere between thirty-seven and fifty-seven. Artificial menopause occurs when the uterus is removed (hysterectomy).

The menopause can come on suddenly or steal up slowly with variable menstruations, on and off for a period of six month to three years or even as high as five. For some, the symptoms can be mild and of short duration, for others, intense and long. In general, for most they are mild to moderate.

Misconceptions: even in this age many women still believe some antique and untrue concepts such as: The onset of menopause will immediately begin to whiten the hair; the menopause signals the loss of mental powers and the arrival of old age; sexual abilities decline and enjoyment of love-making wanes, femininity begins to disappear.

The appearance of grey hair has no relationship to the menopause. Some women don't turn grey until their late fifties, while others begin in their thirties. Sexual ability and enjoyment actually often increase, now that the risk of pregnancy no longer exists. Femininity is a personal characteristic that each women can keep until she dies.

The danger: The danger is mostly psychological, for the body soon adjusts to a lower hormonal state. Each woman must learn to accept advancing years as a part of life.

Symptoms: In some women the onset of menopause is not heralded by any symptom. In others, however, such symptoms as hot flushes and tingling and chills occur. Sweating and headache are common, as is fatigue, frequent urination, giddiness, a slight puffiness, a temporary rise in blood pressure, palpitations, insomnia, some loss of appetite, dyspepsia, nausea, nervous irritability, emotional instability, crying bouts, and periods of depression and anxiety. Any combination of the above symptoms and a few new ones can occur.

Treatment: If symptoms are severe, a gynaecologist should be seen. The administration of female hormones, notably oestrogen, is most often the treatment employed, but it requires medical expertise. Although oestrogen can be beneficial, it can also have side effects, such as bleeding, high nervous tension, abdominal bloating, uterine cramps, sore breasts, nausea and vomiting. A history of breast or genital cancer precludes the use of these hormones.

In addition to oestrogen and sedatives, diuretics can help in reducing puffiness. For those women suffering from serious depression, amphetamine is sometimes given. If symptoms are extensive, it is always advisable for the patient to have a medical examination to rule out kidney disorders, high blood pressure, thyroid disorders, bladder problems, and so on. In some cases, psychotherapy is necessary.

Outlook: The menopause in itself produces no fatalities. Everyone learns to live with it.

VAGINAL AND UTERINE INFECTIONS
Vaginal inflammations 222
(leucorrhoea, vulvitis, vaginitis)

Vaginal inflammation is characterized by a white discharge from the vagina. Sexual intercourse becomes painful. The cause is usually one of the following disorders:

Trichomoniasis **213**.

Candidiasis (moniliasis): a yeast (fungus) infection, candidiasis may develop after the subject has been taking a broad-spectrum antibiotic for a long time, killing off the bacteria but not harming the fungus. The fungus now has the field to itself and takes over and multiplies. It is a good idea for such patients to take nystatin (which kills fungi) along with the antibiotics. The *Candida albicans* fungus causes a white discharge and considerable itching.

Senility: in advancing age when the vagina is no longer resistant to infection, a discharge with severe itching occurs. Treatment consists of the administration of female hormones, but the dosage must be carefully monitored since it can cause bleeding.

Nonspecific vaginitis: a result of poor feminine hygiene, nonspecific vaginitis is characterized by a discharge and severe itching. Treatment includes the internal application of a sulpha cream plus rigid attention to cleanliness.

Diabetic vulvovaginitis: an inflammation of the vulva and vagina in diabetic women that is characterized by itching, this disorder requires treatment of the diabetes as well as localized symptomatic relief of the affected area.

Cervicitis 223

The cervix, the lower neck of the uterus

that expands into the rear of the vagina, has no sense of feeling; consequently, when the surface of the cervix is broken or infected it cannot be felt. The only symptoms of cervicitis, an inflammation of the cervix, are a discharge, bleeding or heavy menstrual flow, and some discomfort or pain, which are particularly manifest immediately after intercourse. Occasionally there may be an ache in the pelvis and low back, particularly before menstruation.

Cauterization is often employed to close the broken area. In severe cases, D & C (dilatation and curettage), a surgical procedure in which the cervix is expanded and the residual tissues are scraped off the uterus, and excision of the infected tissues may be necessary.

STRUCTURAL DEFECTS
Prolapsed uterus 224

When the muscles and ligaments that hold the uterus in place become stretched and weakened because of many pregnancies, advancing years, or an inborn congenital weakness, the uterus (womb) may prolapse (drop), penetrating into the vagina and, often, protruding from the vagina, making it visible. Other symptoms are pain on walking and often a vaginal discharge, cramps in the lower abdomen, painful sexual intercourse, pain in the vagina, and urgent, frequent urination.

A chronic heavy cough, straining at stools, overwork, tumours, or lifting heavy weights the wrong way can worsen a prolapsed womb or even be the cause of it (see *Table 15: How to lift a heavy weight*).

Temporary relief can be obtained by wearing a pessary, a vaginal device worn as an abdominal support (also as a contraceptive measure). Surgery, which is quite safe, is the only permanent answer.

(See *Part 3, Early warning signals, Prolapsed uterus* **224**.)

Cystocoele and rectocoele 225

A cystocoele is a sagging bladder that presses down on the roof of the vagina; a rectocoele is a part of the rectum that presses up into the floor of the vagina. The causes are the same as in *Prolapsed uterus* **224**.

These two disorders produce symptoms only when they are advanced. In cystocoele the woman may have difficulty in completely emptying her bladder and often loses some control of urine when sneezing, laughing, coughing, or mounting stairs. She is also vulnerable to bladder infections. In rectocoele, she may develop some form of constipation and is often obliged to press the floor of the vagina with her fingers in order to effect a proper bowel movement. She may also experience pain in the vagina.

A temporary treatment involves the insertion of a pessary into the vagina. The proper permanent procedure is vaginal plastic surgery to reconstruct the weakened muscles and ligament. Surgery is safe and successful, requiring, however, six weeks of convalescence.

TUMOURS AND CYSTS

The genital area in women is a common site for various cancers, cancer of the cervix, of the uterus, and choriocarcinoma (a rare but very malignant form of cancer). These diseases as well as breast cancer are discussed in *Chapter 23, Cancer*.

Fibroid tumours 226
(myoma of the uterus)

Fibroid uterine tumours are almost always benign and usually multiple, growing on the walls of the uterus and often reaching the size of tennis balls. When large enough, they press against the bladder, inciting pain and can cause

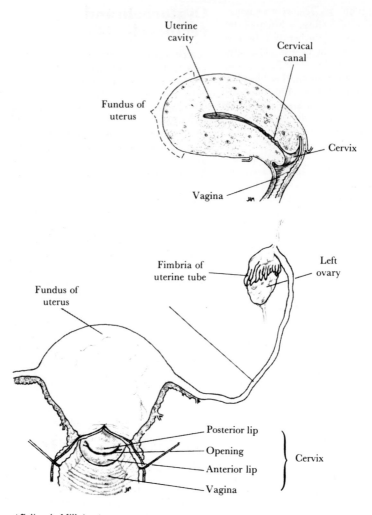

Uterine
cavity

Cervical
canal

Fundus of
uterus

Cervix

Vagina

Fimbria of
uterine tube

Left
ovary

Fundus of
uterus

Posterior lip

Opening

Anterior lip

Cervix

Vagina

(*Julian A. Miller*)

pain in the vagina as well. Often the area has impaired circulation. They occur within the age range of the active reproductive years. The cause is unknown.

There are three types: submucous, or under the lining of the uterus, in which the primary symptom is bleeding between menstrual periods or prolonged heavy periods; intramural, or within the muscular wall of the uterus; and sub-serous, or under the covering of the uterus.

Large fibroid tumours can prevent pregnancy and cause abortion and excessive menstrual bleeding to the point of anaemia.

If bothersome the tumours should be surgically removed without a hysterectomy (removal of the uterus). Very large tumours occasionally require a hysterectomy but this is often not necessary.

Ovarian tumour 227

A tumour of the ovary can become grossly large, often reaching the size of a small cantaloupe. It may begin as a benign growth and later become malignant (about fifteen per cent are initially malignant). It may appear at any age, from the teens to beyond menopause.

Symptoms: Unfortunately, ovarian tumours are frequently asymptomatic, subjective complaints occurring only after complications arise or in the case of malignant tumours after the spread of the disease. Specific symptoms will depend on the size, location, and type of tumours as well as the presence of such complications as twisting, haemorrhage, infection, or rupture. The most common subjective symptoms are low abdominal pain or discomfort together with distension and the presence of an abdominal mass. There may be abnormal menstrual periods in one-third of the cases. Feminizing tumours often produce menstrual irregularities during the reproductive period. After the menopause, a recurrence of bleeding or increased oestrogenic activity may be a sign. Masculinizing tumours may produce an early cessation of menstruation, defeminization, and virilization, such as the appearance of a deep voice, hairiness, and enlargement of the clitoris.

Treatment is surgical removal of the tumour in almost all cases.

Benign cystic tumour of the breast 228

Of unknown cause, hard, lumpy cystic tumours are usually felt in the upper, outer sections of the breasts. They become larger during menstruation and then diminish in size. They can remain stationary, requiring no treatment if the gynaecologist is convinced they are not cancerous or precancerous. If the tumour shrinks after menstruation or after heated moist applications (several times daily), it is probably cystic and not malignant. To be on the safe side, lumpy breasts should be re-examined every six months. If there is doubt, a mammography (x-ray) and/or thermography (device for detecting heat variations) should be done.

Benign cystic growths are never the forerunners of cancer; however, a woman can develop a series of benign cysts and then develop an unrelated carcinoma. Every new lump must be checked. Cancer of the breast is curable if discovered early (see *Breast cancer* **420**).

SEXUAL MALFUNCTION
Sterility in women 229

There are two kinds of sterility in women: absolute sterility, caused by a known faulty structure of the generative organs, and relative sterility, in which the structure is working so that the condition is correctible, at least potentially.

In addition, a good percentage of sterility in women is due to psychological distress, often manifest in dyspareunia (pain during intercourse) and vaginismus (closure of the mouth of the vagina preventing entry). Both disorders curb the frequency of intercourse and thus curb the opportunities for conception. Other factors in which the mind, the psyche, in some totally unknown way impedes conception include over-anxiety, intense desire for children, fear of children, fear of pregnancy, and many others.

General treatment: Some defective structures can be repaired surgically and some are beyond human help. Some specific factors include:

Any infection of any part of the interior genitalia can obstruct the egg. Treatment: most infections can be adequately handled by a gynaecologist.

A blockage of the fallopian tube that prevents the egg from reaching the uterus. Treatment: the fallopian tubes may be blown open, widened, or reconstructed.

Ovarian cysts or tumours can interfere with ovulation. Treatment: most of these growths can be removed, often without damage to the ovary.

A hormonal imbalance caused by disorders of the responsible glands (ovary, pituitary, thyroid, adrenal) can interfere with menstruation and ovulation. Treatment: many of these disorders can be corrected by appropriate medication and hormone therapy.

An absence of ovulation because of a thick ovarian capsule. Treatment: a wedge resection of the ovary.

The sterilization effect of some toxic substances. Treatment: many substances, known and unknown, can interfere with normal fertilization. A few known substances include carbon tetrachloride (cleaning fluid), barium, benzine, quinine, scopolamine (used in many nonprescription tranquillizers), and so on. If the offending drug can be found, conception usually becomes possible.

High acidity of the vagina. Treatment: proper topical or systemic medication will reduce the acidity so that the sperm can survive.

Polyps on the cervical canal (between vagina and uterus) can totally block the entrance to semen. Treatment: polyps can be removed surgically.

Large fibroid tumours can block the passageway for semen. Treatment: if not too large, the tumours can be removed without affecting the uterus.

Ectopic pregnancy (fertilization and growth taking place elsewhere than in the uterus). Treatment: the pregnancy must be interrupted, but future pregnancies are not impaired.

Effects of x-ray. Treatment: most of the time nothing can be done once destruction of the ovarian function has taken place through radiation.

Incompatibility of the sperms and the vaginal secretions. Treatment: artificial insemination using the partner's sperm.

In many cases knowing precisely when the woman ovulates can make the difference, so that sexual intercourse can have optimum effect. The advised procedure is no intercourse for three days prior to ovulation so that the man's sperm can be plentiful, followed by intercourse at proper intervals guided by the basal body temperature charts.

In situations where the man is a premature ejaculator or the woman suffers from dyspareunia, artificial insemination is advised with the partner's semen. For those who are willing, if the partner's semen proves incompetent, artificial insemination with donor semen has been successful.

See also *Sterility in men* **256**.

Frigidity 230

Frigidity, a coldness and indifference to sex, results when a woman cannot respond to sexual intercourse, even though she may wish to, or when she finds it repugnant. Occurring in varying degrees, frigidity can become a socially significant disorder when it interferes with normal sexual relations. Often a frigid woman, in order to sustain her marriage, will simulate interest and go through the motions, but even the most gullible man soon becomes aware of her real feelings.

The causes are overwhelmingly psychoneurotic. Some of the more common causes include:

● A young girl growing up in a household where sex is represented as something sinful and shameful will not shed her induced inhibitions easily after the marriage ceremony.

● A brutal or callous husband can become so repugnant to a woman that she soon hates and avoids sex.

● Bad timing on the part of an insensitive man can also drive a woman towards frigidity, for it often takes longer for a woman to become aroused than a man.

● A woman is left unfinished and unfulfilled by a careless husband who attains orgasm before she does. If this becomes a pattern, her deep frustrations soon lead to frigidity, which is really a defence against being hurt.

● The constant onslaught from a husband who is either impotent or who ejaculates prematurely will also create a frigidity defence.

● Fear and anxiety about disease, pregnancy, and children can also drive a woman closer to this insidious disorder, as well as too long a period of chastity, virginity, or not being loved, or anger at men, or some past sexual misadventure.

• A small percentage of women become frigid because of obesity, overexposure to x-rays, and diabetes.

The danger: Socially destructive relationship, break-up of the family.

Symptoms: Neurotic patterns, premenstrual tensions, dyspareunia, vaginismus, inability to achieve orgasm, drying up of precoital fluid, and, of course, a repugnance for sexual intercourse.

Treatment: Professional and friendly counselling, enlightenment as to the true cause, sex education, and intensive psychotherapy have often been effective. The use of nonexistent so-called aphrodisiacs, such as cantharides (Spanish fly), is not only valueless, it is also highly toxic. The administration of female hormones has not been helpful. There are no medications to alleviate this condition with the exception of some alcoholic beverages before intercourse, which can relax the woman and perhaps minimize some of her inhibitions.

If the husband is responsible, he should be interviewed and instructed. The family doctor is often ill-equipped to advise on this disorder, and specialists trained in this field should be consulted. A form of the Semans technique has a high degree of success (see *Table 17*).

Outlook: All cases of frigidity can be helped. The need is for a willing pupil as well as a good therapist. There are many clinics and family planning centres specifically designed to help frigidity and impotence.

Painful sexual intercourse and vaginal spasm 231

(dyspareunia and vaginismus)

Dyspareunia, which is painful or difficult

sexual intercourse, and vaginismus, the contraction of the mouth of the vagina, making entry of the penis extremely difficult or impossible, are almost always of psychoneurotic origin. A rape, for example, or a repugnant husband might predispose a woman to these disorders. Other psychoneurotic causes include: a religious or rigid upbringing that considered sex shameful; a fear of sex; a defence mechanism against pregnancy; extreme over-anxiety to have children; prudery; a woman's counteractive response to a husband whose body odour, bad breath, callousness, or insensitivity is odious; an impotent or over-anxious husband who infects her with his troubles.

Several physical determinants induce this condition as well, such as the improper insertion of a diaphragm or intra-uterine device (IUD); a prolapsed uterus or ovary; the remains of a hymen; the results of a bad abortion; a marked disproportion of penis and vagina; old vaginal tears and scarring from childbirth; the presence of disease, such as infection, endometriosis, fibroid tumours; dryness of the vaginal mucosa resulting from lack of hormones or of proper stimulation; smegma (an ill-smelling, white, cheeselike substance found around the external genitalia); and a loss of vaginal elasticity after the menopause. In addition, a simple ignorance of sexual anatomy and function may provoke either disorder.

Symptoms: The major symptom, which leads to irritation and pain, is a lack of lubrication (precoital fluid) that is normally produced when a woman is aroused, making entry of the penis smoother and easier for both partners. The precoital fluid also lowers the acidity of the vagina so that the sperm can survive. The classic symptom is, of course, failure to achieve orgasm.

Treatment: Physical causes should, of course, be corrected. If the disorder is due to ignorance or insensitivity, the only answer is frank discussion or family counselling. If the causes are psychoneurotic, marriage counselling or professional therapy is well advised, particularly if the disorder is long-standing.

In mild cases, soothing ointments, sitz baths, and the use of a mild lubricant are effective. Feminine hygiene, which includes cleanliness and being clean-smelling, is essential for good health and physical attractiveness. If the labia are inflamed they should be kept clean and dry.

In general, intercourse should be suspended until all scars, inflammations, and irritations are healed.

Orgasmic failure in women 232

A woman's failure to have an orgasm is as unnatural and as gloomy as is a man's. It is perhaps even a greater failure, since she is perhaps better equipped for this phenomenon than the male. The clitoral system, most of which lies hidden underneath the genital area, is generally larger than the penis, its male equivalent. The tiny clitoris itself is only the small exterior periscope. Fifteen to twenty per cent of all women are capable of having multiple orgasms at each session, the man only one. His single orgasm concludes the act but not necessarily for her.

The danger: A woman who does not have an orgasm, because of her own shortcomings or because of male ineptitude, will suffer psychological harm as well as physical upset from unrelieved congestion of the genitalia. Such continuous frustration can have a serious effect upon her psyche, character, and well-being.

Treatment: The underlying cause must be frankly discussed. Family counselling and professional consultation are always strongly advised. The Semans technique can often restore this function (see *Table 17*).

Contraception 233

Conception can be avoided by a variety of ways – none is perfect, some are dis-

satisfying, some are unreliable, and some have side effects.

Coitus interruptus: undoubtedly the most widely used method, in which the penis is withdrawn from the vagina before ejaculation, coitus interruptus is not only dissatisfying and frustrating, it requires a tense alertness on the part of the man to withdraw fast enough and completely. This practice eventually has a harmful effect upon the long-suffering prostate gland.

The rhythm method: once a month, a woman ovulates, that is, an egg is released for fertilization – the period to abstain from sexual intercourse, the fertile period. The so-called safe period begins ten days before menstruation and should last until the tenth day of the cycle. Theoretically, the rhythm method should work, but, unfortunately, menstrual cycles vary with each woman and can vary in the same woman from time to time. Some women become impregnated on the eighth and twenty-second day of their cycles. Illness and emotional upsets can hasten or delay ovulation. There is no way to ensure safety. Determining the occurrence of ovulation by daily temperature readings, although more accurate, also has too great an error factor. (The basal body temperature is determined by taking one's temperature several times a day for several months. At the time of ovulation the temperature will drop several tenths of a point. Twenty-four hours later it will rise abruptly several tenths of a point above the basal body temperature. In this way the ovulation period can be predicted.) The rhythm method has no side effects except occasional pregnancy.

Chemical contraceptives: antispermicidal foams, jellies, pills, suppositories, all have a moderate effectiveness. The new aerosol form seems to be more competent.

The condom: a condom is a rubber covering that goes over the penis to contain the sperm. With care, this is one of the safest methods, but it does curb the pleasures of the sex act. The rare failure takes place when the condom slips off or a break occurs in the thin rubber as a consequence of age or faulty construction.

The diaphragm (pessary): the diaphragm is a rubber disc that fits over the mouth of the uterus. It must be fitted by a doctor and should be used with a spermicidal cream – messy but safe (about six pregnancies to every ten thousand occasions).

The intrauterine device (IUD): a small plastic loop permanently fitted inside the uterus, the intrauterine device is available in several varieties, some copper clad. Under ideal circumstances it can last a long time. It is as effective as the diaphragm but may have side effects for some women, such as bleeding, cramps, and occasional perforation of the uterus, which can be serious.

Douching: douching, the washing of the vagina with a syringe, is useful if done immediately after intercourse. Although it cuts down the possibility of fertilization, the pregnancy rate is still high.

Vasectomy: in this surgical procedure the vas deferens (the tube that transports the sperm from the testes to the urethra) is cut and tied, thus preventing the sperm from being ejaculated. A minor operation, which in no way interferes with a man's potency or enjoyment, vasectomy is 100 per cent safe, but is irreversible.

Tubal ligation: basically similar to vasectomy but not quite as minor an operation, tubal ligation involves the tying of the fallopian tubes, through which the egg is carried to the uterus, thus making conception impossible. Tubal ligation does not impair a woman's sexuality nor her hormonal flow, but it is almost always irreversible.

The 'pill': the most widely used of all mechanical contraceptives, the prevention of conception by taking the contraceptive pill requires a rigid adherence to the schedule – a daily pill for twenty-one days, no pill for seven days, to be repeated as long as contraception is desired. If strictly followed this method is quite reliable.

However there are dangers. Those about to begin taking the pill should first have their blood pressure checked and then checked again every six months. (Pre-existing high blood pressure completely interdicts its use.) This prudence can save many women serious repercussion, especially those suffering from any kidney disorder.

There are other minor as well as significant side effects. Minor conditions will disappear in a few months, such as nausea, heavy breasts, some puffiness, weight gain (about twenty-five per cent gain weight), vaginal spotting, and even a slight loss of libido.

Significant side effects, which should *not* be ignored, develop in a small percentage of women – a blood clot in the veins, disturbances of metabolism, complications in the liver, severe headaches, dimming of or double vision or temporary blindness, and loss of balance and co-ordination.

Women who develop or have the following conditions should get off the pill and find some other means of contraception: headaches when headaches have been uncommon in the past (a characteristic headache is one that appears in the morning with some general body puffiness); visual disturbances; *Phlebitis* **141** or *Varicose veins* **143**; high blood pressure (the pill will probably make it go higher – those with normal blood pressure will not be affected); fibroid tumours; obesity; breast cysts that have been made worse by the pill. Pill users also often become deficient in vitamin C and vitamin B_{12}.

Occasionally women remain infertile for varying lengths of time after they have stopped the pill; others conceive immediately. However, the pill does not cause cancer. On the contrary, investigators have found evidence that it prevents cancer of the cervix and uterus.

In general, among the large majority, serious side effects are not common. But every woman should be on the alert to the possibility of their occurrence.

PREGNANCY
Detection of pregnancy 234

The first indication that conception has

taken place is a missed menstrual period. Additional signs may be slight; they include fuller, heavier, often tingling breasts, larger, darker, more sensitive nipples, more frequent urination, and drowsiness.

The best-known laboratory test is the Ascheim-Zondek (A-Z) test in which the potentially pregnant woman's urine is injected into a rabbit or a mouse. Faster and newer tests include the chorionic gonadotropin test, which detects the presence of a pregnancy-indicating hormone, or the commercial screening test preparations, either Pregnosticon or Gravindex.

The date of delivery is determined by counting back three months from the *first* day of the last menstrual period and adding seven days. Example: If the first day of the last menstruation was 1 January, the due date would be 8 October. This system is reasonably accurate but can vary as much as a week or even ten days because of the variabilities within the woman herself.

Minor disorders of pregnancy 235

As soon as a woman becomes aware of her pregnancy she should see a doctor for essential advice and counsel. The minor disorders of pregnancy include:

Constipation, flatulence, heartburn: the pressure of the growing foetus on the intestines is usually the cause of these discomforts. Constipation should never be relieved by strong laxatives but rather by drinking plenty of fluids and eating fruits, particularly figs and prunes. Moderate, regular exercise can help greatly. Gassy and fatty foods should be avoided.

Headache: if minor, vague, transient, headaches should be ignored; if severe, the doctor should be consulted.

Backache: usually due to abnormal balance because of the heavy abdomen and/or stretching of the uterine ligaments, backache can be minimized by wearing low-heeled shoes during the

pregnancy. The knee-chest position at night is relieving.

Slight shortness of breath: the iron going to the unborn child cuts down on the number of oxygen-carrying red blood cells allocated to the mother and results in breathlessness. If it is really annoying, a gynaecologist should be consulted (see *Dietary deficiencies in pregnancy* **236**).

Varicose veins: if varicose veins are already present, the condition will be aggravated by pregnancy. Varicosity can also develop in the legs, pelvis, and vulva. A circular garter can induce varicose veins in a pregnant woman where none existed before. Tight clothing should be avoided. Supportive stockings are beneficial. Rest will reduce the prominences. In bed, the lower limbs should be raised with a pillow under the hips.

Haemorrhoids: occasionally the strain on the anal area from the engorged, heavy genital organs will produce haemorrhoids. Constipation and straining at stools should be avoided. Ointments and wet compresses are effective.

Toothache: the unborn child is taking away some of the mother's calcium. Her diet should be supplemented with more calcium-containing foods (see *Dietary deficiencies in pregnancy* **236**).

Excessive salivation: if not relieved, excessive salivation can cause stomach disorders. Proper oral hygiene and an alkaline mouthwash plus vitamins will help.

Itching: a consequence of the stretching of the skin around the abdomen, breasts, and vulva, itching eventually disappears.

Dietary deficiencies in pregnancy 236

A pregnant woman requires additional protein, calcium, and iron – about one and a half times her normal needs. If she doesn't increase these needed substances, she can suffer from anaemia, fatigue and breathlessness. Iron shortage means less haemoglobin and fewer red blood cells to carry oxygen, hence breathlessness.

Protein is easily available in meat, fish, fowl, and eggs. Additional calcium can be obtained by drinking two extra glasses of milk daily (skimmed milk preferred). Iron is found in molasses, kidney, liver, oatmeal, whole wheat, apricots, almonds, raisins, currants, and dates, to name a few.

A pregnant woman should avoid fatty, spicy, and gas-forming foods.

Hidden syphilis and gonorrhoea in pregnancy 237

In women the symptoms of syphilis and gonorrhoea are often hidden; frequently there are no signs at all. Consequently, every pregnant woman should be tested for venereal infection. Either disease can cause havoc in the unborn child.

Drugs and medication in pregnancy 238

A woman's body changes when she becomes pregnant. Whereas before she could absorb all kinds of medication, now even the mildest can affect her and, more importantly, the child she is carrying. All medication, no matter how innocuous, should be avoided. 'Harmless' drugs like aspirin or antacids are no longer harmless. Even an overdosage of vitamins A, C, D, B_6, and K, as well as antibiotics, most tranquillizers, sulphur drugs, and hundreds of others, which before had no adverse effect upon her, may now commit mischief upon the child, either immediately or months after its birth.

The rule should be no sleeping pills, no laxatives, no anti-nausea compounds, no sedatives, no drugs of any kind unless so instructed by a doctor.

Smoking, too, is dangerous during pregnancy. Records show an increase in foetal fatalities among smoking mothers.

X-ray in pregnancy 239

X-ray and any other form of radiation are always serious hazards for the unborn child. Even a normally low dosage can do irreparable harm. No pregnant woman should be x-rayed unless *absolutely essential*.

Vaginal examination during pregnancy 240

Some doctors avoid vaginal examination during pregnancy because of the risk of infection, most especially in the last months, not to mention the possibility of causing a miscarriage. Unless the life of the child or the mother is at stake this procedure is interdicted. However, if done aseptically, important information can be gained with this procedure when necessary.

The Rh factor in pregnancy 241

About fifteen per cent of all people do not have the Rh factor in their blood – they are called Rh negative. Problems arise during pregnancy only when the mother is negative and the father is positive (if both parents are negative or both are positive or if the mother is positive and the father negative, there are no difficulties). The first and second child will usually experience no trouble. During the first or second pregnancy, however, the mother develops antibodies against the Rh-positive child. During the third pregnancy, if the foetus is again Rh positive, the antibodies suddenly increase in huge numbers and act against the baby's blood, causing its destruction. The baby may be born severely anaemic and require exchange transfusion, a procedure that has saved a countless number of such infants.

Production of antibodies may arise not only during pregnancy but also when an Rh-negative woman receives an Rh-positive blood transfusion (in an emergency situation when Rh factors are not normally checked) or when she aborts.

A recently discovered vaccine that is now given to the Rh-negative mother at the delivery of her first child promises to do away with the need for transfusion of the third infant.

Miscarriage 242
(spontaneous abortion)

A third of all women have at least one spontaneous abortion. Actually, the incidence is really much higher, since most miscarriages occur within the first month and are usually symptomless.

The cause of most miscarriages is unknown; they are not induced by sexual or physical activities or emotional upsets. The few known conditions that can precipitate it include acute infections, glandular disorders, x-rays, exploratory surgery, the use of instruments in vaginal examinations, and various drugs, including antibiotics. Seventy-five per cent of all miscarriages occur in the first three months.

On the other hand, if the foetus survives the first three months, it can hold on with remarkable tenacity. One pregnant woman was obliged to parachute from an aeroplane to save her life. Not only did she survive but her baby was born a few months later as healthy as could be.

Miscarriages are not always tragic. When something has gone amiss, nature often decides to terminate a pregnancy for the good of the race and of the foetus, which might have been born with some major defect.

The danger: Not only death to the foetus but occasionally dangerous haemorrhage for the mother.

Symptoms: Miscarriage is characterized by bleeding, the passage of bits of tissue (clots), and cramps in the lower abdomen ranging from annoying to painful.

If clots are not passed, the foetus can sometimes be saved with immediate

medical care. If the foetus is dead or has developed in a way that is incompatible with survival, abortion is inevitable. Pain and bleeding will increase until the foetus and the surrounding tissue are expelled. If the spontaneous abortion is not automatically completed, usually signified by the continuance of bleeding and pain, a D & C (dilatation and curettage), a surgical procedure in which the cervix is expanded and the residual tissues are scraped off the uterus is necessary. In either case, sexual intercourse is forbidden for the next few weeks.

Treatment: Immediate bed rest is advised at the first sign of bleeding. Any physical activity at this stage can complete the threatened abortion. If there is no passage of clots, the pregnancy can often be saved. Large doses of progesterone can often turn the tide. Hormones, sedation, and rest may be prescribed for quite a while. Sexual intercourse is inadvisable until the baby's first movements or heartbeat is noted.

Septic abortion: usually a result of a bad job done by a careless abortionist or a quack, an abortion that becomes septic, that is, in which the lining of the uterus becomes highly infected, requires an immediate high dosage of penicillin and possibly a blood transfusion. Within twenty-four hours a D & C should be performed, along with constant heavy antibiotic therapy until the patient is out of the woods.

Habitual abortion: three or more consecutive miscarriages are considered habitual. Such patients require a full physical examination to determine the cause or causes, which could include tumours, polyps, lesions, malformations, and so on. Hormonal therapy including thyroid may be indicated.

In many cases there is no specific cause. Occasionally, a woman of this type can be nursed through a pregnancy by continuous bed rest, medication, and abstinence from sexual or physical activity. (Normally, sexual intercourse is allowed until four weeks prior to delivery.) Patients who habitually abort are often advised to refrain from trying to become pregnant for a year in order to give their bodies a chance for self-correction.

Morning sickness 243

Morning sickness is the term used to describe the feeling of nausea that occurs in the early weeks of pregnancy. Only a third of the women escape some form of this disorder; about half require treatment.

Symptoms: Occuring during the first three to six weeks of pregnancy, the discomfort can range from mild nausea to pernicious vomiting. Usually the symptoms disappear in three weeks.
Treatment: Eating before getting out of bed in the morning will sometimes help. If she cannot manage a full breakfast, tea and biscuits will do. Instead of three regular meals, many small ones are suggested. After eating, the pregnant woman should lie down for twenty minutes.
The pregnancy should be terminated if the vomiting becomes intense and intractable, if bleeding retinitis appears, or if there is a severe loss of weight, jaundice, and a rapidly rising heart rate.
Outlook: In the vast majority, morning sickness is a mild disorder in early pregnancy that disappears in a few weeks.

German measles in pregnancy 244
(rubella)

A mild viral infection in children, *German measles* **371** in a pregnant woman can be a disaster, especially if contracted in the first three months. The child may be born deformed, mentally retarded, or with a damaged heart or cataracts. German measles can also induce miscarriage.
The current method of circumventing this affliction is to inoculate every child before puberty with a recently developed vaccine. The vaccine should not be used, however, in adult women just before or during pregnancy.

Tubal pregnancy 245
(ectopic pregnancy)

Occasionally, the egg, on its way from the ovary to the uterus, becomes fertilized by the sperm in the fallopian tube and implanted there. Inevitably, between the fourth to twelfth week an abortion occurs. The symptoms include a missed menstrual period, severe one-sided abdominal pain, and staining or bleeding. The condition can become serious; surgery is essential to save the woman's life. The fallopian tube and even the ovary can be removed without affecting the other ovary and tube; pregnancy, therefore, is still possible. Tubal pregnancies are not common.

Toxaemia of pregnancy 246
(preeclampsia and eclampsia)

Preeclampsia is a toxaemic disease of pregnancy that occurs at the beginning of the last three months of term. If not arrested, the next stage is eclampsia, which produces violent convulsions, coma, and frequently death.
The cause is unknown, but those suffering from high blood pressure, diabetes, and nephritis are far more susceptible. The disease occurs in seven per cent of all pregnancies, mostly before age thirty, and usually during the pregnancy of the first child.

The danger: Foetal death in the last four to six weeks of pregnancy. If allowed to go on to eclampsia, the death rate is thirteen per cent for the mother (a third of all pregnancy deaths). The foetal death rate for women with eclampsia is fifty per cent.
Symptoms: The early symptoms of preeclampsia are mild – an uneasy, sick feeling, some headache. Later the disease strikes harder, with considerable swelling of different parts of the body and a large gain in weight, about a pound and a half

more each week. Symptoms are extensive with severe, persistent headaches, violent vomiting, dimming of vision, spots before the eyes, double vision, even blindness, pain in the abdomen, dizziness, amnesia, jaundice, rapid pulse, and drowsiness.

The oncoming eclampsia is heralded by twitching, followed by convulsions and coma. Although the attack lasts only a few minutes, the convulsions can become so intense, with the patient thrashing wildly, that some have suffered broken bones. The patient may seem to be dying but almost always recovers from the immediate convulsion. If labour is not spontaneously induced by the convulsion, it is often artificially induced to prevent injury to the child and danger for the mother. Strangely enough, if the child survives, he is not affected by the disease.

The disease disappears when the baby is born, but on occasion there can be residual complications, such as detached retina and a susceptibility to pneumonia. **Treatment:** Magnesium sulphate, bed rest, and mild sedation should be given. Salt and all forms of sodium must be avoided, including sodium bicarbonate and *all* packaged, prepared foods. Diuretic drugs to reduce water in the tissues are advantageous. The daily regimen should include ten hours of sleep nightly with several hour-rests during the day.

If conditions become worse – weight gain, rising blood pressure, complete suppression of urine, visual disturbances, jaundice, and a rapid rise in the albumin in the urine – hospitalization is vital. This is a *Medical Emergency*. Labour should be induced; if delivery is more than six weeks away, a caesarean section is performed. Pregnancy is often terminated to save the mother's life.

Medically, blood pressure and albumin are reduced; drugs are administered to head off convulsions. When convulsions do occur, the patient must be closely watched to prevent her from falling off the bed or injuring herself. A large spoon wrapped in cloth can save the tongue from being bitten.

Prevention: A good obstetrician with a watchful eye on blood pressure, urine and weight can stave off the disease before it happens (See also *Part 3, Early warning signals, Toxaemia of pregnancy* **246**)
Outlook: Preeclampsia is a comparatively mild disease and can be stopped. Eclampsia is very serious, but if treated promptly it can be contained and cured. If the respiration rate (inhalation and exhalation count as one) is more than 40 a minute, the pulse more than 120, and the temperature 39·4°C, 103°F or more, the disease can go on to convulsions, coma, and death unless drastic action is taken by the obstetrician.

Childbed fever 247
(puerperal sepsis)

Once the greatest single cause of death in pregnant women, childbed fever is now a medical rarity because of sterile conditions in hospitals. A streptococcal disease, instantly controlled today by sulpha and antibiotic drugs, it has, nevertheless, not been totally wiped out – the illegal abortionist and those who attempt self-abortion keep the calamity going.

The symptoms include chills, very high fever, fast pulse, abdominal distress and vomiting, and vaginal discharge.

The outlook is excellent if a doctor is called in time to administer continuous, heavy doses of antibiotics and fluid and electrolyte replacement. Prevention means staying away from quacks and ignorant midwives.

Placenta praevia and abruptio placentae 248

Placenta praevia is due to the placenta (afterbirth) being implanted at or near the cervical os (the opening at the neck of the uterus), inducing a tear in the placental tissue and bleeding when the cervix is stretched (one in every two hundred births). Placenta praevia can often indicate a breech birth or other malpresentation, so that the obstetrician is forewarned. Bleeding can continue even after delivery (postpartum), at times necessitating ligation (tying) of the uterine artery or hypogastric artery, or even a hysterectomy.

In abruptio placentae, the placenta separates prematurely, causing bleeding and abdominal pain. If the separation is small, it will often heal without complications, although repeated separations are quite common. In such cases, the patient should be within easy, quick reach of the hospital. From then on, douching and sexual intercourse are not permitted. However, even though the bleeding may have stopped, labour should be induced to save the baby's life if there is no foetal heartbeat, if it is unduly slow or irregular, or if the area of separation is more than one-third of the placental area. Under such conditions, the infant will not survive for long.

Usually, however, the first bleeding attack is serious – a *Medical Emergency*. Often the mother will require a blood transfusion. In recent years, although fatalities for the mother have been vastly reduced, the fatality rate for infants remains very high, ranging from 10 to 100 per cent.

Both disorders occur late in pregnancy, mostly among older women and those who have had more than one child.

14 The male sexual system

Gordon D. Oppenheimer
with
John G. Keuhnelian

Nature is sometimes thrifty – the penis serves a dual purpose, urination and sex, a combined function that unfortunately produces a greater disease relationship between the urinary and reproductive systems.

Nature can also be incredibly extravagant, expending 300 million sperm in a single volley so that a random *one* will reach and fertilize an egg. Even so, a large number of such volleys are often required. For an average man, perhaps only three or four of the 2 trillion (2,000,000,000,000) spermatozoa he discharges in his lifetime will do the trick.

The testicles (testes) manufacture the spermatozoa, which are then passed through the epididymis to the vas deferens, where new fluids are added by the seminal vesicles to energize them. Then the prostate gland takes over, adding its own fluids, which contain several vital substances, one of which coats the sperm with a wax-like material so that it can survive in the otherwise lethal high acidity of the vagina and another which is a nutrient that feeds and sustains the sperm in their incredible journey to the egg. The prostate and the muscles around it provide the expelling power to eject the ejaculate.

The journey of a single spermatozoon can be likened to a man swimming five miles or more in a sea that would kill him on contact if the waxy liquid he is coated with wears off. He is swimming blind, not knowing where he is going. Only a few thousand ever reach the uterus, only a dozen reach the egg, and only one can fertilize it.

If the ejaculate (normally 300 million sperm, often more) contains 100 million

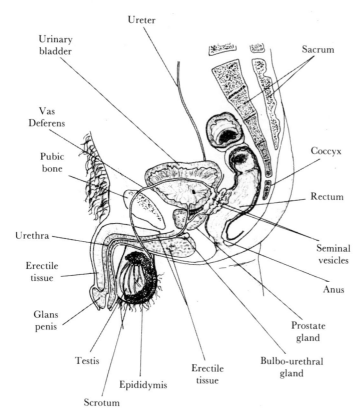

Ureter

Urinary
bladder

Vas
Deferens

Pubic
bone

Urethra

Erectile
tissue

Glans
penis

Testis

Epididymis

Scrotum

Sacrum

Coccyx

Rectum

Seminal
vesicles

Anus

Prostate
gland

Bulbo-urethral
gland

Erectile
tissue

Male sexual system. (*Julian A. Miller*)

sperm or less, the chance that one might reach the egg is so slim as to consider the man sterile.

Masturbation in the absence of female availability is normal and far better than the unreleased tension that must be endured from the constant driving male need.

THE PROSTATE
Prostatitis: acute and chronic 249

An inflammation of the prostate gland with consequent inflammation of the urethra as well, prostatitis has a particularly high incidence in men under thirty-five years of age. The causes can be gonorrhoea, trichomoniasis, and other infections carried by the blood such as sinusitis, tonsillitis, and infected teeth.

The danger: If not adequately treated, the acute form can develop into chronic prostatitis with frequent attacks or cause stricture (closing) of the urethra, blocking urine and requiring dilatation or surgery. Blood poisoning (septicaemia) is a lurking potential.

Symptoms: In slowly developing cases, the signs can be mild and overlooked – low-grade fever, urinary frequency, mostly at night, and not being able to

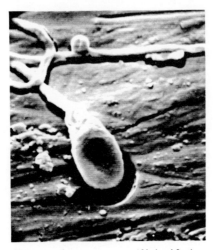

Human male spermatozoan. (*National Institutes of Health*)

fully empty the bladder. More often the onset is suddden, with a sharp pain radiating from the area between the scrotum and anus into the testicles. Sitting is painful; other symptoms are swelling of the prostate, chills and fever, and difficult, burning urination with an occasional show of blood at the beginning or end of the act.

In chronic form there is usually no fever but a great frequency of urination, loss of libido, and bouts of impotence.

Treatment: Sedatives or opiates if pain is intense, along with bed rest, broad-spectrum antibiotics if the infective agent is unknown, and several hot sitz baths daily.

The discharge should be cultured to determine the organism so that a specific medication can be administered. Rectal massage of the prostate may worsen the inflammation and spread the infection; it should be delayed until acute symptoms have died down. The patient's sexual partner should be examined and treated. Plenty of fluids are prescribed but no alcoholic beverages of any kind. Sexual intercourse is not allowed until the infection has been eliminated (about six weeks). Since potency is often limited in this disease, celibacy is no hardship.

Prevention: (See *Part 3, Early warning signals, Prostatis* **249**)
Outlook: Antibiotics will usually cure the acute disease within six weeks.

Enlarged prostate 250
(prostatism)

A disease of advancing years, an enlarged prostate strikes one out of three men over fifty, and nearly one out of two over sixty, half of whom show symptoms. Although the enlargement may be either benign or malignant, and the symptoms may be similar, there is no connection between the two diseases – a benign enlargement does not turn malignant (See *Cancer of the prostate* **424**).

Until recently the cause of prostatism was unknown. In the opinion of some authorities, however, a new understanding of the disease seems to point to the social patterns of contemporary life. Besides some obvious but minor causes, such as an overuse of diuretic drugs and the long retention of urine common to pilots, truck drivers, taxi-drivers, and similar jobs that require constant sitting with no easy access to a urinal, there are the social patterns of sexuality. Prostatism often has its roots in youth when sex stimulation is high and relief is low. Petting, for example, over-extends sexual tension without normal release within a reasonable time, thus keeping the prostate in an overworked state for too long and too often. Continence may be even more injurious to the prostate. The manufactured sperm is retained with no place to go, putting an additional burden on that gland.

This concept has not been fully accepted by the medical profession.

The danger: If unattended, prostatism can have many dire consequences, including stones in the kidney or bladder or ureter, inflammation of the bladder, nephritis, kidney failure, and uraemia. It is not a disease to ignore.

Symptoms: Pain in prostate region, discomfort on sitting, urination is burningly painful, frequent, and urgent, particularly at night. The bladder cannot be fully emptied. Urination often requires straining (the stream can become feeble to the point of dribbling); often there is a show of blood or semen in the urine, pain during ejaculation, unexplained bouts of impotence or premature ejaculation, along with low back pain.

The condition of the prostate can be checked by finger examination inside the rectum. A rise in blood pressure and signs of uraemia are also indicative.

Treatment: The unpassed urine, which has been blocked by the enlarged prostate and collected in the bladder, must be removed by catheter (rubber tube). This should only be done by a urologist.

The urge to urinate must be obeyed immediately; the bladder should not be allowed to become too full, or it may be injured. Prostatic massage is of limited value. If the prostate is very enlarged, removal of all or part of the gland is essential.

In milder cases treatment is palliative – the patient should avoid chilling, forgo long trips in cars, trains, or planes, avoid damp places, and use hard seats on chairs. Sexual activity should be kept at a low level, alcohol and spices held in moderation. Antihistamine and anticholinergic drugs (atropine, belladonna, scopolamine) should be avoided.

Prevention: All viable males need to have periodic release of sperm. Years of such abuse can have an effect later in life.

Outlook: Either conservative treatment or surgery most often results in a diminishment of symptoms, if not a cure, with attendant improvement of general health.

THE TESTICLES
Undescended testicle 251
(cryptorchidism)

A condition in which one or sometimes both testicles fail to come down into the scrotum at birth, an undescended testicle is usually arrested somewhere between the abdomen and the scrotum. The reason remains unknown.

The danger: Since sperm cannot be produced at normal body temperature and needs the cooler environment of the scrotum, sterility will result if both testicles are undescended. The patient is also susceptible to a high incidence of tumours, and hernia is also found in ninety per cent of the cases.

Symptoms: Pain is felt in the undescended testicle, usually a result of its being in a vulnerable position.

Treatment: Care should be taken in determining that the condition is definite. A young boy in cold weather or under excitement or great activity will retract one or both testicles. This is a temporary condition; the testicle can be brought down in a bath of warm water.

Most undescended testicles will come down by puberty as a consequence of increased hormonal flow, but by then the testicle may be permanently damaged. The usual procedure is to administer male hormones before the age of six or seven, usually around four, the earlier the better. Hormones will induce descent about twenty per cent of the time; otherwise surgery is essential. (An undescended testicle cannot be manipulated into the scrotum.) Occasionally the undescended testicle will prove to be permanently defective, but this is more likely to happen when both are undescended.

Additional danger of torsion: Torsion is a twisting of the spermatic cord that holds the testicle. The cord is made up of muscles, ducts, and blood vessels; twisting it will cut off the blood supply and result in gangrene of the testicle. Usually the cause is strenuous exercise or a sudden twisting in bed. The excruciating pain is accompanied by nausea, vomiting, and fever. This is a *Medical Emergency*. Immediate surgery is vital to straighten out the cord and restore circulation. If the testicle has become gangrenous, it must be removed.

Outlook: Recognized early and treated

quickly, the outlook for an undescended testicle is good if the organ is not congenitally defective. A prophylactic surgical fixation of the opposite testicle is in order.

Scrotal cysts 252
(hydrocoele, spermatocoele, varicocoele)

A hydrocoele is a cystic collection of fluid in the scrotum around the testes, which quite often disappears in childhood. If the hydrocoele sac becomes acute, infected, or extensive, it should be removed surgically.

A spermatocoele, a cystic collection of semen in the epididymis, resembles a hydrocoele except that it lies above the testis. It should be left alone. Excision is indicated if it becomes cumbersome or otherwise symptomatic.

A varicocoele is a collection of congested, easily palpable varicose veins in the scrotum. Rarely symptomatic, it usually does not require surgical correction. Occasionally a varicoele may cause certain forms of infertility which can be reversed by surgery. However, the majority of men with varicocoele are not infertile.

All these swellings need examination by a doctor who most often will leave them alone if they are not troublesome. The only condition of serious consequence is the varicocoele, which can cause sterility.

Orchitis 253
(mumps orchitis)

Orchitis, an inflammation of the testicles, can be caused by an accidental blow, an infection (most usually venereal), or mumps. About twenty-five per cent of the cases beyond puberty are caused by mumps. Mumps orchitis can seriously affect the testicles.

The danger: Sterility and degeneration of the testicle.

Symptoms: Swelling of the testes and scrotum, great pain, chills and fever, hiccups, and vomiting. In mumps orchitis there is often swelling of the salivary glands.

Treatment: Antibiotics, if the cause is not mumps; if it is mumps, intramuscular injection of mumps-convalescent serum or mumps-immune gamma globulin may be helpful and offer some protection. In addition, bed rest, scrotum support, icebags, and medication for pain are advised.

Prevention: Prophylactic immunization with mumps vaccine or acquiring mumps before puberty, that is, before it can attack the gonads, is the best way to avoid orchitis.

Outlook: Less than a third of the patients develop permanent sterility of the infected testicle but without loss of masculine hormones. Prompt and vigorous treatment may reduce that percentage.

Epididymitis 254

An inflammation of the spermatic cord and tissues, epididymitis is usually secondary to an infection of the prostate. This is most often caused by gram-negative bacteria. Occasionally tuberculosis may be the agent. *Orchitis* **253** may occur with epididymitis. The epididymus does not become involved with mumps orchitis. The disease is characterized by a swelling of the scrotum, sickening pain, and fever and chills. Treatment consists of bed rest, scrotal support, ice packs, antibiotics, special enzymes, and medication for pain.

Epididymitis is a disabling disease. Prompt treatment can reduce convalescence by half.

Inguinal hernia 255

Inguinal hernia is a particularly male disease, although it is not uncommon in females. The tissues or muscle at the lower end of the abdominal cavity is either congenitally weak or becomes weak from lifting, coughing, or straining at stool, so that it loosens, leaving an opening through which a loop of the intestines protrudes. Often this condition is unnoticed and is only discovered by routine examinination of the doctor. It is, nevertheless, always dangerous.

The danger: A hernia that becomes strangulated (tightly constricted) can cause gangrene and lead to death. A strangulated hernia is a *Medical Emergency*.
Symptoms: A lump, either small or as large as an egg, under the pubic hair indicates inguinal hernia. Often the lump will disappear when lying down as the loop of the intestines falls back into the abdominal cavity. Exertion can bring on pain in the groin that sometimes radiates to the testes.

When the blood supply of the intestinal loop is cut off, the hernia becomes strangulated and results inevitably in gangrene if not immediately corrected. The signs are a sudden pronounced bulging, severe abdominal pain, collapse, faintness and vomiting.
Treatment: Temporary relief can sometimes be obtained by manipulating the loop in the intestines back to where it belongs. The opening in the abdominal wall remains, of course. For the very young and the old, when surgery can be dangerous, a truss is worn to keep the hole blocked off. Generally, for all those who are strong enough, an operation is the only successful treatment. Although surgery is not minor, it usually effects a complete cure. The convalescent period can be long.
Prevention: Avoid lifting heavy packages from high places, and lift things from the floor in the proper way (*Table 15*).

THE SEXUAL FUNCTION
Sterility in men 256

Male sterility means the inability of the sperm to fertilize the female egg. Of the ten per cent of all marriages that are sterile, forty per cent are of male origin. One of the most common and least understood causes is an insufficiency of sperm ejaculated. The normal output of a healthy male is 300 million to 400 million spermatozoa; half that number should be capable of making the long journey to the fallopian tubes. Yet if a man's output is only 100 million and even though the sperm are healthy, the percentage of any of them reaching the egg is too small. Such a man is classified as sterile.

Other causes include low motility and energy in the sperm, an undescended testicle, atrophy of the testes (from mumps or other causes), varicocoele, the effect of over-exposure to x-rays upon the genitalia, the toxic effects of some drugs, such as arsenic compounds, carbon disulphide, cocaine, stilboestrol (see also *Impotence* **257**), excessive heat around the testes (from long exposure to heat or wearing tight, heavy jockey shorts, which retain heat), some chronic diseases, malnutrition, glandular disorders, senility, prostatitis, impotence, and premature ejaculation.

Treatment: General health should never be ignored; infections should be cleared up, most especially of the prostate gland, and overweight reduced. Large doses of vitamin B complex may be beneficial. Men with low sperm yield should avoid all drugs and medication unless absolutely essential. Hormonal therapy has proved disappointing. Thyroid replacement has been effective if the cause (not common) is a malfunctioning thyroid gland.

In addition, it would be well to analyse sexual techniques; the wife's fertile period should be clearly defined (see *Contraception* **233**). Coitus should not be engaged in for four days prior to this period so that the man can deliver the best and most viable sperm at this optimum time for her.

Frequent intercourse does not insure a greater opportunity for pregnancy since too much of it depletes the quantity of sperm, and thus far fewer sperm than the necessary quota are delivered.

Artificial insemination with the husband's sperm has often worked when direct insemination has failed.

Outlook: The causes are numerous and the search may be long. A good specialist in this field, however, can often mean the difference between a barren marriage and a fruitful one.

Impotence and premature ejaculation 257

Impotence has nothing to do with sterility; it means that the man is incapable of performing the sexual act because of failure of erection. The cause is overwhelmingly psychosomatic. In about ten per cent of the cases, however, the cause is physical, such as an abnormally small penis, orchitis, prostatic failure, diabetes, x-ray exposure, heavy drinking, anaemia, leukaemia, multiple sclerosis, or any major chronic disease. In addition, impotency as well as sterility can be caused by such drugs and medication as morphine, heroin, most tranquillizers (Thorazine, Compazine, etc), all antidepressants such as Nardil, Marplan, Parnate, and others, and nitrofurantoin (a common drug in extensive use against urinary tract infections and prostatitis). Deficiencies in vitamins A and C can also precipitate impotence, but a shortage of vitamin E, despite popular belief, has no effect.

Premature ejaculation means the emission of semen before penetration has taken place.

Generally a man's problems with living, or his inability to cope with these problems, are often expressed in his sexuality as well. His non-erect penis or failure to achieve proper coitus is often an expression of his anguish, anxiety, general frustrations, or his abhorrence or resentment of his partner. Sex is the microcosm of the larger world he faces outside the bedroom – a man's sexuality reflects his thrust for life. The change from flaccidity to hardness is not a skill but a natural, instinctive response to stimulation. His failure to achieve erection is not the fault of the organ but of the psyche.

Treatment: If the cause is physical, the underlying disorder should be exposed and treated; if his hormonal output is low, a *careful* use of testosterone can be of great aid (overuse may cause cancer of the prostate). Anaesthetizing lotions are often employed to dull sensation in the penis in order to delay premature ejaculation. However, it should be remembered that the function of the penis is to feel. Interfering with this function creates new and often greater problems than it solves. Basically, an attempt should be essayed to reconstruct the subject's lifestyle with a new and more salutary evaluation of the enjoyment of life. Psychiatry has helped a large number of men, and a modified form of the Semans technique (see *Table 17*) has had a rather good percentage of success for both impotence and premature ejaculation.

Advice and counsel on this disorder is usually not within the province of most doctors. Rather, marriage counsellors, psychiatrists, and clinics at many hospitals can be far more constructive and even remedial.

Phimosis and circumcision 258

Phimosis is a common abnormality in which the foreskin envelops the penis so tightly that erection, if possible, is very painful. Often the condition is not discovered in a young boy before puberty unless an infection gets in under the foreskin and causes a painful infection.

Circumcision is the surgical removal of that part of the foreskin that covers the glans (head) of the penis, thus allowing for better personal hygiene and less chance of infection. Cancer of the penis is unknown among men who have been circumcised since childhood.

Circumcision is best done when the boy is an infant, a procedure that has been practiced by Jewish people since the days of Moses.

15 The joints, bones, and muscles

Robert Lee Patterson, Jr

THE JOINTS
Rheumatoid arthritis (RA) 259

Rheumatoid arthritis, or RA as it is commonly known, is a chronic disease that can affect any and every joint in the body – fingers, wrists, elbows, knees, ankles, toes, hips, neck, and jaw. The cause remains unknown, although many authorities now believe it is an autoimmune disease (the body either panics or malfunctions, attacking its own tissues as if they were some invading organisms).

The disease usually appears in the thirties, but preadolescent children are also subject to this ailment (*Juvenile rheumatoid arthritis* **260**) and women outnumber men by two to one.

Rheumatoid arthritis can be triggered by some major physical or psychological disturbance, such as death of a relative, divorce, a car accident, giving birth, and others. It is suspected, though not clearly established, that inheritance can be a factor. The incidence of this disease seems to be far higher in cold, wet climates, although moving to a warmer, drier climate after acquiring the disease will not help.

The danger: If RA is not properly cared for, the result may be a crippling deformity of the joints and may also affect the heart, blood vessels, and lungs.

Symptoms: Before the disorder strikes fully, early warning symptoms appear weeks or months in advance. Unexplained weight loss, fatigue, evanescent pains in some of the joints, a stiffness in the joints in the morning upon awakening that disappears when activity and exercise are resumed.

Pain in the joints can vary from mild to very sharp, but the common complaint is a burning sensation, with some swelling in the surrounding tissues. The onslaught in the majority of cases usually begins in the fingers, most often symmetrical, that is on both hands at the same time, usually the middle joints. After a while, the fingers look like cigars. It can start in a joint,

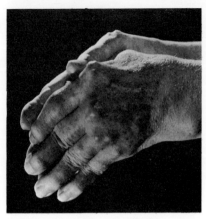

Arthritis. (*National Institutes of Health*)

remain there for a long time, and then, without known cause, spread to many other joints.

The intensity of the disease is variable; some days are worse than others. The first attack is usually short, but arthritis is more than likely to keep returning, each time for a longer period.

Other attendant symptoms are a varying fever, sweating palms of the hands and soles of the feet, anaemia, loss of appetite. The skin over the affected joints becomes smooth and shiny; often the nails may appear to become brittle.

Later, if the disease is allowed to develop, deformity can set in, following bone shrinkage from loss of minerals, atrophy of the muscles, and adhesion of the connective tissues (which have become fibrous) to the bone. The final result, before arthritis burns itself out, can be deformed, twisted fingers, knobby, swollen knees, and lumpy nodules under the skin around the affected joints.

Treatment: It is advised that the earlier this disorder is treated the easier it is to arrest and control. However, this is a moot point. Contrary to popular belief, nutrition is not important. Bed rest is advisable during an acute attack, but prolonged rest can do harm. Those who let themselves sink into invalidism have a very poor prognosis. Atrophy of muscle and stiffening of joints can be prevented by appropriate and constant exercise, as well as massage and warmth applied locally or in the form of hot baths. Basically, major therapy depends on exercise of the joints.

Generally, the patient should have at least ten hours of bed rest nightly with one or two hours of utterly relaxed resting during the day.

By far the best and most reliable medication is aspirin, which reduces not only the pain but also the inflammation. However, aspirin taken in large doses for long periods of time can become toxic. More than eight pills daily (5 grains each) can be dangerous and cause bleeding in the stomach or gastrointestinal tract, anaemia, and iron deficiencies (see *Table 21*).

For severe cases, gold salts are sometimes given intramuscularly. The patient must realize that there may be some side effects, such as skin changes. Reaction to the gold salt may not take place for a long time after use. Indomethacin and antimalarial drugs have been found effective, but they can produce eye damage and blindness. Phenylbutazone is most in use but side effects are common, such as peptic ulcer, bone marrow damage, and hepatitis.

Steroid therapy and ACTH (adrenocorticotropic hormone), although highly effective, are dangerous in the long run. Women are more sensitive to ACTH, and older people respond badly to it. The side effects can be emotional upsets, peptic ulcer, and diabetes.

Articular support, such as braces, special shoes, canes, and crutches, is often very beneficial. Early surgery, such as synovectomy (removal of the membranous lining of the joint), is employed only to avoid serious damage to the joint.

Heat is an excellent means of obtaining temporary relief – dry heat through lamps, electric pads, and hot water bottles and wet heat through fifteen-minute hot baths and wet packs. Physiotherapy is time well spent.

The use of splints for particularly badly inflamed joints, although it will minimize the pain, can hasten the atrophy of muscle and the destruction of cartilage.

The course of rheumatoid arthritis is always unpredictable. Treatment, unfortunately, is not curative but palliative, requiring a specialist who will encourage the frequent remissions characteristic of the disease.

Differentiation from other diseases:
● Gonococcal arthritis: although identical in symptoms, the gonococcal form responds to antibiotics, which effect a complete cure.
● Rheumatic fever: although joint symptoms are similar, identification can be made by observing the additional symptoms of rheumatic fever, such as sore throat, pancarditis, and St Vitus's dance (chorea).
● Osteoarthritis: the osteoarthritic patient rarely has fever; he is usually overweight, over forty, and the attack is most frequently in a joint that has been injured.
● Systemic lupus erythematosus: very difficult to differentiate, lupus should be suspected if the patient is a young woman with other systemic symptoms such as pericarditis, pleurisy, and renal disturbance.

Prevention: The chronic state of this disease, contractures (the permanent contraction of a muscle), can often be prevented if deformities and such are caught in the very early stages and treated.

Outlook: Rheumatoid arthritis is one of the hopeful ailments: more than fifty per cent of the patients have remissions, which can occur at any time. Three-quarters of all patients will improve in the first year with appropriate care and proper exercise. For information, write or phone The British Arthritis and Rheumatism Council, Faraday House, 8–10 Charing Cross Road, London WC2H 0HN. Tel 01–240 0871.

Juvenile rheumatoid arthritis 260

Juvenile rheumatoid arthritis usually occurs between the ages of two to five years and nine to twelve years; by the time the child has reached sixteen he has frequently outgrown the disease. Juvenile RA is much the same as adult RA with a few specific differences.

The danger: *Iritis* **26** is a frequent symptom and can lead to serious eye impairment. Oddly enough, children with the least severe symptoms of arthritis are the most susceptible. Iritis may even antedate the appearance of arthritis.

Symptoms: Before the advent of the joint pains, the patient suffers from high fever and a repeated transient rash appears on the trunk. Usually a single joint is more apt to be affected than a group of joints at one time. Iritis is frequent and recurrent and carditis is not uncommon. Juvenile RA can be distinguished from rheumatic fever by a multitude of other symptoms only characteristic of the latter disease, such as migratory joint pain, chorea, rapid pulse, and pancarditis.

Treatment: No drug should be tried until after eight weeks of treatment with aspirin unless pancarditis or iritis is present. The medication used for adults is employed (*Rheumatoid arthritis* **259**). Steroid therapy is particularly effective in children; however, many doctors will not use it because it interferes with growth, causing short stature, *Osteoporosis* **655** and cataracts.

Antimalarial drugs are effective but dangerous for the eyes. Indomethacin (Indocin) is also effective but its value is diminished by nausea and vomiting. The patient should be encouraged in all non-contact sports such as swimming. Rest and exercise are basic therapy. Eyes should be examined every three months. Any physical or occupational therapy which will prevent or correct deformity is advised. Heat lamps, and heating pads are not recommended.

Prevention: (See *Part 3, Early warning signals, Juvenile rheumatoid arthritis* **260**)

Outlook: Generally quite favourable. Complete remissions run about fifty per cent. A new and promising drug is D-penicillamine.

Degenerative joint disease 261
(osteoarthritis)

A mild disease ordinarily, degenerative joint disease is usually considered a part of the ageing process (after fifty-five) and is hastened by overweight or brought on by an injury. It affects mostly the weight-bearing joints in the knees and hips, although it can also occur in the neck and spine. It is a more frequent disease than rheumatoid arthritis, affecting men and women equally; menopausal women are most vulnerable.

Symptoms: Unlike rheumatoid arthritis, the pain is more pronounced after vigorous exercise; that does not indicate, however, that exercise should be avoided. On the contrary, limited moderate exercise is essential to keep the joints from becoming stiff. Morning stiffness usually diminishes by afternoon. Pain varies but is never really severe. One of the characteristic symptoms is Heberden's nodes (bony lumps around the inflamed furthest joints of the fingers), found more frequently in women. The joints usually ache in inclement weather.

Treatment: Weight reduction to lessen the load on the joints is essential. To alleviate Heberden's nodes in the hands, contrast baths (the hands are placed in hot water for three or four minutes, then in cold for one minute several times a day for fifteen minutes at a time) are prescribed. Otherwise treatment is the same as in *Rheumatoid arthritis* **259** with the main emphasis on aspirin. The use of a cane or braces can be advantageous in cases involving the lower extremities.

New technologies have made it possible to do joint replacements, especially in the knee, the hip, or the small joints of the hands and fingers. People previously confined to crutches or other supportive apparatus because of osteoarthritic changes in the hips or knees, have been relieved of their pain and made ambulatory by the surgical replacement of joints with various prostheses.

Prevention: Since this is a wear and tear

disease, reducing obesity can be very effective.

Outlook: Although osteoarthritis is a progressively degenerative disease, it does not cripple or deform as does rheumatoid arthritis. Most of those afflicted have learned to live with it, learned to be more cautious in their movements so that they might avoid a fall or injury.

Gonorrhoeal arthritis 262

An acute infection from gonorrhoea that settles in a single joint, gonorrhoeal arthritis is more prevalent among women since in women the gonorrhoeal symptoms are often missing or hidden, thus delaying treatment and allowing the disease to spread.

The danger: If not quickly attended to, gonorrhoeal arthritis can destroy the infected area and result in a completely stiff joint. If neglected in the female, gonorrhoeal arthritis can lead to sterility.

Symptoms: The general arthritic aches characteristic of the disease are succeeded by the festering of a single joint, with lumps around it, most likely the knee, wrist, or ankle. The infected joint, surrounding tendons, and soft parts are red, hot, extremely tender, and painful on movement. They also ache in bad weather. Urethritis is always present. In males, the symptoms are of prostatitis. In females, there may be pain in the lower abdomen, more severe on one side, tenderness around the ovarian area, and a vaginal discharge.

Treatment: The liquid in the infected joint may be withdrawn by needle, an outpatient procedure if care is taken in regard to sterile conditions. The fluid is sent immediately to a laboratory for a smear and culture. The joint is then filled with penicillin, followed by large doses of penicillin intramuscularly.

Prevention: It cannot be repeated too often that all venereal disease should receive immediate medical attention.

Outlook: Although somewhat slower acting in the joints than elsewhere, antibiotics are still totally effective.

Bursitis 263
(painful shoulder, tennis elbow, housemaid's knee)

A bursa is a sac lying between two structures, such as between skin and bone, between bone and tendons, and so on. Anything that irritates a bursa such as a calcium deposit, a blow on the side of the hip, the improper grip on a tennis racket or the improper use of a screwdriver (tennis elbow) may produce bursitis. Housemaid's knee is due to constant kneeling and bruising over a long period of time, which irritates the bursa just below the kneecap.

The most common area is the bursa about the shoulder. In most cases a calcium deposit is seen in one of the tendons that elevates the arm when putting on a coat or reaching in a back pocket or combing the hair. The calcium may remain in the tendon, producing pain off and on, for a long time, but in the majority of cases it will soften and rupture into the bursa to produce an acutely painful shoulder.

Treatment: Sedatives and a sling with ice packs seem to help. Steroids and phenylbutazone given by mouth have been helpful in easing the pain. The calcium will be absorbed in about eighty per cent of the cases, but it may take as long as seven to ten days.

A needle inserted into the bursa by a doctor often relieves the acute tension by creating a sensation of pain. If the calcium remains hard and occurs in several areas, surgical removal of the calcium is indicated. It takes time for nature to heal these tendons after such removal, but the best news is that in the end most of these patients get well.

Good physical therapy after a rupture or after surgical removal of the calcium is very important to obtain a normal, functioning shoulder.

Prevention: Neither the formation of

calcium nor the resulting bursitis can be prevented. However, since painful joints can be caused by a variety of ailments, an x-ray to establish a correct diagnosis should be taken before attributing a pain to bursitis.

Outlook: Cure is the rule after considerable discomfort and pain.

Gouty arthritis
See **Gout 334**

THE BONES
Tuberculosis of the joints and bones 264

Fortunately, tuberculosis of the joints and bones has been almost eliminated in the United Kingdom. Better living, better environmental conditions, and better food have all helped in conquering this horrible disease.

A chronic destructive abscess in the joint or on the bone, the disease is caused by the tubercle baccillus, usually, but not always, stemming from a lung infection. It mainly affects the spine and knees; when uncontrolled, it may cause a humpback or even paraplegia (paralysis of the legs and lower part of the body).

TB of the joints and bones can be an insidious disease, because the swelling in the joint or bone can be slow with little heat or pain. However, the disease will limit motion rather early, which might prompt the patient to seek advice. If it strikes the hip it will cause weakness, stiffness, and a limp; if in the back, it will make the spine rigid and change the victim's posture. TB of the joints and bones is not continuous; there are spells of illusionary remissions, which can cause irreversible damage, for the disease, though silent, is still being destructive.

As in other forms of tuberculosis, the symptoms include a rise in temperature at night and night sweats. Night cries (crying out in pain without waking up) are common in children when an unprotected extremity is moved.

Treatment is the same as in *Pulmonary tuberculosis* **112** – the famous triad of medication, streptomycin, isoniazid, and para-aminosalicylic acid. The abscess is surgically removed whenever possible. Occasionally the spine is fixed in a cast to prevent damage to the weakened bones while therapy is in progress. Also, spine fusion may be necessary to stabilize the spine and allow healing.

Osteomyelitis: acute and chronic 265

Osteomyelitis is an inflammation of the bone by invading bacteria (most usually staphylococcus), transmitted by the bloodstream (haematogenous) from a distant infection (inner ear, a boil, a carry-over from pneumonia) or directly derived from a bone injury. Osteomyelitis caused by infection occurs mostly in children, while that caused by bone injury primarily affects adults.

The danger: Loss of bone, blood poisoning (septicaemia), and death. In children, a retardation of growth results when the epiphysis (growth centre) is involved, producing the shortening of a long bone or another deformity.

Symptoms: In the acute haematogenous form, the affected bone is subject to deep pain; the patient sweats profusely as his temperature rises to 40° or 40·5°C, 104° or 105°F plus. The overlying muscles are swollen, rigid, festered, and painful to the touch. The pus from the bacteria can very easily destroy the joint cartilage if the infection has an opening into a joint.

In the chronic state, a discharge of pus from an opening over the infected bone usually occurs, and painful flare-ups are frequent. Parts of the infected bone become necrotic and result in a sequestrum (a piece of dead bone that has become separated from sound bone).

Treatment: If the disease has been recognized as osteomyelitis of the haematogenous type, before the causative germ has been identified and even before all tests and x-rays have been completed, a wide-spectrum antibiotic is immediately administered in massive amounts (an insufficient dosage can mask the symptoms without fully destroying the germ). The sooner bone infections are attacked the better. Bone that has become necrotic is difficult to deal with. Ordinarily, bone areas that are most commonly infected are not well supplied with blood, so that they cannot be reached too well with antibiotics. Sequestrum provides a haven for bacteria and remains a constant threat of infection.

The abscess should be removed by needle suction or by incision; the affected bone should be immobilized (usually by a cast) until the active infection is over. In the meantime the germ must be identified so that the precise antibiotic can be employed.

In chronic osteomyelitis, the removal of sequestra is vital although difficult, requiring many operations and often months in the hospital.

Prevention: All bacterial infections should be treated promptly and vigorously, for their tendency is to spread to other parts of the body where they are often difficult to reach and destroy.

Outlook: Once a highly fatal disease, haematogenous osteomyelitis has dropped to one per cent mortality because of the modern treatment of the complications of an upper respiratory disease (tonsillitis, middle-ear infections, mastoiditis) with antibiotics. However, chronic osteomyelitis is still a problem in compound fractures, gunshot wounds, and automobile injuries.

Osteoporosis of the spine 266

When the bones become porous and brittle because of a loss of calcium and a weakening of the struts in the bones of the spine, osteoporosis occurs, most often in postmenopausal women, including those who have undergone an artificial menopause following a hysterectomy. Although actually a disorder of the natural ageing process, it is thought to be hastened by years of poor diet and/or poor assimilation, years of inactivity, immobilization from prolonged bed rest, or a deficiency in hormones.

Symptoms: Osteoporosis is characterized by back pain, a chronic aching in the spine, round shoulders, height loss, and extreme fragility of the bones – a vertebra can break at the slightest provocation, such as bending down to pick up an object, sneezing, or coughing.

Treatment: When there is a deficiency in the oestrogen hormone, it must be supplied to promote calcium retention. A proper diet is advised with appropriate minerals and medication to aid in the assimilation of calcium and protein (this programme requires medical expertise to prevent kidney trouble). Additionally, with a careful eye on the patient's fragility, increased activity, such as walking about a kilometre or mile a day, will strengthen the bones, as will vitamin D and calcium supplements. Analgesics are administered to reduce pain, thus allowing more activity and greater mobility in physiotherapy.

Paget's disease 267
(osteitis deformans)

A mysterious disease of which nothing is known but its manifestations, Paget's disease affects people over thirty, the older the more likely. Three per cent of all men and $1\frac{1}{2}$ per cent of all women have it or have had it in varying degree, often without knowing it. The bones involved are the lower spine, pelvis, legs, and skull. New bone grows around the old, but the new growth is soft, thick, and deformed. The disease is not virulent, taking twenty to thirty years to develop fully, when the victim may become invalided.

The symptoms include intermittent shifting bone pain, spontaneous bone fractures, a grotesque enlargement of the head, impaired hearing, and height loss. In addition, the possibility of a secondary disease (cancer) exists; the patient requires medical supervision.

There is no known treatment. Orthopaedic exercises are often helpful to stave off invalidism. Research in metabolism and the use of certain drugs are being fully studied – the future may be promising.

Cancer and tumour of the bone:
See **Bone cancer 418**

THE BACK
Low back pain 268
(lumbago)

A most common complaint, pain in the lower back can range from sudden, acute, and agonizing to low-keyed and chronic.

Often difficult to treat because of its bewildering variety of causes, among the known common factors are tension, sedentary occupation, menstruation, pregnancy, kidney infection, prostate trouble, rectal disorders, arthritis, slipped disc, flu, and obesity. A great majority suffer from a sprain, from lifting the wrong way, from an unexpected awkward turn, a mild injury or abuse of the body during some sport.

Any effort to treat this ailment must begin with some understanding of whether the cause is physical or psychogenic. Psychogenic factors can produce just as painful symptoms.

Symptoms: The onset can be dramatic – bending down and being unable to straighten up again – or mundane – a slow-growing chronic pain in the small of the back. The ache may occur only once or it may be frequent and chronic.
Treatment: Bed rest in the position the patient finds most comfortable but on a hard, flat mattress with a board between it and the spring. The application of hot wet packs, aspirin, and a muscle-relaxing drug, are sometimes helpful. Massage is salutary. Occasionally steroids may be injected into the area. If the patient is obese, losing weight is essential; the musculature in the lower back may not be able to sustain the extra load.

Housewives, people who lift and carry, and clerks sitting at a desk all day long should find time several times a day to relax and carry out a few basic stretching exercises (see *Table 14*).

Long years of poor posture, creating strains on muscles and organs, is another significant cause of low back pain. Good posture can be gauged by standing against a wall. Only the shoulder blades and the buttocks should touch the wall. Sitting up properly is far less fatiguing than slouching or slumping.

If a low-back syndrome becomes chronic, a properly fitted back-lace corset is indicated to help take the strain off the back during waking hours, while at the same time exercises are instituted to improve muscle tone.

Slipped disc 269
(ruptured disc)

Between the bones of the spine are discs made of cartilage. If a disc ruptures or slips out and presses against an adjacent nerve root emerging from the spinal cord, the pain can be intense, not only in the back but also in the buttocks and legs.

The discs, which act as shock absorbers, begin to lose some of their suppleness around middle age; they can be kept in good condition, however, if the subject spends a few minutes every day doing stretching exercises (*Table 14*). Disc troubles are due to back strain or injury, noted or unnoted, or for no reason at all except wear and tear.

Symptoms: Early signs are stiffness and pain in the lower back. If the disc protrudes and presses on a nerve, the symptoms may be limited to the area supplied by that nerve, namely the buttocks and/or posterior thigh or thighs or the calf and below the knee to the ankle. A list to one side may be present. Often the patient is unable to straighten up.

Treatment: Most patients (seventy-five per cent) can be treated conservatively without resorting to surgery. Absolute bed rest for up to three weeks or more is more effective than immobilization in a cast. Hot wet applications to the small of the back are beneficial. Many patients are not allowed out of bed until they can raise the leg forty-five degrees from the bed without undue pain. (A chiropractor or osteopath can sometimes induce temporary relief, but their manipulations can often cause significant damage.) As the patient progresses, mild abdominal and back exercises should be instituted.

If conservative treatment fails, an orthopaedic surgeon or a neurosurgeon should be consulted about excision of the troublesome disc. Since the disc is cartilage, it cannot be seen on routine x-rays. One test that may be necessary in diagnosis or in localization of the area of rupture is called myelography, a form of x-ray in which fluid is withdrawn from the spinal canal and an opaque dye inserted. This test does not require general anaesthesia, but it does require two days of hospitalization.

Prevention and outlook: A stiff, unsupple disc is far more liable to injury. Long rides of any kind should be broken up to allow stretching and unstiffening of the spine. If the disc is to be removed, the surgeon must advise whether the patient will have some stiffening of the spine (fusion).

Spinal curvature 270
(round shoulders, scoliosis, lordosis)

A deformity of the backbone, spinal curvature can range from mild and unnoticeable to severe distortion. It takes several forms, round shoulders, scoliosis (a side twist of the spine), and lordosis, sometimes called sway-back, which is a bend in the forward curve at the lower spine. There are many reasons for this condition, such as rickets, bad posture from infancy, and polio, but the most common cause is idiopathic (without recognizable cause).

If caught early enough, some help can be obtained, mainly from appropriate exercises and by employing a remedial brace. Later, when the child has grown, corrective changes are far more difficult to accomplish. More than eighty-five per cent of scoliosis cases occur in girls from the tenth to the thirteenth year. Since a family history of curvature was elicited in twenty-six per cent of the cases studied, scoliosis of unknown origin may be inherited.

Since surgical treatment may produce rigidity of the back, it is only employed when the deformity is severe.

THE NECK
Stiff neck 271
(wryneck, spasmodic torticollis)

Most of the time a stiff neck is a mild disorder resulting from a muscle cramp precipitated by a chill, sleeping in a cramped position, tonsillitis, unaccustomed exercise, or a sudden twisting of the neck while backing a car. This variety of stiff neck can usually be managed with such home remedies as hot wet packs, hot showers, massage, and aspirin.

Other varieites of stiff neck, such as a disc problem or arthritis, need professional help. In spasmodic torticollis, a form that is difficult to treat, and the origins of which are usually known, the head becomes abnormally twisted to the side and twitches but without pain. Occasionally it may be helped if a local anaesthetic is injected into the tender areas (trigger points). Although the cause is unknown, many authorities believe it is psychogenic in origin.

In infants, a stiff neck may be caused by an abscess in the back of the tonsils or by diphtheria.

Whiplash 272

Whiplash is a neck injury commonly sustained in an automobile accident in which the car the victim is sitting in is hit from the rear. His head is snapped back, then forward, like a whip. The injury occurs in the lower level of the neck vertebra where the muscles and ligaments are strained or torn. Whiplash can also be suffered when landing on the feet or buttocks.

Symptoms: Stiffness or pain in the neck is noticed several hours after the accident. The pain can be mild or so severe that any motion of the neck is agony; it can radiate to the hands, causing a tingling and numbness. Additional and seemingly unrelated symptoms are pounding headaches and disturbed vision. Very severe injuries can produce intracranial lesions.

Treatment: The application of heat, gentle, regular massage, and aspirin are prescribed. In more acute cases the patient wears a sponge rubber collar around his neck for several weeks. Highly-strung people seem to take longer in healing.

THE SHOULDER
Frozen shoulder 273

Aptly named, a frozen shoulder is an adhesion of the joints that limits motion. Frozen shoulder can ensue from bursitis or from an injury, such as an incomplete tear of the shoulder cuff, but more often from unknown factors.

Symptoms: The pain is deep inside the shoulder and sometimes involves the arm, the chest, or the back. The shoulder is sensitive to touch. But the basic symptom is pain which is worse at night, plus a disabling limitation of motion. The patient can't lie down.

Treatment: After sufficient rest, appropriate exercises are advised. An anaesthetic is injected into the shoulder and external heat frequently applied. At first progress is quite slow, but after half the

normal range of movement has returned, improvement is rapid. The shoulders and arm must be kept in action.

In stubborn cases, the orthopaedic surgeon will occasionally manipulate the shoulder and loosen the adhesions, using suitable anaesthetics. Improper manipulations can injure the muscle and blood vessels.

Outlook: Almost all cases clear up after six months to a year. Some patients become impatient after a month or so and seek further care. A full explanation should deter 'shopping around'.

Dislocation of the shoulder 274

A shoulder can become dislocated in a singular incident and this can also become periodic, precipitated by some strong activity, such as swimming or other sports. With some people, however, it can occur from nothing more strenuous than getting into a coat or rolling over in bed at night. A dislocation can be as bad as a fracture and may often take longer to heal. If the first dislocation takes place prior to age twenty, the chances of recurrence are about ninety per cent regardless of the treatment.

The danger: A dislocated shoulder can rupture a tendon, which, in turn, can lead to significant disability or a bruising of the axillary nerve, which circles the head.

Symptoms: The normal roundness of the shoulder disappears, the shoulder looks disjointed, and any motion is painful. The arm affected seems longer or shorter than the other.

Treatment: The patient must be anaesthetized and the shoulder joint put back. Three to four weeks are required for healing. If motion of the shoulder movement is allowed too soon, healing will not occur and will create a predisposition to repeated dislocation. A sling and bandage are applied for three weeks and a simple sling for another week. The fingers and wrist are exercised as soon as possible and the swinging of the arm in a small circle is initiated soon after the sling is removed. Stretching the shoulder is contraindicated since this may do further damage. If repeated dislocations occur, operative intervention gives excellent results and usually allows the patient to assume a normal existence.

THE HIP
Congenital dislocation of the hip 275

An infant may be born with one or both hips out of socket or the socket may be so shallow as to allow the hip to subluxate (dislocate) outward and upward. It occurs in girls five times more frequently than in boys and more often on the left side than on the right. Previously this unfortunate condition was picked up only after a child started walking with a waddling gait (pain is absent until adulthood), by which time correction was often difficult and very unsatisfactory. Today, however, the condition can be recognized when the infant is examined soon after birth. Or an alert parent will notice an additional fold of the skin in the posterior thigh when the baby is on his stomach. The extra fold may be from a shortened limb resulting from the dislocation.

The longer a congenital dislocation of the hip is ignored, the harder it will be to restore the hip to its normal position. If only partially seated, *Osteoarthritis* **261** is the end result, usually occurring after the age of thirty and very disabling, requiring extensive and tedious treatment involving casts and weights.

Legg–Perthes' disease 276

Legg–Perthes' disease is a condition in which a disturbance in the blood supply to the head of the femur (thighbone) occurs, resulting in the degeneration of the femur and a progressive worsening of the hip joints. Without early diagnosis and treatment, it results in deformity of the head of the thighbone in the hip socket. It occurs mostly in boys between the ages of three and nine and may involve both thighs.

Symptoms: The child may walk with a limp or he may complain of a pain in the leg or a mild pain in the hip, but usually in the groin. Often the only symptom is a pain in the knee (the hip joint and the knee joint have the same nerve supply). If nothing is found wrong with the knee, attention should be concentrated on the hip.

Long before changes observable by x-ray occur, an irritation of the hip socket may be manifested by a swelling of the lining of the joint and increased fluid. At this stage the child should be confined to absolute bed rest. The irritation may clear up spontaneously or progress to the Legg–Perthes' stage.

If x-rays show that changes are taking place in the head of the bone, bed rest is a must. The patient should not be allowed to put any weight on the leg until restoration has occurred, which may take one to two years. Various braces available may be helpful. If weight bearing occurs too soon, before restoration takes place, the head of the femur will flatten and *Osteoarthritis* **261** may develop later in life.

Infinite patience, both on the part of the child and of the parents, is required for treatment of this condition.

THE WRIST
Ganglion of the wrist 277

Although ganglion has many quite diverse meanings, a ganglion on the back of the wrist is actually a cyst connected with a joint or a sinew (tendon), a painless bump or lump that often disappears on its own. Its removal can be hastened, however, by a sharp blow, as from a heavy book, which will break the cyst and disperse the fluid. It may recur, but the problem remains minimal.

Occasionally the cyst may be part of a tumour from some serious underlying disease such as tuberculosis. An x-ray will usually define it accurately. Aspiration and injection with a steroid has been satisfactory.

Sprained or strained wrist 278

While a sprain is a severe stretching or a tearing of a ligament (the strong connective tissue attached to the bone), a strain is simply a wrenching of a muscle or tendon.

Symptoms: Bleeding into the wrist joint and the surrounding soft parts occurs, causing reddish-blue bruise marks, swelling, and considerable pain.

Treatment: The wrist should be immobilized by an elastic roller bandage, which gives both support and pressure. To avoid cutting off the blood supply, a figure-eight bandaging is used. The swelling can be reduced by ice packs over the wrist during the first twenty-four hours, followed by soaking in hot water or hot moist packs for a half hour several times a day. Gentle exercises should be initiated to prevent adhesions as soon as the patient can tolerate them.

Note: most so-called sprains are really fractures. Every sprain should be examined for a hidden break, especially if the swelling or pain does not abate within a few days. A good practice is to say that 'there is no such thing as a sprained wrist in an adult.' With this approach, fractures of the small bones of the wrist will not be missed.

THE KNEE
Trick knee 279
(locked knee, semilunar cartilage injury)

The knee, the largest and one of the most

complicated joints of the body, is extremely vulnerable to damage. A 'trick knee' is due to an injury that occurs on either side of the knee, producing a tear in one or both of the cartilages lying between the two major bones. Even so, the knee can function normally until a bit of the torn cartilage gets caught between the joint's surfaces, causing it to lock or making the knee suddenly give way.

Treatment involves manipulation, splinting, or needle suction of the knee joint to remove some of the bloody fluid. If the cartilage has been torn, surgical removal of the bits of cartilage (gristle) and repair guarantees against recurrence and is, by far, the most advised course. The outlook is good and the risk of operation small. A great deal of the 'guess' has been taken out of cartilage surgery in the last few years by the use of an arthrogram, a contrast medium injected into the joint that outlines the cartilages. With proper interpretation, the accuracy of diagnosis can be as high as 90 to 95 per cent.

Housemaid's knee:
See **Bursitis 263**

THE ANKLE AND FOOT
Sprained ankle 280

The general concept among orthopaedic surgeons is that a sprained ankle is generally worse than a fracture. Torn ligaments take a long time to heal, and behind every recurrent sprain there is a history of an improperly treated initial injury.

The three kinds of sprain include mild (stretching but not tearing a ligament), moderate (the incomplete tear of a ligament), and severe (a full tear of one or more ligaments). Oddly enough, the mild sprain can be more painful and produce greater swelling than the severe form.

However, the mild form is the only one that does not require a cast. If the ligament is torn, a walking cast is essential for six weeks (anything less will surely cause a recurrence). After that, the ankle is taped for two weeks. Next, the ankle is treated to hot soakings. The patient must not engage in any sports or activities that would put any strain on the ankle for at least another three weeks, not until all stiffness and sensitivity has disappeared. Generally, a period of about three months is required before the ankle can be considered back to normal. Any period of less duration increases the likelihood of recurrence. Surgery may be indicated when stress x-rays show a complete tear of the ligament. This is particularly true in young adults.

Flatfeet 281
(fallen arches)

An abnormal flatness of the soles and arches shows up when the natural arch of the foot, the springy understructure that supports the whole weight of the body, has lost its curvature because of the weakness of its many bones and ligaments.

A flatfoot is not necessarily a serious malformation; many famous athletes have flatfeet. The feet of the newborn are flat, but as they grow and begin to be normally active, their feet begin to shape into proper arches. However, the normal arch can be impeded by shodding the child with shoes too soon or putting him into ill-fitting shoes during his growing years.

Children with flatfeet or a tendency towards flatfeet should not wear tennis shoes, sneakers, sandals, or any shoe without a proper arch, especially when walking or playing on concrete or any hard surface.

Symptoms: Often no symptoms occur at all, nor is there any interference with walking. More often, a pain originating in the arch radiates to the calf muscles and even up to the lower back. Early fatigue in walking or running may be experienced. A frequent symptom of foot strain is night cramps. Walking all day on improperly balanced feet throws a strain on the calf muscles so that after going to sleep one may be awakened by spasms in the calves of the legs.

Treatment: Arch supports should be worn for only a temporary period; long-term use can do more harm than good, since supports weaken the muscles. Care is advised in selecting such supports, so that they will adjust to the shape of the feet in walking as well as in standing still.

For those suffering foot aches and pains, alternating hot and cold foot baths bring relief, while a frequent resting of the feet and appropriate exercise will reduce the discomforts and also help create a more normal arch. The subject should spend five or ten minutes a day walking on the outer rims of his feet, picking up marbles or pencils off the floor with his feet, standing and walking about on tiptoe, bending the feet sharply upward while sitting. Walking barefoot and walking long distances on sand are also excellent exercises.

Prevention: Infants should be allowed to go barefoot as long as possible. Posture should be carefully watched and corrected, if necessary, in childhood. Bad posture can produce flatfeet. Both children and adults should wear properly fitted and properly arched shoes. Those who stand on their feet all day should either change jobs or take frequent rests and keep their feet well exercised. Obese people must reduce their weight, for overweight not only puts an undue strain on the arch, it also causes the person to distribute his weight abnormally over his feet.

Bunion 282
(hallux valgus)

A large outcropping bump on the inner border of the big toe joint that inclines the toe towards the small one, bunion occurs mostly in women, usually on both feet and almost always due to ill-fitting shoes. A bunion is really an inflamed bursa that can result in septic inflammation of the affected bursa. There is usually pain in the joint and walking can be impeded. Putting wads of cotton wool or rubber pads between the big toe and the next toe to correct its incline is of no value. Although a little late, a change to proper, comfortable shoes can still be of help. An operation called the Keller Method, although complex, is completely curative.

Plantar wart 283

Plantar is a Latin word meaning sole of the foot. The consensus of medical opinion is that this yellowish wart is not caused by stepping on a frog but by a virus that enters through a minor break in the skin. A plantar wart can make walking difficult and painful, for, unlike other types of warts, it is not a numb callous. If it can be ignored, it will eventually go away, but more often than not, it requires treatment.

Surgical excision is not advised because it will produce scars, which in themselves can be painful upon pressure. X-rays are also ill-advised, since they can cause disabling burns on the soles. The appropriate curative measures require the wearing of a pad over the wart with a hole in the centre so that no weight is put on the wart itself for the duration of treatment. The surrounding callus is carefully

trimmed with a knife and the base of the wart is carefully and slowly cauterized with acid or an electric needle once a week for six weeks or more. The full co-operation and patience of the patient will eventually bring about full healing without scars.

Ingrowing toenail 284

An ingrowing toenail is caused by constricting shoes and the improper cutting of the big toenail (cutting it too round or too low; toenails must be cut straight across, no curves). What happens is that the edges of the nail become overlaid with tissue, which becomes granulated, infected, painful, and somewhat purulent. A piece of cottonwool soaked in castor oil is slipped under the edge of the ingrowing nail to keep it pointing upward and out. The nail should be free of pressure with a pad of cotton wool over it.

Treatment consists of soaking the toe in warm salt water, removing the dead granulated tissue with scissors, wearing a cutout shoe, and painting the ingrowing part of the nail with a one per cent solution of gentian violet (non-prescription drug). Taking off the toenail is an easy procedure, but recurrence rates are extremely high. Amputation of the nail bed is an extremely successful operation. A coloured nail can always be painted on.

16 Allergies and the skin

Herbert John Spoor

An allergy is an exaggerated response of the body to what would be usually a minor stimulus. Inhaling an otherwise harmless pollen causes some individuals to respond as if the pollen were a highly toxic substance. The allergic response varies with each individual. One person can enjoy a dish of oysters, while another can become ill from the same food. Since a significant segment of the population suffers in varying degrees from some allergy, the subject is of universal interest.

The allergen (the offending cause) can run from ragweed (an inhalant) to food, such as strawberries (an ingestant). Along with the respiratory system, the eyes, and the gastrointestinal tract, the skin, a prime responder to allergens, can react to an allergic substance in several clearly defined ways.

Some common causes of the allergic reactions are:
• Inhalants: pollen from ragweed, grasses, trees, hair (dog and cat hair), animal dander, dust from particulate matter expelled from factories as smoke, house dust, feathers, moulds (spores from mildew, plant rust, and smut).
• Contactants (objects that touch the skin): wool, some synthetic materials, dyes of many kinds, certain plants, cosmetics, jewellery, household cleansers, industrial chemicals, and so on.
• Drugs: many useful and essential drugs, such as penicillin and animal serum, can set off serious allergic reactions in a few specifically sensitized individuals. An allergic response to ingested medicine is still too frequent a medical problem. A careful history of prior experience

413

should precede the use of any medication. The potentially good results must be always weighed against the theoretical potential danger. The risks can run from a minor upset to catastrophe – sudden death. One must never be an indiscriminate swallower of medicine.

Almost any drug can cause hives in sensitized individuals. Other frequent offenders are sulpha drugs, phenacetin, and antitoxin serum. Practically every drug can induce an adverse reaction in some people even though it may have been harmless at one time.

● Chemicals: not only industrial chemicals but also those used at home, such as disinfectants, insecticides, and detergents.

● Food: almost any food can cause an allergic reaction, but the better known culprits are fish, shellfish, strawberries, eggs, wheat, chocolate, tomatoes, nuts, and occasionally, milk, pork, and some cheeses.

● Cosmetics: fairly common producers of allergic reactions (2·5 reactions to every million units sold), such cosmetics include hair dyes, hair bleach, nail polish, lipstick, rouge, creams, and essential perfume oils (0·2 reaction per million units sold).

● Sunlight: too much sunlight can cause a skin disorder and in many cases skin cancer, particularly in relatively non-pigmented skin.

● Heat and cold: occasionally some people will have an allergic response to heat and cold. Aside from hives (urticaria), some individuals can go into shock and unconsciousness from plunging into cold water. Cases of sudden death from drowning have been attributed to this cause.

Helpful drugs for allergic individuals include antihistamines and steroids; desensitization programmes of graduated injections of the allergen itself are of particular value in respiratory allergies. So is the patch test in which a suspected allergenic substance is placed on a small piece of cloth that is applied to the skin and fastened with adhesives. Another substance, not suspected, is similarly applied to the skin. Both 'patches' are removed after twenty-four hours. If only the suspected substance shows irritation, the subject is sensitive to it.

Important note: the removal of possible allergens, such as dust catchers, flowers, wool blankets, and occasionally rubber pillows, is vital in preventive therapy.

A person suffering from one allergy may develop multiple allergies. A hay fever sufferer, for example, is more vulnerable to other allergenic inhalants than the average individual. He must therefore be more alert and take more elaborate precautions, such as avoiding many kinds of pollinating flowers in his home, particularly in his bedroom, keeping his living quarters free of such dust gatherers as curtains, rugs, and pictures. All blankets and pillows should be of cotton or synthetics – no feathers or goose down. Wherever possible, all pets and animals should be kept at a respectful distance and certainly out of the sleeping quarters.

An allergic patient must always advise his doctor of his allergies so that he will be guided in the administration of any drug. He should always wear a wristband or other identification with this allergic information written on it in case of accident. It can save his life.

Hives 285
(urticaria)

A sudden outbreak of hives is caused by an agent such as strawberries, shellfish, nuts, insect bites, jellyfish sting and medications, sensitivity to sunlight, and parasitic, bacterial, or viral infection from hepatitis and other underlying diseases. Mechanical irritations, a belt or collar-type metal watchband worn around the neck, can lead to hives and swelling around the pressure sites. Anxiety and dust are also implicated. Often, however, the cause is unknown.

The danger: On rare occasions severe allergic hives (angioneurotic oedema) can cause difficult breathing to the point of asphyxiation.

Symptoms: The primary symptom is severe itching with the appearance of wheals (large, red, raised patches), ranging from the size of a 1p to a 10p coin and even larger.

Treatment: Prompt medical care is advisable. The doctor may employ antihistamines or inject small quantities of epinephrine (adrenalin).

The acute form may last from a few hours to weeks. Treatment is dependent upon the severity of the case. In the chronic type the itching and the wheals come and go. The allergic agent should be sought, identified, and removed. Drugs such as headache pills, sedatives, laxatives, and sleeping pills should be under suspicion. The search for the responsible cause may be long and arduous and in many cases the trigger remains elusive.

Contact dermatitis 286
(cosmetic dermatitis, housewife's eczema)

Contact dermatitis is due to an irritation or an allergic reaction to any of a large number of substances. It can occur at any age and on any part of the body subject to exposure. Every active person is in daily contact with hundreds of potentially sensitizing chemicals; a large number of ingredients in cosmetics can cause dermatitis; household detergents are well-known offenders, especially on hands that have become dry-skinned from too frequent immersion in water, especially in the allergy-prone individual (classic household eczema); and metal polishes and materials made of nickel are quite allergenic.

The danger: Often the reaction will spread far beyond the limits of contact by a process known as autoeczematization, which may make the subject quite ill for an extended period of time.

Symptoms: At the site of contact, a transient redness develops that then swells and itches. Blisters may appear, small ones in clusters and large ones that rupture, ooze, and crust. Scratching can produce secondary bacterial infection.

Treatment: The offending allergen should be found and removed. If it cannot be determined by history, a patch test of various suspect agents should be done after the acuteness of the attack has died down.

Compresses of salt water (one teaspoon per pint of cool water) for ten to thirty minutes three times daily plus a topical medicament are prescribed. If the hives appear to be infected, a doctor should be seen. Calamine lotion is the preferred medication for home remedy. In any but the most minimal problems one's own doctor or a dermatologist should be consulted.

Serum sickness 288

An allergic reaction to an injection of animal serum (for example, horse serum for tetanus), serum sickness manifests itself in measles-like hives with considerable itching. About a third of the patients develop a mild fever; in severe cases the temperature may run to 40° or 40·5°C, 104° or 105°F and last for more than a week. Swelling usually occurs around the injection site. The additional involvement (swelling) of the lymph nodes may extend widely over the lymph system. The joints can also become inflamed.

Although serum sickness is self-limiting, a doctor should be consulted. Antihistamines and steroid ointments are effective. Calamine lotion and zinc oxide are employed to reduce the itching.

Allergic drug reactions 289

An allergic reaction to a drug can be due to overdosage (too much at one time or one too many regular doses) or to the body's instant rejection of an irritating drug on initial administration. The following drugs are common allergens:

- Barbiturates and sulpha drugs can produce all kinds of skin eruptions and rashes.
- Iodides (thyroid medication) may cause small and large blisters.
- Heparin (an anticoagulant) has been reported to induce falling hair.
- Chlorine, fluorine, and iodine can bring about acne-like skin eruptions.
- Chlorpromazine (tranquillizer) can instigate jaundice and liver damage.
- Mercurial medications can initiate kidney damage.
- Chloramphenicol (antibiotic), arsenical medication, and analgesics can give rise to anaemia.

The patient himself must be the detective in trying to identify the agent causing a possible drug reaction. He must know all the drugs he has taken.

Readministration of a drug to determine whether it is the cause of an allergy should only be essayed by expert hands and only when the initial reaction has been quite minor. In severe reactions readministration can be catastrophic.

When an allergic reaction occurs, all suspected drugs should be withdrawn immediately. Steroid therapy can be vital.

Physical allergy 290
(hypersensitivity to cold and heat)

The hypersensitive body's response to cold and heat is an outbreak of *Hives* **285** limited to the area of exposure (for example, the hands or the face in cold air). If the whole body is involved, however, as in swimming in cold water, the hives can be general and fatal in reactive cases since there may be a drop in blood pressure, rapid pulse, and loss of consciousness. Needless to say, individuals suffering from cold allergy should not try swimming in cold water even if it's shallow. Response to cold can be tested by placing an ice cube on an arm. If reactive to cold, the skin will produce hives on the spot within a few moments.

Heat sensitivity will cause itching and hives.

Treatment is by antihistamines, steroid ointments, and avoidance of the physical allergen in any form, such as drink, food, or cold showers.

General neurodermatitis 291
(atopic dermatitis)

A chronic, complex skin disorder, general neurodermatitis begins early in life, often with a family background of asthma, hay fever, or migraine. Basically, the sufferer is of a nervous temperament and has dry skin and a disposition towards developing many aggravating problems.

Symptoms: The areas usually affected are around the elbows, knees, neck, and face. The eruption appears as dull red, scaly patches of thickened skin covered with blood crusts from scratching. The itching is intense. Characterized by frequent remissions, the disease generally persists into adult life. The most severe flare-ups occur in winter, and the continuous irritation eventually hardens the skin.

Treatment: Most forms of medication are effective for a while but soon lose their usefulness, so that new drugs are constantly necessary. The most effective medications are topical steroid ointments and lotions, while antihistamines will relieve the itching.

Anaphylactic shock 292
(hypersensitivity to insect sting, penicillin, anaesthesia, and serum)

A *Medical Emergency*. A sting from a bee, wasp, or hornet will cause pain and a little swelling, which will shortly subside – most of the time. Some individuals, however, respond most violently to a sting and go into anaphylactic shock. Known deaths occur from insect stings yearly;

but many are unrecorded, labelled, instead, as death from heart attack; and, of course, those who narrowly escape death are not listed at all. The same anaphylactic shock can result from anaesthesia and injection of penicillin or a foreign serum. The response is so quick and so overwhelming that even if a doctor is present he would need all his wits to inject Adrenlin fast enough to prevent death.

The danger: Convulsions, loss of consciousness, and death.

The catastrophic reaction rarely, if ever, happens on the first bee sting, but the second or later stings can set up a fulminating reaction. Gaint hives break out all over the skin, breathing quickly becomes obstructed with asthmatic attacks, swelling occurs over the entire body, accompanied by a rapid pulse and a plummeting blood pressure. When a victim goes into anaphylactic shock he can be dead in minutes.

Treatment: Any person allergic to bee stings, that is, anyone who has had an un-

usual or particularly bad reaction when stung, should carry an antihistamine.

All sting-sensitive people should wear medical identification tags, which can be obtained from a supply such as The Medic Alert Foundation, 9 Hanover Street, London W1.

Note: insect repellents are not very effective against bees even though they deal appropriately with other stinging insects. The bee bite is a defensive reaction, not a response to hunger.

Allergic rhinitis
See **Hay fever and allergic rhinitis 65**

Bronchial asthma
See **Asthma 108**

Allergic conjunctivitis
See **Acute conjunctivitis 21a**

17 The skin and connective tissue

Herbert John Spoor

The human skin, the largest body organ, covers and protects the tissues, organs, and bones and acts as well as a thermostat, a waste disposal unit, a defensive wall against invasion, and a storehouse for fats, sugar, and salt.

As the skin most often absorbs the first blows from the outside world, it is, therefore, subject to many disorders. It often acts as a barometer, indicating the age of the body, and to the keen eye, its state of health. Additionally, it is often the first part of the body to manifest systemic disease occuring elsewhere.

SKIN DISEASES, GENERAL
Acne 293
(common acne, acne vulgaris)

Although no one suffering from acne dies or is often hospitalized, it is not a minor disease, for it can be not only disfiguring, but also embittering, altering the personalities of many sensitive young people. Acne affects more than eighty per cent of all teenagers in varying degrees of severity, striking hardest at those who have the misfortune of inheriting an oily skin.

The basic cause is a step-up in the production of androgen (male) and oestrogen (female) in maturing teenagers. The increased production of these hormones stimulates the sebaceous glands of the skin to produce an over-supply of sebum, an oily substance that keeps the skin normally pliable and healthy. The sebum plus other biochemical factors clogs up the pores, resulting in blackheads and whiteheads (a blackhead is not dirt but the result of oxidation of the skin and oil). Acne has no relation to sexual indulgence or lack of it; nor will sexual intercourse cure this disorder.

Although not as deeply implicated as once thought, such foods as chocolate, nuts, milk, and so on are still a factor in a majority of cases. For girls, menstruation can be an aggravating factor.

The danger: Besides the possibility of scarring and pitting, severe acne can cause psychological problems, affecting social development.
Symptoms: The lesions appear on the face, neck, shoulders, upper chest, and back, presenting a crop of pimples, blackheads, and whiteheads ranging in size from pinhead to a small pea. Some lesions develop into abscesses and cystic masses, which hang on for a month or more until they finally rupture and heal, leaving scars and pittings. The skin becomes flabby, without tone, and remains oily.
Treatment: The face must be kept clean, washed daily with soap and water and carefully dried. There are numerous special soaps designed to reduce the oiliness. Scrubbing should be thorough but not to the point of abrasion, unless so directed by a doctor.

Removal of pimples or blackheads by finger squeezing can only bruise the skin, making it more vulnerable for spreading infection than ever.

Ultraviolet lamps and sun lamps should be used only under medical directions, because of the potentially harmful effects on certain skins if misused.

Tetracycline (250mg daily before meals for a month or more) and other antibiotics can be very helpful. Hormone treatments are sometimes valuable but need careful administration.

For home treatment there are a large number of lotions and ointments that can be bought over the counter, that cause a mild degree of peeling, loosening the hardened sebum. Benzoyl peroxide, sulphur compounds, Resorcinol, and vitamin A acid have been proven useful.

For best results, a dermatologist may help in arriving at a good regimen, which most often will include medication available only on prescription and must often be revaluated as the condition changes. As in all skin disorders, therapy must be individualized for each patient.
Prevention: Acne cannot be prevented, but constant, energetic treatment will

noticeably reduce its severity. The use of greasy make-up on a skin condition can only worsen it.

Outlook: Usually the patient has one bad year. Inevitably, however, acne disappears. After twenty-five it is much less common.

Rosacea 294
(acne rosacea, rum nose, whisky nose)

Rosacea has two major characteristics, a blush or redness (rash) in the middle third of the face – the nose, adjacent parts of the cheeks, chin, and the centre of the forehead – and a rhinophyma, or so-called 'rum nose' (an unfair designation since many patients are teetotallers), in which the nose becomes bulbous and red. Additionally, there is a characteristic dilation of capillaries, pimples, and overgrowth of tissue, dandruff, and occasionally ulceration of the cornea of the eye.

In some patients, it appears that certain foods, such as coffee, tea, nuts, chocolate, hot peppers, alcohol, and spices, can exacerbate this skin condition by their ability to cause vasodilation, but the role of diet is still controversial. Those who believe that diet indiscretion is a cause relate rosacea to gastric hypochlorhydria (diminished secretions of hydrochloric acid in the stomach).

Therapeutic measures may include antibiotics (tetracycline, 250mg daily), topical preparations, and, in severe cases, electrosurgical removal of tissue.

Psoriasis 295

A tenacious, recurring, unsightly disease affecting approximately 5 to 7 per cent of the population, psoriasis involves mostly adults between the ages of twenty and fifty. Despite intensive research, the cause of this disease remains unknown. The few good things that can be said about it is that it is neither a threat to life and health nor contagious; but it remains, however, a very distressing ailment because of its unsightliness and discomfort.

The danger: Psychologically only, except for occasionally associated arthritis.

Symptoms: Psoriasis first appears as small dull red patches (rash) covered with dry, silvery, or asbestos-like scales. The definitive symptom is a tiny bleeding point under a scale. The areas most affected are around the elbows, knees, low back, ears, and scalp. The small patches tend to coalesce into larger ones. The lesions heal without scarring. There may be itching. Fingernails are often affected. The nails may be split, cracked, discoloured, pitted, and separated from the bed.

Treatment: Psoriasis is controllable but not curable. Remissions, which may last from weeks to months to years, occur about twenty per cent of the time. More than half the remissions occur in the summer, generally a good period for this disease.

Although no specific treatment is available, a large number of different procedures are employed. The most consistently beneficial treatment, more than any other, is full body exposure to sunlight. Such topical measures as steroid creams and coal tar derivatives are often effective. Recently medications derived from drugs used in cancer therapy (antimetabolites) have been administered internally but are dangerous except in very expert hands. Steroids taken internally are usually contra-indicated because of their frequently dangerous side effects.

Psoriasis is an erratic disease that responds and behaves differently with different individuals – a medication that will help one patient will do very little for another.

Outlook: Modern methods of treatment have somewhat improved the outlook for psoriatic patients. Many patients have spontaneous remission, which may last for a prolonged period of time even after the disease has had many years of duration.

Lichen planus 296

The cause of the itchy skin eruption lichen planus still defies the medical profession. Its occurrence has been noted more frequently among highly-strung, tense personalities, especially after an emotional upheaval, between thirty and sixty. There is some possibility that the source of this disease might be viral, although the theory of a psychological cause is still the most accepted.

The danger: None.

Symptoms: Pimple-like violet lesions, which are flat and angular with a distinct sheen that glistens, varying in size from pinhead to tackhead, often coalesce to form larger patches on the wrists, trunk, legs, male genitals, vagina, and the mucous membrane of the mouth (see *Oral lichen planus* **83**). On the legs the eruption can become quite large and warty (verrucous). Any minor injury, such as a scratch, produces new lesions. Itching can become quite severe and is difficult to control.

Treatment: Topical steroids. For relief of itching, mild tranquillizers or antihistamines are prescribed. Large local lesions are often injected with steroids.

Outlook: An erratic disease, the course of lichen planus is difficult to determine, for it is often marked by remissions and exacerbations. Although it rarely clears up in under six months, it leaves no injurious permanent effects.

Pemphigus 297

An uncommon but serious skin disease, pemphigus is characterized by large water blisters called bullae. Although a majority of the patients have been thought to be Jewish, the disease has been seen in various other population groups as well, especially Greek, Italian, Arab, and East Indian.

The danger: Untreated, pemphigus is fatal.

Symptoms: Blisters appearing on the mouth rupture quickly, leaving an eroded and quite painful base. Blisters on the rest of the body usually break, leaving areas of denuded raw skin. Anaemia is a usual symptom. Untreated, death can come from secondary bacterial infection of the lesions or septicaemia from these infections. Severe protein loss also occurs because of the loss of body fluids into the blisters.

Treatment: Steroid therapy and/or antimetabolite drugs, if started early, seem to be the only medication that can arrest the progress of pemphigus. Prolonged treatment with steroids is a risk, but there is no alternative therapy for this disease. Often steroids can effect a complete cure; however, the more likely prospect is control not cure of the disease.

Vitiligo 298
(piebald skin)

Vitiligo has no other symptom but the loss of pigmentation in patches of the skin, with the affected parts becoming more vulnerable to sunlight and, consequently, burning more quickly.

The area may be a single patch or a number of patches of any size with sharply demarcated lines. Often a permanent condition, vitiligo is usually slowly progressive.

Generally there is no specific medication except protective ointments or lotions against the sun.

Baldness 299
(alopecia)

The only cure for male pattern baldness (hereditary) is a toupee or hair transplant. The latter is unpleasant, tedious, and expensive, involving the transplanting of each individual hair by punch graft from a thick spot to the bald area. Despite years of research and large expenditures of money to cure this affliction all that has been learned so far is that it is not an affliction – it is the same as inheriting blue eyes or a long neck or pointed ears.

There is some small solace believed by

many, including some authorities (perhaps they are bald themselves), that bald men with heavy beards also enjoy a superior virility, noting that such men have a higher output of male hormones. Eunuchs, they argue, are known to have a heavy head of hair and little or no beard. The validity of this concept has not been thoroughly investigated.

Male pattern baldness can start in middle age or in youth, often as early as in the late teens.

Patchy baldness (alopecia areata), ranging in size from a 1p to a 10p coin or larger, is a different matter. After a few weeks or months the hair returns as mysteriously as it disappeared. No one seems to know much about it.

Women do not suffer from hereditary pattern baldness. They can and do lose some of their hair, but it is usually in late middle age and follows a less definite pattern. However, hair loss earlier in life does occur, resulting from specific causes, such as pregnancy (the hair will return after the child is born). Other conditions that can produce some degree of baldness in both sexes are high fever, syphilis, TB, and infectious diseases. If and when the underlying condition is removed, the hair usually returns.

Hair loss in women is more often due to abuse – dousing the hair with rinses, bleaches, hair dyes, none of which does the hair the slightest bit of good.

BACTERIAL SKIN DISEASES
Erysipelas 300
(St Anthony's fire)

An acute streptococcal infection often induced by an open wound, erysipelas is now rare, since the advent of sulpha drugs and antibiotics, but is still occasionally seen among the elderly and the debilitated.

The danger: The basic danger is septicaemia (blood poisoning). Other serious complications are notably pneumonia, nephritis, and rheumatic fever.

Symptoms: The skin (most particularly the face) is painful and warm. The rash, which is raised, varies from dull red to scarlet with advancing margins. The most tender spots are immediately beyond the margins. The rash can also appear on the legs. Attendant symptoms are chills and a very high fever, with severe, intense, intermittent headaches plus nausea and vomiting as the body tries to fight off septicaemia. The face can become badly swollen, often closing up the eyes. The lymph nodes also become swollen and painful.

Treatment: Oral penicillin is highly successful against this once very dangerous disease. A cold compress of magnesium sulphate is both therapeutic and soothing. Since erysipelas is highly infectious, proper care and sterilization of clothing are necessary.

Boils and carbuncles 301
(furuncles)

An inflamed, infected lump on and under the skin, boils and carbuncles are results of infection from the ever-present staphylococcal germ, which lies in wait on the skin to take advantage of lowered resistance and weakness.

A boil is a local skin infection based in a hair root, usually found in the neck but also on the face, armpits, back, and buttocks. A carbuncle is a close collection of boils filled with pus, with the communicating channels several centimetres across.

The danger: Carbuncles can be dangerous to life by infecting the bloodstream with staphylococcal germs and their toxins; they can also cause infection of the bone (osteomyelitis). Diabetic and debilitated people seem to be more prone and are far more seriously affected. Boils inside the nose or in the central facial area are particularly hazardous, since they can cause meningitis as well as blood poisoning.

Symptoms: The inflamed area is hard, dark red, swollen, hot, tender, and quite painful. Eventually, if unassisted, the carbuncle will come to a head and break, exuding pus. Additional symptoms are a high fever and occasionally prostration from toxicity in the blood.

Treatment: The staphylococcal germ must be identified in a laboratory so that the resistant germ can be destroyed with a very specific antibiotic. All carbuncles must be treated by a doctor. This is no disease to ignore or self-treat.

A single boil can be treated by intermittent moist heat and antibiotic ointment. But when it is in the nose or on the face it will also require systemic antibiotic pills as well as careful direct treatment.

Usually the doctor will incise the carbuncle to hasten the drainage of staphylococcal pus. The carbuncle and the area around it should be washed with an antibacterial soap and then rubbed with a seventy per cent solution of alcohol to kill off any remaining bacteria, thus preventing new outbreaks from forming nearby.

Impetigo 302
(impetigo contagiosa)

An infection of the skin that affects mostly infants and children but can also strike young adults, impetigo is caused by the staphylococcus germ or a combination of the staphylococcus and streptococcus germs.

Contagion: Very high. Impetigo patients should be kept far away from other children. Towels, clothing, even the sink, should be scrupulously sterilized and washed with a germicide. Outbreaks occuring in infant wards in hospitals need strong hygienic prophylactic measures to keep the disease from spreading.

The danger: Untreated impetigo can often engender fatal systemic infection in infants; in children and young adults it will cause ulcers and cellulitis.

Symptoms: Red patches, which soon turn to watery blisters, appear around the face. A small crop of blisters forms around

the mouth and nostrils, encircled by a red ring and looking very much like ringworm. Impetigo can also appear on the scalp and even on the arms. The blisters enlarge and finally break, exuding a straw-coloured liquid. Yellowish crusts form, which look as if they have been pasted on. Removal of these crusts creates new ones unless medically treated. Itching can be considerable.

Treatment: First the crusts must be washed off with bacterial soap and water. If the crusts do not come off easily, they should be soaked with a warm saline solution. After they have been stripped, the application of an antibiotic cream or lotion will efficiently attack the now exposed bacteria.

At all times complete hygiene must be observed, such as the thorough washing of the hands, separate towels, and the avoidance of direct contact.

Very severe cases are treated with additional systemic antibiotics.

Outlook: Impetigo usually responds to treatment and the application of proper antibiotic creams and lotions.

VIRAL SKIN DISEASES
Shingles 303
(herpes zoster)

An acute outbreak of blisters on reddened skin along the path of a nerve, shingles is caused by the same virus that causes chicken pox. Shingles can be incurred at any age.

The danger: Among the elderly, the pain can persist for months, even for as long as a year, and require strong analgesics. There may be a residual scarring of the skin.

Symptoms: Before the skin erupts the patient may suffer from mild flu-like symptoms. Shortly afterwards, a line around the body – chest, back, or neck – becomes reddened and burning with a sudden crop of painful, small blisters. The string of blisters is only on one side of the

body, usually going from the back around to the abdomen, following the path of a nerve. The blisters soon dry, become crusty, and disappear within three weeks.
Treatment: In mild cases with little pain, no treatment is indicated except for the application of calamine lotion several times daily. Idoxuridine is the treatment of choice. In very painful cases, codeine, or any strong analgesic is needed. Therapy is based on preventing secondary infection, although some success has been achieved with large doses of B_{12} vitamin. One attack usually gives the patient immunity against another.

Herpes simplex 304
(cold sores, fever blisters)
A recurrent skin eruption around the lips but occasionally also occurring elsewhere, herpes simplex is manifested by a group of small blisters on a slightly raised, reddened surface; it is triggered off by exposure to strong sunlight, a respiratory infection, physical or emotional distress, or a gastrointestinal upset – the virus waits for an opportunity to attack.

The danger: Herpes simplex can be a serious disease in infants, when the virus enters the bloodstream to cause viraemia, a form of blood poisoning that is occasionally fatal.

Patients with *General neurodermatitis* **291** are especially vulnerable to herpes simplex, which can result in quite serious complications. This mild disorder can also cause corneal involvement with impairment of vision.
Symptoms: The onset is marked by tingling and itching at the site, followed by the sudden appearance of a group of blisters on a reddened patch around the corners of the mouth. After several days the blisters dry up and form a yellowish crust.
Treatment: Moist areas delay healing. Drying lotions, such as calamine or plain alcohol (seventy per cent), are effective. Zinc oxide on the crusts will hasten recovery. If recognized early, the attack

can be staved off by bathing the area with very hot water. Herpes simplex can recur again and again.
Outlook: Mostly curable. (See *Part 3, Early warning signals, Herpes simplex* **304**)

Warts 305
(verruca vulgaris)
Warts are small growths on the skin that range in size from pinhead to small bean. They are caused by a virus and are quite contagious, occurring frequently in children and uncommonly among the aged.

Symptoms: Generally greyish and firm and irregular in shape (although a few are quite flat), with a rough warty consistency, warts sit placidly on the skin without causing a ruffle or inflammation around them. Their course is erratic; they can disappear spontaneously or hang on for years. The incubation period is from one to six months. Painless (except for the *Plantar wart* **283**, on the sole of the foot), their usual haunts are the backs of the hands, fingers, soles, and elbows.
Treatment: Individual, unbothersome warts are best left alone; if uncomfortable or unsightly, they can be removed by acid, topical agents, electric needle, and freezing with liquid nitrogen. Strangely enough, children can lose their warts by painting them with special 'magic' paint or employing mumbo jumbo. Removal by surgery is not too successful and may induce new growths.

Pityriasis rosea 306
A common disease of young adults, pityriasis rosea is now mostly considered to be viral despite the fact that no virus has, as yet, come into focus. Although a serious-appearing disease, it is actually quite innocuous and disappears within two months.

Symptoms: Pityriasis rosea appears suddenly – a single, large, oval or circular, raised, red, somewhat scaly patch, looking very much like ringworm. This solitary patch, called the herald patch or mother patch, soon gives birth to a multitude of itching smaller ones, usually five to ten days later. They are spread over the body but rarely above the neck or below the knee or the elbow. Occasionally there is a mild headache and a mild malaise.

Treatment: The condition is not contagious; the itching is generally light. Steroid creams are beneficial, and recovery is often hastened by exposure to sunlight.

FUNGAL SKIN DISEASES

Ringworm 307

All forms of ringworm (scalp, body, groin, nails) are highly contagious. The carrier can be human or animal, a dog, a cat, or a horse, for example. Ringworm of the scalp, a childhood disease, can be acquired by borrowing an infected cap, comb, or brush or rubbing against a pet animal – all of which can transmit the disease. In the scalp form, the hair falls out, leaving unsightly patches of baldness.

Symptoms: Ringworm is easily identified by its ring formation of blisters, a red eruption that grows ever outward. Healing takes place in the centre of the ring while the infection spreads on the periphery; scaling, itching can be intense. Ringworm will cause a nail to become dull, grey, brittle, fragile, and ultimately to disintegrate.

Treatment: Topical treatment by itself does not do much good. Griseofulvin, an antibiotic for fungal infections, is quite effective. It is taken systemically, often for as long as two months for stubborn cases. The topical application of salicyclic acid (Whitfield's ointment, for example) is often used in conjunction with a griseofulvin or other oral medication.

Athlete's foot 308

Nine out of ten men have athlete's foot at one time or another, and women are by no means immune. Whenever the space between the toes remains moist for a long period (hot-weather sweating, swimming), the fungus, which is everywhere in the environment, establishes a home for itself. The infection can be caught more quickly by walking barefoot in gyms and locker rooms. Basically, however, the contracting of athlete's foot is determined by each person's vulnerability to the fungus.

Symptoms: In mild cases, itching, redness, and cracking of the skin occur; in severe cases, the skin becomes decomposed, scaly, and cracked with white patches, which can blister and become subject to bacterial infection. The entire foot and nails may be involved.

Treatment: The foot should be bathed many times daily with soap and warm water or in a solution of potassium permanganate (one 120mg tablet in 1 litre, 1 quart of water), thoroughly dried, and well sprinkled with Desenex or Tineafax. The socks should be sprinkled as well. Additional treatment consists of applying benzoic and salicylic acid preparation. If possible, the foot should be exposed to air by walking about in sandals. In severe cases the doctor will prescribe the antibiotic griseofulvin to be taken orally.

Anyone who gets this infection is usually quite vulnerable to the fungus and must take extra precautions by keeping his feet dry and occasionally using foot dusting powders that contain zinc – even in the absence of symptoms.

PARASITIC SKIN DISEASES

Scabies 309
(the itch)

An extremely contagious skin disease, scabies is caused by a mite, barely visible to the naked eye, which is just as well since it is a rather horrid-looking parasite. The female burrows under the top surface

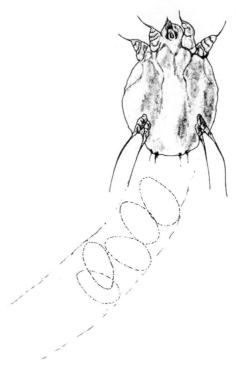

Scabies mite laying eggs. (*Julian A. Miller*)

of the skin to lay her eggs, leaving a wavy line. At the point of entrance, a pimple or blister appears. The eggs hatch in four to eight days. The sites most affected are the webs of the hands, elbows, skin folds, genitalia, buttocks, and under the arms, but rarely on the face.

Symptoms: Intense itching. Pimples, blisters, and grey lines as long as three-eights of an inch. A dermatitis from the irritation may cover up the initial lesions, especially if the infestation has persisted for two weeks or longer.

Treatment: A prolonged hot bath in which the patient scrubs himself with a nailbrush and soap. This will remove the coverings of the burrows. The entire body is then covered with an application of a sulphur ointment or any of the newer drugs, such as crotamiton (eurax) or gamma benzene hexachloride (quellada) (these need a prescription). This appli-

cation is repeated again in eight to twelve hours. All clothing and bed linens should be thoroughly laundered.

Prevention: Physical contact with unwashed, unhygienic people or clothes is always unwise. The effects of poverty and carelessness are catching.

Lice infestation 310 (pediculosis)

Lice are rarely found where good hygiene is practiced. War and overcrowding are frequent breeders of the parasitic insect. Transmission is by personal contact or by the use of borrowed combs, brushes, hats, clothing. The white nits (eggs), which are tenaciously attached to the hair and clothing, mature in three to fourteen days.

The danger: Body lice may be carriers of typhus.

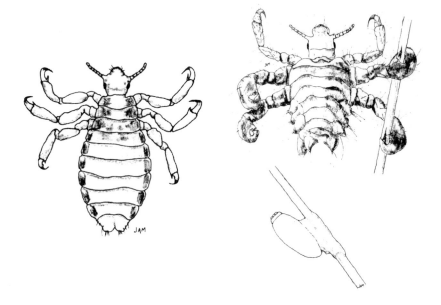

Left: Louse. The body louse and head louse belong to different races, the body louse being the larger of the two. Magnification: approximately 25 times for body louse. *Right:* Crab louse and white eggs or 'nits'. The nits are attached to human hairs with a blob of adhesive material secreted by the female louse. Magnification: approximately 100 times. (*Julian A. Miller*)

Symptoms: Severe itching. Tiny red marks from the actual bite of the louse. Occasionally the lymph nodes swell, and small wheals appear. The lice and nits are visible to the naked eye but can be better seen with a small magnifying glass.

Treatment: A safe insecticide in cream or lotion should be applied to all hairy surfaces and rubbed into the scalp at night, followed by a shampoo in the morning. This treatment should be repeated in a week to catch any nits that have survived and matured. Secondary bacterial skin infections should be treated with an antibiotic ointment.

Prevention: Members of the family should be scrutinized for any signs of lice. All clothing, hats, brushes, and combs should be sterilized or discarded.

Crab louse 311
(phthirus pubis)

Infesting the pubic hair area, crab louse causes pale blue spots on the skin and considerable itching. The nits are usually attached to the skin at the base of the hair roots. This louse is larger than the others and rather easily seen.

Transmission is through personal contact, through sexual intercourse. 'The crabs' can also be acquired innocently from a toilet seat and clothing. Treatment consists of rubbing the hair and area with appropriate ointment, one of the commercial preparations such as carbaryl (Carylderm) or malathion (Prioderm) or gamma benzene hexachloride (quellada).

PHYSICAL CONDITIONS THAT AFFECT THE SKIN

Frostbite 312

Frostbite is always a *Medical Emergency.* The most vulernable parts of the body are the toes, fingers, ears, and nose – places that have the lowest degree of circulation. The people most affected are the very young, the very old, and those with circulatory troubles. However, extreme, prolonged cold can affect everyone.

The danger: Gangrene of the part involved and amputation.

Symptoms: Advance warning of oncoming frostbite is a tingling, numbing sensation in a toe or finger. The skin becomes painful and red to violet red. Burning, itching, swelling may develop. When the finger loses all feeling and becomes dead-white it is completely frostbitten. Pain will occur on rewarming.

Treatment: The frostbitten area must absolutely not be rubbed with snow – or anything – for it will cause permanent injury. Thawing at room temperature is too slow to save the damaged tissue from gangrene. The best procedure is to immerse the affected part in warm water between 39·4° and 41·5°C, 103° and 107°F. Less will not be effective, more might do further harm.

Hot beverages, such as tea or coffee, can help. Whisky is even more preferable – anything that will dilate the blood vessels (smoking contracts them). When thawing has been accomplished, raising and lowering the frozen part will stimulate further circulation. In severe cases a doctor will administer anticoagulants to reduce the possibility of developing gangrene. Any pressure on the frostbitten area must be avoided.

While waiting for help to arrive, a frozen hand should be kept warm by placing it between the thighs or under the armpit. Prompt and correct treatment can save a finger or toe.

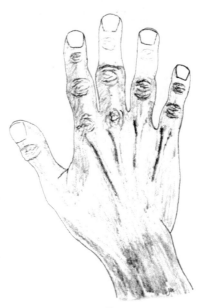

Frostbite. (*Julian A. Miller*)

Chilblains 313

Chilblains, a common complaint, is not due basically to subzero temperatures but to the low state of health or poor circulation of the subject, especially if he is given to wearing tight clothing or is suffering from poor nutrition. In fact, the weather need not be terribly cold. However, in really cold weather chilblains can become frostbite if not treated.

Symptoms: The affected extremity (fingers, toes, ears, nose, feet) develops an itching, burning sensation. Shortly afterwards, it becomes red and swollen. Blisters may form and break, an event to be avoided because cold injuries take a long time to heal.

Treatment: Calcium lactate (two 5-grain tablets taken 3 times daily) may be helpful.

Prevention: A few simple rules can reduce the occurrence of chilblains: improvement of general health, warm, loose clothing, and vigorous exercise in cold weather.

Sunstroke 313a
(heat stroke, hyperpyrexia)

Prolonged exposure to high temperatures or the expenditure of great effort in extreme heat can result in a breakdown of the body's mechanism for heat regulation, or sunstroke. Lying in a hot sun for too long can do the same. Older people are far more often subject to this disorder.

The danger: This is always a *Medical Emergency*. Sunstroke is a very serious threat to life. Mortality is high, especially when treatment is delayed. A body temperature that reaches 42°C, 108°F, even if the patient survives, will damage his brain.

Symptoms: Beginning with headache, dizziness, nausea, collapse, sunstroke is characterized by little or no sweating, a flushed, hot, dry skin, a racing pulse, often as high as 160 beats per minute, a respiration of 20 to 30 times a minute, and a temperature of 41°C, 106°F or more. The subject is usually confused and his behaviour erratic. If the body temperature is not *quickly* brought down, profound shock, convulsions, delirium, coma, and death can occur.

Treatment: A doctor or ambulance should be called at once. In the meantime dynamic action should be taken. The patient should be placed in a bath of ice water and the skin rubbed until the temperature drops. (Sponging with alcohol or ice water is not sufficient in serious cases.) A rectal temperature should be taken every ten minutes until the critical figure of 38·9°C, 102°F is reached. Cooling should then be stopped. If the temperature continues to drop nevertheless, the patient must *now be kept warm*. Massaging must be continued, no matter what, to prevent the blood vessels from constricting.

The patient should be placed in a cool, well-ventilated room, possibly with an electric fan. The return of a high temperature must be prevented. If his temperature goes up again, the patient should be returned to the bath of cold water.

After the immediate danger is over, the patient must be kept in bed for several days – longer if he has any organic disease.

Prevention: No strenuous work in high temperature should be undertaken until the body has adjusted to the heat; a head covering should be worn in very hot weather; salt and water should be taken freely (in any form); clothing should be clean and unstarched.

Outlook: If treatment is prompt and correct and if the subject is under care for the next few days, total recovery can be achieved.

Heat exhaustion 313b

A comparatively minor disorder, heat exhaustion, although similar to sunstroke in some respects, such as dizziness and headache, is unlike the more serious ailment in other ways. Whereas in sunstroke the skin is flushed and hot, in heat exhaustion it is clammy and cold. Whereas in sunstroke there is no sweating, in heat exhaustion it is profuse. The pulse rate is never high, nor is there any significant rise in temperature. A sudden feeling of faintness warns the subject to get into the shade and stop all activities. Other advance symptoms are weakness and a dimming or blurring of vision. Occasionally there is muscular cramp.

Treatment consists of lying down in a cool place with the head lower than the body and replenishing lost fluids and salt by slowly sipping water for a half hour and ingesting salt tablets.

The condition is transient (See *Part 3, Early warning signals, Heat exhaustion* **313b**)

Sunburn and sunlight 314

Sunbathing in mild, judicious amounts is no doubt a salutary practice. However, dedicated sun-worshippers do themselves considerable harm. Fair-skinned people burn more quickly and more severely than others. Most blondes and

429

redheads cannot tan at all but break out in freckles.

There are many illusions about sun-bathing. A hazy or even cloudy day can still deliver a serious burn. Thin clothing does not shield from the burn-producing rays of the sun but ordinary plate glass will. The effects of sunshine are multiplied by reflection from water or from snow. Snow blindness, which is a burn on the cornea of the eye, can be excruciating.

The danger: Besides the obvious burn of the skin, sun-worshippers would do well to examine the following facts about their dedication. Tanning causes premature ageing of the skin, induces wrinkles, and destroys the tone and elasticity of the skin. Chronic exposure to sunlight will also produce the hard, dark grey, horny lesions called keratosis, which are precancerous.

Symptoms: In mild cases, overexposure causes redness, itching, and mild pain. Nothing need be done about it. In severe cases, the skin becomes angry red, with a large number of large blisters, and the victim experiences chills, fever, headaches, often nausea and vomiting, with weakness and even shock. These symptoms can last a week and are followed by considerable peeling.

Treatment: A soothing steroid ointment or a cold compress of whole milk or a compress of saline solution (one teaspoon to a pint of cool water) is applied to the affected area. Preparations containing an anaesthetic should be used with extreme caution and be used only once, for the anaesthetic, benzocaine or similar drugs, is toxic to the skin.

Severe cases with much blistering should be treated by a doctor to prevent secondary bacterial infection.

Prevention: The first day of exposure to sunlight should never exceed a half hour. Each succeeding day an additional seven or eight minutes is more than enough until the skin has sufficiently thickened and tanned. Late mornings to midafternoon (10 to 4) are the periods of most intense sunshine. Proper suntan lotion applied before exposure can help in reducing skin tightness and in keeping the skin area moist and loose. Pre-exposure application, however, will not totally protect against sunburn.

A large number of commercial creams and suntan lotions are available, some good and some quite expensive. *Table 18* has some formulas for creams and lotions that are effective, much cheaper, and can be made up by any pharmacist. (Note: many pharmacists, however, are loath to compound nonprescription items today.)

VARIOUS OTHER SKIN DISORDERS
Moles and birthmarks 315
(naevi, angiomas)

Birthmarks (angiomas) such as strawberry marks and port-wine stains are utterly harmless and should be left alone. No treatment is necessary nor is any treatment of any value.

Moles may be congenital or acquired in the early years of childhood. They have a great range in size and shape and range in colour from pale to mostly dark brown and black. They may be raised or flat, smooth, hairy, or warty.

Moles rarely become cancerous (hairy ones seldom); nevertheless, this can and does happen. There is usually ample warning. If a mole suddenly begins to grow (normal however in pregnancy), to ulcerate, bleed, or itch, or suddenly develops a halo of colour or nodules around its base, or if a neighbouring lymph node swells or hardens, a doctor should be consulted immediately.

If the mole is situated in an area of irritation, such as under the arms or under the breasts, or is cosmetically disfiguring, it should be surgically removed.

Dandruff 316
(seborrhoeic dermatitis)

A mild but chronic inflammation of the

scalp, dandruff is innocuous but unsightly; the flaking of the skin surface falls like snow on the shoulders.

Mild treatment with various shampoos is only mildly helpful. However, a preparation with selenium compound can be far more effective (Selsun). The hair should be shampooed with the preparation and left on for five minutes, making sure that none of it gets into the eyes or mouth since it is toxic. Afterwards, another shampoo with soap and water will wash away the toxic ingredients. The hands and fingers should be scrubbed clean.

Corns and calluses 317

Corns are usually caused by tight-fitting shoes; calluses are often due to excessive use of an area. Hard corns are conical in shape, extending downward into the skin. Soft corns lie between the toes and are kept soft by moisture.

Treatment of a corn consists of soaking it in warm water for more than fifteen minutes, applying a ten per cent solution of salicylic acid in collodion, and covering it with a corn pad for four days. The corn is then soaked again and will now come out easily.

Calluses can be removed with an application of ten per cent salicylic acid and then pared down. The subject will know immediately when he has cut into live flesh. A bottle of iodine should be kept handy. If possible, corns and calluses that are really troublesome should be treated by a chiropodist. Diabetics and those suffering from circulatory disorders *must never* treat their own feet. Their care should be taken over by a doctor.

Bedsores 318
(decubitus)

Large sores that develop on bedridden patients at points of long-sustained pressure, usually the buttocks, heels, elbows, shoulder blades, and bony prominences, bedsores can usually be avoided with meticulous nursing.

Bedsores begin as areas of reddened, shiny skin that have no sensation. At this point they can be stopped if an alert nurse will wash, dry, and powder the area and rearrange the position of the patient, or place a sponge rubber doughnut over the affected area, so that the potential sore does not touch anything.

If untreated, the skin surface breaks down and sloughs off, leaving a large, ugly ulceration, which can become infected and even gangrenous. Bedsores are very slow to heal and difficult to get rid of after they have appeared; they can often turn out to be worse than the original disease, requiring additional months in the hospital. Treatment of bedsores is rather complex, involving all kinds of medication, surgical excision of necrotic (dead) tissue, stimulation of circulation, application of antibacterial lotions, and coating the skin with protective compounds.

Body odour 319
(bromhidrosis)

Body odour, or BO as it is commonly known, is due to the action of bacteria on sweat. Washing under the arms plus the use of a topical antibiotic ointment (neomycin solution 0·5 per cent) is by far the best deodorant known.

Daily bathing with soap and water (that is, a very thorough washing) is not as healthy as it seems. The natural body oil, which lubricates and protects the skin, is washed off, leaving the more tenacious germs behind. Bathing twice a week is sufficient to get rid of grime and dirt. The parts that do need washing are the rectal and genital areas, occasionally the feet, and occasionally under the arms when there is excessive sweating. The use of commercial deodorants, which also prevent perspiration, is similar to using medication to prevent the kidneys from getting rid of waste products. Also, some deodorants can cause contact dermatitis.

Normal body odour not changed by the

action of bacteria or yeasts on sweat is not only not offensive but attractive to the opposite sex.

CONNECTIVE TISSUE DISEASES
Lupus erythematosus: discoid and systemic 320

Really two diseases, discoid lupus erythematosus is generally a benign disorder affecting only the skin, while systemic lupus erythematosus (known as SLE) is a grave, intractable ailment affecting not only the skin but many vital organs – the heart, lungs, spleen, and kidneys – as well.

Young women are most affected by this disease, the cause of which is still unknown. Many believe it to be an auto-immune disorder in which the body mistakenly manufactures antigens to attack its own connective tissues.

Identified by lesions on the skin, it is quite often precipitated by exposure to sunlight, submission to x-ray, or the result of a highly emotional crisis. It can also be brought on by the following drugs: Ten per cent of those who take hydralazine (lowers blood pressure) will contract lupus. Isoniazid (an important medication in treating TB) and all anti-convulsant drugs will, on some occasions, induce lupus.

The danger: Discoid lupus can cause baldness; SLE has become less fatal with modern medical treatment; life is considerably prolonged.

Symptoms: A patchy, red, skin rash, roughly resembling a butterfly, appears on the cheeks, bridge of the nose, and elsewhere. As the old butterfly patches heal, new ones form. These lesions itch and form scales.

In the deadlier SLE, besides skin rash, the patient suffers from severe arthritic joint pains, lung inflammation (*Pleurisy* **118**), and heart involvement. Inflammation of the kidneys (*Nephritis* **197**) is the most serious life-threatening complication. The patient is usually feverish, emaciated, and anaemic. Any number of odd, unrelated symptoms can suddenly show up.

Treatment: The benign form, discoid lupus, will respond to the administration of antimalarial drugs plus steroid therapy. In the systemic form antimalarial drugs are less effective but steroids may be vital in keeping the disease in check until the severity has passed.

The elimination of stress, anxiety, tension, fatigue, and overwork is good therapy in any disease but particularly so in SLE. The patient is weakened and especially subject to all kinds of transient infections. The various organs that are attacked or inflamed should also be treated directly as well.

Outlook: No two patients have the same outcome of this harassing disease. Much depends upon which organs have been involved. Those who develop nephritis or lung involvement have a less favourable outlook than those in whom lupus is limited to the skin and the joints. SLE is a chronic disease with years of remission but also, unfortunately, many relapses. Rarely, however, does it follow a fulminating path and end fatally in a few weeks. Occasionally remissions are permanent.

Scleroderma 321 (hidebound skin)

Scleroderma is a progressive disease of the skin and connective tissues that causes a thickening, hardening, and rigidity of the skin and involves some of the internal organs as well, such as the gastrointestinal tract, lungs, kidney, and heart. Women of middle age are more often affected.

The onset is gradual with some swelling of the skin, which becomes mottled, shiny, and red, beginning with the hands and feet and spreading over the rest of the body. The face becomes masklike (from the effect upon the connective tissues) and the hands often clawlike. Later the joints are painful because of the calcium deposits. Kidney involvement can raise the

blood pressure. Swallowing may be difficult; heart involvement may cause malfunctioning.

There is no specific medication for
scleroderma.

If the skin involvement is only in one
local area, the chances of recovery are
very good. Spontaneous recovery is not
uncommon. Generally the progress of the
disease is quite slow.

18 Blood and lymph diseases

Julian B. Hyman

Anaemia 322
(iron-deficiency anaemia)

Anaemia is a condition in which there are fewer than the normal number of red blood cells or less than the normal amount of haemoglobin. The red blood cells cannot carry oxygen to the cells of the body without adequate haemoglobin. In iron deficiency anaemia the body has an insufficient supply of this essential mineral, leading to a diminished number of red blood cells, and, consequently, a shortage of oxygen that results in shortness of breath and all the other symptoms of anaemia.

The two basic causes are a nutritional deficiency of iron, found most frequently in infants kept too long on a milk diet, or in a growing child on an improper diet, or in a woman during pregnancy; and chronic blood loss (often hidden), such as peptic ulcer, in which bleeding may be slow and unnoticeable but steady. Other more apparent causes are obviously bleeding ulcers, haemorrhoids, heavy menstrual flow, bloody diarrhoea, tapeworm, hookworm, which live on the blood of the host, or any disorder that causes a loss of blood. A search must always be made for the underlying disorder.

Although the diet may include enough iron, the body may be unable to absorb it because of a lack of copper or cobalt, which are essential for the absorption of iron.

The danger: A shortage of iron leading to anaemia can cause heart failure. If the anaemia is severe enough, blood pressure may fall, often to dangerous shock levels.

Symptoms: Besides the basic signs of pallor, breathlessness, fatigue, weakness, and palpitations, additional signs may appear, depending upon the degree and type of anaemia. Pallor can often go unnoticed because some people are naturally pale, but the whites of the eyes may have a touch of blue, the gums and mucous membranes will be pale, as will the fingernail beds and the inside lids of the eyes. Pallor means less than normal redness everywhere, the consequence of a diminished number of red blood cells.

In an infant, additional signs may be irritability and holding his breath. In adults, the tongue can become large, flabby, and pale, showing teeth marks. Drowsiness, vertigo, a pounding, rapid heartbeat, and noises in the ear can occur. The fingernails may become longitudinally ridged and spoon-shaped. There is loss of libido and the hair takes on a dry, lustreless appearance.

In severe cases the signs may include sore tongue, jaundice, numbness of limbs and some loss of their control, great thirst, and shock. The memory may be poor, breathing is weak and shallow. There may be nausea and diarrhoea as well.

Treatment: The source of the anaemia must first be found. Mild cases are put on an iron-rich, protein-rich diet. Foods that contain iron include meat, especially liver, eggs, spinach, raisins, turnip tops, beet greens, whole wheat bread, and molasses. Copper, which is equally essential, is found in the same foods; cobalt, necessary for the absorption of iron, is found principally in vitamin B_{12}. Zinc, considered to be another factor in the absorption of iron, is found in iron-rich foods, particularly leafy vegetables, herring, and maple syrup.

In addition to vitamin B_{12}, medication includes ferrous sulphate or ferrous gluconate (0·3 grams orally 3 times daily after meals) to avoid abdominal disorders. If the patient cannot tolerate iron medication, it can be administered by injection. The amount of injectable iron must be carefully weighed since too much can be toxic.

Severe cases often require blood transfusion after the cause is established.

Outlook: If the underlying disease can be found, the prognosis is excellent.

Pernicious anaemia 323

Pernicious anaemia is due to the lack of an intrinsic factor made in the stomach, an enzyme essential for the absorption of vitamin B_{12} and folic acid. Pernicious anaemia victims also suffer from insufficient hydrochloric acid, which is normally found in the stomach and is vital in the assimilation of iron.

While adult men and women are equally prone to this form of anaemia, it is rare among children and young adults. Occasionally the disorder is hereditary.

Until recently, pernicious anaemia was a fatal disease. Since the discovery of the missing enzyme, the intrinsic factor, however, and the method of overcoming its absence by the injection of vitamin B_{12}, life expectancy has been brought up to practically normal.

Symptoms: Besides the usual anaemic symptoms – pallor, weakness, shortness of breath, and palpitations – additional symptoms include nosebleeds, a tingling and numbness of the hands and feet, general pain, a sore or burning tongue, which is smooth and red, loss of appetite, considerable weight loss, and a yellowish-lemon colour of the skin. If the anaemia is severe, there may also be cardiac failure, degenerative changes in the nervous system, including the pins and needles sensation in varying places, and difficulty in walking, especially at night. Impotence and frigidity are common. Sometimes there is nausea, vomiting, and diarrhoea. Mental confusion is a frequent sign.

Treatment: Vitamin B_{12} is the answer, in comparatively large doses, given intramuscularly twice weekly until the major symptoms have abated, followed, generally, by 100mcg twice a month thereafter. This medication will bring a dramatic about-face for the patient – from serious illness to health. Symptoms respond dramatically to treatment.

Prevention: None.

Outlook: Untreated, the disease is fatal; with treatment, the given name 'pernicious' is no longer applicable. To maintain normal health a patient will have to remain on B_{12} for the rest of his life – a very small price to pay considering the alternative.

HAEMOLYTIC ANAEMIA 324

When the spleen begins destroying red blood cells faster than they can be produced, the process is called haemolytic anaemia. While the condition can be hereditary, other indicated causes are malaria, mismatched blood transfusion, Rh-blood incompatibility, and a large number of chemicals and medications, such as benzine, naphthol and Lysol (antiseptic disinfectants), nitrites (food preservatives), quinine (antimalarial), resorcinol (antiseptic), sulpha drugs, phenacetin (analgesic and fever reducer), and phenol (extensive antiseptic agent).

The danger: If not treated, severe cases may result in shock or death.
Symptoms: Besides the typical anaemic symptoms, jaundice, faintness, dizziness, weak, rapid pulse, rapid respiration, as well as breathlessness also occur. In addition there may be chills, fever, aches in the extremities and abdomen, and a painful enlargement of the spleen. The patient may be very sick.

In the hereditary form, there are periods of dangerous crises, which may last for several days with an increased severity of all symptoms.
Treatment: Whenever possible, the causative factor must be eliminated. Transfusion is given, if essential. Often the recourse is surgical removal of the spleen, particularly in the hereditary form, which leads to complete control of anaemia.

In the acquired form the red blood cells are coated with an abnormal protein antibody that provokes the spleen to destroy them. In the congenital form the body attacks itself (another autoimmune disease), as if the red blood cells were foreign invaders. In such situations, removal of the spleen is only occasionally remedial. Cortisone is more effective.

Outlook: In the acquired form removal of the blood-destroying element can bring about a cure, but in the congenital form the condition remains chronic for life.

Sickle cell anaemia 325

Sickle cell anaemia attacks the black population almost exclusively, and is inherited when both parents carry the hereditary tendency to it. As yet, there is no known cure or specific medication, although there has been some breakthrough – cyanate therapy holds the possibility of some medical solution.

For some strange reason, the normally round red blood cells take on a sickle shape, which makes the blood thicker, thus clogging up the capillaries and re-

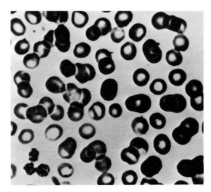

Top: Normal red blood cells. *Below:* Red blood cells in sickle cell anaemia. (*National Institutes of Health*)

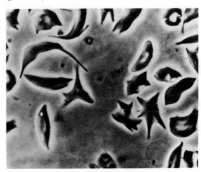

ducing the blood supply to the vital organs as well as the oxygen supply to the cells.

The danger: Only fifty per cent of the victims survive until age twenty and none to the fortieth year. Many of the patients, weakened by the disease, succumb to intervening infections, such as TB, pulmonary embolism, and heart failure.

Symptoms: Generally, the same symptoms as in severe anaemia, accompanied by jaundice, joint pains, and fever. In infants, the first appearance of the disease, at the age of six to twelve months, may be painfully swollen hands and feet. The patient is usually poorly developed with long arms and legs, a short trunk, an enlarged heart, and a prominent skull. In addition, because many vital organs are affected, the patient may suffer the symptoms of a multitude of other diseases. The disease attacks in sudden bouts – a series of severe crises with extreme pain. It frequently mimics acute abdominal disease.

Treatment: At the present time, the only form of treatment is to alleviate the pain and help the patient through a bad period with supportive therapy. Occasionally transfusion is necessary during a crisis. Cyanate and urea therapy may be the answer in the near future. Removal of the spleen is never indicated. The spleen is usually small in this disease.

Prevention: This dread disease can be prevented by ensuring that carriers do not marry. If the sickle cell trait is carried by only one parent, each child born to them will have an even chance that he will carry the trait but no child will actually have the disease. However, if both parents carry the trait, 50 per cent of their children will carry the trait, 25 per cent will be normal, and 25 per cent will have sickle cell anaemia. Such parents should think twice about having children and seriously consider adoption as an alternative.

Aplastic anaemia 326

Aplasia means arrested development.

Aplastic anaemia occurs when the bone marrow's ability to make red and white blood cells and platelets is arrested, a condition caused by some chemical medications, including benzine, arsenic compounds, gold medications, fluorides, sulphapyridine, sulphathiazole, quinacrine (antimalarial), chloramphenicol (antibiotic), as well as various insecticides (especially DDT), radiation, and last but hardly least, x-ray.

The danger: If the toxic agent or cause is not discovered, the disease is fatal. Blood transfusion is only a delaying tactic.

Symptoms: The disease can creep up slowly, becoming obvious only weeks or months after exposure to the poison, or it can break out with sudden violence. Aplastic anaemia presents all the symptoms of severe Anaemia **322**. Ancillary signs are brown pigmentation on a pale, waxy skin, bleeding from the nose and mouth, and black and blue marks. The debilitating effects of this disease make the patient fair game for various infections, because of the deficiency of the white blood cells.

Treatment: The patient is given blood transfusions to keep him going until the bone marrow resumes its normal function. Transplantation of bone marrow has been disappointing, because of the body's normal rejection of any foreign living substance; it fights it as strongly as it would fight foreign bacteria. The only successful form of treatment is discovering the toxic agent and removing it. Often the disease is idiopathic, that is, of no known cause, but many haematologists believe there is always a hidden toxic agent.

Medications of some value are B_{12}, folic acid, steroid, and testosterone (male sex hormone). Testosterone derivatives are proving somewhat more effective.

Polycythaemia 327
(polycythaemia vera)

The opposite of anaemia – too many red

blood cells – polycythaemia occurs mainly in middle age and later years and has a predilection for attacking males, Jewish people, and whites more often than blacks. It is often associated with gout and frequently with hypertension, although the actual cause remains unknown.

The danger: A slowly developing disease that usually culminates with fatal results from cerebral haemorrhage or coronary thrombosis. After many years it quite often leads to leukaemia.

Symptoms: The initial symptoms include constant dull headaches, itching skin, dizziness, fatigue, shortness of breath, and bluish-red skin chiefly on the face and extremities, often cyanotic spots in the fingernail beds, fiery or purple tongue and ringing in the ear (tinnitus). As the disease progresses bleeding occurs in the swollen blood vessels of the gastro-intestinal tract causing blood to appear in the stools. As blood clots form in the veins, the disease may lead to strokes.

Treatment: Some measures for controlling the disease are available but no known cure. Since the number of red blood cells is often twice as high as it should be, the doctor will frequently bleed the patient, an old form of general treatment. Polycythaemia is a quasi-cancerous condition and similar forms of therapy are often employed, such as nitrogen mustard and x-ray. Radioactive phosphorus can help suppress the overproduction of red blood cells.

Outlook: Polycythaemia is controllable with vigorous treatment; life can be prolonged with a reasonable degree of comfort for ten to fifteen years.

Purpura 328
(idiopathic thrombocytopenic purura – ITP)

The tiny red spots, purpura, that appear all over the body and eventually become black and blue marks are often a symptom of disease rather than a disease itself. Basically, purpura is a form of bleeding into the skin or mucous membrane resulting from the fragility of the capillary walls. Ordinary purpura can be a symptom of scurvy, meningitis, and streptococcal blood poisoning, as well as scarlet fever, typhus, and other diseases with high temperatures.

However, there is also a specific purpura disease, idiopathic thrombocytopenic purpura (ITP), which means an abnormal decrease in platelets without known cause, an autoimmune disease in which the spleen unaccountably destroys its own platelets. (Platelets are colourless blood cells that plug up wounds to prevent bleeding.) If a cause is known, such as a chemical poison or x-ray exposure or the presence of a known disease that leads to purpura, the disorder is called symptomatic or secondary purpura and not ITP.

Women between twelve and twenty-five are most often affected.

The danger: Occasionally, especially without medical help, a patient can bleed to death. Cerebral haemorrhage is the most severe complication.

Symptoms: Small red or reddish-blue spots, which often run together making larger ones, appear. There may be bleeding from the mouth or mucous membrane on slight injury, pain in the abdomen and joints, a slow clotting of blood from cuts and wounds, and black and blue marks. Remissions and relapses are common. Traces of blood in the stools are frequent.

Treatment: When too much blood is lost, transfusion is necessary. Iron, calcium, and vitamins are administered in large doses. Steroid therapy can be effective. If the cause of ITP cannot be found and the disease fails to abate, removal of the spleen may be necessary. Over seventy per cent of those who undergo this surgery are cured or are greatly improved. Removal of the spleen does not seem to interfere with a normal life and normal longevity.

Haemophilia 329

A hereditary disease in which the blood fails to clot, haemophilia is extremely variable, ranging from an inconvenience to a deadly ailment, in which a slight scratch might mean hospitalization. Spontaneous bleeding is a constant danger. The disease is due to a deficiency in the blood of a special coagulating substance, antihaemophilic globulin (factor eight). The trait is carried by the female but only affects her male offspring.

The danger: In severe cases, invalidism and massive fatal haemorrhage.

Symptoms: Haemophilia is characterized by an inability of the blood to clot properly or at all, with an abnormal tendency to bleed. The joints may become painfully swollen. Bleeding into the joints causes deformity. Extreme cases of haemophilia usually die in infancy from uncontrollable bleeding. A few, however, survive into adulthood but only with extraordinary care. Occasionally there are remissions.

Treatment: In moderate cases the patient can often help himself when bleeding occurs by applying thrombin directly on the wound and Oxycel (oxidized cellulose). If these do not help, he must be injected with AHF (antihaemophilic factor, a special blood-clotting substance). Patients must always be properly prepared for elective surgery.

Prevention: A good safety precaution is for all haemophiliacs to carry a card or a wristband indicating that they are bleeders in case of an accident.

Outlook: Research indicates that a medical breakthrough is quite possible.

Lymphangitis 330

An infection mainly of the streptococcal variety, lymphangitis is spread through the lymph channels from an infected toe or finger.

The danger: Septicaemia (blood poisoning) is a constant and serious threat.

Necrotic tissue can develop along the lines of the infected channels.

Symptoms: The patient experiences chills, a high fever ranging from 38·9° to 40·5°C, 102° to 105°F, a swelling of the lymph nodes, a general aching all over, and headache. Pink or red lines or streaks extend up the arm or leg from the primary infection towards the lymph nodes in the groin or armpit.

Treatment: First, the basic infection should be treated, usually with an antibiotic. The affected part should be elevated and hot, dry or wet dressings applied along the red streaks.

Outlook: The prognosis is dependent upon the virulence of the infection and the patient's ability to resist and his response to treatment. The disease is more difficult to overcome among the very young, the aged, and the debilitated.

Lymphadenitis 331

An inflammation of one or more lymph nodes, lymphadenitis is usually a progression from lymphangitis. Often there is no primary source of infection. Any organism can produce this disease (bacteria, viruses, fungi), but streptococci and staphylococci are most frequently responsible.

Septicaemia (blood poisoning) is often present. The lymph nodes are enlarged, palpable, tender, and often painful. The overlying skin becomes red and tender as well; it may abscess.

Treatment consists of first removing the underlying cause, often with the aid of a specific antibiotic. Alternating hot and cold moist compresses will help relieve the pain. Abscesses should be incised and drained.

Often, despite massive and acutely inflamed lymph nodes, the disease may subside completely, but not infrequently sufferers will be left with unsightly scars from infected lymph nodes. The outlook is dependent on the virulence of the infection and more importantly on the resistance of the patient. Adequate treatment is essential.

19 Metabolism and the endocrine glands

Benjamin N. Park

METABOLISM

Diabetes 332

(diabetes mellitus)

Diabetes results when the islet cells of Langerhans in the pancreas fail to produce the hormone insulin. Without insulin the body is unable to metabolize carbohydrates, fats, and proteins. In addition, when diabetes occurs, the util-ization of glucose (sugar) is blocked, with the consequence that glucose accumulates in the blood (hyperglycaemia) and spills into the urine (glycosuria). Furthermore, fat and protein are broken down excessively, sometimes resulting in an acute medical emergency called diabetic ketoacidosis.

With the discovery of insulin in 1922 by Canadian scientists Sir Frederick Banting, Charles Best, and John Macleod, diabetes ceased to be a dreaded fatal dis-

440

ease and became a manageable ailment. However, there is, as yet, no cure for this ailment and patients may succumb to its complications. Indeed, the greater threat to a well-controlled diabetic is the complication of premature coronary heart disease, stroke, kidney failure, or blindness, rather than ketoacidosis.

The disease is more frequent in women than in men, and the incidence increases with age. Two types of diabetes are recognized: the juvenile-onset and the adult-onset.

The juvenile-onset is a more severe form with a great deficiency of insulin. The patient is more prone to develop diabetic ketoacidosis as well as other complications. Most will require insulin for treatment.

Adult-onset diabetics generally have a milder disease, and many of them can manage without insulin therapy. They are usually able to produce insulin but in inadequate amounts. Obesity is present in more than half of these patients.

Although separation of these two types is generally useful and valid, there are exceptions. Some juvenile diabetics have a mild form, and many adults may develop a severe type.

The exact cause of diabetes remains undiscovered, although it is generally agreed that an absolute or relative lack of insulin is the underlying mechanism. Heredity is an important factor, as is evident by the frequent occurrence of diabetes in the same family. Exactly how the disease is inherited is not known.

In a small number of cases, destruction of the pancreas by tumour, inflammation, infection, and alcoholism have been shown to be responsible. In patients with acromegaly and Cushing's syndrome, an excessive secretion of growth hormone and adrenal steroid hormones produce diabetes because of their insulin counter-acting property. Obesity can precipitate diabetes in susceptible persons, because insulin is less effective in obese people. Other precipitating factors include drugs (steroids, thiazide diuretics), pregnancy (gestational diabetes), and stressful conditions.

The danger: The diabetic runs two kinds of risks: the first is acute complications, such as diabetic ketoacidosis and hypoglycaemic coma; and the second is chronic complications, such as premature coronary heart disease, stroke, kidney failure, and blindness.

Before insulin became available in the 1920s, ketoacidosis was the leading cause of death in diabetic patients. Now death from uncomplicated diabetic ketoacidosis is rare, although the condition still requires emergency treatment in a hospital. Severe hypoglycaemia, resulting from the excessive administration of insulin or hypoglycaemic agents, can result in permanent brain damage, coma, and death. Every diabetic and his family should be aware of this problem and know how to handle such a possibility. The chronic complications of diabetes, which are described below, are generally related to the duration of the disease.

Symptoms: The classical symptoms of diabetes are excessive thirst, excessive urination, and excessive hunger, but despite increased food intake, weight loss is common. Generalized weakness, lassitude, and a tendency towards frequent skin disorders, especially boils, and vaginal infections, especially of the fungus type, are common. Blurred vision, numbness, dry mouth, tingling, cramps in the legs, and impotence are frequent symptoms. Delivery of a large baby may be the first sign of the disease.

When the disease is suspected, medical diagnosis is easily made by measuring the glucose level in the blood. If the fasting blood glucose level is borderline, a glucose tolerance test can give a more definitive answer. This is done by administering glucose (usually 100 grams, about $3\frac{1}{2}$ ounces, by mouth) and measuring blood glucose response.

Treatment: Proper diet, exercise, and medication (hypoglycaemic agents or insulin) are the basic fundamentals of treatment. In mild diabetes proper diet and regular exercise are sufficient, but in the severe form insulin is mandatory.

1. Diet: the goal of the diabetic diet is to bring the body weight to an ideal level

as well as to provide balanced nutrition. Carbohydrates, particularly in the form of refined sugar and concentrated sweets, are restricted, because they are poorly handled in the diabetic. Reduction of weight to the proper level is important because obesity reduces the effectiveness of insulin. In patients on insulin small amounts of carbohydrates between meals are necessary to avoid hypoglycaemia.

2. Exercise: because exercise promotes the utilization of glucose in the muscle, a regular workout frequently improves control of diabetes and decreases the requirement for insulin and hypogly-caemic agents. However, since extensive exercise can produce hypoglycaemia, small amounts of carbohydrates are recommended during or after a heavy session.

3. Hypoglycaemic agents: when diet and exercise are inadequate to control the symptoms of diabetes, and insulin treatment is not practical or applicable, oral hypoglycaemic agents are used. There are two groups of hypoglycaemic agents on the market: the sulphonylurea group (Rastinon, Diabinese, Daonil, and Tolinase), which acts by stimulating the pancreas to secrete more insulin, and the phenformin group, which acts by stimulating the metabolism of glucose directly in the cells and not by stimulation of the pancreas. One drug from each group is sometimes used in combination.

4. Insulin: if diabetes cannot be controlled by diet or by the addition of oral hypoglycaemic agents, insulin therapy becomes necessary. There is a variety of insulin preparations, which produce action of different duration. When the prompt action of insulin is required as in diabetic ketoacidosis, short-acting insulin (regular or crystalline insulin) is used.

For an intelligent treatment of diabetes, the patient should test his own urine daily for sugar. If sugar is present in large quantities, the urine should be tested again for ketones. Sugar and ketones can easily be detected with the use of commercially available test tapes and tablets (abstix). The presence of large amounts of sugar

and ketones is usually a sign of keto-acidosis and requires prompt action (a doctor should be called at once). The administration of extra insulin can offset dangerous ketoacidosis.

The prediabetic: the tendency towards diabetes occurs among those whose are born of diabetic parents, overweight people over forty, women who have delivered large babies (nine pounds or more), and women who have repeated miscarriages. (There are, however, many diverse reasons for miscarriages, some of which have nothing to do with diabetes.)

Diabetic ketoacidosis (*diabetic coma*): when there is a severe lack of insulin, glucose accumulates rapidly in the blood, causing marked hyperglycaemia and glycosuria. In addition, fat is broken down, with an accumulation of its metabolic products, known as ketone bodies. Since ketone bodies are acids, their accumulation produces acidity of the blood (acidosis). When a large amount of glucose is spilled into the urine, large amounts of water and salts (sodium, potassium, and so on) are also lost and severe dehydration results. The acidosis makes the patient breathe rapidly and deeply, as if he were hungry for air. Nausea, vomiting, dizziness, and abdominal pain are common. Acute dehydration leads to sunken eyeballs, poor skin tone, and low blood pressure. Eventually, shock, stupor, and coma may result.

Diabetic ketoacidosis is a *Medical Emergency* requiring immediate treatment in a hospital. Large amounts of insulin, fluid, and electrolytes are frequently required to correct the situation.

Ketoacidosis, which is frequently precipitated by stressful conditions, such as infection, heart attack, and emotional crisis, can be prevented in many cases by testing the urine daily. The most common immediate cause of diabetic ketoacidosis is the failure of the patient to remain on insulin. This usually happens when he is unable to eat anything because of nausea and vomiting. Even if a diabetic cannot eat or fails to eat, his body still requires insulin. Insulin should never be stopped without the explicit advice of a doctor. Insulin reaction (*insulin shock*): in patients on insulin, serious hypoglycaemia will appear when excessive insulin is taken. Hypoglycaemic symptoms include weakness, confusion, nervousness, trembling, sweating, and hunger sensations. When severe, it can produce fainting, prolonged loss of consciousness, and coma. Oral hypoglycaemic agents, particularly Diabinese, can also produce hypoglycaemia if too much is taken. Because this complication can cause serious brain damage and even death, prevention and prompt treatment of hypoglycaemia is important. Diabetics, especially those taking insulin, should carry an identification card describing their condition. Mild hypoglycaemic reactions can be treated by drinking a glass of orange juice or eating sugar. In more extreme cases injection of glucagon (a hormone that releases glucose from the liver) or the intravenous administration of glucose is necessary.

Chronic complications of diabetes

Kidney involvement: in patients with a long duration (fifteen to twenty years) of diabetes, kidney involvement is a serious complication. In ten per cent of juvenile-onset diabetes, kidney failure is the cause of death.

Eye involvement: diabetes is the third leading cause of blindness in the western world. This is due to damage of the retina as well as the result of an increased incidence of cataract and glaucoma. Again, the duration of diabetes is an important factor.

Cardiovascular disease: premature hardening of the arteries (atherosclerosis) is a serious complication of diabetes. Diabetic women are particularly vulnerable.

Gangrene: diabetics are more prone to develop gangrene in the toes and feet because of poor circulation in the legs. As a consequence, amputation of the legs is more frequent in diabetics than in non-diabetics.

Nerve and muscle involvement: dia-betes may involve nerve and muscle tissue, producing pain, a decreased sensation in the legs and hands, and a wasting of the muscles. Because of the deficiency in sensation, diabetics with nerve involvement are prone to develop traumatic injuries and burns. When there is involvement of the autonomic nervous system, impotence and intractable diarrhoea may cause much distress.

Infection: diabetics are more susceptible to infections, particularly if their disease is inadequately controlled. This may result in frequent disorders of the skin, vagina, and urinary tract.

Prevention: (See *Part 3, Early warning signals, Diabetes* **332**)

Outlook: Although diabetic patients can now enjoy a near normal lifespan, serious disability may arise because of the chronic complications of the disease. As yet, no definitive procedures are available to prevent these complications. Good control of diabetes is desirable, although there is no firm proof that this will prevent additional problems. Conditions that contribute to kidney damage, coronary heart disease, and gangrene should be corrected. Thus, high blood pressure, hyperlipidaemia, and kidney infections should be promptly and vigorously treated on discovery. Particular attention should be given to foot care to prevent ulceration and gangrene. Obesity and cigarette smoking must be avoided.

Hypoglycaemia 333

Glucose is an important substance in the body economy because it provides ready energy for all the tissues. It is especially important for the brain, because that organ is almost totally dependent on glucose for its energy need. Normally, the glucose level in the blood is maintained at a fairly constant range (between 60 to 100 mg per 100ml), despite many events that tend to affect this equilibrium. When carbohydrate is consumed, it is converted into glucose; excess glucose is stored in the liver as glycogen. As various tissues utilize glucose and thus decrease its blood level, glycogen is changed back into glucose and released into circulation. If the supply of glucose from glycogen is inadequate, glucose is made anew from other materials in the liver. These regulatory processes are primarily governed by hormones. Insulin is the most important hormone in this respect; it promotes the formation of glycogen and suppresses its breakdown. Insulin also inhibits the formation of an oversupply of glucose, thus decreasing the blood glucose level. Other hormones, such as glucagon, the growth hormone, and adrenal steroid hormones, have the opposite effect, tending to increase the glucose level. When there is a disturbance of these regulatory processes, the blood glucose level drops below normal and produces symptoms of hypoglycaemia.

Two of the many causes of hypoglycaemia are too much insulin, as in the case of patients with a rare insulin-secreting tumour of the pancreas or in diabetics with an overdose of either insulin or oral hypoglycaemic agents, and too little of the insulin-counteracting hormones, as in those suffering from hypopituitarism or adrenal insufficiency. Hypoglycaemia also appears in a case of severe liver disease when that organ is unable to produce glucose. In children, a deficiency of enzymes, which are involved in the production of glucose from glycogen, is an important determinant of hypoglycaemia (glycogen-storage disease). In infants and children, a sensitivity to fructose (a carbohydrate, which is present in large quantities in fruits and honey) and galactose (a carbohydrate, which is present in large quantities in milk) is an occasional cause of hypoglycaemia. These are all familial disorders which, fortunately, tend to become less acute with age. The most common type of this disease in the adult population is reactive hypoglycaemia, most often affecting patients with a history of stomach surgery or with an early mild diabetes. An attack typically occurs several hours after meals rich in carbohydrates, brought on by an imbalance between glucose and insulin metabolism.

Most often, however, there is no known underlying cause, and reactive hypoglycaemia appears without any apparent reason. This is especially true in young women who tend to be tense or who are under emotional strain.

Symptoms: Hypoglycaemia can present many diverse symptoms, depending upon the rapidity and the extensiveness of the disorder. Episodes of severe weakness, dizziness, palpitation, shaking, sweating, blurred vision, and headache are common. Blackout spells, an inability to concentrate, bizarre behaviour, and various psychiatric symptoms are frequent. In severe hypoglycaemia, convulsions and coma are not unusual.

Hypoglycaemia is easily diagnosed by measuring the blood glucose level. For reactive hypoglycaemia, a determination of the blood glucose level following a high carbohydrate meal (usually a drink of glucose solution) is necessary to demonstrate hypoglycaemia. Once the presence of hypoglycaemia is established, it is important to find the cause.

Treatment: Hypoglycaemic symptoms are relieved promptly by the administration of carbohydrates. When the patient is conscious, he can take a sweet, orange juice, or biscuit. In patients with more severe hypoglycaemia who are unconscious and unable to take anything by mouth, intravenous administration of glucose is necessary. The injection of glucagon is useful when facilities for intravenous therapy are not immediately available.

The definitive treatment of hypoglycaemia depends upon its cause, once the acute form of hypoglycaemia is corrected. If there is a tumour on the pancreas, surgical removal is curative. In hypopituitarism and adrenal insufficiency, replacement therapy with adrenal steroid hormone is usually adequate. Patients with a sensitivity to fructose and galactose must avoid the offending substances. Frequent high carbohydrate feedings are recommended for those with glycogen-storage disease. For patients with re-active hypoglycaemia, a diet high in protein and low in carbohydrate taken at frequent intervals in small servings is generally effective. If hypoglycaemic reactions occur because of an overdose of insulin or oral hypoglycaemic agents, the dosage must be decreased.

Outlook: Hypoglycaemia is a chronic disease. The prognosis is varied and guarded, but the disease can be kept under control.

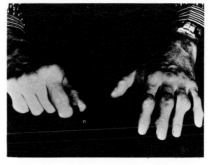

Gouty arthritis. (*National Institutes of Health*)

Gout 334

Gout is a relatively common disease, which has been recognized from antiquity, and mainly affects middle-aged men (only five out of a hundred patients are women). In many cases, gout is hereditary.

The immediate cause of gout is an excessive accumulation of uric acid in the body. Both increased uric acid production and decreased excretion may be responsible. In such conditions as leukaemia, lymphoma, and polycythaemia, increased production of uric acid sometimes results in secondary gout.

The danger: Kidney failure is the most serious complication of gout, occurring in about ten per cent of the patients. Chronic arthritis and the destruction of bone in the hands and feet are also important complications.

Symptoms: The initial attack is usually sudden in an otherwise healthy person. Nine times out of ten the attack is on the joint of the big toe, although it can occur on the wrist, ankle, and thumb joints. The toe becomes shiny, red to purplish red, swollen, and excruciating to the touch so that even the weight of the lightest clothes cannot be tolerated. (Ordinary arthritis produces pain that is deep and aching; in gout the pain is sharp and agonizing.)

There may be fever and chills, with a rapid pulse. The first attack can last from one to four days; later attacks may not be as intense but will last longer. As the disease progresses, the attacks tend to become more frequent. The arthritis is due to the deposits of uric acid crystals in the joint.

Uric acid can also be deposited in other parts of the body, such as the earlobes, and in various joints and tendons, producing hard, painless tumours (tophi). When uric acid crystals are deposited in the kidneys, serious kidney damage can follow. In addition, an excess spillage of uric acid into the urine may produce kidney stones (in 10 to 20 per cent of the patients). Gout is readily recognized when tophi are present or when typical attacks of arthritis occur. Demonstration of uric acid crystals in the joint fluid or urine confirms the diagnosis. A high uric acid level in the blood is presumptive evidence of gout.

Treatment: Regular, daily, consistent, exercise will decrease uric acid in the blood. The affected part of the body should be cradled, wrapped in cotton, and kept immobile.

An effective medication, colchicine, made from the autumn crocus, was discovered by some unknown Egyptian genius in 500 B.C. and has been in steady use ever since. No one knows why or how it works, but it does bring relief within a comparatively short time. Since colchicine has no effect on any other disease, it provides confirmation of the diagnosis. But it is very strong medicine and can cause nausea and vomiting and other side effects. For those who cannot tolerate colchicine, an effective substitute, phenylbutazone, is somewhat less toxic.

In patients with prominent tophi, drugs such as Benemid, which increase the excretion of uric acid, are in wide use. More recently, allopurinol, which blocks the formation of uric acid, has been successfully used to reduce the uric acid level. To prevent the formation of uric acid stones in patients excreting large amounts of uric acid, the alkalinization of urine is induced (uric acid is soluble in an alkaline environment) by the administration of sodium bicarbonate. Drinking large amounts of water is also helpful. Moderation is recommended in the consumption of foods that produce large amounts of uric acid, such as liver or kidney. Contrary to popular belief, alcohol is well tolerated in most cases.

Prevention: (See *Part 3, Early warning signals, Gout* **334**)

Outlook: The condition is chronic, but it can be reversible. Much depends on the patient's following the daily regimen advised by his doctor. The inter-critical period (the silent period between attacks) when he is symptomless may lull the patient into overlooking essential adherence to diet and medication. It is during this silent period that much of the damage of gout takes place. Simply, the outlook is mostly up to the patient.

Hyperlipidaemia 335
(hyperlipaemia, hypercholesterolaemia)

The fat level in the body has received increasing attention in recent years because persons with a high fat level are more prone to develop hardening of the arteries (atherosclerosis). Thus coronary heart disease, stroke, and peripheral vascular disease are several times more common in those people than in the general population. In this respect, among many different classes of fat (lipid), cholesterol and triglyceride are the more important. Hyperlipidaemia literally means the elevation of lipid in the blood. This may be due to the elevation of either cholesterol or triglyceride or both. Five different types are recognized.

Hyperlipidaemia may occur as a hereditary disease (familial hyperlipidaemia; primary hyperlipidaemia) or as a complication of other disorders (secondary hyperlipidaemia). Secondary hyperlipidaemia occurs in diabetes, obesity, hypothyroidism, primary biliary cirrhosis, and certain types of kidney disease (nephrotic syndrome and chronic kidney failure). Contraceptive pills, steroid drugs, and excessive alcohol intake can also cause hyperlipidaemia in susceptible people. Dietary factors greatly influence blood lipid levels. Foods containing large amounts of cholesterol and animal fat increase cholesterol levels, while a high carbohydrate diet may greatly increase triglyceride levels in susceptible people.

The danger: Arterio-atherosclerosis, with its train of diseases, most notoriously coronary occlusion, is often the end result of hyperlipidaemia.

Symptoms: Obvious outward symptoms specifically related to hyperlipidaemia may not be evident. However, there are certain signs that indicate the presence of high blood lipid levels. The deposition of cholesterol as painless yellow lumps (xanthoma, xanthelasma) is frequently seen around the eyelids, palms, knees, elbows, buttocks, and tendons of the legs and hands. In some cases, acute pancreas inflammation may develop as a consequence of an extremely high triglyceride level. Not infrequently symptoms and signs of atherosclerosis (coronary heart disease, stroke, and poor circulation in the legs) at a relatively early age may be the only signs. *Arcus senilis* **42** may be another symptom but only significant when it appears in those under forty.

Treatment: A proper diet is the primary and essential treatment for all types of hyperlipidaemia. Weight reduction to an ideal level is an important manoeuvre, which will of itself often lower blood lipid levels significantly towards the normal range.

Dairy fat, eggs, and milk, which are high in cholesterol, and animal fats should be avoided or sharply curtailed, since they will elevate the blood cholesterol level. But vegetable oils, such as corn or safflower oil, are recommended, since they lower the cholesterol level. Patients with a high triglyceride level are particularly sensitive to carbohydrates (especially those contained in concentrated sweets); their diets should have a significant low carbohydrate content. For some patients fat intake must be drastically curbed.

When dietary measures are not sufficient to completely normalize lipid levels in the blood, several different drugs are administered, depending upon the type of hyperlipidaemia. Currently, the most commonly used drugs are clofibrate and cholestyramine.

In secondary hyperlipidaemia, successful treatment of the underlying disorder will often correct the hyperlipidaemia.

Prevention: Because of the adverse effect of hyperlipidaemia on arterio-atherosclerosis, efforts should be made to detect and treat hyperlipidaemia as early as possible. Thus every person with evidence of atherosclerosis and a family history of hyperlipidaemia should have his blood lipid levels checked. Patients suffering from disorders that cause secondary hyperlipidaemia also should have their lipid levels determined.

ENDOCRINE DISORDERS

The endocrine glands are small ductless glands scattered throughout the body that perform the vital function of producing hormones, which are discharged directly into the bloodstream. Although all the endocrine glands together weigh no more than two ounces, they are, nevertheless, essential for life. Every aspect of life is greatly influenced by hormones – growth, reproduction, sexuality, general metabolism, and mental function are under their control. Any over-production or underproduction of hormones results in a disordered condition of the body.

The endocrine glands of clinical importance include the pituitary gland, thyroid gland, four parathyroid glands, pancreas, two adrenal glands, and two sex glands.

The pituitary is the master gland in the body; it elaborates not only its own unique hormones, such as growth hormone, vasopressin (helps to maintain blood pressure and controls the regulation of water balance in the body), and many others, but also influences the hormonal production of other glands – the thyroid, adrenal, and sex glands, and to a lesser extent, the pancreas – by controlling their activity. The pituitary is the size of a hazelnut and is located in the base of the brain; it is divided into a larger anterior part, where most of the pituitary hormones are produced, and a smaller posterior part.

The activity of other endocrine glands, which are under the control of the pituitary gland, have an important influence, in turn, on the pituitary gland.

The thyroid gland is a butterfly-shaped gland astride the windpipe; its hormones are manufactured from iodine and have an important influence on the body's consumption of oxygen and on basal metabolism.

The parathyroid glands (located around the thyroid gland) are extremely small in size, comparable to rice grains. They are essential for the proper metabolism of calcium and phosphorus in the body.

An adrenal gland sits atop each kidney and weighs less than 5gm, a sixth of an ounce. The outer part (the cortex) of the adrenal gland produces a number of steroid hormones, the glucocorticoids and the mineralocorticoids. The glucocorticoids (such as cortisone) have more influence on general body metabolism, while the mineralocorticoids (such as aldosterone) have a greater influence on salt metabolism. The inner part (medulla) of the adrenal gland produces the well-known hormone epinephrine (adrenalin) and its closely related hormone norepinephrine (noradrenalin).

Epinephrine provides for a sudden burst of energy when needed, increasing both heart and breathing rate and raising the blood sugar level for additional energy; it also constricts arteries and quickens the clotting of blood to prevent rapid bleeding in case of injury.

The pancreas is a unique gland, composed of both an endocrine gland (ductless, discharging its secretions into the bloodstream) and an exocrine gland (discharging into a duct and not directly into the bloodstream). The endocrine pancreas (a collection of cells known as the islets of Langerhans) produces insulin and glucagon, which play important roles in carbohydrate, protein, and fat metabolism in the body.

The sex glands are the ovaries and the testes, producing female hormones (such as oestrogen and progesterone) and male hormones (such as testosterone) respectively, and thereby controlling sexuality and reproduction. The diseases involving the sex glands are described in *Chapters 13* and *14.*

(*Pituitary gland*)
Acromegaly and pituitary gigantism 336

When the pituitary gland produces too much growth hormone, acromegaly or pituitary gigantism results, depending upon the age of the patient. The overproduction of the growth hormone is usually due to a benign tumour in the pituitary gland.

The danger: When the pituitary tumour becomes enlarged, it may destroy the surrounding tissues in the base of the skull and produce visual disturbances. In addition, high blood pressure and heart failure can complicate the disease. Since the growth hormone counteracts the action of insulin, diabetes is present in about half of these patients.

Symptoms: In growing children, the growth hormone stimulates linear growth. When there is an overproduction of growth hormone, a spurt of excess growth results, producing a tall stature and, in a small number of cases, towering giants. Some of the legendary giants undoubtedly

had pituitary gigantism, although excessive growth hormone secretion is not always found in giants. When this excessive hormone production occurs in adult life, after cessation of the growth period, acromegaly, the overgrowth of hands, feet, and face, rather than gigantism, is the result. In patients with acromegaly, the face becomes coarse and large with a prominent nose and jaws, the hands and feet become large and stubby. Also affected are internal organs – the heart, liver, and kidneys – which may become enlarged. Additionally, there is an impairment of mental ability and a loss of libido. Because of the thickening of the vocal cords, the voice often becomes low and husky. Severe headaches, excessive sweating, and pains and aches in the joints are also common symptoms. The typical patient with acromegaly is easily recognized because of his distinctive features. The definitive diagnosis can be made by measuring the growth hormone level in the blood.

Treatment: The usual treatment consists of either surgical removal or x-ray irradiation of the tumour. When there is extensive tumour involvement of the pituitary gland, the whole pituitary gland, including the tumour, may have to be removed.

Hypopituitarism 337
(Simmonds' disease, Sheehan's syndrome, pituitary dwarfism)

Hypopituitarism is a condition resulting from the malfunction or destruction of the pituitary gland. Since the pituitary gland controls the activity of the thyroid, adrenal, and sex glands, poor functioning of these glands frequently accompanies hypopituitarism.

The most common cause of pituitary gland destruction is the aftermath of a difficult childbirth during which there has been severe haemorrhage. Other causes in the adult include tumours, infections, cysts, an overgrowth of fibrous tissue, basal skull veins inside the skull.

The danger: In children, if treatment is not started promptly, a permanent stunting of growth and dwarfism will result. Although hypopituitarism is an uncommon cause of dwarfism (accounting for approximately ten per cent), every effort should be made to determine the exact cause of growth retardation in a child. In adults, because of the usually insidious nature of the disease, diagnosis and treatment are frequently delayed. Severe hypoglycaemia and shock at times of stress are potentially fatal complications of the disease.

Symptoms: In children, hypopituitarism frequently results in stunted growth and dwarfism because of the lack of growth hormone secretion. Unlike other dwarfs, the pituitary dwarf has a well-proportioned body and his intelligence is normal.

In adults, the symptoms of hypopituitarism usually develop slowly. Common signs include easy fatigue, intolerance to cold, scanty menstruation, and diminished libido. Patients may have a poor appetite, lose weight, and become apathetic. In postpartum hypopituitarism, failure to lactate may be the first symptom. The skin is usually thin, cool, pale and sallow with fine wrinkles. Pubic and axillary hair may become sparse or even absent. The pulse is slow and feeble; blood pressure is low. A low basal metabolism rate and hypoglycaemia may occur. When there is indication of multiple glandular failure, diagnosis is established by measuring the adrenal, thyroid, and sex gland functions as well as the growth hormone level.

Treatment: When a tumour is responsible, surgical removal or x-ray irradiation are the usual methods of treatment. Since the thyroid, adrenal, and sex glands are frequently underactive, replacement of the hormones produced by these glands is necessary. In children, the growth hormone can be given to promote growth, although at the present time, unfortunately, this hormone is expensive and not easy to obtain, because of the difficulty of its extraction.

Diabetes insipidus 338

Diabetes insipidus (no relation to diabetes mellitus) occurs when there is a lack of the antidiuretic hormone vasopressin (Pitressin), which is normally produced in the hypothalamus and stored in the pituitary gland before release. It maintains the water content of the body by limiting urine formation in the kidneys. Any destructive lesion of the hypothalamus or the pituitary gland (tumour, infection, or traumatic injury) can cause diabetes insipidus. In a small number of cases, it occurs as a hereditary disorder. In about ten per cent of patients, the disease occurs not because there is lack of the antidiuretic hormone but because the kidneys cannot respond to the direction of the hormone.

Symptoms: The cardinal symptom is the excretion of large volumes of dilute but otherwise normal urine. The total urine volume may reach many litres a day, and the patient is often awakened at night to relieve himself. Unlike patients with 'sugar diabetes' (diabetes mellitus), there is no sugar in the urine and the blood sugar level is normal. Because of the large loss of water in the urine, patients invariably feel very thirsty and have to drink large quantities of water. This thirst should be quenched to avoid severe dehydration and shock.

Treatment: The use of the hormone as a nasal spray or an injection corrects the symptoms. In mild cases, chlorpropamide (Diabinese) can be used.

Outlook: This is a chronic disease, controllable but not really curable.

(*Thyroid gland*)
Hypothyroidism 339
(myxoedema, cretinism)

The underproduction of the thyroid hormone produces hypothyroidism. If the disease occurs during foetal life or in a growing child, severe impairment of mental and physical development results (cretinism). The disease occurs in women far more often than in men. Hypothyroidism may be either primary (failure of the thyroid gland itself) or secondary (failure of the pituitary gland). Primary hypothyroidism is the more common of the two. A lack of iodine is an important cause, particularly in children. Large numbers of hypothyroid patients are seen in the areas of the world where the supply of iodine is limited, notably in inland areas. Hereditary disorders that interfere with production of the thyroid hormone can also result in this disease.

In adults, the most common cause of spontaneous hypothyroidism is a shrinking of the thyroid gland by an unknown cause. Some defect in the body's immunological mechanism has been blamed, because of the frequent discovery of thyroid antibodies in the blood of patients with this condition. Another source of hypothyroidism is the destruction of the thyroid gland following surgery or radiation therapy for hyperthyroidism. Paradoxically, too much iodine has also been implicated. Finally, certain drugs and foods (such as cabbage and soybeans) are thought to induce hypothyroidism in a small number of susceptible patients.

The danger: If cretinism is not diagnosed and therapy is not begun immediately, permanent physical and mental retardation may occur. In patients with severe hypothyroidism (myxoedema), psychosis (myxoedema madness) and coma (myxoedema coma) are frequent. Heart failure, bowel obstruction, and serious respiratory depression are additional complications of severe hypothyroidism.

Symptoms: Hypothyroidism impairs physical and mental development in children; they are short, stocky, and dull with occasional goitre and swollen feet. Their faces are coarse, with thick lips, protruding eyes, and broad, flat noses; the skin is rough and dry and the muscle tone is diminished, resulting in pot-bellies and hernias. Their temperature is lower than

normal, 35·5°C, 96°F or less. Their skeletal growth, as well as their intellectual growth, is retarded, classifying these children as cretins.

In adults, hypothyroidism produces a soft goitre and results in apathy, sluggishness, and increased sensitivity to cold. In addition, the skin becomes dry, cool, and rough, the hair brittle, and the voice low and husky. Frequently the hands, face, and eyelids become puffy, the fingernails discoloured, and the muscles weak. The pulse rate and reflexes become slow. Weight gain is common, as are heavy menstrual periods, constipation, and anaemia. The normal temperature may drop below 35·5°C, 96°F. In a typical case, recognition of this condition is not difficult. In a mild case, measurement of the thyroid hormone level in the blood and the capacity of the thyroid gland to absorb the iodine are helpful diagnostic tests. A low basal metabolism rate and a high blood cholesterol level are also helpful signs. In secondary hypothyroidism, evidence of failure of other endocrine glands (such as the adrenal glands and sex glands) may be evident.

Treatment: The daily administration of the thyroid hormone preparations is an effective form of treatment. In regions of severe iodine deficiency, filling this lack has eliminated the incidence of this disorder.

Outlook: If caught early and treated properly, growth in children may become normal, and great improvement in mental status can be achieved.

Hyperthyroidism 349 (Graves' disease, thyrotoxicosis)

Overproduction of the thyroid hormone causes hyperthyroidism. Two types are recognized: one is associated with a diffuse enlargement of the thyroid gland (exophthalmic goitre: Graves' disease) and the other with the growth of multiple small tumours (toxic nodular goitre: Plummer's disease). Hyperthyroidism is much more common in females than in males, by a ratio of five to one, and occurs predominantly in young women. The exact cause of Graves' disease and Plummer's disease is unknown. Although the pituitary gland can stimulate the thyroid gland, an overactive pituitary gland is not the cause of hyperthyroidism.

The danger: One of the complications of severe hyperthyroidism is thyroid storm, in which the patient may lapse into high fever, dehydration, shock, and coma, a *Medical Emergency* requiring immediate hospitalization. Thyroid storm is more likely to appear during such stressful conditions as surgery, trauma, or infection. Untreated, it is usually fatal.

The patient with protruding eyeballs (marked exophthalmos) runs the risk of eye infection, ulceration of the cornea, and prolapse of the eyeballs.

Older patients frequently suffer the complications of irregular and rapid heartbeats and heart failure if the disease is not controlled.

Symptoms: Common symptoms include enlarged thyroid gland, increased nervousness and emotional outbursts, excessive sweating and feeling too warm in normal weather (intolerance to heat), and hyperactiveness. Frequently, there is muscle weakness, fatigue, and a loss of weight despite a healthy appetite. Menstruation becomes scanty and infrequent, hair becomes thin, and the patient may suffer from frequent loose bowel movements. The skin is invariably warm, moist, and smooth. Tremors of the outstretched hands may be evident, as well as emotional instability. The pulse is rapid; the heartbeat so strong and pounding that it may shake the body. In patients with Graves' disease, the eyes become prominent (exophthalmos) and there may be visual disturbances. In severe cases the eyeballs bulge (often giving the appearance of alarm or rage) to such a degree that the eyelids cannot be completely closed, which may result in injury and eye infection. Full-blown cases are not hard to recognize. When there is a suspicion of hyperthyroidism, the diagnosis is established by measuring the thyroid hormone level in the blood. Because iodine, the building block of thyroid hormone, is taken up by the thyroid glands in increased amounts in hyperthyroidism, measurement of the thyroid uptake of iodine is a useful test.

Treatment: The most commonly employed procedures are surgery and radiation. Surgical risk and the danger of complications are minimal in competent hands. Usually only three-quarters of the gland is removed. Radiation is more commonly used for children, for young women who wish to become pregnant, and for elderly people who are poor surgical risks. Radioactive iodine is employed for radiation, because it selectively destroys the thyroid gland. Medical follow-up is important.

Prevention: (See *Part 3, Early warning signals, Hyperthyroidism* **340**)

Goitre 341

A goitre is an enlargement of the thyroid gland, a condition that may be accompanied by either hyperthyroidism (a toxic goitre), hypothyroidism, or a normal functioning of the gland (a nontoxic goitre). If the goitre is very large, it compresses the oesophagus and the trachea (the windpipe). As a result, difficulty in swallowing and breathing may arise. When the goitre is relatively small, the administration of thyroid hormone can shrink the enlarged gland to normal size. If the goitre is large and is causing compression symptoms, surgery is the best treatment.

(Parathyroid glands) Hyperparathyroidism 342

The result of the overproduction of parathyroid hormone, primary hyperparathyroidism is due to a benign tumour of the parathyroid gland in the majority of cases. Other instances are due to either a diffuse enlargement of the glands or a malignant tumour. A chronic failure of the kidneys stimulates the parathyroid glands and may produce clinically significant hyperparathyroidism (secondary hyperparathyroidism).

The danger: The most serious complication of this disease is kidney failure as a consequence of calcium in the kidneys and repeated urinary tract infection. Peptic ulcer and inflammation of the pancreas also occur more commonly in hyperparathyroid patients than in the general population.

Symptoms: The production of kidney stones is an important sign of hyperparathyroidism. When an overproduction of parathyroid hormone occurs, excess calcium is mobilized from the bone; the excess calcium accumulates in the blood (hypercalcaemia) and spills into the urine, which causes deposits of calcium in the kidneys and the formation of kidney stones. As calcium is being mobilized rapidly, bone destruction may result.

Another form of this disease will produce another set of symptoms – muscle weakness, loss of appetite, nausea, constipation, excessive thirst, and excessive urination.

The diagnosis of hyperparathyroidism is made by measuring the calcium level in the blood. Although hypercalcaemia is not always caused by hyperparathyroidism, in the absence of other causes of hypercalcaemia, an elevated calcium level in the blood is presumptive evidence for hyperparathyroidism.

Treatment: Surgical removal of the tumour is the treatment of choice. If a diffuse enlargement of the glands is responsible, three of the four parathyroid glands are removed.

Outlook: Surgery can mean full recovery, depending on the extent of kidney damage.

(*Adrenal glands*)
Cushing's disease 343
(Cushing's syndrome)

First described in 1932 by the famous

Boston neurosurgeon Dr Harvey Cushing, Cushing's disease is due to an overproduction of the adrenal steroid hormones. The disease is due to either a tumour of the adrenal glands (usually benign) or to a diffuse overgrowth of the glands through excessive stimulation by the pituitary gland. In the latter situation, tumour of the pituitary is sometimes responsible. Excessive use of steroid hormone can also cause Cushing's syndrome.

The danger: Bone fractures, particularly of the spine, resulting from a thinning of the bone (osteoporosis), high blood pressure, and diabetes are not uncommon. The patient is also more susceptible to infections.

Symptoms: The most familiar symptom is weight gain and obesity. Typically, increased fat accumulates in the trunk, back (buffalo hump), and face (moonfaced). Excessive hair growth and acne are usual. Patients bruise easily, cease to have regular menstrual periods, and have muscle weakness.

The diagnosis is made by measuring the adrenal hormones in the blood and their metabolic products in the urine. Sophisticated tests have made it possible to determine whether the disease is due to a tumour in the adrenal gland or to an overactive pituitary gland.

Treatment: If a single adrenal tumour is responsible, removal of the tumour is curative. In cases in which the pituitary gland is primarily responsible, with secondary enlargment of the adrenal glands, surgical removal of both adrenal glands is the prevailing treatment. Such radical surgery always requires the daily administration of adrenal steroid hormone.

Adrenal insufficiency 344
(Addison's disease)

In 1855, Thomas Addison, a famous London physician, first described adrenal insufficiency as a result of the underactivity of the adrenal glands. In the past, tuberculosis was the most common cause of adrenal insufficiency; now, a spontaneous wasting of the adrenal glands from unknown causes is most frequently responsible. Less commonly, destruction of the glands can occur from haemorrhage, tumour, and infection. Failure of the pituitary gland may also result in adrenal insufficiency (secondary adrenal insufficiency). A prolonged use of adrenal steroid hormones can occasion atrophy of the glands and produce symptoms of adrenal insufficiency when the use of the hormones is suddenly discontinued.

The danger: A severe deficiency of adrenal steroid hormones can produce a *Medical Emergency* called adrenal crisis (Addison's crisis), which is usually precipitated by such stressful conditions as infection, surgery, and traumatic injuries. The classic symptoms of adrenal crisis are severe weakness, lethargy, nausea, vomiting, abdominal pain, dehydration, high temperature, and a drastic drop in blood pressure. Ultimately, vascular collapse, coma, and death may follow.
Symptoms: The onset of the disease is usually slow. The predominant symptoms are easy fatigue, fainting spells, loss of appetite and weight, nausea, vomiting, and abdominal pain. Frequently, patients become irritable, depressed, and emotionally unstable. Dark pigmentation in the skin over the knees, elbows, and knuckles is a prominent sign. Pigmentation of the lips and gums is quite frequent. Other symptoms are a craving for salt, anaemia, low blood pressure (hypotension), and a low blood glucose level (hypoglycaemia).

As in Cushing's disease, the diagnosis is established by measuring the adrenal hormone level in the blood, as well as the metabolic products of the hormones in the urine.
Treatment: Adrenal insufficiency is successfully treated with the daily use of adrenal steroid hormones, such as cortisone and prednisone. In adrenal crisis, these hormones must be given intravenously, as well as fluids with salts.

Patients taking steroid hormones should never discontinue them. Furthermore, the maintenance dosage of steroid hormones should be increased to prevent adrenal crisis in any case of undue stress. Every patient who has adrenal insufficiency should carry an identification card describing his condition and providing the name and telephone number of his doctor.

Primary aldosteronism 345
(Conn's syndrome)

Aldosterone, one of the steroid hormones normally produced by the adrenal glands, is responsible for the accumulation of salt in the body. Primary aldosteronism, an excess production of aldosterone, was first described by Dr Jerome Conn, an endocrinologist at the University of Michigan, in 1954.

A single benign adrenal tumour is the most common cause (eighty per cent of reported cases). Less commonly, a diffuse enlargement of the adrenal glands or a malignant tumour may be responsible.

Symptoms: The most usual symptoms are fatigue and muscle weakness. Other signs are numbness and tingling; occasionally, increased thirst and urination may be noted. The elevation of blood pressure is frequently present.

Although primary aldosteronism is an infrequent cause of high blood pressure (accounting for perhaps one per cent), it is important to consider the existence of this condition in all patients with hypertension because the treatment of aldosteronism will correct hypertension. Because some drugs used for the treatment of hypertension (such as thiazide diuretics) can lower the blood potassium level, a low potassium level should be interpreted with caution in patients taking these drugs. In such a case, a repeat evaluation of the blood potassium level when the medication has been stopped is required. Measurement of the blood levels of aldosterone and renin (a hormone closely related to aldosterone) will confirm the diagnosis.

Treatment: Removal of the responsible adrenal tumour is the treatment of choice. In mild cases, aldosterone antagonist (Aldactone) may be employed.

Phaeochromocytoma 346

The inner portions of the adrenal glands (adrenal medulla) normally produce small amounts of epinephrine (adrenalin) and its closely related hormone, norepinephrine (noradrenalin). Phaeochromocytoma is a tumour arising from the secretion of excessive amounts of these hormones by the adrenal medulla. Less frequently, phaeochromocytoma may arise in other parts of the body, such as the abdominal cavity, chest, and bladder. Most phaeochromocytomas are benign, but occasionally they are malignant.

Symptoms: The symptoms include pounding headaches, sweating, palpitations, tremulousness, flushing of the face, and nausea and vomiting. The most important sign is high blood pressure, either sustained or paroxysmal. Although phaeochromocytoma is a rare cause of hypertension (0·1 per cent), recognition of the disease is important because its treatment also cures hypertension. The diagnosis is usually made by measuring the metabolic products of epinephrine and norepinephrine in the urine. In a few cases in which the phaeochromocytoma is only intermittently active, manoeuvres to stimulate the tumour may be necessary.

Treatment: Surgical removal of the tumour is the advised treatment. Prior to surgery, drugs blocking the action of the hormones are used to control the symptoms. These drugs are also employed in cases where the patients have inoperable malignant tumours.

20 Nutritional and deficiency disorders

Louis Arnold Scarrone

Obesity 347

Anyone twenty per cent beyond the average weight for persons of his height, sex, and age is considered obese. Although more common in females up to middle age, obesity is common to both sexes thereafter – and although gaining weight in middle age is normal, so is death. The first can be avoided, the latter delayed. Staying alive and healthy as long as possible can best be accomplished by not being obese. Between the ages of forty and fifty, 4·5kg, 10lb of overweight increase the mortality rate by 3 per cent; 9kg, 20lb by 18 per cent, 14kg, 30lb by 28 per cent, and 23kg, 50lb by 56 per cent. The mortality rate is lowest among those who weigh 5 to 10 per cent below average.

The overwhelming cause is obvious – eating more than is necessary. The basal metabolism rate is usually normal among the obese, attesting to the fact that it is not organic. Appetite has engulfed hunger – we eat not to satisfy our hunger but our appetite.

Other causes include such glandular factors as a diminished output of sexual hormones, the removal of the testes or ovaries, adrenal overactivity, or rarely, hypothyroidism. Too much insulin, resulting in hypoglycaemia, will induce greater hunger and consequently greater consumption. In addition, obesity often results from bad habits of overeating developed in childhood by overeager mothers; a lack of exercise to burn up excess food; enforced inactivity because of prolonged illness; the use of food as a release from nervous tension; the substitution of the pleasure of eating for the lack of other pleasures or unsatisfied sexual needs; and overconsumption following pregnancy (undetermined whether of psychological or hormonal origin).

The danger: If obesity is present for months or years, the incidence of heart and kidney disease rises considerably, as well as that of diabetes, high blood pressure, liver disorders, arthritis, and leg ulcers. An obese person is generally more prone to disease, especially gallbladder diseases and appendicitis and is, in addition, more susceptible to post-operative complications. Overweight women have a greater tendency to serious complications during pregnancy than their thinner sisters.

Symptoms: The basic sign, of course, is fatness. In extreme cases there is also shortness of breath, fatigue, aching back, legs, and feet, signs of high blood pressure, heart failure, diabetes, and arthritis.

Treatment: The ideal daily intake of food is nine calories per pound of ideal body weight as indicated in *Table 13.*

Medication is generally not advisable. The drugs in use are mainly amphetamines, which can cause insomnia, high blood pressure, and heart disease. Other drugs are no less harmful, and their effectiveness in keeping weight off for any length of time is minimal. Any thyroid medication in the absence of thyroid disorder can be quite hazardous. Drug therapy should never be considered without a doctor's advice.

Crash diets are very dangerous. Too rapid a loss of weight may be damaging to the heart, gastrointestinal tract, and normal metabolism. When rapid weight loss is essential, it is best carried out at a hospital. Rocking between gaining and losing weight is equally bad, upsetting body metabolism and possibly inducing atherosclerosis.

Innumerable diet plans, touting a dramatic loss of weight are, in the main, hazardous to health. Some of these diets advocate an unlimited intake of saturated fats and cholesterol-rich foods but avoid carbohydrates. Carbohydrates are essential foods, while saturated fats and cholesterol-laden foods are damaging to the heart and blood vessels.

The ideal body weight indicated in *Table 13* is not always as ideal as claimed. Ten per cent overweight for some might be healthier than the ideal weight. Violent efforts to reduce this weight can often do more harm than good.

Dr Jean Mayer of Harvard believes the best way to determine obesity is to measure the thickness of a skinfold between the shoulder and the elbow point (the triceps) between two fingers: For young boys, the proper thickness should be 12mm, or somewhat less than half an inch; for girls, 14mm, or slightly more than half an inch; for men, 23mm, or about an inch; for women, 30mm, or about a scant one and a quarter inches. The best results are obtained with calipers especially made for measuring the thickness of skin, along with a precise chart for different age groups.

The best regimen is not to limit the diet to special foods but to eat all nourishing foods – only a little less of them. A glance at the calorie chart (*Table 24*) clearly shows that a piece of cantaloupe is nearly four times less fattening than a banana; mushrooms are nearly thirty times more slenderizing than fried potatoes; codfish is not only healthier but provides more than five times less weight gain than hamburgers.

Hundreds of books have been written on how to lose weight, each one with its special secret on how to do it easily. Unfortunately, facts are stubborn things. Weight is arithmetic. Adding 2 and 2 will always make 4.

Certain gimmicks in these books are basically dishonest. For example, sweating, hot saunas – besides putting a strain on the heart and lowering the volume of the blood, the weight loss is only water and will positively return within the week. No amount of massage will take off a gram of weight. Calories do count. Skipping a meal or two will most likely add more weight because of the ravenous hunger developed by the next mealtime.

The only effective way to lose weight and keep it off is a slow, mild change of eating habits. If one is accustomed to eating three slices of toast in the morning and two eggs, cutting down to two slices or cutting out one egg is no really great hardship. If one is in the habit of having two teaspoonfuls of sugar in a cup of coffee, eliminating a half teaspoonful is not difficult. In restaurants it is advisable to have the salad brought first instead of filling up on bread and butter. Substitutions should not be hard but easy – eating whitefish instead of salmon, cottage cheese instead of Cheddar, lean corned beef instead of hamburger, tea instead of cocoa. More fish and less meat means fewer calories and far less cholesterol.

In six months, the sly dieter has eaten 68kg, 150lb less without feeling it. And if he walks an extra mile a day he will lose an additional 2·5kg, 5lb in the same period. In six months he will have reduced his weight considerably without trauma or agony and better still without regaining it. This method will afford him all the vitamins of a well-balanced diet without having to resort to pills.

The benefits of not being overweight are immense, such as removal of strain from the heart and glands, easier breathing, less of a load to carry around, less fatigue, more joy of living, improved physical appearance, less susceptibility to disease, less likelihood of diabetes, varicose veins, and high blood pressure, and less possibility of serious complications in pregnancy.

Vitamin A deficiency 348a

Vitamin A is perhaps the most abundant nutrient found in nature. Any coloured vegetable or fruit, particularly yellow, as in carrots, as well as green and red, contains carotene, a form of vitamin A. It is also available in eggs, liver, and kidneys. Fish liver has the highest content.

Boiling can destroy vitamin A, especially after long cooking in open vessels.

Vitamin A is essential for growth, eyes, cell functioning, a healthy skin and mucous membranes.

Another cause of vitamin A deficiency, besides incredibly poor nutrition, is the malfunction of the body so that it is unable to utilize the vitamin even when it is available. This systemic fault is due to such diseases as sprue, cystic fibrosis, cirrhosis of the liver, ulcerative colitis, bile duct obstruction, pneumonia, scarlet fever, rheumatic fever, diabetes, and hypothyroidism.

The danger: A greater susceptibility to infections and serious eye defects, including destruction of the cornea, which can often lead to blindness if not corrected.

Symptoms: Retarded growth, night blindness, inflammation of the kidneys, horny layers on the skin, dryness of conjunctiva (the eye), ulceration of the cornea.

Treatment: Vitamin A is administered in large therapeutic doses, plus improvement in the diet, under the watchful eye of a doctor. Prolonged large dosages should be avoided because of the considerable danger of *Vitamin A toxicity* **384b**.

Outlook: Usually excellent if the condition is caught early.

Vitamin A toxicity 348b
(hypervitaminosis A)

A rare condition resulting from an overenthusiasm for vitamin A by food faddists (consuming 80,000 units a day or more), vitamin A toxicity is characterized by a loss of appetite, falling hair, pain in the joints, irritability, and headaches. Overdosage can retard growth in children and mimic brain tumour by increasing the fluid pressure inside the skull.

Treatment obviously consists of the elimination from the diet of excessive vitamin A. The recommended daily allowance for infants is 1,500 IUs, up to 3,500 for children, 5,000 for adults, 6,000 for pregnant women, and 8,000 for nursing mothers.

Vitamin B₁ (thiamine) deficiency 349

(beriberi)

Beriberi, the severe form of thiamine deficiency, is no longer a significant disease in the western world, although isolated cases still occur. The disease occurs mostly among people who have taken to eating polished rice when natural rice is the staple food (thiamine is in the husk, not in the grain). A mild thiamine deficiency is fairly frequent, however, particularly in alcoholics, patients with hypothyroidism, chronic diarrhoea, severe liver damage, and pregnant and nursing women who have a greater need for thiamine.

Deficiency in vitamin B₁ is usually found in those people who have a high intake of sugar and processed cereals and a very low intake of protein and fresh green vegetables. Vitamin B₁ is plentiful – whole grain cereals, all meats (organ meats in particular), eggs, vegetable greens, fowl, and nuts.

The danger: Vitamin B₁ deficiency can occasionally cause death from beriberi and heart disease unless promptly treated.
Symptoms: Beriberi begins with a loss of appetite and weight, followed by neuritis (a prickling and numbing sensation in the legs and feet and other parts of the body), emotional instability, cramping pains in the legs, a difficulty in walking, a rapid heartbeat, difficulty breathing, and fatigue.

Later symptoms are swelling and the collection of fluids in the tissues (wet beriberi), congestive heart failure, or a depressed appetite causing severe emaciation (dry beriberi).
Treatment: Vitamin B₁ orally from 10 to 100mg. If there is serious heart involvement, the vitamin is given by hypodermic injection.
Outlook: If the disorder has not been current for too long, the outcome is excellent. Symptoms can be reversed with time and a good diet and supplements. The recommended daily allowance of vitamin B₁ is about 1·5mg for both children and adults.

Vitamin B₂ (riboflavin) deficiency 350

A deficiency in vitamin B₂ is no longer common except in cases of severe malnutrition, diseases of the liver, or chronic diarrhoea. Riboflavin is essential for well-being, vigour, growth, and healthy skin and eyes. Foods that contain riboflavin are liver, brewers' yeast, milk, vegetable greens, beef, pork, eggs, and fowl.

The danger: Serious eye disease.
Symptoms: Vitamin B₂ deficiency is characterized by glossitis (the tongue may become large, inflamed, reddish to reddish purple, and fissured), chapped lips or cracks around the corners of the mouth, and dry, scaly, red skin around the nose, ears, and scrotum. The eyes, however, present the most significant symptoms – cloudy or ulcerated cornea, impairment of vision, photophobia, and a burning sensation in the conjunctiva. Additionally there is general body weakness.
Treatment: The administration of riboflavin (10 to 25mg daily in several equal doses, tapering off to 3mg until full recovery) along with other vitamins to help in its absorption. The recommended daily dosage is around 2mg for both children and adults.
Outlook: If treatment has not been delayed too long, a full cure is usual.

Vitamin B complex (niacin) deficiency 351

(pellagra)

Although niacin is plentiful in most foods, niacin deficiency is still prevalent in most areas of the world, occurring principally where diets are high in corn. Niacin is found in liver, whole grain cereals, lean meats, fish, fowl, peanuts, milk, potatoes, and leafy vegetables.

Niacin is not only essential for the proper utilization of carbohydrates, the metabolism of tissue, and the maintenance of a healthy skin, but also for the well-being of the nervous system. A severe deficiency of this vitamin results in pellagra and produces neurological, gastrointestinal, and skin disorders.

The danger: Serious gastrointestinal disorders and brain lesions. Before the discovery of this vitamin, two-thirds of pellagra patients died.

Symptoms: The early symptoms are weakness and a loss of appetite and weight. Later there are headaches, gastric disturbances, red symmetrical spots on the skin, which turn brown and become larger and scaly (usually in body areas exposed to sunlight or rubbed by clothing). The margins of the tongue and the mucous membrane of the mouth become scarlet, and salivation is increased. Diarrhoea is an early symptom later becoming more intense and bloody.

The psychological signs may be confined to insomnia, headaches, and poor memory but are more likely to go into irritability, depression, irrational behaviour, dementia, and violence.

Treatment: The daily administration of 300 to 1,000mg of niacin orally in divided doses, plus an improved diet. If there is diarrhoea, the vitamin should be given intravenously. The results are excellent.

The recommended daily allowance is about 13mg for women, under 20 for men, and from 8 to 15 for infants and children.

Vitamin C deficiency 352

(scurvy)

Scurvy, once a serious and common ailment, is now a rare disease. Until the inclusion of lime in the English sailor's diet, British seamen died in droves; hence the name of 'limey'. Today vitamin C

deficiencies are still seen in bottle-fed infants whose mothers neglect to add fruit juices to their diets, people of low income with peculiar eating habits, among pregnant and nursing women, and in those suffering from thyrotoxicosis (an overactivity of the thyroid gland) who have an increased vitamin need.

Vitamin C is found in most fruits, especially citrus, melons, and berries, tomatoes, cabbage, and dark green leafy vegetables (broccoli, green peppers, Brussels sprouts). Vitamin C is basic for the health of blood vessels, teeth, and gums and essential for bones, connective tissue, and cell structure. It is absolutely vital for life, and nature has made it abundant in our food supply.

The danger: Anaemia, internal haemorrhages, coma, and eventual death if not treated.

Symptoms: Scurvy is characterized by weakness, easy fatigue, listlessness, bleeding gums, loose teeth, fragile bones, and bleeding under the skin and in the mucous membrane. In infants the symptoms – a loss of appetite, irritability, failure to gain weight, swollen gums, painful joints and bones – do not appear until after four months of age.

Treatment: High dosage of vitamin C (from 500 to 4,000mg daily) or large amounts of fresh, pure orange or grapefruit juice. The normal daily allowance is about 70mg for children and adults.

Outlook: Treatment is almost always effective.

Vitamin D deficiency 353a

(rickets, osteomalacia)

Unlike other vitamins, vitamin D is not found in abundance in natural foods, although some is provided by fish liver oil (most fat fish), liver, eggs, and food with vitamin D added, as is now customary in the preparation of milk. A source of vitamin D, however, is simply the action of sunlight on the skin. Those persons rarely exposed to sunshine and those with dark skins often need supplementary vitamin D, which is essential for the metabolism of phosphorus and calcium (to maintain bones and teeth).

The danger: Infants with neglected rickets will develop permanent bone deformities.

Symptoms: In infants, rickets is characterized by restlessness, a softening and thinning of the skull and weakness of the bones throughout the body, noted by knock-knees, bow-legs, and pigeon breast. The teeth are badly formed. At the indicated age, the infant can neither walk, sit, nor stand. Later, children develop kyphosis (spinal curvature).

In adults, chiefly women, a vitamin D deficiency can end up in osteomalacia with symptoms of pain in the pelvis, limbs, and spine with progressive weakness.

Treatment: Vitamin D plus additional calcium and phosphorus. Very large doses of vitamin D can be toxic (*Vitamin D toxicity* **353b**).

Outlook: Excellent if too much time has not elapsed.

Vitamin D toxicity 353b
(hypervitaminosis D)

Excessive vitamin D can cause loss of appetite and weight, nausea, weakness, excessive urination, calcium deposits under the skin, hypertension, kidney failure, and death. In pregnant women it has been known to cause a narrowing of the aorta in the foetus.

Of all the vitamins, vitamin D is the most dangerous when taken to excess. The recommended daily allowance is 400 IU for both children and adults. Some people can tolerate high dosages of this vitamin, but many cannot. Damage has been noted in children on a daily dosage as low as 2,500 IU. Overdosage can cause irreversible damage.

Treatment: Instant removal of vitamin D from the diet, which should also be low

in calcium. If calcification has already set in and kidney damage has occurred, the condition is probably irremediable.

Vitamin K deficiency 354
(hypoprothrombinaemia)

Normal blood clotting requires vitamin K, which is produced by the bacteria that permanently inhabit the colon. Since the colon is sterile for the first five days of an infant's life, and a consequent vitamin K shortage exists, circumcision and other operations are often not performed in the first week of life.

Additional vitamin K is obtained from such foods as milk, liver, cabbage, spinach, cauliflower, other green leafy vegetables, soybean oil, and tomatoes.

A deficiency in vitamin K can result from various conditions, including a lack of bile salts, which are essential for the proper absorption of vitamin K by the body; a diminution of the bacterial source of vitamin K in the colon that results when oral antibiotics and sulpha drugs are administered to combat intestinal bacteria; the administration of mineral oil as a laxative, which prevents absorption of vitamin K; such gastrointestinal disorders as ulcerative colitis, regional enteritis, sprue, and coeliac disease; the restriction of the flow of bile salts by an obstruction of the liver or gallbladder; and anticoagulant therapy.

The danger: Bleeding emergencies, especially gastrointestinal and intracerebral haemorrhage.

Symptoms: The failure of the blood to clot will cause bleeding from various organs – the nose, gums, vagina, and stomach. There may also be blood in the urine.

Treatment: Vitamin K in doses as high as 15mg daily, although 2mg is usually effective if it is properly absorbed. An injection of vitamin K in time can save a patient from many complications. The daily requirement remains unknown.

All-vegetarian diet deficiency 355

Pure vegetarians (vegans) are those who do not include milk and eggs in their diet with resultant harm to themselves and their children. They are depriving themselves of vitamin B_{12}, iodine, and often certain essential amino acids not found in fruits or vegetables.

Vitamin B_{12} is absolutely vital for the formation of red blood cells. A deficiency results in anaemia and pernicious anaemia, as well as glossitis (inflammation of the tongue) and such nerve disorders as numbness and twitching. Vitamin B_{12} is found in meat, fish, eggs, and milk. The daily requirements are 5 micrograms.

All-out vegetarians may also deprive themselves of iodine, which is basic to thyroid function.

Vegetarians who also drink milk and eat eggs are not in this category; they may, in fact, be following a very excellent health programme with proven results of a longer, healthier life.

Salt deficiency 356

Five grams of salt are needed daily. This hardly poses a problem in the United Kingdom where the average intake is 12g, ½oz or more (all processed food contains salt). In fact, to our detriment, we eat too much salt. However, salt deficiencies do occur, mostly from over-exertion, such as intense exercising during hot weather, causing a massive loss of sodium chloride through sweating. Chronic diarrhoea and vomiting will produce the same result.

Symptoms include stomach pains, a flabby skin, scanty urine, twitching muscles, apprehension, a faint, rapid pulse, and in extreme cases, convulsions. The administration of salt tablets will alleviate the condition.

Iron deficiency
See **Anaemia 322**

21 Infectious diseases

Randolph M. Chase, Jr

Fungal diseases
Histoplasmosis **393**
Coccidioidomycosis **394**
(valley fever, San Joaquin Valley fever,
desert fever)

(Note: other infectious diseases not listed above will be found under the specific category involved such as *Meningitis* under *The brain and nervous system, Gonorrhoea* under *Venereal diseases*, and so on.)

Not so long ago – and still true in many less advanced countries – life expectancy for the majority, because of the toll of infectious disease, was not more than thirty years. Today, thanks to the magnificent advances in this field of medicine, the overwhelming majority, wherever modern medical aid is available, survives into middle and old age. The control of infectious diseases is perhaps man's finest achievement in the ceaseless war against disease.

All infectious diseases derive from five major sources: bacteria, viruses, parasites, rickettsiae, and fungi.

Bacteria: antibiotics and sulpha drugs have provided a means of effectively dealing with these diseases.

Viruses: a variety of chemical agents have become available for specific viral diseases; the major thrust against these ailments has been the development of vaccines.

Parasites: most of the major parasitical diseases have been prevailed over with new drugs that either inhibit or destroy particular parasites.

Rickettsiae: antibiotics and sulpha drugs work on rickettsiae as well.

Fungi: the majority of fungal infections can now be controlled and often cured by newly developed drugs, but a few remain that are resistant.

BACTERIAL DISEASES
Whooping cough 357
(pertussis)

Caused by *Bordetella pertussis*, whooping cough is characterized by a paroxysmal cough with a whooping sound. A most serious infection in the first six months

of an infant's life, it is responsible for more infant deaths than diphtheria, scarlet fever, and polio combined, with half of all cases occurring before the age of two. All ages are affected, however, those most susceptible and in the greatest danger being the extremely young and old.

Contagion: Highly contagious, the disease is transmitted by airborne droplets from an infected patient, who remains infectious through the eighth week of illness.

Incubation: From 5 days to 2 weeks with a maximum of 21 days.

Duration: Average is about 6 weeks – 2 weeks' incubation, 2 weeks' full-blown illness, and 2 weeks' convalescence.

The danger: In infants there is danger from asphyxiation, pneumonia, and cerebral complication resulting in death; it ranks first in infant mortality. The complications of bronchopneumonia can be fatal in the elderly. Whooping cough can also precipitate permanent damage of the lungs in the forms of chronic bronchitis and emphysema. In older children the disease is not generally serious.

Symptoms: Beginning like a cold – runny nose, sneezing, tearing, small hacking cough, loss of appetite (usually no fever or very low) – the characteristic 'whooping' cough develops later. The paroxysmal cough – coughing a dozen times or so in one breath with the final catching of breath in a whooping or crowing intake of air – is repeated many times with only a few normal breaths in between. It produces a thick gagging phlegm, which in children is usually swallowed, causing vomiting. The white blood cell count is high.

Frequently this disease is difficult to distinguish from bronchitis or flu; a microscopic examination of a smear will reveal the causative organism.

Treatment: A beneficial effect is attained with immune globulin used intramuscularly in conjunction with one of a variety of antimicrobial agents (ampicillin, tetracycline) for patients under two years of age and other patients with severe whooping cough.

Since seriously ill infants can frequently choke to death, they should be hospitalized where emergency treatment – suction of phlegm, the administration of oxygen, and even tracheotomy – is available. At home an electric suction apparatus should be kept on hand for emergencies. Cough medicines are valueless and can even cause further vomiting.

Occasionally convalescence may be delayed with persistent heavy coughing. The child should be carefully watched and protected against other respiratory infections during this period.

Prevention: All exposed infants and susceptible persons should be given immune globulin and removed from the premises in which someone is ill with whooping cough.

All infants are normally routinely given DPT (diphtheria, pertussis, tetanus) vaccine by the fourth month, followed by two more injections a month later, unless considered unsuitable.

Outlook: With prompt and effective medical care, fatalities among very young infants, which can run as high as 25 per cent, can be reduced to 1 per cent. One attack usually confers lifelong immunity. In older children and adults the disease runs a troublesome but generally benign course.

Diphtheria 358

Fast-moving, dreaded diphtheria, which once proved fatal for one-third of its victims, has been almost completely eradicated, but not quite – it still presents a threat. The causative bacteria, *Corynebacterium diphtheriae*, produces an exotoxin, a deadly poison, that destroys tissue, attacking the mucous membrane of the throat and sometimes the nose and larynx. Although it strikes children from one to ten for the most part, adults are not immune.

Contagion: Extremely contagious, diphtheria is transmitted by air and contact with secretions from the nose and mouth of a patient or an asymptomatic carrier and by infected milk. All patients must observe the strictest quarantine until full recovery. All susceptible persons, the very young and the old, should be removed from the vicinity and their immune status should be determined.

Incubation: From 2 to 5 days.

Duration: A week of active symptoms, usually followed by long, slow recovery, often quite prolonged if there are complications.

The danger: If antitoxin is administered late, there can be heart damage, pneumonia, and nerve palsies. Death can occur from airway obstruction, heart failure, or paralysis of the respiratory muscles.

Symptoms: Diphtheria may begin with a deceptively mild sore throat, followed by fever, headache, vomiting, and foul mouth odour. The telltale sign is a greyish false membrane appearing in the throat or nose, which is firmly attached and causes difficult breathing. The voice is husky, respiration noisy, swallowing difficult, throat swollen. In extreme cases, there may be prostration, difficulty in breathing, and cyanosis. Paralysis may involve the palate, the nerves of the eye, the larynx, or any part of the body to which the toxin has been carried by the bloodstream.

Treatment: In severe cases this disease presents a *Medical Emergency*. The patient should be hospitalized where treatment is available for such sudden emergencies as total obstruction of the airway (requiring tracheotomy), heart failure from the toxin affecting the heart muscle, or complications from pneumonia or central nervous system involvement.

Antitoxin (hyperimmune globulin) and penicillin should be administered as early as possible – on the very first day even if the diagnosis of diphtheria has not been fully determined. This cannot be stressed too strongly. If the vaccine is not given early, the morbidity and mortality rate rises precipitously, despite massive doses later. Penicillin eradicates the bacteria; the antitoxin neutralizes the unbound or loosely bound diphtheria toxin.

Diphtheria antitoxin is available as horse serum or human hyperimmune globulin. Since reaction to an animal serum can often be extreme, preliminary tests are essential; if the patient is sensitive to the vaccine, it can be delivered in a number of small shots of gradually increasing amounts.

Recovery from diphtheria is slow; too early a resumption of normal activities can be fatal if the patient has developed toxic myocarditis (inflammation of the heart muscle). During the illness the patient should be watched constantly for airway obstruction. Bed rest is absolutely essential.

Prevention: All infants should be routinely given DPT (diphtheria, pertussis, tetanus) vaccine followed by two more injections a month apart, and a booster injection one year later. Additional booster injections are given on entry into school. The Schick test will indicate whether the child is susceptible to diphtheria.

Failure to provide a child with these shots can be tragic. Most of the deaths from these diseases are a result of negligence in taking these simple precautions.

Outlook: No patient is considered cured until two throat cultures taken two days apart are negative. Recovery without residual effect is usual.

Scarlet fever 359
(scarlatina)

Caused by Group A streptococcus, scarlet fever is defined by a red rash over the entire body. Persons of both sexes and all races and ages are susceptible, although the incidence is lowest in infancy, rises thereafter, and peaks before adolescence; it is rare in the tropics. One attack usually confers immunity. Although the virulence of scarlet fever has diminished in recent years it remains a serious ailment, the major threat being its complications.

Contagion: Although contagion is very high, some patients will develop only a mild case and others will be asymptomatic carriers. Scarlet fever is airborne by droplets or by close contact with the patient. All patients should be kept in isolation.

Incubation: From 1 to 4 days, appearing abruptly.

Duration: From 1 to 2 weeks.

The danger: With the advent of antibiotics, the dangers of complications – inner-ear infections resulting in permanent deafness, nephritis, pneumonia, meningitis, encephalitis, and rheumatic fever – have been minimized, but they still exist.

Symptoms: The disease appears abruptly with frequent vomiting, a fever as high as 40·5°C, 105°F, and a red, raw, swollen sore throat. The characteristic symptom is a heavy, white, furred tongue with enlarged red papillae (white strawberry tongue). This layer soon peels, revealing a bright all-strawberry colour. Pinpoint scarlet spots appear on the already inflamed palate. There may also be a yellowish grey exudative membrane over some of the inflamed areas of the mouth or pharynx.

On the second day a collection of tiny, red, densely packed dots, which blanch when pressed, spreads over the body, beginning at the neck and chest. Darker red lines appear over the rash at the skin folds. The face is deeply flushed except around the mouth (a prime characteristic of this disease). Enlarged lymph nodes appear in the neck.

After the eighth day, the skin in the area of the rash begins to peel, a process that can persist for weeks. The urine is highly coloured and scanty. The white blood cell count is high.

Treatment: Penicillin should be administered promptly, even before full identification is made. *Important note:* even in the mildest cases antibiotics should be maintained for a minimum ten days to forestall rheumatic fever.

Continued bed rest is governed by the patient's condition. Good nutrition is important. Fever can be controlled by tepid water sponge baths (aspirin for older patients). A painful swollen neck can be relieved by hot or cold compresses. A constant watch should be maintained for infectious and noninfectious complications.

Prevention: Complete prevention is not presently possible because of some healthy-appearing carriers. School-age children should avoid scarlet fever patients. (See *Part 3, Early warning signals, Scarlet fever* **359**.)

Outlook: Prompt medical care can make this a comparatively benign ailment.

Blood poisoning 360
(septicaemia, bacteraemia, sepsis)

Blood poisoning occurs when bacteria get into the bloodstream and spread to distant parts of the body. It indicates that the body is unable to contain the organisms at the site of infection. Blood poisoning can follow a tooth extraction, tonsillectomy, carbuncle, and even minor scratches, cuts, or burns. Most deaths from illegally performed abortions are due to blood poisoning, because of aseptic conditions.

The danger: An untreated or unresponsive septicaemia (from poor or impaired resistance) can prove fatal from either damage to vital organs or from general toxaemia resulting from toxins in the blood. Death can occur in two days if not treated, especially in children or the elderly. Early recognition of the symptoms can preserve life.

Symptoms: Blood poisoning is characterized by a severe shaking chill; an irregular, variable, and intermittent fever; severe headaches; temporarily acute diarrhoea; periods of profuse sweating, especially when the fever falls; skin rashes, with minute or extensive haemorrhages into the skin turning black and blue, and pustules and blisters as well.

Vascular collapse (failure to supply body tissues with a sufficient supply of blood) is most common.

Treatment: Large doses of a bactericidal antibiotic (usually penicillin) are indicated, coupled with other supportive measures as determined by the patient's condition. Cure is indicated by the absence of bacteria in blood samples and the eradication of the seeding focus (the site of the original infection).

Prevention: All wounds should be cared for as soon as they are recognized. If there is an inordinate purulence on the skin or an unusual reddening around the injury, a doctor should be consulted at once.

Outlook: The chances for full recovery are best with vigorous and prompt medical treatment.

Tetanus 361
(lockjaw)

A grave acute infection (causative bacteria *Clostridium tetani*), which affects the central nervous system and causes acute muscular contraction, particularly of the jaw and neck, tetanus attacks males three times more often than females.

The *Clostridium* genus of bacteria is probably the most devastating lethal microorganism that afflicts man, causing *Botulism* **165** and *Gas gangrene* **362** as well. The organism is found in the soil everywhere in the world, in the manure of grass-eating animals, and in the stools of most mammals. Injuries on the farm are potentially more dangerous than elsewhere. The two characteristics that make this bacteria particularly deadly are its anaerobic nature, which means they thrive in the absence of oxygen, and its toxins, which are the most potent poisonous substances known. Any deep though minor-appearing injury, such as stepping on a nail or a tack or even being pricked by a thorn, which can seal itself, thus making the wound airless, provides this organism with the proper environment to multiply and produce its toxins. This toxin attacks the nerves, resulting in spasms and convulsions. Tetanus is easy to prevent but difficult to cure.

The common belief that the offending agent must be a 'rusty' nail is important only as an indicator of a lack of cleanliness – dirt not rust is the bacterial medium. Tetanus can occur from shrapnel wounds, lead pellets, bullets and postpartum injuries; drug addicts who use unsterilized needles are particularly susceptible.

Incubation: From 3 to 12 days but can range up to 20 or more.
The danger: The lower the incidence of disease the better. Adequately immunized people never get the disease. About forty per cent of all unimmunized victims of tetanus die either of paralysis of the diaphragm (respiratory failure), heart failure, asphyxiation, exhaustion, or starvation.
Symptoms: Onset usually begins with headache, low-grade fever, irritability, apprehension, and restlessness. The first real sign of tetanus is a stiffness of the jaw and difficulty in opening the mouth. Muscular stiffness can also develop in the neck and elsewhere. The patient yawns frequently. The disease may come on rapidly. Muscle spasms can also occur in any skeletal muscle in the body. Most agonizingly, the patient remains alert. He cannot open his mouth or swallow; his eyebrows become raised; the corners of his mouth become upturned, giving the appearance of a perpetual grin. By the third day any minor event, such as a sudden noise, a jar of the bed, or a light touch, may set off excruciating violent spasms lasting for fifteen minutes. As noted, throughout the convulsive muscle contractions, the patient remains alert and aware. (Strychnine poisoning can produce similar symptoms.)
Treatment: This is a *Medical Emergency.* Early hospitalization is essential. Much depends on the early administration of tetanus antitoxin (preferably human hyperimmune globulin). Although antitoxin cannot neutralize the toxin already bound to the nerves, it can render harmless the newly produced unbound toxin.

Local reaction at the site of the original wound is usually nil. If the original wound

can be found, it should be reopened if it has healed and the dead tissues surgically removed. Additional treatment is supportive and directed at controlling the convulsive reaction with the use of muscle relaxants and sedation. Continuing nursing care is vital. Tracheotomy is usually necessary in moderate to severe cases.

Although antibiotics have no effect on the toxins, they are nevertheless given simultaneously to eradicate the bacteria. In non-allergic patients penicillin is the treatment of choice for all clostridial strains.
Prevention: Today tetanus appears only as a result of gross neglect. The routine administration of DTP (diphtheria, pertussis, tetanus) vaccine in infants and tetanus toxoid in adults is 100 per cent effective in producing immunity.
Outlook: A lack of sleep and nourishment can make the patient susceptible to other diseases and great care should be taken during the period of convalescence to guard against complications. Survivors generally suffer no permanent ill effect. Illness, however, does not confer immunity. Immunization procedures are imperative.

Gas gangrene 362

Like tetanus, gas gangrene is caused by a member of the *Clostridium* genus (*Clostridium perfringens*). The anaerobic bacteria enter the tissues from deep, penetrating wounds. Once established, they multiply rapidly and produce the toxins that kill the surrounding tissue and the red blood cells. Gas gangrene is particularly seen in auto accidents, where tissue is damaged by broken glass and infected by dirt, and in illegal abortions performed in unsterile conditions. The disease can strike quickly; the patient may go into shock and die before a doctor can evaluate the extent of the injury.

Note: gangrene itself is not a bacterial disease; it is the death of tissue, the physical change that occurs when the blood supply is cut off. Gangrene can appear in strangulated hernia, in acute appendicitis, in a pedunculated (on a stalk) tumour, in frostbite, and in many other conditions. Although gangrene should be distinguished from gas gangrene, which is caused by bacteria and extracellular toxins, the results are the same.

Incubation: Gas gangrene strikes quickly, often in as little as six hours after the initial wound or injury.

The danger: Gas gangrene and gangrene are very grave disorders, which may end in amputation and death. This is always a *Medical Emergency*.

Symptoms: The site of the wound becomes very painful and tender. Pressure at the margins of the wound will produce gas bubbles emanating from the pinkish fluid oozing from the injury. A characteristic crackling sound can be elicited when the area is rubbed or pressed with the fingers (the gas moving in the tissues). The skin around the wound becomes dusky, bronze-like, dark, and then black. In severe cases there may be prostration, delirium, and coma.

Treatment: A polyvalent antitoxin (serum) is available and often used, although thought to be of questionable value by some authorities. The accepted procedures are surgery, antibiotics, and more recently, the use of hyperbaric oxygen (oxygen under pressure). Treatment must be swift. Amputation is often a desperate but life-preserving measure when the local removal of dead tissue does not stop the progression of the disease.

Prevention: All deep, dirty wounds, particularly those with damaged blood vessels, must be seen immediately by a doctor.

Typhoid fever 363

A severe, highly infectious systemic disease, typhoid fever is caused by the bacillus *Salmonella typhosa*, which lives in human faeces and is spread by flies, contaminated sewage, and careless infected food handlers. Contaminated water,

milk, and shellfish are other prime sources; outhouses and toilet facilities situated too near wells and sources of drinking water also contribute to its incidence.

Incubation: About 2 weeks is average but may vary from 1 to 3 weeks.

Duration: Typhoid may persist for 5 weeks or more.

The danger: Most of the fatalities are due to complications, such as inner-ear infection, bronchitis, and pneumonia. The major complications include intestinal haemorrhage and/or perforation leading to *Peritonitis* **179**. A sudden drop in temperature within the first two weeks does not mean improvement but may herald perforation – a *Medical Emergency*.

Symptoms: Beginning like the flu, with a frontal or bitemporal headache that lasts well over a week, the fever increases day by day, reaching 40·5°C, 105°F and levelling off at that figure for a week. During this period of high fever, the patient is often half conscious and in a muttering delirium. The fever tends to be lower in the morning and higher at night. Nosebleeds are frequent, rosy spots appear mostly on the trunk and abdomen; the abdomen is very distended, a slight cough is common, the pulse is slow, the tongue is coated white or brown with reddened edges, and constipation is usual but may give way to bloody diarrhoea. When diarrhoea appears, it may become dominant (six times a day or more), which may indicate a gastrointestinal complication, making this a *Medical Alert*. Relapses are frequent, but the duration of a second attack is usually shorter.

The abrupt appearance of typhoid with immediate, severe symptoms usually means an early convalescence. Ambulatory typhoid, with symptoms so minor that the patient refuses to stay in bed, is insidiously dangerous – the patient is a sitting duck for intestinal perforation.

Treatment: Antibiotics are the basic medication (ampicillin, chloramphenicol) and should be administered for a full three weeks to lessen the incidence of relapse. Blood in the stools and urine should be guarded against. The patient should be constantly observed for complications. Haemorrhage and excessive diarrhoea are ominous signs and require hospitalization.

Bed rest during the acute illness is vital. The long siege requires provision against bed sores (air mattresses can save much grief). Patients who are delirious must not be allowed to leave their beds for any reason because of the hazards of complications. Scrupulous attention should be paid to faeces and urine disposal. All possibly infected clothing and articles must be sterilized.

Prevention: Although vaccines are available none are totally protective. Everyone should beware of 'typhoid Marys', asymptomatic carriers who shed typhoid organisms in their stools. Travellers to endemic countries are well advised to avoid the water, ice, unsterilized milk, and shellfish.

Outlook: Prompt antibiotic treatment has cut the mortality rate down from a high of 14 per cent to a low of less than 1 per cent. The recurrence of fever (without other symptoms) during convalescence may not be signs of a relapse but merely due to some slight stress. Guarding against complications during recovery is an effort very well spent.

Cholera 364
(Asiatic cholera, epidemic cholera)

Although today cholera occurs rarely in the Western world, this infamous worldwide disease is still an active pestilence that is capable of exploding into a full-fledged epidemic wherever sanitation is poor. An overwhelming infection caused by a bacteria that looks like a comma (*vibrio comma*), cholera is characterized by massive diarrhoea, dehydration, and collapse.

Contagion: Extremely contagious, cholera is spread by water and food contaminated by the faeces of those ill with the disease. Persons with mild infections

or asymptomatic carriers are often instrumental in the epidemic dissemination of this pestilence.

Incubation: From a few hours to 6 days; the average is 3 days.

The danger: Death occurs within a few days if not hours in 60 per cent of untreated cases. Treatment reduces mortality to 5 per cent. The victim must survive dehydration and salt depletion from diarrhoea and vomiting or have salt and water effectively replaced.

Symptoms: Onset is sudden and extreme with constant diarrhoea (the patient can lose as much as ten litres, twenty quarts of fluid a day). The stools are of rice-water consistency and voluminous. Other symptoms include severe stomach and leg cramps, violent but effortless vomiting without nausea, an intense thirst, a cyanotic, cold, clammy, wrinkled skin, and total collapse.

Treatment: Although the body is able to kill off the bacteria rather quickly, survival is dependent on resupplying the incredible fluid loss caused by the toxins produced by the bacteria. Antibiotics are of limited value; the basic procedure is to replace the great loss of fluids by saline solutions given intravenously, rather than to destroy the bacteria. On occasion, the quantity of fluids replaced has been staggering, amounting to twice the body weight of the patient. In addition, iced drinks, frequent drinks of glucose water, and keeping the body warm with blankets and a hot water bottle are helpful.

Prevention: A visit to cholera endemic countries should be preceded by immunization. Careful hygiene, however, provides the only sure protection against cholers.

Outlook: If a resupply of fluids can be achieved and maintained, loss of life can be prevented and recuperation assured.

The plague 365
(bubonic plague, 'black plague', Black Death

One of the most devastating bacterial disseases, 'black plague' killed 100 million people in one epidemic and in another three-fourths of the population of France. Fatalities in the various forms of the disease run from 30 per cent to 90 per cent. The *Pasteurella pestis* bacterium is conveyed from rodent fleas (the rat in particular) to man and in the pneumonic (respiratory) variety from man to man. The disease, however, is quite rare except in tropical countries particularly India, and has been seen in the United Kingdom as a laboratory infection.

Incubation: From 2 to 5 days.

The danger: If untreated, death will occur in most cases from widespread bacterial damage to the brain, kidneys, and lungs or from shock in three to six days. In the pneumonic form the toll is ninety per cent in three days, with death occurring in many instances within hours after onset.

Symptoms: The onset is sudden. The patient experiences chills, very high fever, rapid heartbeat, a staggering gait, stupor, and prostration. The most important sign is the development of buboes (inflamed lymph nodes) in the groin, axilla, and other areas. Ranging in size from crab apple to apple, the buboes may become filled with pus and drain. The minute bleeding spots into the skin, which turn black, have given the disease the name Black Death. Final stages are shock and coma.

Treatment: Antibiotic therapy (streptomycin and tetracycline) is the medication to combat this disease. A heat-killed vaccine is available for persons of high risk and will produce protective immunity.

Bacillary dysentery 366
(shigellosis)

A highly infectious disease of the large colon, which is caused by the *Shigella* bacteria, bacillary dysentery occurs in big city slums, overcrowded communities where sanitation facilities are poor.

Incubation: From 1 to 4 days.

Duration: Usually 4 to 8 days, but in severe cases 3 to 6 weeks.

Contagion: The faeces of infected subjects harbour the bacteria. The disease is transmitted by careless infected food handlers and flies.

The danger: In previously healthy adults, bacillary dysentery is a self-limiting disease. The mortality in children in the United States is less than one per cent. Malnutrition is a main factor in higher incidences of mortality.

Symptoms: The onset of the disease is sudden, with constant diarrhoea and soft liquid stools. The fluid loss is considerable. Other symptoms are abdominal pain, thirst, nausea and vomiting, and a constant urge to defecate without results. The characteristic sign is blood, pus, and mucus in the stools after three days. Relapses and reinfection are frequent.

Differential diagnoses: Such diseases as salmonella gastroenteritis, ulcerative colitis, sprue, coeliac, and amoebic dysentery often have similar symptoms. A rectal swab sent for culture can identify the organism and the disease.

Treatment: Antibiotic therapy has been questioned since this is a self-limiting disease; however, ampicillin, chloramphenicol, and tetracycline are effective. Sulphonamides are no longer in use. Fluid and electrolyte replacement is the most effective method of restoring the patient's well-being. Relieving agents are a hot water bottle and paregoric.

Prevention: All food should be protected from flies. Windows should be screened. All exposed clothing and towels must be disinfected. Good personal hygiene is essential.

Outlook: If treatment is prompt and thorough, recovery is excellent.

Traveller's diarrhoea 367
(Montezuma's revenge, la turista)

No one knows much about this disorder, but it is usually mild and of bacterial origin. Some people are more affected than others. In the more advanced countries the dangers are not any higher than in the United Kingdom, but in less developed lands, especially in small towns, villages, and out of the way places, the traveller would be well advised to avoid milk, cheese, yogurt, and local highly spiced dishes. Eating bland foods and not overeating can often prevent this disorder. Drinking water, water used for brushing the teeth, even ice, should be boiled first or treated with water purification tablets. Eating uncooked food or fruit and vegetables that cannot be peeled is risky, as are unbottled soft drinks.

When visiting doubtful countries the traveller should be certain he has taken required immunization.

Commercial preparations of kaolin and pectin can be included in the traveller's medical kit for mild cases. For a more serious attack a local doctor should be consulted.

Safe foods: well-cooked meats, bread, peelable fruits, alcoholic drinks, beer, wine, bottled mineral water.

Leprosy 368
(Hansen's disease)

Leprosy is no longer the dread ailment it once was. Although it is contagious, it is the least contagious of all infectious diseases – only prolonged, intimate contact with someone who has the active form of the disease will allow infection to occur. The organism, *Mycobacterium leprae*, is similar to the TB germ, which also has the waxlike coating, making it difficult to kill. Leprosy is found worldwide, but is rare in the UK.

Incubation: From 4 to 20 years; usually requiring close and prolonged contact.
The danger: Disfigurement, loss of sensation, destruction of tissue and bone, and loss of hair. Death can occur from other intercurrent infections (TB or pneumonia) after long years of the disease.
Symptoms: The onset is insidious. Red or brown patches that develop white

centres appear on the skin. The patches grow in groups, enlarge, and spread, often enveloping the face and giving the patient a leonine appearance. Small, hardened nodules appear on the legs, feet, or face. A loss of feeling occurs in various parts of the body, which is noticed only after that part is injured by trauma. A loss of feeling occurs in the coloured patches and often in a complete extremity, a hand or a foot. The voice becomes hoarse, body hair falls out, notably the eyebrows and lashes. Additionally, there may be a painful neuritis, a wasting of the bone, open sores that penetrate deeply into the tissues, causing deformity and loss of toes and fingers (spontaneous mutilation), nose bleeding, and atrophy of the muscles (the wasting of muscles in the hand produces a clawhand).
Treatment: Persons long associated with lepers should be closely examined for the presence of the bacteria. Often the germ cannot be found, however, and the symptoms are the only means of identification. The earlier the treatment the better the chances of recovery.

The sulphones (not the same as sulpha drugs) have been effective but not totally satisfying. Rifampicin has been demonstrated to be a worthwhile agent and is currently recommended in conjunction with sulphone (dapsone).
Prevention: Isolation of the bacterial-positive untreated patient is warranted. The guidelines for postexposure prophylaxis in highly susceptible contacts (children) have not been established. However, the separation of children from lepromatous parents who are under effective treatment may no longer be necessary.

Relapsing fever 369

Relapsing fever is endemic in Southern Europe, in Africa, especially Ethiopia, in the Middle East, Northern India, Central and South America, Western USA and Canada, but not in the United Kingdom. It is a recurrent infectious fever transmitted by lice or ticks. The spirochete bacteria (same family as syphilis) enter the abraded skin from infected blood or body fluids released from a crushed louse or from a tick bite.

The danger: The mortality rate in the general population is less than five per cent, although it is higher among the very young, the old, and the debilitated.

Symptoms: The disease is characterized by chills, high fever, rapid heartbeat, severe headaches, vomiting, muscle and joint pain, profuse sweating, and a rose-coloured rash on the trunk and extremities. Jaundice may also appear.

The distinguishing symptom that differentiates relapsing fever from similar diseases, such as malaria, yellow fever, smallpox, and typhus, is the symptom that named it, the recurrent nature of its attacks. Relapsing fever can abate, dropping to a normal temperature only to appear again and again with concomitant high fever. The duration of each attack ranges between two and three days with intervals of a week between. Its behaviour is much like a bouncing ball, dying down a little with each bounce. The disease spends itself after three relapses.

Treatment: Bed rest and broad-spectrum antibiotics (tetracycline) will hasten recovery. Codeine is advised for severe headaches.

Prevention: All tick bites should be considered dangerous; they can produce other, even more serious, diseases. A tick must never be removed forceably (*Table 19: Wood ticks: how to remove them*). Louse control and tick control will, of course, reduce disease incidence.

VIRAL DISEASES
Measles 370
(morbilli)

Measles, a supposedly benign disease, is not so benign. It is a highly contagious generalized infection characterized by a rash involving the entire body. Children are primarily affected, but adults contract measles more often than suspected.

Contagion: High; spread by droplets from nose, throat, or mouth.

Incubation: From 7 to 14 days.

Duration: From the first catarrhal symptom, measles will persist for ten days.

The danger: Although the disease itself is not very serious, the patient can become susceptible to additional viral and bacterial diseases such as pneumonia tuberculosis, middle-ear infection, and the dreaded measles encephalitis. *Acute encephalitis* **8** is a serious, potentially crippling and fatal complication that occurs in 0·1 per cent of measles cases. The most frequent period of encephalitis onset is usually between the second and sixth day after the rash has appeared, but it can also occur during the pre-rash or post-rash period. Most complications usually develop after the rash fades. If the disease lasts longer than the indicated time, a new disorder may be developing.

Symptoms: Beginning like a cold, with runny nose, the temperature skyrockets and is difficult to bring down. It is accompanied by a harsh hacking cough. On the second day the eyes become bloodshot, conjunctivitis appears, and the patient is troubled by photophobia. On the third day the first telltale sign, Koplik's spots (white spots surrounded by a rosy area on the mucosal inner surface of the cheeks), appears. On the fourth day (or any time from the third to the fifth day) the rash appears, first on the scalp and temples, then the neck and over the entire body. The brownish pink, slightly elevated spots, which run into each other, begin to disappear after two or three days, although a brownish pigmentation can remain for several days.

Treatment: Nonspecific, but the patient should be kept in complete isolation for two weeks. The high fever can be brought down by tepid sponging baths or aspirin. Dark glasses should be provided for acute photophobia. Bacterial infections should be appropriately treated with antibiotics. Parents should maintain a watchful eye for any signs of complications.

Human gamma globulin (convalescent serum) can often prevent or check the disease after known exposure.

Prevention: An effective measles vaccine is available and provides sound immunity. Immune globulin is also of great value in the unvaccinated exposed child. The clinically involved child should not be allowed to return to school in less than fourteen days from the appearance of the rash; an exposed child in not less than sixteen.

Outlook: One attack usually confers a life-long immunity.

German measles 371
(rubella, three-day measles)

In children this is a mild viral illness with a well-known rash, but in pregnant women rubella is a very serious illness with serious consequences (*German measles in pregnancy* **244**). About 70 per cent of the cases occur in children from ages three to twelve years; 25 per cent range from twelve to forty.

Contagion: High. The disease is spread by droplets from the nose and mouth.
Incubation: From 14 to 21 days.
Duration: About a week. The rash usually disappears in three days.
The danger: A woman who contracts German measles during early pregnancy is in a hazardous situation. The danger to her unborn infant is great enough to warrant terminating the pregnancy, because of the risks of stillbirth, crippling heart malformation, retardation, permanent deafness, or cataracts.
Symptoms: The disease begins with a slight fever and a slight runny nose and sore throat. Then a light rose-coloured rash appears, beginning on the face and neck and finally covering the entire body. The specific sign is swollen lymph nodes behind the ear and in the neck just below the back of the head. There may also be some stiffness in the joints. In adults lassitude and a slight headache occurs. The rash disappears in two to three days.
Treatment: None is necessary except for pregnant women who have never had the disease and have been exposed to it in the first three months of pregnancy. The doctor may advise a gamma globulin injection or if warranted, interrupt the pregnancy.
Prevention: Rubella vaccine should be given routinely to all young girls long before childbearing age. An adult woman who receives the vaccine must wait at least two months before becoming pregnant.

Chicken pox 372
(varicella)

A mild viral disease with a distinctive eruption involving the entire body, chicken pox most often affects children but adults are not exempt. By the time a child has reached fifteen there is a seventy-five per cent chance he has had the disease. Infants are immune for the first six months.

Contagion: One of the most contagious of all the infective diseases, the infectivity of chicken pox is strong from the first sign until after the outbreak of the blister-like spots (vesicles). It is usually contracted by direct contact with someone who has the disease or by droplet from the nose or mouth.
Incubation: Average 13 to 17 days, but can stretch to 21.
Duration: About two weeks.
The danger: Secondary infections, often serious, from scratching the vesicles. Occasionally there may be ear involvement and inflammation of the kidneys.
Symptoms: The itching skin eruption begins as a spotty rash (macula), which soon develops into raised pimples (papules) and then into teardrop blisters (vesicles), which finally crust. Several of these stages can exist at the same time. The transition from rash to scab takes about four days. A particular feature of this disease is its severity in adults, when it causes headache, backache, high fever, chills, and a high incidence of complication.

Chicken pox is a self-limiting disease.
Treatment: Rest is advised until all the

blisters have crusted. When *only* crusts remain, the patient is no longer contagious and can be freed from isolation. Scratching should be restrained. In younger children where this is not feasible the child's hands should be kept scrupulously clean and the nails cut very short.

Basic treatment includes alleviation of itching, which can best be accomplished by calamine lotion or zinc oxide with starch and bicarbonate of soda in equal parts made into a paste with water. Bathing in water in which starch has been added can greatly reduce the itch. (Water will not aggravate the rash or blisters.)

The need for a doctor is indicated when the temperature goes above 39°C (102°F) or if the skin lesions become infected or haemorrhagic. There are no vaccines for chicken pox. One attack confers permanent immunity.

Prevention: (See *Part 3, Early warning signals, Chicken pox* **372.**)

Outlook: Always full recovery.

Smallpox 373
(variola)

Smallpox is a highly contagious viral infection with epidemic potential, affecting all ages and races. During the Middle Ages, epidemics of this infection killed off as much as a quarter of the population of Europe. Now comparatively rare in developed countries, it is, nevertheless, still a serious threat in the poorer lands of the world. Those who survive acquire permanent immunity. (Alastrim, also known as whitepox or milkpox, is a mild, nonfatal form of smallpox.)

Contagion: Extremely high. The patient remains very infectious until the *last* crust disappears. Transmission is by droplets from the nose and throat or by any contact with the patient, including the handling of *any* material touched by the patient, such as clothes, books, silverware, and other innocent objects. All persons in contact with the patient should be immune or vaccinated.

Incubation: From 1 to 2 weeks.

Duration: The acute illness from 2 to 3 weeks, convalescence another 2 to 3 weeks.

The danger: In untreated cases, death is the frequent termination in the severe form of this disease. The battle is a fight against permanent disfigurement from pockmarks, which occur from the larger blisters. Mortality remains high in the very young and the old. Other complications are gangrene of the skin, iritis, nephritis, and pneumonia.

Symptoms: Starts suddenly with very high fever and violent frontal headaches. There is intense backache, muscle pain, convulsions in children, occasional nausea and vomiting, delirium, and a rapid pulse.

On the third day large crops of small reddish pink spots (maculae) appear, spreading over the face, forearms, and the rest of the body. In severe cases the crops become massive. Within a few hours they become pimples (papules). By the fifth or sixth day they have blistered to about the size of tack heads. The blisters (vesicles) are surrounded by a red area, are dimpled, and will not collapse when pricked. On the ninth day the fluid in the blisters becomes pustular; the blisters soon dry into foul-smelling scabs (crusts), which are contagious. The crusts finally drop off in three to four weeks.

The differentiation between chicken pox and smallpox can be determined by the fact that in chicken pox all four stages of skin eruption can appear at the same time, while in smallpox each stage appears uniformly and at one time, tending to relatively spare the trunk and concentrate on the extremities, head, palms, and soles, more intensively.

Treatment: This is a *Medical Alert.* The patient should be in an isolation hospital, so as not to infect his contacts and where his chances of recovery are also much greater. Antibiotics are often used to treat secondary bacterial infection of the blisters to avoid additional disfigurement. All substances in contact with the patient must be considered contaminated. Treatment is basically supportive and symptomatic with care in preventing the disease from getting worse. Early vaccination will accord five to seven years' immunity.

Prevention: The best and only real prevention is vaccination. However, vaccination should not be performed during pregnancy, general viral illness, or if a diffuse skin rash exists. The use of steroids or immunosuppressive therapy is also a contra-indication to vaccination.

Vaccine immune globulin, if available, should be used in conjunction with vaccination in susceptible contacts. Methisazone (Marboran) has been employed in prophylaxis of those exposed persons who cannot be vaccinated.

Outlook: The disease is now so uncommon that routine vaccination has been discontinued. The risks of vaccination outweigh the possibilities of acquiring the disease in the United Kingdom.

Polio 374
(poliomyelitis, infantile paralysis)

A viral infection caused by one of three distinct types of polio virus that attacks the central nervous system and can result in muscle paralysis, polio can strike at any age, although children are most often affected. There are two forms of the disease; the minor illness (abortive polio), which is nonparalytic, has only mild symptoms, and lasts only a few days, and the major illness, which involves a weakening and paralysis of the muscles. Many people have the mild form without ever knowing it. They are fortunate in that immunity is acquired as in the major illness.

Polio is endemic throughout the world. The disease is milder in the epidemic form than in isolated cases. The development of the Salk and Sabin vaccines has practically reduced the incidence of polio to zero for those who avail themselves of this therapy.

Contagion: Dissemination was thought to occur by the spread of droplets from nasal secretions. Present evidence indicates, however, that polio is spread by the anal-oral route, by faecally contaminated water, food, flies, and other insects.

Incubation: Average, 7 to 12 days, but can range from 3 days to a month or longer.

The danger: In the major illness about half those infected will suffer weakness and paralysis of the muscles and occasionally death from paralysis of the respiratory muscles. Prompt treatment, possibly a tracheotomy, and respiratory care can prevent death.

Symptoms: The onset is abrupt – high fever, severe headache, sore throat, and fretfulness on the first day. The patient will resist sitting up unless the legs are flexed. In the mild form these may be the only symptoms, and the child may seem to get well. However, this can be a most critical period. If the patient is allowed to get up and go about his normal routines, he may relapse into the major illness. Complete bed rest is vital since there is a close correlation between physical activity early in the major illness and the incidence of subsequent paralysis.

The symptoms on the second day or so are more specific – stiff neck, deep muscle pain, severe weakness, prostration, tremors and twitching of the muscles and paralysis in the legs, arms, and body. Early signs of bulbar (brain stem) involvement are difficulty in swallowing and a nasal voice.

Treatment: Once the disease has taken hold there is no specific treatment. In the paralytic form there are some procedures that can lessen the damage to muscles, such as the use of hot water packs on the affected muscles and early physical therapy – the earlier the institution of physical therapy the greater the return of muscle facility. For a patient with respiratory muscle damage, the use of a mechanical respirator can save his life. Tracheotomy has often been employed when pharyngeal muscle failure has caused air obstruction or when coughing is impaired by weakened muscles.

Prevention: Polio is preventable but not curable. Either the Salk (inactivated) vaccine or the Sabin (live attentuated) vaccine given early in infancy confers immunity. The disease can be totally prevented by universal vaccination.

Mumps 375
(epidemic parotitis)

A very common generalized viral infection that encompasses the salivary glands, mumps, in adults, can also affect the testicles and less commonly the ovaries. Children between five and thirteen years are most vulnerable. A mild disease in childhood, beyond puberty mumps can be quite serious.

Contagion: High. By droplets from infected saliva – sneezing, coughing, breathing – or by coming in contact with any contaminated article handled by the patient.

Incubation: Average, about 17 to 18 days but can vary from 12 to 26.

Duration: After the appearance of the first symptom, mumps persists for approximately three weeks.

The danger: In males beyond puberty mumps can cause *Orchitis* **253** with atrophy of the subjected testicle. Mumps can have an adverse bearing on other organs, including the heart, thyroid, and central nervous system, as well as predispose towards *Acute pancreatitis* **166**. In the first four months of pregnancy mumps can lead to deformity of the foetus.

Symptoms: A moderate to high fever appears shortly after the onset of the swelling of the salivary glands under the jaw or in front or below the ear, bilaterally or unilaterally. Swelling and pain may be considerable.

A simple test before distinctive symptoms have appeared is to have the patient eat a pickle or suck a lemon. If this act is very painful or impossible the disease is suggested. Pain may increase on opening the mouth or swallowing.

Saliva is usually scanty but can also be excessive; it is, however, never normal. The mouth is dry, the tongue is furred, and the lymph nodes in the neck are enlarged. Swelling usually disappears by the tenth day.

Treatment: There is no specific treatment. The patient should be isolated and kept at rest for eight days. A good mouthwash is helpful, as is a soft or liquid diet to avoid painful chewing and swallowing. Hot or cold compresses over the affected areas give some relief. If the testicles are affected, *Orchitis* **253** describes the proper treatment.

Prevention: Children would do well to contract mumps early in childhood. After puberty, males who have not had the disease and have been exposed to it should be immunized. Passive immunization with mumps immune gamma globulin is of questionable value. Live attenuated mumps vaccine confers transient immunity (four years) but should not be given to pregnant women or to those who are allergic to eggs or to neomycin; it has been successfully combined with measles and rubella virus vaccine in terms of immunity and safety.

Outlook: One attack of mumps confers a lifelong immunity in greater than ninety-five per cent of all cases.

Flu 376
(influenza, grippe, intestinal flu)

A severe but ordinarily short-lived disease, flu is a respiratory infection caused by three groups of viruses identified as A, B, and C (Asian flu is type A). Each group has a number of different variants, but each variant produces a similar disease that differs only in its intensity. Very young children usually escape this ailment during an epidemic, but young adults in good health seem prone to attack. Flu can strike in epidemic explosions anywhere, anytime.

Contagion: Very high. Spread by droplets from sneezes and coughs.

Incubation: From 1 to 3 days.

Duration: The acute phase of the illness runs for 4 to 5 days, but lassitude and fatigue can persist for weeks or even months.

The danger: The complications of pneumonia among the old or those weakened by a chronic or debilitating ailment, as well as bronchitis, sinusitis, and inner-ear infection, are all frequent consequences of the flu.

Symptoms: Flu comes on abruptly with chills, considerable fever, severe head pain, and aches in the back, muscles, and joints. Weakness to the point of prostration, excessive fatigue, and sweating are common. There are mild cold symptoms, such as runny nose, sneezing, sore throat, dry or hacking cough, conjunctivitis, and a flushed face.

If gastrointestinal symptoms, such as vomiting or diarrhoea, are present, the disease is often called intestinal flu.

Treatment: Although no specific treatment is available, rest in bed will diminish the intensity and duration. Isolation, if possible, is advised because of the great infectiousness of the disease. Flu vaccines are available but are specific for a particular virus strain. Each epidemic usually heralds the emergence of another type, making control of this disease quite difficult.

If fever, cough, and sore throat continue for longer than three or four days, the likelihood of bacterial pneumonia is considerable, in which case the cough may worsen and be coupled with shortness of breath and other signs of respiratory insufficiency. This can be a particularly vicious form of pneumonia with a very high and rapid mortality among elderly patients with pulmonary or heart disease.

No person can be considered cured until he no longer suffers from weakness or fatigue.

Prevention: The old, the debilitated, those with serious cardiac, pulmonary, or chronic disorders should be vaccinated with the specific type of flu that is prevalent. This may require yearly boosters, but it can be lifesaving. During outbreaks, those most susceptible should avoid crowds, and not allow themselves to become overfatigued, making sure they get plenty of rest.

If it is necessary to be in close contact with a flu patient, a strict sterilization programme should be followed regarding clothes, towels, dishes, and napkins.

Outlook: In uncomplicated flu, full recovery is usual. If bacterial pneumonia develops, antibiotics appropriately prescribed can almost always result in control and cure.

Infectious mononucleosis 377 (glandular fever)

A seemingly mild viral illness affecting mostly young adults from the ages of 15 to 21 infectious mononucleosis is rare after thirty-five. It is often an elusive disease to diagnose, its symptoms ranging from being barely noticeable to a severe, debilitating illness. Diagnosis is made by finding atypical lymphocytes (a type of white blood cell) and employing a special serum check called the Paul-Bunnell test.

Contagion: Little is known about how this disease is transmitted. It is often called the kissing disease but how true this designation is no one can say with assurance. The patient remains infectious for seven days after fever and the swelling of the glands have subsided.

Incubation: From 5 to 15 days from contact.

Duration: From 2 weeks to 2 months. The fever may last 3 weeks; weakness and debilitation may last for weeks and even months.

The danger: The patient should be alerted to the fact that his spleen is highly vulnerable to easy rupture by trauma, a dangerous development. During the acute illness no heavy exercise should be limited.

Mononucleosis may affect the liver and present a picture of infectious hepatitis.

Symptoms: The onset is sudden or insidious with fever, headache, and sore throat. The major symptom is a painful swelling of the lymph nodes under the jaw, which usually occurs on the second or third day. Lymph nodes in the axilla (under the arm) and in the groin can also become inflamed and swollen. Weakness and fatigue are characteristic of mononucleosis. The patient is listless, has no appetite, gets recurrent daily headaches, and often daily low-grade fever, all of which may continue for weeks or months.

A generalized rash occurs in about ten per cent of the cases, and there is occasionally jaundice. The patient may feel unwell for from two to six months.

Treatment: There is no treatment for the disease itself, only for each symptom. If mononucleosis is severe and accompanied by thrombocytopenia (an abnormal decrease in blood platelets), steroid therapy may be justified.

Relapses do occur. Bed rest during the active stage is wise.

Prevention: Mononucleosis shows up more frequently among those with histories of physical excesses or those who are suffering from exhaustion. No organism has been isolated, but a viral agent is presumed to be the factor.

Outlook: Total recovery is the rule.

Rabies 378
(hydrophobia)

Rabies is a dread viral disease caused by the bite of a rabid animal. It is rare in the UK but has been seen recently when quarantine laws for animals have not been observed.

The virus is in the saliva of the animal. In furious rabies it is due to the bite of an animal maddened by the disease; in dumb (paralytic) rabies it may be due to licking by a pet with characteristic excessive saliva. In dumb rabies, although the animal does not bite, *the disease is transmitted just the same.*

Incubation: About 40 days, although extremes may run from 6 to 180.

The danger: Untreated rabies is 100 per cent fatal.

Symptoms: The bite usually heals, but the site remains red and inflamed. The patient is at first depressed and irritable

but soon becomes excitable and wild. Salivation becomes profuse; drooling occurs because of the inability to swallow. Although the patient may be thirsty, he cannot drink because of agonizing pain; his reaction is one of fear at the sight of water, hence the name hydro (water) phobia (fear). Finally, paralysis, coma, and death. Treatment with vaccine seems to be the better way.

Treatment: In addition to a local cleansing with soap and water, flushing with benzalkonium chloride (a surface disinfectant), and a deep swabbing of the wound, it should be infiltrated with rabies antiserum to mechanically remove viral particles.

Systemic antirabic treatment is accomplished by the administration of either nervous tissue (NT) vaccine or duck embryo (DE) vaccine. Either course of therapy is protracted and includes fourteen daily injections and boosters on the tenth and the twentieth day after the two-week series. The vaccine has serious side effects on the nervous system, but reactions are less severe with the duck embryo vaccine.

Bites around head, neck, or face need a quicker determination regarding the administration of the vaccine, since the virus has a shorter distance to travel to reach the brain.

Yellow fever 379
(yellow jack)

Once a deadly affliction, decimating populations of cities over the world, yellow fever is now rare but still exists in tropical and subtropical areas.

The disease is transmitted by the infected *Aëdes aegypti* mosquito (Greek *aëdēs* means unpleasant).

Incubation: From 3 to 6 days after the bite, but may be longer.

The danger: In isolated cases the disease is comparatively mild, but in epidemic form it can be raging with fatalities running from 50 to 85 per cent.

Symptoms: The disease has two stages.

The onset is sudden, with fever, prostration, severe headaches, pain in the back and limbs, flushed face, and scanty urine. On or about the second day the fever falls and convalescence seems to begin. But around the third day the disease returns with a recurrence of the fever and the other symptoms, along with jaundice and the vomiting of black blood. The pulse rate is slow in relation to the fever. The symptoms may persist for as long as a week. In the extreme form, bleeding from the nose, mouth, and gastrointestinal tract can occur.

Treatment: There is no specific treatment. Bed rest and good nursing are most important. If vomiting is intense, intravenous replacement of the lost fluids and control of the nausea are essential. Vitamin K is administered in haemorrhagic conditions.

Prevention: Vaccination confers immunity up to ten years. Those travelling in sub-Sahara Africa and southeast Asian countries are required to be vaccinated.

Dengue fever 380
(breakbone fever)

A common viral disease of warm countries, dengue fever is transmitted by mosquito and is very rarely fatal.

Incubation: From 5 to 6 days, ranging from 3 to 16.

Duration: Several weeks with attendant weakness and fatigue after the acute phase.

Symptoms: Dengue appears suddenly, with chills, high fever, and severe headaches. Pain is felt in the back of the eye when the eyeball is moved. Pain in the muscles and joints can be so severe as to cause prostration, hence the name 'breakbone fever'. The fever drops and the symptoms disappear, but this period of calm lasts for only a day or so, when symptoms return with a lower fever and the onset of a measles-like rash.

Treatment and outlook: There is no specific therapy. Treatment consists of taking plenty of fluids, complete bed rest, and the liberal use of aspirin. Complete recovery is the rule.

Common cold
See **Common cold 63**

German measles in pregnancy
See **German measles in pregnancy 244**

PARASITICAL DISEASES
Malaria 381

The most widespread infectious disease of mankind, resulting in high morbidity and mortality, malaria is caused by four species of *Plasmodium* parasites, which produce various forms and degrees of the disease. Infection is transmitted to man by infected female *Anopheles* mosquitoes. On a worldwide basis, several hundred million people are affected at any given time. The disease is often seen in soldiers and travellers returning from tropical foreign lands.

Contagion: Malaria is caused by a protozoan that lives in the red blood cells of humans. The parasite leads a most complicated life. It begins its life cycle as an undeveloped parasite in the abdomen of the *Anopheles* mosquito, migrating to the salivary glands. When the mosquito bites a human being the parasite is released into the bloodstream and then to the liver where it matures. It returns to the bloodstream where it attaches itself to a red blood cell and multiplies. The life cycle is continued when the infected person is bitten by another *Anopheles* mosquito.

Malaria has also been contracted by blood transfusion in which the donor fails or forgets to notify the doctor of previous malarial infection and by the common use of syringes (drug addicts who have had malaria can transmit the disease in this manner).

Incubation: From 10 to 35 days after the mosquito bite.

The danger: Death from malaria is rare except in that form caused by the parasite *Plasmodium falciparum* or in malaria complicated by other infectious disease.

Symptoms: The disease has three distinctive phases: severe teeth-chattering chills, which last from ten to thirty minutes; extremely high fevers, as much as 40·5°C, 105°F, with severe headaches, vomiting, diarrhoea, rapid pulse, and rapid breathing, which last from four to six hours; and following the fever's decline, a drenching sweat.

The bouts of fever return in intervals, ranging from one to four days, depending upon the type of parasite involved. Malaria can become chronic; relapses are common, the disease reappearing from time to time, especially with *Plasmodium vivax* parasite. Eventually, malaria burns itself out. Frequent attacks or severe disease can cause progressive anaemia.

Treatment: Chloroquine is most effective except in the deadly, resistant *Plasmodium falciparum* variety, in which case quinine or pyrimethamine are used. Another useful medication is primaquine.

Prevention: Prevention of malaria is dependent on the individual and mosquito control. The World Health Organization has demonstrated that the mosquito can be exterminated (as has been done in many countries) by vigorous eradication efforts, including the spraying of breeding places and the drainage of large and small stagnant pools.

Amoebic dysentery 382 (amoebiasis)

Amoebic dysentery is caused by *Entamoeba histolytica*, an amoebic parasite that invades the intestines. It exists in two forms, the active free state and the encysted state, in which they are excreted in the stools. Ten per cent of the world's population is said to harbour these parasites. Although typically a tropical disease, amoebic dysentery is more related to poor hygiene and inadequate sanitation than climate.

Contagion: Spread by sewage-contaminated drinking water, the transmission of the amoeba from human faeces to food by flies and insects, and food handlers who are negligent about their toilet habits, but is almost never contracted in the United Kingdom.

The danger: Severe amoebic dysentery can be a serious threat to life. Untreated, the disease can give rise to liver abscess, severe dysentery progressing to bowel perforation, peritonitis, and death.

Symptoms: In the mild form there may be irregular bowel movements with nausea, headache, and flatulence. Ulceration of the bowel results in amoebic dysentery of variable intensity. In the more common form, there is extreme diarrhoea (from ten to twenty bowel movements daily). The stools can be either fluid or semifluid with mucus, pus, and blood. Other symptoms may include abdominal pain, usually on the right side, weight loss, prostration, and deep fatigue, often coupled with chills and fever.

Treatment: In severe cases bed rest with support and fluid replacement to offset losses from diarrhoea. A battery of amoebicidal drugs is available, the most effective being metronidazole (Flagyl), which is the treatment of choice as well for amoebic liver abscess, coupled with surgical intervention where indicated.

Amoebic dysentery has a tendency to relapse; no one should be considered free of the disease until three separate examinations of the stools reveal no amoeba.

Prevention: The elimination of amoebic dysentery is dependent upon strict sanitary control, strict personal hygiene, and adequate sewage disposal, which should be remote from sources of drinking water. Travellers in suspect countries should boil all drinking water and avoid raw fruit and vegetables. Acceptable fruits are those that can be peeled. Particular care should be practised in countries where human excrement is used for fertilization of the soil.

Bilharziasis 383
(schistosomiasis)

Bilharziasis is a major world health problem, particularly in the Near East, Africa, the Caribbean, and South America. There is no risk of transmission in Europe, but the disease may be imported. The disease is caused by an extremely tiny flatworm, which spends part of its life cycle in the snail and the other part in man. Man becomes infected by swimming or bathing in snail-infested streams or rivers or working in rice paddies in which the free-swimming cercarial worm, having left the snail, enters the body of man, penetrating the skin, invading the bloodstream, and travelling to the liver, where it matures and mates. The fertile female penetrates the mesenteric veins and deposits eggs. The eggs are sent out into the world through the walls of the intestines and bladder into the faeces and urine.

The danger: Repeated infections proceed to ulcerations of the intestines and liver, biliary tract disorders, and anaemia.
Symptoms: A temporary smarting redness where the worm enters the body, followed a month or so later by abdominal pains, skin rash, a swelling of the face, limbs, and genitalia. Later a loss of blood and a reaction to the eggs in the organs result in the changes associated with bilharziasis, anaemia, chronic fatigue, and general ill health.
Treatment: A number of antimony drugs are competent against the parasite, but they have serious side effects. A newer drug, niridazole (Ambilhar), has been demonstrated to be effective. Cure is determined when eggs are no longer evident in the stool, urine, or tissue.
Prevention: The proper disposal and sanitation of human excreta is basic. Prevention depends upon breaking the infectious cycle. Snail control has yet to be proved effectual.

Toxoplasmosis 385

A serious parasitic disease affecting the central nervous system, the lymph nodes, and the spleen, toxoplasmosis results from eating undercooked pork, beef, and mutton. The high infection rates in cats implicates this domestic animal, which excretes the parasite *Toxoplasma gondii* in its stools, but rodents, cattle and other animals also transmit the disease.

The danger: The severe congenital form can be fatal in early infancy.
In a pregnant woman toxoplasmosis is particularly dangerous and can result in spontaneous abortion; if the child survives, the disease can cause brain damage, retardation, hydrocephalus, and blindness.
Symptoms: The patient is subject to body rash, chills, high fever, inflammation of the heart muscle, swelling of the lymph nodes, severe headaches, hepatitis, and enlargement of the spleen. The subacute form mimics *Infectious mononucleosis 377*.
Treatment: The recommended therapy is pyrimethamine (Daraprim) in conjunction with sulphadiazine.
Outlook: For those patients in whom the disease has been detected early and treated, the outlook is good, but for those who have reached a chronic phase, the prognosis is poor.

Trichinosis 386
(trichiniasis)

Trichinosis acquired from ingesting insufficiently cooked pork, is due to the parasite *Trichinella spiralis*, a slender roundworm barely visible to the naked eye. The worms mature quickly, mate, and within a few days give birth to live young, which travel throughout the body and eventually encase themselves inside the muscle fibres.

Incubation: From 7 to 15 days after eating contaminated insufficiently cooked pork.
The danger: Frequently trichinosis in

the severe form can result in pneumonia, auditory disorders, meningitis, and a more serious and often fatal possibility, the invasion of the brain or of the heart muscle, which can give rise to heart failure. However, most infections are minor and many people have no symptoms at all.

Symptoms: A swelling of the face, particularly around the eyes, upper eyelids, and forehead, occurs, accompanied by a high fever, a soreness to acute pain and swelling in the muscles of the body invaded by the parasites (especially in the respiratory and swallowing muscles). Profuse sweating is common; headache is frequent. In the very early stages of the disease there is usually gastric distress, nausea, and diarrhoea. In severe cases, if the parasites have invaded the respiratory muscles (diaphragm and chest wall), there is great shortness of breath.

Treatment: Thiabendazole (Mintezol), a broad-spectrum antihelminthic, may be helpful, but has not been demonstrated effective against encysted larvae. The disease, however, most often is self-limiting. Steroid therapy is best for relief in the severe form of the disease and in central nervous system infestation.

Prevention: Uncooked or poorly cooked pork should not be eaten. With effective meat inspection and laws to prevent the feeding of garbage to swine, trichinosis can be eliminated.

Outlook: Recovery is the rule.

Roundworm 388

(ascariasis)

One of the largest parasites, the roundworm often measures 35cm in length. It looks like an earthworm with tapered ends. Ascariasis is caused by faecal contamination of the soil. The eggs enter the body through contaminated water, food, or by soil-contaminated hands. When the parasite reaches the intestines, it develops into a full-fledged worm and lays eggs.

Incubation: From 6 weeks to 3 months in the human body; one year in the soil.

The danger: Roundworms can cause mental retardation in children.

Symptoms: Vague colicky pains in the abdomen, loss of weight, and malnutrition. There may also be easy fatigue, irritability, skin rash, abdominal swelling, diarrhoea, and the pulmonary symptoms associated with worm migration.

Treatment: Piperazine (Antepar) is the curative treatment, or Bephenium granules (Alcopar) in a single dose.

Prevention: Proper sanitation and good personal hygiene will help avoid this disease. The use of human excrement for fertilizing vegetation remains a worldwide problem. Pet dogs that have worms should be kept away from children until treatment is completed.

Threadworms 389

(enterobiasis)

Infection caused by the threadworm is found throughout the world. Less than a half inch in length, it lives in the lower part of the small intestine and the upper part of the colon. During sleep, the female emerges from the anus and lays her eggs in numbers approaching 10,000, causing severe itching in and around the anus.

Threadworm. (*Julian A. Miller*)

Incubation: From 3 to 6 weeks.

The danger: Although believed by many doctors, the theory that threadworms cause appendicitis remains unsubstantiated.

Symptoms: The infection is characterized by painful itching, restless sleep, poor appetite, and a failure to gain weight. The worms can be seen in the stools as small wriggling white threads.

Treatment: Since each female lays about 10,000 eggs, which are microscopic and very light, the disease is difficult to control because the eggs are spread everywhere. The intense itching causes the patient to scratch, getting these tiny eggs under his fingernails and eventually to his mouth, where the cycle begins again. The eggs are also found in clothing, bed sheets, and even in the air.

Piperazine (Pripsen, which also contains standardized senna) or Viprinium (Vanquin) is very effective and can be taken in a single dose. Equally essential are daily showers to wash away the eggs and washing the hands and nails before every meal.

Prevention: Meticulous personal hygiene. All infected material, pyjamas, bedclothes, underwear, should be washed with soap and hot water daily.

Tapeworm 390

Not as common as threadworm infestation but still quite common, infection caused by tapeworm occurs from eating improperly cooked meat (beef, pork) or fish (fresh water) contaminated with tapeworm larvae. The worm settles in the intestines, eating the food it finds there and sucking blood. Some tapeworms can measure ten feet or more in length.

The danger: In fish tapeworm severe pernicious anaemia (B_{12} deficiency) is a significant consequence.

Symptoms: The patient suffers abdominal pain, diarrhoea, mild toxaemia, exhaustion, and a loss of appetite rather than the common belief of a voracious appetite. Segments of the worm are seen in the stools.

Treatment: A new drug, niclosamide (Yomesan) rendered in a single dose. This should be followed by a saline purge of magnesium sulphate (30ml).

Prevention: All beef, pork, or fish should be thoroughly cooked. Eating steak tartare is living dangerously, especially in communities where the incidence of tapeworm occurs.

RICKETTSIAL DISEASES

Neither bacteria nor a virus, the micro-organism known as rickettsia is much smaller than bacteria and larger than a virus.

Typhus 392
(epidemic typhus, European typhus, louse typhus; also murine typhus)

An infamous, deadly, worldwide affliction, which killed three million people in eastern Europe at the end of World War I, typhus is a disease of epidemic proportions, constantly threatening to break out, especially in wartorn countries and wherever poverty, famine, or disaster occurs. It is transmitted by body lice. (Murine typhus is a disease of rats, transmitted from rat to rat by the rat flea, which has no hesitation about biting man and giving him the disease as well.)

Incubation: From 6 days to 2 weeks.

The danger: Mortality can be very high in epidemic typhus, rarely, if ever, in murine typhus. The aftermath can cause pneumonia and nephritis.

Symptoms: The characteristics of the disease include a high fever (up to 40·5°C, 105°F and lasting ten days), severe headaches, body aches, prostration, a furry white tongue, a flushed or dusky face, and bloodshot eyes. In four to five days a rash, dark to pinkish red mottlings, appears over the body with pinpoint bleeding under the skin, which turns purple. The face is usually not affected. When the fever breaks, profuse sweating occurs.

The pulse is rapid and weak; the headache is a characteristic sign; stupor may change to delirium and coma. The pupils may be contracted with muscular twitching, and the urine may be highly coloured and scant. Vascular collapse and renal failure are usually terminal events.

Treatment: Broad-spectrum antibiotics (especially tetracycline) are most successful but should be administered early in the illness. Chloramphenicol is indicated for gravely ill patients. The fever can be controlled by sponging. The patient should be kept in strict isolation, and all his clothing should be disinfected.

Prevention: Meticulous cleanliness in overcrowded, impoverished areas and war zones, along with louse control and immunization, with killed rickettsial vaccines are indicated. These vaccines, however, do not protect fully.

Outlook: Those treated early survive, usually with no aftereffects, although the convalescent period may be long.

FUNGAL DISEASES

Systemic fungal infections can run the gamut from quite mild to deadly. The fungi include not only mushrooms and toadstools but also very tiny organisms such as moulds and yeast.

All fungal infections respond well to amphotericin B, a specific agent used for the treatment of systemic fungal infections. Some fungal diseases were considered hopeless and untreatable until amphotericin was developed. The side effects of the drug, however, are appreciable.

Histoplasmosis 393

The droppings of pigeons, chickens, and bats provide an optimal environment for the growth of the spores of the soil fungus *Histoplasma capsulatum.* Histoplasmosis, which is acquired by the inhalation of the spores, is most apt to occur in rural, humid areas.

The danger: Although the acute form of the disease in endemic areas is either undetectable or present as a mild respiratory disease, the severe form, progressive disseminated histoplasmosis, can be fatal and tends to affect infants of both sexes and old men more commonly.

Symptoms: About a third of the patients develop ulcerations on the tongue, palate, larynx, or other gastrointestinal sites. The fever is irregular and there may be ulcerations of the stomach, with vomiting, diarrhoea, and black tarry stools. Weakness, emaciation, and the involvement and swelling of the lymph nodes, liver, and spleen are common findings.

A chronic form simulates TB of the lung with chronic cavitation.

Treatment and outlook: The mild form is usually benign; the progressive disseminated form if untreated is inevitably fatal. Amphotericin B reduces mortality in this form significantly.

Coccidioidomycosis 394 (valley fever, San Joaquin valley fever, desert fever)

Coccidioidomycosis is nowhere near as obscure as its complicated name suggests. A highly infectious fungal disease, it occurs via inhalation, with the highest incidence around new housing developments or wherever contaminated soil is excavated. There are two forms: primary, which is a benign self-limiting, respiratory infection, and progressive, a malignant, chronic, often fatal variety.

Incubation: From 1 to 3 weeks.

The danger: The progressive form will kill the patient if not treated; even with treatment, the fight for survival is difficult.

Symptoms: In the primary form, about sixty per cent show no symptoms at all; the disease is discovered by accident. Those who do present symptoms indicate a low-grade fever, pleurisy, a cough, and malaise. The progressive form occurs in one out of four hundred cases of this illness among whites and one out of ten among dark-skinned races. Additional signs are great weakness, loss of weight, cyanosis, shortness of breath, and occasionally the spitting of blood.

Treatment: Early treatment with amphotericin B, despite its dangers, provides a better chance of survival.

Outlook: The primary form runs a benign course. The progressive form has a high incidence of fatalities.

22 Paediatrics

Charles Henry Bauer

(For all the other childhood diseases see the chapters on the specific category involved, such as *Chicken pox* in *Infectious diseases*.)

The human infant is among the weakest and certainly the most dependent (for the longest time) of all animal young. The number of disorders and mishaps to which children are susceptible is immense – yet, somehow, millions of children grow up happily and become healthy, productive adults. This section is concerned with the major disorders of childhood not covered in other chapters (infectious diseases, for example, were covered in Chapter 21).

Good paediatric medicine is preventative as well as curative. The important aspects of a healthful life for children include the following: *adequate nutrition* (a diet high in proteins for growth and carbohydrates and fats for energy, but not so much as to cause overweight); *physical exercise and play* (stimulate growth and development, improve resistance to illness, and allow the acquisition of life skills); *intellectual stimulation* (toys, games, educational materials, contact with people and places, good schooling, books, and so on); *protection from accidents and proper medical care* (regular check-ups, immunizations, prompt treatment of illness and injury, emergency care); and an *emotionally secure, loving, supportive, nurturing, relaxed homelife.*

Infant – when to call the doctor: if the baby is not looking or acting well; if he is pale, bluish, or yellow; is behaving oddly – listless, lethargic, over drowsy or excessively irritable, or unconscious; is having convulsions or is obviously in pain and cannot be comforted; has severe diarrhoea or is vomiting persistently or coughing; is bleeding from the nose, ears, mouth, or navel or shows blood in his urine, stools, or vomit; has lost his appetite for more than a few feeds; or has injured his head and is not back to normal in ten or fifteen minutes – call the doctor.

Child – when to call the doctor: if the child is bleeding a great deal or has bleeding that cannot be halted; is inexplicably dizzy or unconscious; has a high fever (more than 38·9°C, 102°F); has lost his appetite for more than a day; has suffered a burn that is more than slight or localized; has a respiratory disorder that persists more than a week; shows a radical alteration of behaviour, becoming either extremely overactive or inactive or behaving oddly or atypically; or if the child has any significant accident even if no symptoms of injury are evident (see *Accidents* **408**).

Sign of orthopaedic problems: typical orthopaedic signs are a wryneck, an obviously curved spine, an oddly shaped chest, a lump in the spine, uneven skin folds at the buttocks, an extraordinary stiffness or looseness of any joint; a tightness of the skin in certain places, a redness, swelling, or pain in one or more joints, or an obvious defect such as clubfoot.

Additional orthopaedic signs include difficulty in walking or an odd walk (toe-in or toe-out, flatfeet, knock-knees, bowlegs, limp, a pelvis rotated forward with buttocks out); bad posture (one shoulder higher than the other, curved back, slumps continually); pains in feet, shoulders, legs, hips, or back; excessive falls, incoordination, unathletic, frequent self-injuries; inability to touch toes, bend freely, or stretch normally, or other signs of muscle imbalance; foot trouble despite properly fitted shoes (shoes for children must be broad and flexible, offering protection but allowing the feet room to spread out and also to grow). 'Toe-ing in' in an infant or young child may mean a bone abnormality in a child's leg; orthopaedic consultation should be obtained.

Birth defects 395

The term birth defects refers to an astonishingly broad variety of structural and metabolic disorders, malformations, syndromes, and other abnormalities present at birth and caused by genetic and/or environmental (prenatal) factors, including such disorders as muscular dystrophy, cleft lip and cleft palate, cerebral palsy, cystic fibrosis, clubfoot, congenital hip dislocation, Down's syndrome (mongolism), brain damage, and certain forms of blindness, deafness, and retardation. In virtually all of these cases, modern medical research has demonstrated that the earliest possible detection and treatment of birth defects offer the best chance for complete correction or a significantly reduced severity of the disorder. Further, a large number of preventative measures, tests, and procedures have been developed, of which every potential parent should become aware.

The effects of a birth defect may range from the mildest of orthopaedic or cosmetic problems, which the person may barely notice throughout a completely normal lifetime, to the most deadly of crippling, degenerative disorders. The specific dangers, symptoms, and treatments for each of the major birth defects will be dealt with separately. Preventative measures, however, are common to all birth defects and should be studied carefully by all prospective parents.

Prevention: Prior to conception, all prospective parents should receive genetic counselling if there is a history in either family or any hereditary disorder or other birth defect. The ideal age for a mother is between twenty and thirty-five; if younger than eighteen or older than forty the chance of having a child with birth defects is increased. *It is imperative that every woman make sure that she has had rubella (German measles) or has been effectively immunized against it at least two months before becoming pregnant.* Rubella in a pregnant mother can cause serious defects, including deafness, eye defects, physical and mental retardation, and heart abnormalities, in fully *fifty per cent* of those infants whose mother had the disease in the first month of pregnancy when the disease may not even have been noticed by her (see *German measles in pregnancy* **244**). Thus all women who are contemplating becoming pregnant and have not had German measles should be immunized so that they will not contract this mild, yet terribly destructive, disease.

Prospective mothers with the Rh-negative blood factor must make sure that their doctor has taken the necessary steps to avoid Rh-factor incompatibility disease in any future children. Today this is done by the administration of a vaccine following every Rh-positive birth and every miscarriage and abortion if the mother has not been immunized. With the appropriate precautions, virtually all of these defects due to Rh incompatibility can be prevented.

During pregnancy, regular antenatal care is essential. The pregnant woman should keep herself in excellent health throughout the pregnancy and avoid all contagious diseases – *especially* during the first three months. A nourishing diet is important, high in proteins, vitamins, and minerals, with an adequate caloric intake. (The ideal weight gain over the course of a pregnancy is somewhere between 9 and 9·3kg.) *No drugs or medications of any kind* should be taken without the direct and express prescription of a doctor who is aware of the pregnancy. This warning includes pills of every kind, aspirin, sleeping pills, tranquillizers, laxatives, douches, or even being near insecticides. Many of these substances can be transmitted to the foetus during the very fragile prenatal period, irreparably damaging its growth and development. Undercooked red meat should be avoided, as well as contact with unfamiliar cats (danger of toxoplasmosis). No x-ray should be allowed except in absolutely essential emergencies. Every caution should be taken to *avoid prematurity*, which includes extra protection against illness. *Low birth weight* **396** increases the likelihood of almost all the major birth defects.

At birth, good obstetrical care in a modern, well-equipped hospital is of prime importance. Many serious defects are caused by, or associated with, prolonged and difficult labour, complicated delivery, or delay in breathing after birth. Modern equipment and professional care reduce the chances of any birth-related defects, which include cerebral palsy, mental retardation, and neurological abnormalities.

Outlook: Tremendous progress has been made in the last decade, and continues to be made, in the prevention and treatment of birth defects. Advances in paediatric surgery, the detection and control of chemical and metabolic disorders, the development of vaccines and amniocentesis (the extraction of small amounts of fluid from the uterus that enables the detection of certain defects early in the pregnancy), and ongoing research have all contributed to a steadily improving outlook.

Low birth weight 396

Prematurity was formerly defined by birth weight, that is, less than 2·5kg, 5½lb, regardless of the length of pregnancy. Today, regardless of the birth weight, the gestational age determines the maturity of the baby. This is determined by maternal history, laboratory tests during the mother's pregnancy, and physical as well as laboratory tests on the newborn child. If the gestational age is less than 38 weeks, the baby is known as preterm; if it is more than 42 weeks, the baby is known as post-term. Between 38 and 42 weeks, the baby is known as term.

If the weight, regardless of the cause, is lower than would be expected from the gestational age, the baby is known as a 'low-birth-weight infant'. Thus an infant may be mature but weigh only 1,200 grams, 2lb 10oz, a low-birth weight infant. On the other hand, the baby may have a gestational age of 33 weeks and still weigh only 1,200 grams, 2lb 10oz, an obviously immature or pre-term baby. Mature infants who have a low birth weight must be watched carefully for low blood sugar soon after birth.

Between 7 and 10 per cent of all live births are low weight, and these infants are susceptible (in varying degrees, depending upon their maturity) to many diseases, defects, and disorders. Low birth weight can be caused by any of the following: chronic disease in the mother (tuberculosis, diabetes, heart disease); acute infection in the mother; malnutrition of the mother; mother too young or too old; too many children too close together; hereditary factors; mother who smokes a great deal or who takes drugs of any kind (analgesics, sedatives, stimulants, etc); toxaemia of pregnancy; unfavourable living conditions during pregnancy; premature separation of placenta; multiple pregnancy. The low-birth-weight baby may develop perfectly normally or may suffer from any of a wide range of problems – from subtle learning disabilities through severe retardation, blindness, or an ultimately fatal infirmity.

The danger: Low-birth-weight infants are notoriously vulnerable to their environment and survive roughly in direct proportion to their maturity. Thus 50 to 75 per cent of all infants weighing less than 1,500gm, 3lb 5oz at birth have major defects of vision, hearing, or intellectual capacity; less than half of these extremely low-weight newborns survive. Premature babies have a higher likelihood of neurological problems, learning disabilities, and defects of every kind; taken as a group, their IQ is lower than the average IQ of normal-birth-weight children. Other complications of immaturity include respiratory difficulties, a decreased ability to combat infections, a tendency towards rickets, anaemia, nutritional disturbances, poor appetite, and haemorrhagic diathesis (an excessive response to trivial injury).

Symptoms: Inactivity, weakness, feeble crying, irregular breathing, a large head with prominent eyes, a protruding abdomen, a lack of subcutaneous fat are all common concomitants of low birth weight and/or early delivery.

Treatment: In order to ease the transition from the uterus to the harsh external environment, treatment for low-birth-weight infants attempts to provide aspects of the uterine environment and only 'wean' the infant from them as he is ready. Thus *warmth* (an incubator temperature of 30° to 32°C, 88° to 90°F), *humidity* (55 to 65 per cent or higher), *easily digested food* (sometimes fed directly to the stomach by means of catheter), *adequate oxygen* (airways kept clear, oxygen artificially administered only if necessary), and *prevention of infection* (the protected environment of an incubator) are the major aspects of treatment. Minimal handling and exposure, expert nursing care, and a vitamin-supplemented special diet are also required. The first twenty-four hours of life are the most critical, and the second twenty-four hours are next in importance.

Prevention: Excellent prenatal care, including the good health and nutrition of the mother, favourable living conditions during pregnancy, and no smoking or drugs constitute the major preventative measures.

Outlook: The survival chances of the low-birth-weight infant are directly related to maturity. The lower the gestational age, the higher the mortality. Immature babies generally show a slower growth and development than full-term children and tend to lag physically for two years at least but overcome most of their deficits by school age. Competent medical care and a loving, protective home are the two most important factors in enabling the low-birth-weight baby to grow into a healthy, normal child.

Cleft lip and cleft palate 397

Cleft lip occurs when the sides of the upper lip fail to grow together properly before an infant is born. Cleft palate is a similar defect affecting the roof of the mouth, such that a split or opening exists between the two sides. In forty-five per cent of the cases both the lip and palate are involved. Some cases are caused by a defect in the intrauterine environment early in pregnancy, while others are hereditary. The disfigurement is immediately apparent at birth; modern surgical methods, however, have rendered cleft defects far less serious than they were in the past.

The danger: An immediate and urgent feeding problem exists, because infants with cleft defects often cannot suck or swallow properly. Later on there are likely to be speech problems and hearing defects (caused by infections of the middle ear to which these children are extremely susceptible) in approximately half of all cleft cases. Other complications include pneumonia, bronchitis, other respiratory infections, and dental problems.

Symptoms: Obvious physical malformation, the inability to suck or swallow, ear infections, dental problems, and a nasal voice.

Treatment: The primary treatment is surgery, performed immediately after birth or at a weight of 3·6 to 4·5kg, 8 to 10lb in the case of cleft lip (which effectively closes the gap between the two sides of the upper lip), followed by cosmetic surgery during the second year of life. Cleft palate surgery is usually performed after the first year. Other treatment involves revised feeding techniques (including the possible use of prosthetic devices), speech therapy, regular ear examinations, and treatment of infection. The services of a paediatrician, oral surgeon, plastic surgeon, audiologist, orthodontist, otolaryngologist, and speech therapist may all be required in the effective treatment of these defects.

Prevention: See *Birth defects* **395**, *Prevention*.

Outlook: With early treatment and surgery, the child with cleft defects will reach school age with only the most minimal disfigurement or impairment of function.

Sudden infant death 398
(SID, sudden unexplained death)

The reason for the sudden, unexplained death of an apparently normal, healthy baby remains a mystery. Despite frequent parental guilt, it is extremely unlikely that an infant's death is ever caused by suffocation. SID strikes several babies out of every thousand born, mainly males of lower income families, most frequently in winter and spring, and usually late at night. These deaths rarely occur in infants over six months; the peak is at two to four months. There are some small clues. One is that a third of all SID's are infants with a low birth weight; the other, the evidence is scanty as yet, is that magnesium deficiency in both the diet of the pregnant mother and the infant can induce histaminic shock, which can lead to sudden infant death. There has been no definitive corroboration and investigation is still going on.

Close supervision of the infant for the first six months should be the rule.

Parents must never hold themselves responsible for this incredible disease whose only real and solitary symptom is death.

Roseola 399
(roseola infantum, pseudorubella)

An acute disease of infants characterized by fever and a pink body rash that appears after the fever has dropped, roseola is caused by a virus that has not been fully identified.

The illness begins with a high fever, from 39·4° to 40·5°C, 103° to 105°F, which may last three to four days. When the fever drops (suddenly), the rash appears – profusely over the chest and abdomen and much less on the face and extremities. During the rash phase, the child feels well and normal. The rash may only last a few hours or may run on for several days. It is sometimes not observed by the parents.

The only treatment required is the reduction of the fever if it is very high by tepid sponging.

Breast-feeding 400

Breast-feeding is, of course, the natural means by which an infant receives nourishment. It is, in general, the recommended method, barring certain contra-indicating conditions described below.

Advantages
●Breast-feeding provides the *ideal* food for full-term babies in the first months of life.
●Mother's milk is conveniently available at no cost, at the precisely correct temperature, and free from bacteriological contamination. Feeding problems are much less common among breast-fed babies than among the artificially fed.
●Breast-feeding creates a close bond between mother and child and provides the infant with a sense of security, contact, and affection.

Factors to discourage breast-feeding:
●Acute illness in the mother (tuberculosis, anaemia, heart disease, cancer).
●A mother who is addicted to drugs, taking certain medications, or is malnourished.
●The fissuring or cracking of the nipples, mastitis (temporary contra-indication only).
●An infant who is too weak to suck (immaturity, cleft lip or palate).
●Severe mental disturbances of the mother or a psychological aversion to nursing.

Care of breasts while nursing:
●Nipples should be washed with plain water before and after each feed; they should be washed with soap and water once or twice a day.
●If fissuring of the nipple occurs, the nipple should be kept dry and greased if necessary with Vaseline or cold cream.

●A supportive brassiere should be worn by nursing mothers at all times.

Factors conducive to an adequate milk supply:
●The mother must have a healthy, positive, and relaxed state of mind. Worry, anxiety, and depression decrease the milk supply or may cut it off entirely.
●The mother should maintain excellent health through good diet (sufficient calories and fluids, a high protein, vitamin, and mineral intake, especially calcium) and adequate rest and exercise. All illnesses, however slight, should be treated early.
●The regular and complete emptying of both breasts is the prime stimulus for the secretion of milk; if necessary, the breast should be emptied manually or by mechanical means.
●Certain drugs and medicines taken by the nursing mother can be transmitted to the infant and must be avoided. Some common drugs known to be transmitted through mother's milk include nicotine, salicylates, quinine, iodides, barbiturates, opiates, hormones (as in birth-control pills), sulphonamides, and atropine.
●A deficient milk supply may be caused by pituitary insufficiency, illness, emotional factors, mastitis, malnourishment, anaemia, an interruption of nursing, and birth-control pills.

Feeding techniques:
●The best feeding schedule is one of reasonable 'self-regulation' or 'self-demand' by the infant; however, if this conflicts with the home environment or the mother's schedule, some approximation of three- to four-hour intervals should be established.
●The baby does not need to be encouraged to feed more than it wants; it can be trusted to know its own needs. The baby should be allowed to sleep any length of time between feeds and should not be wakened for a feed.
●The nursing infant should be hungry and dry. A baby can be held in any comfortable semi-sitting position, supported by the mother, so long as the

infant's shoulders are higher than its buttocks.

● Successful breast-feeding is indicated when the baby appears satisfied, sleeps three or more hours after feeding, does not seek to nurse too often, and is healthy.

● An inadequate milk supply is indicated when the baby is not satisfied after emptying both breasts, sucks too hungrily, sleeps restlessly or only for short periods, and does not gain weight, assuming that the baby is otherwise healthy and feeding techniques are good.

● The nursing infant should be burped in the middle and at the end of each feed by holding him over a shoulder and gently patting or stroking his back.

Weaning:

● Weaning usually takes place between six and nine months but should be avoided during very hot weather if possible.

● Daily breast-feeding should be gradually replaced, one breast at a time, with whole warmed milk. Tastes of solid food can be introduced earlier, especially if the baby is hungry.

● Past the age of one year, the mother's milk alone is not adequate to meet the nutritional needs of the infant; unless other foods becomes at least part of his diet, severe deficiencies (including anaemia) may result.

Colic 401

Colic is not really a disease but rather a symptom-complex, or syndrome, involving abdominal pain and excessive crying, usually occurring in infants of less than three months of age. It is not to be confused with normal fretfulness and crying, which every baby manifests. The causes of colic include overfeeding or underfeeding, an intolerance to certain foods, feeding methods that are incorrect (wrong position, wrong schedule, excessive burping), and emotional factors such as worry, excitement, or anger – frequently in response to *parental* anxiety and concern.

The danger: Colic may be indicative of intestinal obstruction, peritoneal infection, dietary insufficiency, or some other undiagnosed illness.

Symptoms: Colic is characterized by excessive, prolonged crying, screaming, and fretfulness, from which the infant cannot be comforted in normal ways; diarrhoea, vomiting, passing gas, and a distended abdomen. The legs may be drawn up and flexed to the abdomen, the hands may be clenched, the hands and feet may be cold and moist, the skin bluish and mottled.

Treatment: A variety of treatments may be attempted, but there is no sure cure. A change of formula, the administration of drugs by the doctor, pacifiers, hot water bottles, burping, comforting, rocking, more and smaller feeds, all are variously recommended. A doctor should be called in extreme cases. A tranquillizer for the parents is frequently a required remedy.

Prevention: Good feeding techniques (content, amount, schedule, burping), the investigation of possible allergenic foods in the child's or the mother's diet, and a relaxed, stable, positive home environment are the best preventative measures.

Outlook: Occasional colic is normal in many infants and usually ends well before the age of six months. The key word is perseverance.

Infant diarrhoea 402

An increased number of unusual stools, together with digestive disruption, indicates diarrhoea. The causes may be foods that are contaminated with viruses or bacteria, too much food, an allergic reaction to certain foods, cystic fibrosis, gastroenteritis, emotional excitement or fatigue, coeliac disease (malabsorption syndrome), dysentery or other infections or irritations of the intestinal tract, or as a complication of infection elsewhere in the infant's system. Soft and even explosive stools *may* be quite normal in the breast-fed baby but are less normal in the bottle-fed.

The danger: In severe or prolonged cases, extremely serious dehydration can occur, which can be fatal. Frequently, serious infectious disorders (such as gastroenteritis) are indicated by diarrhoea. In all but the mildest of cases, a doctor should be consulted.

Symptoms: Infant diarrhoea is characterized by a greater than normal number of watery stools, which are often green, foul-smelling, and contain blood or mucus. There is frequently fever and vomiting.

Treatment: The maintenance of adequate hydration (to prevent water loss), resting the gastrointestinal tract (dietary alterations), and combating infection (through use of antibiotics) are essential. The dietary readjustments generally include a brief period (in the most extreme cases, perhaps a few days) in which all solid food is withheld and the child is given slightly sweet liquids (flat ginger ale, tea with sugar, apple juice). Later food is reintroduced with small, frequent feeds beginning with half-strength boiled skim milk, fruit being the last food added.

If the symptoms are quite severe, however (including a high fever, vomiting, and pus or blood in the stools), or if the child does not respond to treatment within twenty-four hours, a doctor *must* be called. Severe dehydration requires hospitalization and the intravenous feeding of fluids with added mineral content.

Outlook: Generally benign if treated immediately and carefully.

Mental retardation 403 (MR)

Mental retardation is not a single disorder or even a series of disorders; it is rather a description of intellectual functioning that is significantly below normal. This subnormality usually involves aspects of *maturation* (developmental stages such as sitting up, crawling, walking, and talking); *learning* (concepts, numbers, reading, school performance); and *social adjustment* (employment, independence, community living). In terms of IQ (which changes during a person's lifetime and also measures certain types of intelligence), retardation is associated with an IQ score of less than 75. Retarded people have degrees of ability and inability, areas of competence and incompetence, as do all people. Although a child may test extremely low at a certain time in his life, modern educational and medical progress has shown that tremendous improvement in functioning can be engendered with the proper treatment. MR is not a static or incurable condition but rather a diagnosis of the level on which a child is functioning at a particular time.

The factors that determine the level on which a child is functioning, or his functional intelligence, include the genetic quality of the brain; brain injuries that may have been suffered before, during, or after birth; other handicapping physical conditions such as blindness, hearing loss, and learning disability; and such environmental factors as the nature and quality of the child's home life (the intellectual stimulation received at home, the values his culture places upon intellectual development, the emotional climate, and the adequacy of educational resources). Obviously, many of these factors are amenable to change, and thus no child's intelligence can be said to be fixed.

The major physiological causes of mental retardation include infection of the pregnant mother with rubella, syphilis, or toxoplasmosis; toxaemia of pregnancy; birth trauma, injury, poisoning, malnutrition of the mother, asphyxia; disorders of metabolism (PKU, Tay-Sachs disease); and chromosomal abnormalities (Down's syndrome, or mongolism). (Mongolism is an incurable congenital disorder of unknown origin, which marks the infant with mongoloid eyelids, a sloping forehead, flattened bridge of the nose, dwarfed physique, and severe mental retardation. Amniocentesis, the withdrawal of some of the amniotic fluid from the amniotic sac that surrounds and protects the foetus, can, without disturbing the pregnancy, determine whether the telltale enzyme is missing, indicating that the infant will develop Tay-Sachs disease of Down's syndrome. In such a case the pregnancy can be interrupted, preventing suffering and anguish to the child and its parents.)

Eighty-nine per cent of all children diagnosed as retarded are 'mildly' retarded (IQ 52 to 67) and are usually not identified until they fail to perform normally in school. In other respects, they are similar to most other children of their age and are often reabsorbed into the work force and the community when they grow up. Most of these children have no detectable abnormalities of the central nervous system and may be, in fact, only 'socially' or 'functionally' retarded – that is, having a normal intellectual potential that has been delayed by social, cultural, environmental, or emotional conditions.

Another six per cent are considered 'moderately' retarded (IQ 31 to 51) and are also capable, with the proper educational, medical, and social opportunities, of living quite normal and productive lives, although their academic achievement may never reach the average adult level.

The remaining five per cent of all retarded children are 'severely' or 'profoundly' retarded (IQ's below 30) with extremely subnormal functioning. Many of these children also have other physical handicaps and disabilities. None the less, they can all learn, improve, and profit from educational programmes and therapies of various kinds.

The danger: Dependent existence, institutionalization, injury and poor health, and emotional difficulties often result.

Symptoms: At birth: abnormalities of labour and delivery, abnormal size of the head, jaundice, convulsions, low birth weight, a low five-minute Apgar score. In infancy: lethargy, a lack of alertness or responsiveness to the environment, a slow development at feeding skills or other 'milestones' of maturation. Ninety per cent of all children can laugh by 3·3

months, lift their heads at 3·2 months, reach out for an object at 5 months, sit alone for 5 seconds at 7·8 months, say 'mamma' or 'dadda' at 10 months, walk well at 14·3 months, drink from a cup at 16·5 months, throw a ball overhand at 2·6 years, copy a circle at 3·3 years, balance on one foot for 5 seconds at 4·3 years, recognize three different colours at 4·9 years. Obviously, there is a wide variation in patterns of development, but if a child lags *significantly* behind the normal schedule a condition of retardation should be suspected.

Treatment: In some cases, such as retardation caused by thyroid deficiency or PKU, treatment can mean the difference between becoming normal or remaining retarded. In cases of PKU, treatment started after the third year will be of no value. Other conditions, those not amenable to cure, can, nevertheless, be vastly helped by treatment and special programmes. Special educational programmes are a vital part of treatment, and, when possible, efforts should be made to integrate the retarded child into classes with normal children so that social development will not be curtailed. Physical health should be maintained, and emotional security and a stable, supportive, loving home environment provided. Overprotectiveness is to be avoided. Institutionalization is not recommended in any but the most severe cases that require intensive care; even then, institutionalization should not be considered as a permanent 'putting away' but rather as a comprehensive treatment course designed eventually to return the child to community life. Most states now have a broad range of programmes for retarded people of all ages, including special nursery schools and developmental daycare programmes, special classes in regular schools, vocational training, sheltered workshops, and group homes for young adults living in the community. All aspects of the child should be considered in developing a programme of treatment and therapy, including the physical and emotional as well as the purely intellectual.

Prevention: It has been estimated that fully one-half of all mental retardation can be prevented with the full application of all presently available knowledge. Expert prenatal care, the maintenance of the mother's health before, during, and after pregnancy, the reduction of prematurity and birth defects, good medical care for all growing children, the attention and involvement of parents, improved educational opprtunities, and an increased awareness on the part of parents and professionals alike can contribute significantly to the reduction of mental retardation incidence over the next decade and thereafter.

A note to mothers: An infant is not a rattle; shaking an infant with too much enthusiasm can cause brain damage and retardation, especially in the first six months.

Outlook: Extremely promising. The great majority of retarded children, given the right schooling and opportunity, can become productive, self-supporting adults. Many others, although they may never be completely independent, can lead happy, useful lives and work under protected conditions. Many children once thought to be hopeless, incurable cases are being helped and are helping themselves to learn, grow, develop, and function. Research and treatment methods, especially in the educational realm, have improved phenomenally in the last decade and the outlook is good.

Minimal brain dysfunction 404

(learning disability, dyslexia)

Children fail in school for a wide variety of reasons, including emotional problems, subnormal intelligence, physical disabilities (hearing and vision defects, illness), and an inability to adapt to the social and/or cultural demands of the school system. Some, however, manifest learning disabilities attributable to minimal brain dysfunction not related to the factors mentioned above. Minimal brain dysfunctions are minor errors of the central nervous system that may be inherited or develop from injury or illness before, during, or shortly after birth. The dyslexic child is of normal (or even higher) intelligence and his problems and/or behaviour are not due to emotional or environmental factors.

Generally speaking, MBD's involve disorders of perception, language use, conceptualization, learning styles, attention, impulsivity, and motor development. Some of the terms reflecting major types of minimal brain dysfunctions include dyslexia, perceptual handicap, psychoneurological brain disorder, hyperkinesia, primary reading retardation, aphasia, and organic brain damage. At least 7 per cent and possibly as much as 15 to 20 per cent of all primary school children evidence some degree of learning and/or behaviour problems attributable to minimal brain dysfunction. The causes include prematurity, complications of pregnancy and birth, infections and the malnutrition of pregnant mothers, genetic factors, and the range of variation in human brain input systems. Actually, any factor that can affect the brain and central nervous system from conception to early childhood may be responsible for minimal brain dysfunction.

The danger: Academic failure, emotional problems, social maladjustment.

Symptoms: Perceptual problems (errors in judging distance, left-right ordering); specific learning disabilities (markedly uneven achievement in school, typically testing high in some subjects and low in others); language disorders (slow development, mispronunciation, stuttering, difficulty in understanding); disorders of attention (being easily distracted, lack of concentration, short attention span); behaviour problems (hyperactivity, restlessness, purposeless activity, reduced or restless sleep, impulsiveness, recklessness, unpredictability, emotional instability, and explosive rage); poor coordination (clumsiness, confusion of right and left, poor eye-hand coordination) and occasional loss of balance.

Treatment: A multidisciplinary team diagnosis is required in most cases, including the perspectives of parents, teachers, psychologist, paediatrician, and neurologist. Treatment is mainly educational and may include individualized remedial work, speech therapy, and counselling. Medication is sometimes indicated for the hyperactive. The home life of the child and the sensitivity of his educators are critical factors in the successful adjustment of the MBD child.

Prevention: See *Birth defects* **395**, *Prevention.*

Outlook: Given specialized education, accurate diagnosis, and supportive, involved parents, most MBD children can overcome their handicap and become productive, well-adjusted adults.

For further information write to Aphasic, Room 14, Toynbee Hall, 28 Commercial Street, London E1 6LS.

Muscular dystrophy 405

Muscular dystrophy refers to a group of hereditary, noncantagious, progressive disorders involving the degeneration of voluntary muscles and leading to increasing disability and usually death. The cause is unknown but appears to be an error of metabolism in the muscle cell itself.

The danger: Weakness, immobility, infirmity, and death.

Symptoms: In the Duchenne type, which affects only males, the symptoms appear as the child begins to walk. He has difficulty in standing or walking, with weakness of the legs and a waddling gait. He falls frequently, has lordosis and scoliosis, and encounters difficulty in rising. Besides the cramping pains, there is an increase in the size of calves and other muscles.

In the facioscapulohumeral type, the shoulders and upper arms are affected more than the legs, with an inability to raise the arms above the head, and the facial muscles are affected (the face becomes expressionless and mask-like). Usually beginning around adolescence, it later spreads to the pelvis and legs.

Treatment: No treatment has yet been found to cure this condition or to totally arrest its progress. The use of the muscles can be prolonged by exercises, surgery, orthopaedic devices, and encouraged activity.

Prevention: None. However, since patients are frequently from families with a history of muscular dystrophy, genetic counselling may be of some value.

Outlook: The rate of degeneration varies, a more rapid wasting usually being associated with the earlier onset of characteristic symptoms. Death generally occurs within five to ten years after the appearance of the Duchenne type symptoms. Progression of the facioscapulohumeral type takes two or three decades, when the patient finally succumbs from respiratory failure or cardiac involvement. Research in progress is promising.

Cerebral palsy 406

Not really a single disease but rather a groups of disorders in which a child has little control over his muscular motions because of damage to the motor centres of the brain, cerebral palsy is caused by injury to the foetus during the latter part of pregnancy (bleeding, toxaemia, diabetes, placental problems, kidney infections); damage to the infant at birth (asphyxia, breech birth, difficult labour, complications of delivery); and, to a lesser extent, Rh-incompatibility disease, rubella of the mother in early pregnancy, twin pregnancy, excessive radiation, congenital brain malformations and brain damage in early infancy from encephalitis, meningitis, or injury. Early diagnosis is important in the treatment of this disorder; sixty-eight per cent of all cases are detected by the age of twelve months.

The danger: Muscular incoordination can range from slight to the most severe paralysing handicaps. A large percentage of children with cerebral palsy have other related complications, including mental retardation, epilepsy, hearing, vision, and speech defects, learning disorders, and behaviour problems.

The movement patterns of cerebral-palsied children are often distorted, uncontrolled, and extremely difficult. As many as fifty per cent have difficulty speaking. Physical deformities and other orthopaedic problems frequently develop from the defective muscle functions. Social adjustment and self-sufficiency are made more difficult by these deficiencies.

Symptoms: The more severe involvements may be evident from birth as indicated by vomiting, irritability, difficult nursing, susceptibility to infections, jaundice, a low five-minute Apgar score, a need for oxygen, twitching of the limbs, listlessness, or frailty of physique. Milder forms may not become apparent until the child fails to develop normal motor skills at the expected pace (may not sit up until 20 months, may not crawl until 26 months, or walk until 2½ years). General symptoms in infancy include convulsions, twitching, spasticity of limbs, lethargy, excitability, high pitched crying, partial paralysis of the face, a lack of awareness and alertness, and a marked slowness of development. The three major types of cerebral palsy (determined by which part of the brain has been most affected) include the *spastic* (stiffness and great difficulty in movement), the *ataxic* (lacks normal sense of balance and depth perception), and the *athetoid* (constant involuntary writhing and flexion of hands and feet). Frequently these types are mixed and may also include tremor (rhythmic involuntary movement), rigidity, and atonia (a total lack of control of muscular function). Spasticity, however, is by far the most common symptom, appearing in seventy-three per cent of all cases and usually affecting the legs more than the arms. Disturbances of articulation and swallowing are also common. Of all CP children seventy per cent evidence *apparent* mental retardation, although in a large number of cases the inability to communicate accounts for a low test result rather than an actual deficiency of intellectual capacity.

Treatment: Early diagnosis is extremely important. Treatment, of course, varies, depending upon the nature and degree of involvement, but generally it includes physical therapy (muscle re-education, corrective orthopaedic procedures and other training to increase coordination and control of the muscles); special education and vocational guidance; psychological evaluation to insure the healthiest mental and emotional development; speech therapy; and special dental care. The attitude of the child's family is of paramount importance in helping him to achieve his potential of independence and emotional well-being. Realism, acceptance, security, and support are the cardinal virtues of parenthood with respect to the CP child. Many communities provide special workshops and treatment centres designed specifically for CP children.

Prevention: See *Birth defects* **395**, *Prevention.*

Outlook: The outlook for the cerebral-palsied child has improved significantly in recent years and is continuing to improve with new research and new methods of treatment. The child requires a broad range of help, including the active participation of parents and a high degree of self-motivation on the part of the child to develop muscle skills and communication skills that require a great deal more effort than for the normal child. The prospect of normal or near normal functioning for many CP children, given proper care, is very promising.

Cystic fibrosis 407
(pancreatic fibrosis)

Cystic fibrosis, a disease of the young (from infants to young adults), is a non-contagious hereditary disease caused by a generalized dysfunction of the exocrine glands (those that produce saliva, mucus, and sweat), in which an abnormally thick mucus clogs the lungs, obstructs their function, and prevents the flow of certain pancreatic enzymes to the small intestine. It is the prime cause of chronic lung disease in children.

The danger: Three major dangers are associated with cystic fibrosis: (1) chronic lung disease, susceptibility to respiratory infections, and an inability to recuperate from pulmonary disorders; (2) pancreatic deficiency, causing such digestive disorders as diarrhoea, weight loss, malnutrition, and retarded growth and development; (3) abnormally salty sweat, which may lead to dehydration, heat prostration, and even death.

Symptoms: Of the CF children ninety-five per cent are normal and healthy at birth. Thereafter, the disease is signalled by a failure to regain birth weight and grow normally, a ravenous appetite, bulky, greasy, foul-smelling stools, a chronic cough with a rapid respiratory rate, persistent wheezing, a runny nose, and recurrent respiratory disorders such as bronchitis and pneumonia. The child may be continually fussy, may appear to be suffering from asthma, allergy, or coeliac disease, and is very thin with a protruberant abdomen.

Treatment: The four major steps in treatment include: (1) control of pulmonary obstruction through the use of mist tents, aerosol sprays, postural drainage (*Table 8*), and breathing exercises (*Table 9*); (2) control of respiratory infections through antibiotics, maintenance of immunities, and avoidance of exposure; (3) correction of the pancreatic insufficiency by the addition of a powdered pancreatic enzyme preparation that is added to the food at every meal; and (4) dietary adjustment to include vitamin supplements, high caloric content, low fats and starches, and salt tablets (particularly in hot weather).

Prevention: None. However, a family history that includes cystic fibrosis should alert parents to the danger, as one out of every twenty persons is a carrier of the disease. Early screening and treatment is vital in preventing and minimizing complications.

Outlook: Although a dozen years ago most cystic fibrosis babies died before school age, improved treatment has steadily lengthened life expectancy and now three-quarters of those afflicted reach adulthood. The early treatment of lung disorders combined with dietary adjustments can afford a relatively normal, happy life for the CF child. Physical activity and school attendance (with the doctor's approval) can be encouraged.

Accidents 408

Accidents are the largest single cause of death in children over the age of one year. The majority of these disastrous fatalities as well as countless other crippling and disfiguring injuries occur in the home. It is the duty of every parent to be aware of these dire facts and to take every precaution to prevent the occurrence of a serious accident in their household and to their children. However, it must also be recognized that children learn and grow through encountering challenges and obstacles and mastering the skills that a vigorous interaction with the environment requires; a sheltered, overprotected child is ultimately less competent and less confident than one who has had the opportunity to experience the bruises and bloody noses that every healthy childhood incurs. These two considerations must be balanced, but the avoidance of serious accidents is, of course, a parent's prime concern.

The major accidents in which children are involved include falls; swallowing poisons (pills, medicines, cleansing agents, cosmetics, spray can pesticides); burns (scalds, sunburn, electricity); cuts and wounds; concussion; unconsciousness; choking, asphyxiation, and strangulation; swallowing foreign objects (bones, pins, coins, buttons); explosions (fireworks and firearms); electrocution, drowning, and car accidents.

The danger: Death, crippling, disfigurement, permanent handicap, psychological trauma, and pain.

Symptoms: Besides the usual indications of bruises, burns, pain, crying, bleeding, unconsciousness, vomiting, difficulty in breathing, and swelling, there may be, under certain conditions, sudden or radical changes in behaviour. Every parent must consider seriously a child's account of an accidental injury or of swallowing foreign objects or poisons, even if he shows no obvious symptoms at the time. Internal injuries, such as abdominal bleeding, may not be apparent but are none the less quite dangerous (see *Child – when to call the doctor*, pp485–6).

Treatment: Treatment obviously varies with the nature and severity of the accident, ranging from a Band-Aid and a kiss to immediate hospitalization. Every parent should be familiar with first-aid procedures and be able to recognize the signs of serious injury when they appear. In general, the primary life-and-death procedures a parent must know are how to restore breathing via artificial respiration (*Table 22*) and how to prevent or treat *Shock* **133**. Each and every parent should take the time to learn first-aid methods. Knowing what to do can save a child's life.

Prevention:

1 Poisonous substances (most cleansers, kerosine, petrol, pesticides, pills) should be kept in a place that is inaccessible to a child.

2 Eliminate frayed wires in the home; keep the child away from all electric plugs; cover all unused sockets.

3 Do not leave sharp knives, scissors, tools, broken glass, power tools, and other dangerous instruments anywhere in house or yard within reach of a child.

4 Keep on hand a first-aid kit, poison control kit, antidote chart, and emergency phone numbers for doctors, hospital, and police in easily available locations.

5 Be aware of hot liquids; hide matches and lighters. No child should be left alone near a burning fireplace or bonfire.

6 Teach a child safety precautions and repeat them until they are completely understood and ingrained in his head. It is impossible to observe a child every second of the day, but if he is taught how to avoid dangerous objects and situations from the earliest possible opportunity, his chances of avoiding serious accident are tremendously improved.

23 Cancer

David L. Levin
and
Marvin Arthur Schneiderman

Any unusual growth of cells in the body can be called a 'new growth' or 'neoplasm'. Most of these are simple local growths with no serious consequences and are therefore called 'benign'. The common wart is an example of such a 'benign tumour'. Sometimes, however, a 'new growth' becomes malignant, behaving in a very different manner and causing the frightening and serious condition called 'cancer'.

Doctors and laymen alike have often thought of cancer as a single disease. This is true only in the sense that all cancer is characterized by an unrestrained growth of cells. In most cases these cells build up into tumours that compress, invade, and destroy normal tissues and, if untreated, usually lead to death. These 'malignant' tumours generally share some common characteristics, whatever the specific form of cancer involved. These include (1) a higher rate of cell growth (or lower rate of cell death) than the normal tissues from which the cancers are derived, (2) failure to maintain the boundaries of normal tissues and organs, (3) appearance under the microscope which suggests in some way a resemblance to immature rather than mature tissues, and (4) a tendency to spread to parts of the body distant from the original site of the cancer. Not all of these features necessarily accompany every malignant tumour, but they are characteristic of most forms of cancer.

Despite these similarities, most observers are more impressed by the great differences among various forms of cancer. For many purposes it is better to think of 'cancer' as a collection of diseases – skin cancer, lung cancer, leukaemia, and so on. But even these more specific terms, based on the original location of the tumour, include several distinct disease forms.

Over the course of a lifetime, the chances of developing cancer are approximately one in four. If skin cancer is included, the risk is closer to one in three. The risk is higher for men than for women and higher for blacks than for whites.

Not all tumours are cancer and not all cancers are inexorably fatal. Still, cancer is second only to heart disease as a leading cause of death; for women twenty-five to fifty years old it is the number one cause; between the ages of five and twenty-five, cancer is the leading cause of death from disease.

The risk of developing cancer is related to many things: who you are, where you are, and what you do.

Age and sex: cancer, predominantly a disease of middle and old age, is rare in children and young adults (more than half of all cancer victims are over sixty-five). Cancer in women appears earlier – between the ages of twenty and forty cancer is more than three times as common in women than in men. Between the ages of fifty and eighty, men account for more cancer cases than women. Women usually survive longer after the onset of cancer than men do. Total cancer rates for men are rising, while rates for women have been declining, but are beginning

to level off; perhaps they may begin to increase in the future as women experience increased exposure to cigarettes and occupational hazards.

Race and country: While the overall cancer risk is higher for blacks than for whites, the rates vary for different cancers. The incidence rates for whites are higher than those for blacks in the following cancers: colon/rectum, breast, bladder, uterine corpus, leukaemia, lymphomas, and ovary, while blacks have higher rates for cancers of the oesophagus, pancreas, stomach, prostate, lung and bronchus, and uterine cervix, both invasive and *in situ* (cancer that has not spread from its original site).

In a study of twenty-five countries, the United States rated highest in leukaemia, Japan highest in stomach cancer, the Netherlands highest in breast cancer, Scotland highest in lung cancer, and Israeli women lowest in uterine cancer.

The socio-economic status: in general, persons in low socio-economic classes have higher risk of developing cancer. This may be a reflection of conditions, such as working in 'dirty' jobs and being exposed to more environmental hazards. However, there are some higher-income cancers, too, for example, breast cancer, and possibly the leukaemias and Hodgkin's disease.

Environment: urban areas have higher cancer rates than do rural regions, which may reflect differences of exposure to occupational and other environmental hazards. The immense growth of modern industry has brought with it an increasing number and diversity of carcinogenic (cancer-causing) substances, many of which are associated with particular occupations or industries.

The ever-increasing use of large numbers of chemicals is undoubtedly contaminating our environment (both at work and at home) and endangering our health.

The family: familial aggregations of cancer have long attracted attention. Nearly everyone knows at least one person who has had several close relatives with cancer. However, cancer is a common disease and some such 'clustering' of cases would be expected on the basis of chance alone. There does seem to be some increased risks within families for such cancers as leukaemia and cancer of the breast, stomach, lung, and colon. Persons who have already developed a cancer may also have an increased chance of a second cancer, often in the same site.

Whether these increased risks are truly familial (i.e. are in some vague way 'hereditary') or are due to a common environment that family members share is not at all clear. There is probably some of each factor, heredity and environment, at work, but in general the increased familial risk for 'cancer families' is not large.

Are you married?: wedded people generally have a lower risk of many diseases, including cancer. Cancers of the breast and uterus show different patterns in married and unmarried women, which is discussed in more detail later in this chapter.

Contagion: there is no good evidence at this time that one can 'catch' cancer from someone with the disease. A lot of work is being done on the 'virus theory'. So far this work has shown that if viruses are connected with human cancer, they are not the kind of viruses we commonly think of. If they have an infectivity at all, it is very weak; and they may have none. The place of viruses in human cancer is just not known, today.

Smoking: cigarette smoking is definitely associated with an increased risk of developing cancer, and not only lung cancer, but also cancers of several other sites such as bladder, perhaps pancreas, and oesophagus.

Food: food and drink can affect health in many ways. The relationships between diet and cancer are very complex, but some risk factors seem to be generally accepted. Alcohol has been linked to cancers of the oesophagus and mouth. Some foods, especially meats, have been associated with increased risk of colon cancer. Some authorities urge that the use of artificial colouring, flavourings, and pre-servatives be avoided whenever possible.

What to do if cancer is suspected: the fear of cancer is an important factor in delayed diagnosis and treatment. An individual will often ignore his symptoms and pretend the danger isn't there, rather than accept the possibility that he may have a malignancy. Often during this retreat from reality, he will persist in, or even step up, the activity he knows to be harmful. It is only when increasing pain, disfigurement, or other unpleasant symptoms become great enough to override his fear that he seeks professional help. Delay in getting a clinical evaluation of his disease can often mean the difference between a curable case and an incurable one. Most suspected cancers turn out to be a less severe (and less frightening) disease. The best chance for cure depends on early diagnosis. *Many cancers are curable if detected in time.* Cancer *in situ* is most frequently curable. Prompt and careful medical attention to any suspected malignancy is required to reach a proper diagnosis and plan of treatment for each individual patient.

There are no surefire ways of preventing cancer, but there are many ways to increase the chances of avoiding it. And early detection, when the cancers are more capable of being halted or cured, is the best medicine.

1. Smoking is deadly. Cigarette smoking is directly related to risk at several sites, primarily the lungs. In addition, smokers are at a higher risk for other disease such as heart disease and respiratory disease. If one must smoke, high 'tar' brands should be avoided.

2. A suntan may be hazardous. A dark suntan may look 'healthy', but it's not an unmixed blessing; the risk for skin cancer is directly related to exposure to ultra-violet light. Avoiding overexposure means avoiding cancer.

3. Working conditions need vigilance. Occupational exposure to carcinogenic chemicals can be stopped. If possible, a change of jobs should be considered. If one must work with hazardous substances, protective clothing (masks, gloves, and so on) must be worn. Efforts

to clean up the environment need everyone's support.

4. Personal hygiene and cleanliness are essential. Cancers of the mouth are directly related to low levels of oral hygiene. The way in which circumcision in the male protects against penile cancer is not clear, but circumcised men are at lower risk. Part of this protection may be related to cleanliness.

5. Excess alcohol is harmful. Heavy and prolonged use of alcohol is associated with high rates of cancer of the oesophagus, pharynx, larynx, and oral cavity.

6. X-ray and radioactive materials are dangerous. Although x-ray is a magnificent medical tool, everyone should be alert to the danger of overexposure and unnecessary exposure, for excess can cause cancer.

7. Some precancerous conditions can be avoided. Jagged teeth or poor dental appliances in the mouth; black moles that are constantly being irritated by clothing; childbirth injuries that are neglected – all of these may lead to cancer if not corrected.

8. Moderate sexual behaviour is best. The occurrence of cervical cancer may be related to inordinate sexual activity. The risk might be lower for women who start sex life later and have intercourse with fewer partners.

9. The key to prevention is alertness. A doctor should be consulted at the slightest suspicion of cancer. Women should have annual cervical smears and know how to examine their own breasts for possible malignancy (see *Table 20* and *Benign cystic tumour of the breast* **220**). The American Cancer Society has drawn up the following '7 Warning Signals':

● A change in bowel or bladder habits
● A sore that does not heal
● An unusual bleeding or discharge
● A thickening or lump in the breast or elsewhere
● Indigestion or difficulty in swallowing
● An obvious change in a wart or a mole
● A nagging cough or hoarseness

Any one of the above symptoms should be considered a reason for seeing a doctor.

A note on cancer in children: death is a rare event in children and the risk of death resulting from cancer is correspondingly very low. However, cancer is, nevertheless, the leading cause of death resulting from disease in children.

Of the childhood cancers, leukaemia is the predominant form, accounting for almost half of all deaths. But the fact is that leukaemia is far more common among adults than in the very young. Other forms of cancer (*Wilms' tumour* **428**) are exclusively seen in children.

Skin cancer 409
(basal cell carcinoma, squamous cell carcinoma)

Skin cancer is the most common and the most curable cancer to which humans, particularly fair-skinned humans, are susceptible. Skin cancers usually occur where they are easily seen; they are not hard to recognize as something out of the ordinary; and people usually see their doctors in plenty of time. Two of the three major types of skin cancer are almost 100 per cent curable, basal cell carcinoma and squamous cell carcinoma. The third type, *Malignant melanoma* **410**, is quite rare but may be fatal.

Fair-skinned people, especially those who are blonde and blue-eyed, are most susceptible. The Oriental, Latin, American Indian, and Negro people seem almost immune. Sunlight, in particular certain wavelengths of ultraviolet light, seems directly related to the development of this disease. The more intense the sunlight, the higher the skin cancer rates. The intensity of the sunlight diminishes as one moves away from the equator, and skin cancer incidence rates, consequently, are very much higher nearer the equator.

Skin cancer also appears more frequently in persons exposed to too much x-ray, coal tar, beryllium, nickel – all over an extended period of time. The disease usually develops in people past middle age. Senile keratosis (the harsh, dry, horny skin of the aged) is generally considered precancerous dermatosis.

Basal cell carcinoma, which accounts for more than three-fourths of all skin malignancies, almost never metastasizes (the transference of disease from one organ to another not directly connected to it) but may become deeply invasive. Squamous cell carcinoma tends to metastasize more frequently, particularly on the back of the hand and the ear.

Symptoms: Any skin change that does not heal promptly or properly should be brought to the doctor's attention. When a pigmented patch of skin that a person may have had for years suddenly changes appearance, colour, or size, it is particularly suspicious.

Basal cell carcinoma appears first as a pale, pearly, raised, translucent nodule that slowly enlarges and ulcerates. Squamous cell carcinoma is a small raised area or patch that may be dark coloured or reddened and hard. After a period of months or years it may start to grow and form a crusted ulcer. A common site is the lower lip. It can also arise on normal skin.

Treatment: Most of the huge number of skin conditions are not cancerous; a biopsy (excision of a tiny piece of tissue for microscopic examination) will determine the true nature of the lesion. Squamous cell carcinoma calls for wider surgical removal than in the basal cell variety. Both radiation and chemotherapy are also effective.

Where the disease has been neglected, all three therapies are employed, but success in this condition is much harder to achieve.

Prevention: Avoidance of overexposure to sun or unnecessary x-ray or other carcinogenic agents may help to prevent skin cancer. All skin conditions appearing late in middle age require prompt medical attention. Skin cancer becomes a strong possibility beyond age fifty. Any skin condition in this age bracket should be examined medically.

Outlook: Basal cell carcinoma has the best outlook. For both forms, the percentage of cure is high.

Malignant melanoma 410

Although quite rare, malignant melanoma is by far the most dangerous skin cancer. No age group is exempt. The cause is unknown. The tumour is unpredictable; it may grow with great speed and metastasize quickly or move quite slowly. Redheads and blondes are particularly vulnerable. Most malignant melanomas arise from pigmented moles (naevi). The peak incidence occurs in the forty to seventy age range.

The danger: The very frequent fatal outcome of this skin cancer is due to the quick metastasis, before treatment or before delayed treatment can curb it.

Symptoms: Malignant melanoma is signified by a sudden increase in the rate of growth and the darkening, ulceration, and bleeding of a pigmented mole. Moles can change colour, turning reddish to blue-black. Any inflammation or halo of pigment around the base of a mole is also cause for alarm.

Treatment: Surgery as soon as possible to cut out the mole and the surrounding area. In tumours of the face, radiation is sometimes employed to keep scarring and disfigurement to a minimum. Local lymph node dissection is an additional procedure.

In melanomas of the arms and legs with regional lymph node involvement, a new technique using such drugs as hydroxyurea, actinomycin-D, and BCNU, sometimes in combination, has been helpful in 25 to 30 per cent of the cases.

Prevention: At the first indication of change in a mole, a doctor should be consulted without any delay.

Outlook: Untreated malignant melanoma develops swiftly and fatally. Rarely is there spontaneous regression and healing. For those without metastasis, following adequate treatment there is about sixty per cent five-year cure rate (survival beyond five years). With metastasis, the prognosis is very poor.

Lung cancer 411

Cancer of the lung, the most common cancer in men and rapidly becoming more and more important among women, is probably the most preventable of the common cancers. The people who are most likely to develop lung cancer are men over forty-five who are heavy smokers, who work in dirty or dusty occupations, and who live in large cities – but no one is really exempt.

Symptoms: The first symptoms of lung cancer are not dramatic or startling, and they seldom send a person to the doctor. Many people ignore a little chest pain, a beginning mild cough, or a little wheezing and foul breath. Older persons, especially smokers, expect some shortness of breath and often ignore it.

Later the cough becomes persistent and hacking, the shortness of breath becomes more acute, and there is wheezing and fever; there is often a pain in the chest behind the breastbone that may be stabbing or dull. As the disease advances there will be a loss of weight, fatigue, hoarseness, and night sweats.

Coughing up blood is usually a late sign, but in a small proportion of cases it can show up as a first symptom. Repeated bouts of pneumonia or bronchitis are other early warnings.

Treatment: Lung cancer is not an easy disease to treat. Treatment, when it is possible, usually requires pneumonectomy (the removal of a whole lung) or lobectomy (removal of a large segment of a lung). Only about thirty per cent of all cases are operable, however. Irradiation and chemotherapy are given when the disease has spread beyond the lung or when other disease makes surgery too risky. The drugs most frequently used are thio-tepa, cyclophosphamide, and sometimes 5-fluorouracil combined with radiation. Regression of the tumour occurs in at best a third of the patients, and is of short duration.

Diagnosis of lung cancer is made via a physical history, deep cough sputum samples, x-ray studies, bronchoscopy, and always some form of biopsy.

Prevention: The average lethal dose is about one pack of cigarettes a day for thirty years. Men who smoke two packs or more are thirty times more likely to contract the disease than non-smokers. Eighty per cent of lung cancer is attributable to cigarette smoking.

Industrial hazards and air pollution in the form of incomplete combustion of heating systems, untreated smoke from industrial chimneys, car exhaust fumes, dust, and asbestos from asphalt roads are clearly related to the increase of lung cancer. The incidence of lung cancer is higher in large industrial cities.

Those who breathe into their lungs both cigarette smoke and polluted air are far more likely to add to the lung cancer statistics.

Preventive measures include efforts to clean up the air and industrial pollution. (See *Part 3, Early warning signals, Lung cancer* **411**.)

Outlook: When the patient finally consults his doctor, his lung cancer is in most cases already well advanced and has metastasized. Only 5 to 10 per cent are alive five years after diagnosis. If the disease is caught before it has spread, the survival rate is vastly improved. Women do somewhat better than men, but the difference is small. The average survival of a lung cancer patient is well under a year, in men under six months. Some forms of the disease have slightly better survival than others; the so-called adenocarcinomas, which are more common in women than in men, and the squamous cell carcinomas.

Brain cancer 412

Brain cancer accounts for 1 to 2 per cent of all cancers. It occurs slightly more frequently in men, with peak incidence during middle age. In children, brain cancer is responsible for 25 per cent of all cancer deaths under the age of fifteen. The most common form in children is the astrocytoma, a slow-growing and highly curable type. The cause is unknown.

The danger: Any brain tumour is serious. Extension of life depends very much on the nature of the cancer and treatment. Some persons live for twenty-five years or more after removal of a tumour; others die within a year.

Symptoms: Pressure by the growing tumour on the brain produces a wide variety of symptoms: headaches, vomiting, muscle weakness (often limited to one side of the body), failing vision, a lack of balance and coordination, personality changes, drowsiness, lethargy, disordered conduct, and psychotic episodes. Double vision is common.

Treatment: Surgery, with or without radiation, and occasionally with chemotherapy.

Outlook: Survival is better for women than for men. About twenty per cent of all patients survive ten years or more. Early diagnosis and treatment increase the chances for survival.

Malignant tumour of the nervous system 413
(neuroblastoma)

The deadly neuroblastoma of childhood is categorized by its arising from the primitive cells of the nervous system, most often in the nerve cells of the adrenal gland. A major tumour of early childhood, half the cases occur in children two years of age and younger and three-fourths of all cases occur during the first four years of life. The cause is unknown.

Symptoms: The characteristic abdominal mass is usually firm, irregular in shape, non-tender, and crosses the midline of the abdomen. Symptoms produced by neuroblastoma are largely due to pressure on other organs by the primary tumour or by metastasis. Pressure on the urinary system may cause obstruction to the flow of urine. Tumours in the chest may produce respiratory distress. Metastasis often occurs to the bones. There may be periorbital pain with the characistic symptom of discoloration around the eyes. Lymph node enlargement may be the first symptom. Rapid weight loss, anaemia, and fever are additional signs.

Treatment: The most effective treatment when possibly is surgery. Radiation and chemotherapy are also used and are often very effective.

Outlook: Early diagnosis must be accomplished with great speed in order to afford any chance of success with this extremely fast growing tumour. Cure rates (percentage of children alive and free of disease two years after diagnosis) range from 8 per cent for the common adrenal tumour to 61 per cent for the rare pelvic tumour. Children under age two experience longer survival rates than do older children. Spontaneous remissions have been known to occur.

Cancer of the retina 414
(retinoblastoma)

A rare tumour, retinoblastoma is seen almost exclusively in children. The average age at diagnosis is eighteen months. When both eyes are involved the disease is largely hereditary. One-third of all cases show involvement of both eyes (retinas).

Symptoms: The parents are often first to note the abnormality. A whitish pupil (cat's eye reflex) is the usual first sign. Visual changes and loss of vision are often present but not recognized in children except through careful examination. The eyeball may become enlarged.

Treatment: Surgical removal of the eye is indicated when the disease is advanced. Early stages may be treated with radiation therapy without surgery. Chemotherapy is also employed.

Prevention: Since many cases of the disease are inherited, birth control and family counselling are indicated. A family's alertness for symptoms may result in early diagnosis and cure. (See

Part 3, Early warning signals, Cancer of the retina **414**.)
Outlook: The overall death rate is about fifteen per cent. Early diagnosis and treatment can save the patient's vision as well as his life.

Leukaemia 415

The leukaemias are a group of diseases resulting from the uncontrolled production of ineffectual white blood cells. As these abnormal cells increase, other blood elements, particularly red blood cells and platelets, are crowded out. Many of the symptoms of leukaemia are due to the relative reduction in red blood cells (anaemia) and in platelets (bleeding disorders). Although leukaemia in children has received much general attention, the disease is far more common in adults. In children, however, leukaemia is the major cancer.

Leukaemia can be roughly divided into two forms: acute and chronic. Although both forms are seen at all ages, acute leukaemia is primarily a disease of childhood and chronic leukaemia a disease of adults (usually over fifty). The leukaemias are also divided into groups depending on which type of white blood cell (monocytic, lymphocytic, granulocytic) is involved.

Leukaemias in some animals are known to be produced by viruses and a search is under way for human leukaemia viruses. At this time, however, there is no definitive evidence that viruses cause leukaemia in man.

Symptoms: Acute leukaemia in children usually appears suddenly, with symptoms similar to those of a cold, and progresses rapidly. Fatigue and malaise are primary symptoms. The lymph nodes, spleen, and liver may become enlarged, painful, and tender. The crowding out of the red blood cells produces anaemia and considerable pallor. Platelet interference causes general bleeding – nose, gums, into the skin in the form of pinpoint spots – and easy bruising.

(The child often looks as if he has been beaten.) The abnormal function of the white cells causes increased susceptibility to infections. Weight loss is common. Often the first symptom is discovered during dental work when prolonged bleeding is noted. There may be a sore throat and night sweats. Later signs include a rapid pulse, joint pain with feverish periods, and weakness. Chronic leukaemia appears more gradually, but the symptoms are approximately the same. Often fatigue is first noted. Many times the disease is first found during a routine blood examination for other reasons. The only definite way to diagnose either form of leukaemia is through examination of the bone marrow.

Treatment: Much progress has been made in the treatment of this disease with the development of new chemotherapeutic agents. Chemotherapy and radiation therapy are both used.

Prevention: Exposure to radiation is associated with an increased incidence of leukaemia. Prevention, therefore, depends on avoiding unnecessary radiation. Some industrial chemicals can cause this disease. All of these chemicals have not been identified or sufficiently tested.

Outlook: Although leukaemia still remains a serious and deadly disease, the survival rate has been improving as new chemotherapeutic agents are developed. Half of all patients with the acute form have survived between three and four months. Twenty per cent survived one year and 3 per cent survived more than three years. In the more advanced treatment centres, the chances of survival are much better; as many as 50 per cent have lived a leukaemia-free existence for five years, and some doctors now speak of 'cures'. The picture for chronic leukaemia is better. Half of all patients survive more than a year and a half and the ten-year survival rate is 8 per cent.

Hodgkin's disease and other lymphomas 416

Lymphomas, a group of diseases of which

Hodgkin's disease is one, are characterized by the increased production of lymphatic tissue, usually seen as enlargement of the lymph glands. The lymphomas account for 3 to 5 per cent of all cancers. Men have slightly higher rates than women. A rare tumour, Hodgkin's disease is the major cancer of teenagers and young adults.

Although Hodgkin's disease has received much publicity regarding a possibly infectious character, transmission of the disease from one person to another has not been proven. While the disease cannot be prevented, prompt medical treatment can lead to good results.

The danger: Untreated Hodgkin's disease runs a progressively worsening course. In the other lymphomas, untreated malignancies become terminal even more rapidly.

Symptoms: The most frequent first symptom of Hodgkin's disease are painless, enlarged lymph nodes, which may grow to any size. In some cases anaemia may be the first indication of illness. The enlargement of lymph nodes throughout the body from lymphoma can cause varied symptoms, including backache, swelling of the legs, and difficulty in breathing and swallowing. Later symptoms include severe itching, weakness, weight loss, and fever.

Treatment: While some limited surgery is occasionally used, radiation alone or in combination with chemotherapy remains the definitive treatment for these diseases.

Prevention: (See *Part 3, Early warning signals, Hodgkin's disease* **416**.)

Outlook: Women respond better to treatment than do men. The overall survival figures show that half of all patients with Hodgkin's disease survive almost three years. Among patients under twenty-five years of age, half survive more than five years. Most other lymphomas show similar good survival. Recent advances in the treatment of Hodgkin's disease give promise for substantial improvements in survival.

Cancer of the thyroid 417

Cancer of the thyroid accounts for slightly more than one per cent of all cancers. It is seen almost three times more frequently in women than in men and occurs at all ages. Persons with goitre are more susceptible to this cancer than the rest of the population. (It has been found that even moderate exposure to A-bomb radiation has caused this disease.)

Symptoms: Most tumours of the thyroid develop slowly over a period of as long as twenty-five years. The first sign is usually enlargement of the thyroid, which is often discovered by the patient himself. Later symptoms may be hoarseness, difficulty in swallowing and breathing, a sensation of fullness in the neck, vocal paralysis, weight loss, and coughing up blood.

Treatment: Surgery, which removes the thyroid and adjacent lymph glands, is the most frequent treatment. Radiation therapy often administered as radioactive iodine is another successful method of treatment.

Prevention: Since exposure to radiation increases the risk of thyroid cancer, radiation in children should be avoided whenever possible. One form of the disease (medullary thyroid carcinoma, which is often associated with phaeochromocytoma of the adrenal gland) is 'genetic', and members of such a family should be carefully followed.

Outlook: Nearly all patients under twenty years of age are likely to survive more than ten years. Cancer of the thyroid is one of the slowest growing of all cancers and has one of the best survival records.

Bone cancer 418

Although other cancers spread to the bone, the bones themselves are rarely the primary site of a cancer. Those that do occur are usually seen in children or young adults. The major type of bone cancer is osteosarcoma. The cause is unknown.

The danger: Fatalities run very high in this disease, especially in Ewing's sarcoma, a particularly deadly form.

Symptoms: A common symptom of bone cancer is pain, which is sometimes relieved by exercise. The pain is often intermittent. Although pain may develop in any area of the skeleton, the predominant sites are the knee, thigh, upper arms, ribs, and pelvis, often with much swelling.

Treatment: Although the psychological effects of amputation cannot be overlooked, surgery offers the best hope for cure. Combinations of radiotherapy and chemotherapy are also used for some sites and types of bone cancer.

Prevention: Prompt medical attention to symptons is vital to possible cure.

Outlook: The prognosis for bone cancer depends to a large extent on the type of cancer. Survival after the removal of giant cell tumours and reticulum cell sarcomas is relatively good. Ewing's tumour and osteosarcomas have a much poorer outlook. Half the patients with bone cancer survive for more than one and a half years; survival among children is slightly less; patients diagnosed between the ages twenty-five and forty-four show the best survival rates.

Multiple myeloma 419
(bone marrow cancer)

A disease of the bone marrow that forms multiple tumour masses affecting primarily the manufacture of blood cells (all blood cells are produced in the bone marrow), multiple myeloma is predominantly a male disease of the fifty to seventy age bracket. These tumours are rare in children and adolescents.

The danger: Almost always fatal.

Symptoms: The first and early indications are intermittent local pains in the bones that are deep seated and boring. The pain worsens with exercise. As the disease progresses, there may be episodes of very extreme pain followed by collapse. The pain can spread to other areas. There may be a swelling of the ribs and skull, spontaneous fractures, weight loss and severe anaemia. The most common first sites are the thigh, pelvis, and upper arms.

Treatment: Radiotherapy and chemotherapy.

Outlook: Death usually occurs rapidly. Single focus myeloma (occurring in only one area) has a better prognosis with a longer survival rate, but it too eventually is fatal.

Breast cancer 420

Breast cancer is the most common cancer among women in the West. It is almost, but not quite, exclusively a female disease. The incidence in men is less than one per cent. For women aged between 35 and 54 it is the leading cause of death. One woman in 20 will develop the disease and one in 30 can be expected to die of it. Breast cancer is most common in more affluent countries, countries where women have small families and fat-rich diets. The highest rates in the world have been reported in the Netherlands, England and Wales, Denmark, Scotland, and Canada.

Although there is some tendency for breast cancer to 'run in families', it is not inherited in the sense that the daughter of a woman who has the disease is very *likely* to develop it. She may be slightly more likely to contract the disease than her neighbour whose mother, sisters, and aunts have all been free of this affliction, but not overwhelmingly more likely. The women most subject to breast cancer are those who have married late or not at all, who have no children or whose children were born after her thirtieth year, and, some authorities believe, the somewhat overweight woman whose diet has, for a long time, included large amounts of animal fats in the form of meat and such dairy products as butter and cheese.

Variables associated with the risk of female breast cancer

Variable	Risk of breast cancer Lower	Higher
Race	Oriental	Caucasian
Caucasian admixture in Negroes	Lesser	Greater
Ethnic group	Gentiles	Jews
Marital status	Married	Single
Age at first pregnancy	Younger	Older
Number of pregnancies	More	Fewer
Age at menarche	Later	Earlier
Artificial menopause	Present	Absent
Benign breast disease	Absent	Present
Family history of breast cancer	Absent	Present
Socioeconomic status	Lower	Higher
Obesity (high intake of butter, cheese, milk, green vegetables, sugar, fat)	Absent	Present

Breast-feeding or being breast-fed does not seem to alter the chances, one way or another. There is little evidence that trauma, or a blow to the breast, has anything to do with developing breast cancer.

The cause (or causes) of breast cancer is not known. In some laboratory animals a virus has been 'indicated' and probably even proven guilty. If there is a virus involved in the human form, it is not a virus of the type we commonly think of, that is, infectious, or capable of transmitting the disease. There is no evidence whatever of anyone 'catching' breast cancer from anyone else. Hormonal involvement in breast cancer is known, but the exact nature of the involvement has not been worked out. Users of contraceptive pills (which are hormones) do not seem to be subject to any increased risk of breast cancer. One study in this country has shown them to be at reduced risk of benign (non-cancer) breast disease.

The danger: Untreated cases usually end terminally. Early discovery and immediate treatment can save life, and patients should be on guard against recurrences, which are frequent.

Symptoms: Breast cancer is most often discovered by women themselves. Although eighty per cent or more of the lumps, or tumours of the breast are *not* cancer, a women finding a lump in her breast should take medical advice. The cancerous lump is likely to be hard, firm, and not easily movable, usually located in the upper outer quadrant of the breast near the armpit (the most likely site) and growing slowly. But all lumps of any kind must be medically examined.

Retraction of a nipple that has not occurred before, a swelling, an area of 'denting' or indentation of the breast, and certainly bleeding or dicharge from the nipple also requires immediate medical investigation.

Treatment: Breast cancer is a disease that can be treated with success. The earlier in the course of the disease that it is treated, the more the likelihood of success. The major form of treatment is radical surgery – removal of the breast, the pectoral muscles, and the axillary lymph nodes. There has been some medical argument for both more conservative treatment and for more radical treatment. The 'conservatives' argue that if treatment were less mutilating women would be less hesitant in coming to their doctors for diagnosis, and thus would come earlier in the disease for which simpler treatment would suffice. The 'radicals' argue that the disease spreads by way of the lymph node chains and, therefore, every effort must be made to remove any and all tissue that might possibly be involved.

In addition to surgery, patients are often treated with radiation, x-rays, or cobalt therapy, to help 'sterilize' the tissue and kill any cancer cells that the surgeon may have missed. For more advanced disease, or for recurrence after a disease-free interval, there are many other procedures, ranging from surgical or x-ray castration of the ovaries of premenopausal women to the use of drugs and chemicals, such as some of the hormones (both male and female) and cyclophosphamide, thiotepa, and methotrexate. Most recently a combination of these (and other) drugs has been given experimentally with some reports of success. There is much research now going on to find the best treatments for breast cancer.

Prevention: Early detection is the only preventative. This can be accomplished by regular self-examination (see *Table 20*) every month, besides regular check-ups.

New mass screening techniques, particularly the use of mammography (x-ray photograph of the breasts) or thermography (a heat-activated photograph of the breasts), show promise of early detection and hence better chances of cure. Mammography seems to be most useful in postmenopausal women, the age group in which most breast cancers occur. (See *Part 3, Early warning signals, Breast cancer* **420.**)

Outlook: The response to treatment is good; eighty per cent of the patients whose disease has not spread beyond the breast and who have been treated to radical mastectomy live beyond the five-year proof of cure. The wider the spread of the disease at the time of treatment, the poorer the prognosis. Onset during pregnancy or lactation carries an additional risk. The accompanying table is taken from 'Cancer Rates and Risks', a

pamphlet distributed by the United States Public Health Service.

Cancer of the cervix 421

The cervix, the neck of the uterus, is the site of a slow-growing cancer that is the second most common cancer in women. Of forty countries surveyed, Israel has the lowest rate. The disease is rare among nuns, Jewish women, and women whose sexual partners have been circumcised. It is highest among prostitutes and women in low income groups. In Britain in 1976 2200 women died of it.

Cancer of the cervix seems to be related to sexual behaviour in many ways. It is a disease of younger women, very often premenopausal. Women most at risk seem to be those who have had sexual intercourse quite early in their lives, have had many sexual partners, and have had many children.

The danger: Cancer of the cervix has one of the lowest death ratios, about one out of four patients with the condition.

Symptoms: Early indications are a slight watery or bloody vaginal discharge, especially after intercourse, along with irregular menstruation and vaginal bleeding or spotting. Later there may be pain in the lower back, vomiting, constipation, various urinary aberrations, and weight loss.

Treatment: If the cancer has not spread, limited surgery is employed for young women who still wish to bear children. For older women a simple hysterectomy (removal of the uterus) is usually all that is necessary, though on occasion more extensive surgery is performed. Radiation in the form of radium implants or x-ray or cobalt therapy is in wide use since these cancer cells seem to be more sensitive to radiation than normal cells and are more easily destroyed.

Prevention: Personal cleanliness and hygiene (soap and water, *not* the so-called hygienic preparations, which are more than likely to be dangerous) may be preventative. Attention should be paid to obvious signs. An annual cervical smear which takes only a few minutes and is ninety-five per cent efficient, is advised. Early cancer of the cervix can be detected easily and thus is easier to treat successfully.

Outlook: A substantial majority of women who are treated survive beyond the five-year proof of cure. If caught in time, almost all patients can be restored to health.

Cancer of the uterus 422

(cancer of the endometrium, uterine sarcoma, choriocarcinoma

Cancer of the uterus is common, detectable early, curable, and probably preventable. Cancer of the uterus is a disease of older women, usually not appearing until after the menopause. It is closely related to hormonal status, and a higher incidence is associated with late menopause, obesity, hypertension, diabetes, childlessness, previous treatment with x-ray and radiation, and prolonged oestrogen (female hormone) stimulation. Family history may also be a predisposing factor. The disease has no relationship to sexual intercourse. Note: Most tumours of the uterus are benign fibroids (see *Fibroid tumours* **226**).

The danger: Although most uterine cancers are detectable and treatable there is a particularly deadly form, fortunately rare, called choriocarcinoma (chorioepithelioma), which may occur during pregnancy or abortion.

Symptoms: For premenopausal women, there may be several heavy menstrual flows and then none, followed by a resumption of bleeding. For women of all ages any bleeding that occurs at the wrong time needs a medical check-up. Constipation is a usual symptom.

The most common signs are vaginal bleeding and a malodorous, watery vaginal discharge. Later there may be urinary irregularities and general pains in the lower back or abdomen.

Treatment: If the cancer has not spread beyond the uterus, hysterectomy (removal of the uterus) is the treatment of choice. Preoperative radiotherapy is beneficial. Inoperable cases are treated with radiation alone, often with surprisingly good results, since these cancer cells seem more sensitive to radiation than normal cells.

Prevention: Enlargement of the endometrium or endometrial polyps are considered precancerous; persons with either condition must be followed closely. In very early stages the condition can be treated.

Good personal hygiene (soap and water, *no* special preparations as they can be quite harmful) may be preventative.

An annual cervical smear test (ninety-five per cent efficient) can catch this disease before it can take hold; it is an absolute must for all women over thirty-five.

Outlook: An alert and reasonably careful woman will rarely, if ever, succumb to this disease.

Cancer of the ovary 423

Ovarian cancer accounts for five per cent of all cancers in women. They are seen at all ages but are most frequent between the ages of forty-five and seventy-four.

Very little is known about the cause of these tumours.

Symptoms: In general, ovarian tumours grow silently and reach a huge size before causing enough symptoms to prompt the patient to see her doctor. Thus, more than fifty per cent of ovarian cancers are inoperable when first seen. The general signs and symptoms common to all tumours, including benign tumours (five to six times more common than malignant tumours), include lower abdominal pain or backache, an enlarged abdomen, pelvic mass, and abnormal vaginal bleeding. As the tumour grows in size, it may press upon the intestinal and urinary tracts, causing changes in bowel and urinary habits. Tumours in children may cause early sexual development (precocious puberty).

Treatment: Depending on the stage of the tumour, the usual treatment includes the surgical removal of the uterus, fallopian tubes, and ovaries and radiation, either together or separately. Chemotherapy may also be used.

Prevention: Nothing is known at the present time.

Outlook: The survival statistics for patients with cancer of the ovary are variable, depending upon the type of tumour and the extent of the disease at time of diagnosis. Younger patients survive for a longer period of time. For all ages, half the patients survive for a little less than one and a half years or longer.

Cancer of the prostate 424

Prostatic cancer is a disease of the elderly, with over eighty per cent of the cases occurring after age sixty-five.

Although the symptoms of benign prostatic disease (*Prostatism* 250) are the same as those of prostatic cancer, the benign form is not believed to be precancerous.

Symptoms: The symptoms are related to the location of the tumour; some tumours give no early warning, while others encroach on nerves to produce back pain and pain with urination. Since the prostate surrounds the urethra, the key signs are such urinary difficulties as progressive difficulty in urination, diminished stream, increased frequency, and a sense of an incomplete emptying of the bladder. Impotence is characteristic. Blood in the urine may also be seen in a few cases. Since any of these may also result from a benign disorder, a careful medical examination is of prime importance for proper treatment.

Diagnosis is made via digital rectal examination, needle biopsy, and x-ray.

Blood tests have a good degree of accuracy in determining whether metastasis has occurred.

Treatment: Surgical removal of the prostate offers the best chance of cure in cases where the tumour has not spread. Most cases are treated with surgery combined with chemotherapy. Androgen (male sex hormone) control, including both the elimination of testicular androgens by orchiectomy (surgical removal of the testes) or their neutralization through the administration of oestrogens (female sex hormones), may provide dramatic relief of advanced symptoms; but such treatment has many physical and emotional side effects and is often reserved for patients in whom all other treatment has failed.

Prevention: Cancer of the prostate is a penalty of old age. Early discovery means control and longer life.

Outlook: More than half the patients under age sixty-five survive for over five years; half of all patients live three years or more. Since this is a disease of the elderly, long survival rates indicate that many patients live a relatively normal life.

Cancer of the testis 425

Although cancer of the testis accounts for only 1 per cent of cancer in men, it is the most common cancer in the age bracket twenty and thirty-four, and 75 per cent of the cases are seen between the ages of twenty and forty-nine.

Testicular tumours are associated with undescended testes, but it is not clear whether one causes the other or both are the result of hormonal imbalances. Although trauma is often claimed as an initial factor, it is difficult to determine whether the trauma simply called attention to a tumour already present. While these tumours cannot be prevented, prompt attention to symptoms and a close observation of persons with undescended testicles can help identify cases early.

The danger: While there are many forms of cancer of the testis, the worst and deadliest, with the highest fatality rate, is the rare choriocarcinoma, which also strikes women as one of the uterine cancers.

Symptoms: Since testicular tumours often develop slowly and silently, an early symptom may simply be a sensation of discomfort resulting from the weight of the tumour. A soft or hard mass can be felt in the scrotum. A dull scrotal ache or pain may be present. Occasionally there is a backache. Tumours producing changes in hormone level may produce early sexual development in children, feminization of adult men, and other symptoms.

Treatment: The treatment of choice for all testicular tumours is surgical removal of the testes, usually in combination with radiation and often accompanied by chemotherapy.

Outlook: Survival, which has been improving with recent advances in therapy, depends largely on the type of tumour, ranging from a 60 to 70 per cent five-year survival rate for seminomas to the rapidly fatal, but rare, choriocarcinoma.

Cancer of the bladder 426

Bladder cancer is approximately four times more common in men than in women. It is most common past the age of fifty with the peak incidence in the seventies and eighties.

Exposure to chemical carcinogens, especially those in the dye industry, has been associated with high rates of bladder cancer. Long-term smokers also show high rates. A parasitic infection of the bladder, *Bilharziasis* **383** (also known as schistosomiasis), has also been associated with these tumours.

The danger: Untreated or late treated cases end up fatally.

Symptoms: Blood in the urine, often without pain and appearing suddenly, is the usual first sign. Even small tumours may produce large amounts of blood. Although the passage of blood in the urine does not necessarily indicate a malignancy, it is an indication for immediate medical evaluation. Urination is painful, urgent, and frequent.

Treatment: The most commonly used form of treatment is surgery. Radiation therapy, including internal implantation of radioactive sources, is often used. Chemotherapy is used only occasionally.

Prevention: Those who work in dye factories have a maximum time of three years before they are in danger of bladder cancer. Since smoking increases the incidence of this disease, the answer is obvious.

Outlook: The results of treatment depend largely on the stage of the cancer, with survival reported as high as eighty-five per cent for some. Overall, half the patients with cancer of the bladder survive for more than three years.

Cancer of the kidney 427

Cancers of the kidney account for just under 2 per cent of all cancers and approximately 20 per cent of childhood cancers (*Wilms' tumour* **428**). Men are affected twice as often as women and whites slightly more often than non-whites. Approximately 60 per cent of these tumours are seen between the ages of fifty and seventy-four.

Cancers of the kidney have been observed in association with kidney stones and kidney infection. Thus, patients with these conditions should be on the alert for possible symptoms of this disease.

The danger: Untreated, practically all cases of renal cancer end fatally.

Symptoms: Since this disease metastasizes to other parts of the body early, the symptoms may mimic and suggest a diversity of disorders. The classic combination of back pain, abdominal mass, and blood in the urine often indicates cancer of the kidney. Weight loss is inevitable. Less common symptoms are fever and anaemia.

Treatment: About half of all patients are treated with surgery alone. Another ten per cent also receive radiation. Some tumours respond to hormone therapy.

Prevention: None.

Outlook: For patients under fifteen years of age, the five-year survival rate is 41 per cent and the ten-year survival rate is 40 per cent, indicating that if patients survive for five years they will amost certainly survive for ten. The rates for adults are lower and continue to decline. For patients fifty-five to sixty-four years of age the five-year survival rate is 37 per cent and the ten-year rate is 28 per cent. Overall, half the patients with cancer of the kidneys survive for one and a half years or more.

Wilms' tumour 428

A major childhood cancer originating in the kidney, the tumour, which probably begins before birth, grows slowly, with the peak incidence during the third year of life. Boys are slightly more likely to have Wilms' tumour than girls. While the cause is not known and the disease cannot be prevented, early diagnosis can often result in cure.

The danger: Late discovery, late treatment is fatal.

Symptoms: An abdominal mass, limited to one side of the body, is the most common first symptom and is usually discovered by the child's parents. Painful and bloody urination is another frequent first symptom. Later symptoms include pain, anaemia, and weight loss.

Treatment: Responsive to drugs and radiation, Wilms' tumour can best be treated by a well-planned combination of surgery, radiation, and chemotherapy.

Prevention: None.

Outlook: Survival rates as high as ninety per cent have been reported for this tumour, one of the most common but most responsive cancers in children.

Cancer of the oesophagus 429

Reported death rates for oesophageal cancer show remarkable variation in different countries, with high rates reported in Iran, China, and France. The male/female ratio also show wide geographic variation; in the United States the ratio is about three men to one woman. The disease is more common among blacks than among whites. Ninety per cent of all cases occur after the age of fifty. Cancer of the oesophagus accounts for 1 to 2 per cent of all cancers.

Although many factors are suspected in causing this malignancy, none has been definitely proven. Current research is focusing on excessive use of alcohol, hot and spicy foods, air pollution, smoking, and some dietary deficiencies.

The danger: Cancer of the oesophagus has a very high mortality rate.

Symptoms: The early symptoms, which are often ignored, include difficulty in swallowing and a vague feeling of fullness or pressure beneath the breastbone. These are usually followed by a rapid weight loss, emaciation, dehydration, thirst, cough, heavy salivation, flatulence, and occasionally chest pain. As the tumour spreads, anaemia, loss of voice, fever, and a foul-smelling odour of the breath can occur.

Treatment: Radiation therapy is the treatment most often used today. Some tumours, especially those occurring in the lower third of the oesophagus, can be successfully treated by surgery.

Prevention: The avoidance of tobacco and a reduction of alcohol consumption may help. A difficulty in swallowing over a few days' time, especially if accompanied by weight loss, requires immediate medical evaluation. (See *Part 3, Early warning signals, Cancer of the oesophagus* **429**.)

Outlook: Less than half of all patients survive for more than five months; only three per cent live for more than five years. Survival is better for women than men and depends on the specific location of the tumour as well as the degree of spread at diagnosis.

Stomach cancer 430

Twice as common in men, stomach cancer occurs mainly after the age of fifty, with peak incidence in the seventies. The rates of gastric cancer have been declining for several decades in several countries, with US whites having the lowest rate in the world. Japan, which has one of the highest rates, shows no evidence of a decline among men and only a suggestion of decline among women. Migrants to new countries usually show rates between that of their home country and that of their host country.

Persons with blood group A and a history of pernicious anaemia or achlorhydria (the absence of hydrochloric acid in stomach secretions) appear to be at high risk. Although ulcers are not thought to cause cancer, they do delay its diagnosis. Diet is thought to be a significant factor. The Western diet, in contrast to the Japanese, with fresh fruit, vegetables, milk, and so on, seems to have preventive qualities.

The danger: The prognosis is poor unless the disease is detected early.

Symptoms: Heartburn, abdominal distension, a vague sense of heaviness in the upper abdomen, and a rapid satiation at meals are often early signs and, unfortunately, are frequently attributed to other causes. Later symptoms include relatively quick mental and physical fatigue, a sudden distaste for food (particularly meat), gradual weight loss, and anaemia. Occasionally the first sign of disease is a sudden pain, the vomiting of blood, or black tarry stools. When these occur, the cancer is usually already far advanced.

Treatment: Since the disease is usually widespread by the time it is diagnosed, almost half of all stomach cancer patients receive no definitive therapy. Although surgery offers the only chance for complete removal of the tumour, the removal of part or all of the stomach (gastrectomy) is a difficult surgical procedure.

Prevention: Avoiding diets high in smoked meats and pickled foods would be prudent. A sufferer of benign gastric disturbances (which can mask symptoms of cancer of the stomach) should be particularly vigilant, especially beyond the age of fifty. (See *Part 3, Early warning signals, Stomach cancer* **430**.)

Outlook: If the early diagnosis can be obtained, the chances for survival are increased. Only half of all patients survive for more than six months. However, when the tumour is localized at the time of surgery, the five-year survival rate is more than thirty per cent.

Cancer of the pancreas 431

The incidence of cancer of the pancreas is increasing. Almost uniformly fatal, it ranks as the fourth leading cause of death among all cancers, with rates for US blacks among the highest in the world. The disease, which occurs late in life (almost half of all cases reported after age seventy), is slightly more common in men than women. Almost nothing is known about the cause.

The danger: Cancer of the pancreas is one of the deadliest malignancies.

Symptoms: Tumours arising near the bile ducts may cause jaundice, clay-coloured stools, dark urine, and other symptoms mimicking gallbladder disease. Often, however, pancreatic tumours grow 'silently', producing no symptoms at all until the cancer is far advanced. Usually the major symptom besides jaundice is a constant boring pain that extends to the back. Most symptoms that do occur are nonspecific: weight loss, weakness, indigestion, and constipation.

Treatment: By the time the cancer is diagnosed, only twenty per cent of the patients are candidates for definitive therapy, usually consisting of surgery or chemotherapy. Tumours originating away from the intestines and bile ducts are better risks for surgery, but these tumours are also diagnosed late in the course of the disease; such surgery entails high operative risk. Palliative surgery, such as removal of an intestinal obstruction, may also be performed.

Prevention: None.

Outlook: The severity of most tumours at the time of diagnosis accounts for the bleak survival patterns. Less than two per cent of all cases survive three years; half of all patients die within two to three months. Those few patients with operable tumours have the best survival rate, with five-year survival figures as high as ten per cent for selected patients.

Cancer of the gallbladder 432

A rare tumour, cancer of the gallbladder is seen three or four times more often in women than in men and slightly more often in whites than in blacks. It is chiefly a disease of old age and is rarely seen in the young.

Although gallbladder cancer is associated with gallstone disease, it is not known if one disease causes the other or if both result from the same underlying cause. Often not found (or even suspected) until after death or during surgery for benign gallbladder disease, the possibility of cancer is an important reason for removal of the gallbladder at the earliest signs of gallstone symptoms.

The danger: Because the patient presents himself to the doctor at an advanced stage of the disease, the mortality rate is high.

Symptoms: Often nonspecific, the symptoms mimic gallstone disease: a diffuse or sharp pain in the upper right abdomen, jaundice, indigestibility of certain foods, a loss of appetite, and progressive weakness. There may be vomiting.

Treatment: Surgical removal of the gallbladder is the major therapy, although radiation and chemotherapy may also be given.

Prevention: None.

Outlook: A disease of the elderly and diagnosed only in late stages, the survival rates are low, with fewer than half of all patients living four months following diagnosis.

Cancer of the liver 433

Although in the United States and most other Western countries cancer of the liver is relatively uncommon, it is frequently seen in some parts of Africa and Asia. In most countries the mortality rates are higher for men than for women by about four to one. Liver cancer is seen at all ages, though it is more common after the age of fifty.

Several causes are known: persons with long-standing liver cirrhosis are at high risk; infection by certain parasites (common in the Orient and elsewhere) predisposes to cancer; and chemicals such as butter yellow (a dye) and toxins produced by moulds on grain and peanuts have been shown to produce liver cancer.

Symptoms: Symptoms of liver cancer mimic stomach disturbances: nausea and vomiting, a feeling of fullness or pressure in the abdomen, jaundice, constipation, weight loss, and anaemia.

Treatment: If diagnosed early enough, surgery may provide a cure. In three out of four cases, however, surgery is ruled out by the extent of the disease, leaving chemotherapy as the major treatment. Radiotherapy is also used in some cases.

Prevention: Cancer of the liver can be curbed by public health measures to control parasitic and mould growth as well as control of pesticides and a large array of chemicals (such as butter yellow, a dye) known to affect the liver. Alcoholics have a greater disposition to this disease.

Outlook: Survival is poor; half of all patients die within two to three months. Patients under twenty-five years of age at diagnosis may survive longer, but only six per cent of the patients are diagnosed at that early age.

Cancer of the colon and rectum 434

In the United States cancers of the colon and rectum represent the second most common site in women and the third most common site in men, while other countries, such as Japan, show much lower rates. Migrants from one country to another adopt the pattern of their new home. Most tumours occur after age fifty-five, and men experience a slightly higher risk than women.

Persons with a personal or family history of digestive diseases, such as ulcerative colitis, polyposis, or immune deficiencies (failure of the immunity system to create antibodies), are at a higher risk for these cancers. However, environmental factors are probably of more importance; diet may be a critical variable, but the exact factors have not yet been ascertained. Some authorities urge more bulk in the diet, while others suggest that high meat intake, especially beef, may be related to the high incidence of these tumours.

The danger: Without detection and treatment this cancer will terminate fatally.

Symptoms: Any persistent change in bowel habits, particularly a narrowing of the stools, discomfort not relieved by bowel movement, rectal bleeding, unexplained anaemia, pain or difficulty in defecation, and constipation followed by diarrhoea should alert one to the possibility of cancer. Advanced disease is characterized by intestinal obstruction, excess gas, weight loss, and pain.

Treatment: Tumours of the colon and rectum are best treated by complete surgical removal. Although the normal intestine is very sensitive to radiation, radiotherapy and chemotherapy may be used in conjunction with surgery.

Prevention: (See *Part 3, Early warning signals, Cancer of the colon and rectum,* **434**.)

Outlook: Half of all patients survive more than two years after diagnosis. Half of the patients under the age of forty-five at diagnosis survive more than ten years. The long survival rates reflect true cures of cases diagnosed in time to be successfully treated.

Cancer of the lip 435

Usually found on the lower lip, cancer of the lip is far more common in men than in women and occurs predominantly in older age brackets. It is rare in black people. The major cause of this disease is exposure to the sun. Pipe and cigar smoking is also suspect.

The danger: The few deaths from this disease are usually due to inadequate treatment.

Symptoms: Most cancers of the lip begin as a 'sore' or blister at the lip margin that does not heal and bleeds easily. There may be a history of recurrent scabs that finally result in a bleeding ulceration. Usually it is a scaled ulcer where the skin meets the lip and bleeds easily. It can also be in the form of a fissure or a hardened nodule or an irregular, raised, horny surface. Often these symptoms are ignored.

Treatment: Surgery is a major and most successful form of treatment. Radiation alone or in combination with surgery is also employed.

Prevention: For those over fifty overexposure to the sun and frost is ill-advised. Aging pipe smokers are also at risk. Any lesion on the lips that does not show signs of healing within a few days needs medical inspection by a doctor.

Outlook: Because of the accessibility of this tumour to treatment, survival for long periods of time or total cure is the usual outcome.

Cancer of the tongue 436

Occurring most frequently in elderly men, tongue cancer is one of the major cancers in the mouth area. Poor oral hygiene is a major cause of this cancer, as is the excessive use of alcohol, smoking, and chronic irritation (for example, from decayed teeth stumps, sharp protrusions). A high association between syphilis and cancer of the tongue has also been reported. In some parts of the world the chewing of betel nuts has been implicated.

The danger: Untreated cancer of the tongue will cause death.

Symptoms: Often preceded by areas of irritation on the tongue, usually the sides, the cancer often presents itself as a slight growth or a slightly painful area. As the tumour progresses, hard nodules, ulcers, severe pain, and bad breath may be present. Cancer at the back of the tongue will produce pain in the throat or ear.

Treatment: Radiation is the major treatment. Surgery, either alone or in combination with radiation, is also widely employed.

Prevention: The chewing of tobacco or continuous heavy drinking is ill-advised. Avoidance of contracting syphilis in the light of its incredible number of complications seems worth whatever effort necessary. Dental appliances in the mouth should be in good condition.

Cancer of the mouth 437

Including several specific sites, the gums, salivary glands, floor of mouth, palate, and jaw, each cancer of the mouth presents a distinct character and clinical course, is treated differently, and has a different prognosis. Together, these tumours account for nearly two per cent of all cancers, are seen at all ages but primarily among the elderly, and are twice as common in men than in women.

Factors related to these cancers include smoking cigarettes, cigars, and pipes, poor oral and dental hygiene, and high alcohol consumption. In India and several other Asian countries, high rates have been related to chewing tobacco and betel nuts.

The danger: Untreated, these cancers end fatally.

Symptoms: Overt cancer is often preceded in the early stages by the appearance of whitish, thickened patches on the lining of the mouth, which may become hard. They are often noticed by the patient or during a dental examination. Such plaques are not necessarily malignant but do indicate the need for medical survey. In the later stage they may take the form of irregular protrusions or deep fissurelike ulcerations, accompanied by pain, bleeding, bad breath, and a stiffness of the jaw muscles.

Treatment: Combinations of surgery and radiation are employed.

Prevention: Much depends on good hygiene, the avoidance of irritating agents such as tobacco and the overuse of alcohol, and prompt attention to early symptoms. The mouth and teeth, especially among the elderly, should be kept scrupulously clean.

Outlook: Since these tumours are often detected early, a long survival and a high cure rate are possible. Persons who, out of fear or for other reasons, delay seeking prompt medical attention develop widespread disease and contribute to its low survival rate.

Cancer of the pharynx (throat) 438

The pharynx extends from the nasal cavity down the throat to the beginning of the larynx and oesophagus; thus it is subject to both respiratory and digestive assault. Tumours of the nasopharynx are usually seen around the ages of forty to forty-five, while tumours of other parts of the pharynx appear late in life. Men are affected more often than women. Nasopharyngeal cancer is unusually common among the Chinese.

The use of tobacco (in all forms) has been implicated in nasopharyngeal cancer; a possible role of viruses is also being studied. Preventive measures include avoidance of tobacco and prompt attention to early symptoms.

The danger: If cancer of the throat has metastasized the usual conclusion is fatal.

Symptoms: Cancer of the nasopharynx often causes no symptoms, is difficult to detect, and is not suspected until it has spread, causing enlargement of the lymph nodes. If early symptoms do occur, they may include a visible mass in the throat, nosebleeds, a nasal twang in speech, bad breath, difficulty in breathing and swallowing, and throat pain, which later can radiate to the entire side of the face. Symptoms of other cancers within the pharynx depend on their location: tonsillar enlargement may interfere with swallowing, the vocal cords may be affected, earache and sore throat may occur. Later stages of the disease may involve facial nerves, leading to paralysis, sensory changes, and severe pain.

Treatment: Radiotherapy offers the best chance of cure for these cancers, which are usually too widespread at diagnosis to allow for surgical treatment.

Outlook: More than half of all patients survive for longer than one year after diagnosis. Ten-year survival rates are seen in more than 10 per cent of all cases and in more than 20 per cent involving localized tumours.

Cancer of the larynx 439

Ninety per cent of cancers of the larynx are seen in men, the majority between the ages of fifty and sixty-nine. The rates are related to smoking and the use of alcohol.

The danger: As in most cancers, untreated cases have a fatal termination.

Symptoms: The most common early and major symptom is hoarseness, which often becomes progressively worse over a period of weeks. Depending on the location of the tumour, there may be difficulty in breathing and swallowing, bad breath, and frequently a sticky mucus that requires almost constant throat-clearing. While cough is not a common symptom, it sometimes does occur. The spread of the disease and infection in the cancerous tissue can result in enlarged glands in the throat and pain, locally in the throat, as well as in the ear.

Treatment: Treatment is usually a combination of surgery and radiation. Experience and careful technique are required because of the proximity of the larynx to other vital organs.

Prevention: No smoking and a limited use of alcohol among the aging.

Outlook: Half of all patients survive more than four years. Half of those patients diagnosed before the age of forty-five survive more than ten years. Early diagnosis gives the best survival rates.

Part 3
General guidelines

Early warning signals
Tables, tests, and guides
A briefing for good health and long life

EARLY WARNING SIGNALS

Many diseases give early warnings so that often the person can do something if not to prevent it, at least to minimize its onslaught. Despite the occasionally dramatic news of someone dropping dead of a heart attack or suffering a stroke without any previous indication of the disease, the overwhelming majority of such victims have had symptoms and a large number have had very early warnings months or years before.

Glaucoma, for example, although it often steals up treacherously, just as often will exhibit warning signs months or years earlier. Tuberculosis can quite frequently be caught early, before it has had a chance to become entrenched. Another disease, regional enteritis, can often be caught as much as ten years before it becomes a crippling illness. Most forms of cancer produce symptoms while it still can be cured or contained.

Caught early, most diseases can be arrested if not cured.

Early warning signals
(Diseases that often give preliminary warning symptoms)

Epilepsy **2a** (grand mal)
Multiple sclerosis **6**
Meningitis **7**
Encephalitis **8**
Brain tumour **9**
Migraine headache **13b**
Glaucoma **23a** and **23b**
Deafness in infants and
children **48** and **49**
Temporal arteritis **33**
Pulmonary tuberculosis **112**
Heart disease **123**, **124**, **125**, **126**
Stroke **139**

Regional enteritis **168**
  (Crohn's disease, ileitis)
Appendicitis **178**
Sprue **180**
Uraemia **207**
Prolapsed uterus **224**
Toxaemia of pregnancy **246**
  (preeclampsia)
Prostatitis **249**
Juvenile rheumatoid arthritis **260**
Herpes simplex **304** (cold sores,
  fever blisters)
Heat exhaustion **313b**
Diabetes **332** (diabetic coma)
Gout **334**
Hyperthyroidism **340** (Graves' disease)
Scarlet fever **359**
Chicken pox **372**
Cancer
Lung cancer **411**
Cancer of the retina **414**
Hodgkin's disease **416**
Breast cancer **420**
Cancer of the oesophagus **429**
Stomach cancer **430**
Cancer of the colon and rectum **434**

Epilepsy 2a (grand mal): hours, sometimes only minutes, before an epileptic attack the subject will see a flashing light, hear a ringing in his ears, feel a strange tingling or a peculiar warmth in some part of his body. His sense of smell and taste also may become disordered so that he can 'smell the sunshine' or 'smell the rain'. Known incidents can trigger off a seizure, such as high excitement or violent anger.

Knowing in advance of the oncoming seizure, the patient can protect himself with Dilantin or any of the new anti-seizure drugs and avert the attack.

Multiple sclerosis 6: early signs of multiple sclerosis can appear months or even years before the actual advent: inexplicable emotional upsets, giddiness, vague, ill-defined trouble with the bladder, an unexplained unusual fatigue of a limb. If the leg is affected, walking may be difficult. There may also be mild visual disturbances or a fleeting palsy of the eye. A combination of some of these symptoms should prompt the subject to see his doctor.

Meningitis 7: a slight sore throat or minor upper respiratory infection can herald the arrival of meningitis. More definitive tests include extreme tenderness on pressure behind the lower jaw and the flexure of the ankle, hip, or knee when the neck of the patient is bent.

In cerebral meningitis, tapping any bone of the extremities will cause the patient to wince.

When these early signals are noted, the patient should see his doctor.

Encephalitis 8: pain in all the muscles, a feeling of being knocked out, a stomach ache and running a fever that begins to mount signal encephalitis. These symptoms can also indicate a mild virus, of course; however, the key to encephalitis is the sense of great fatigue.

Brain tumour 9: anyone who has never suffered from headaches and then develops a persistent, severe headache should consult a doctor as soon as he can.

Migraine headache 13b: a migraine headache very often signals its arrival minutes or hours before an attack: a tingling of the limbs, noises in the ear, visual distortions (the appearance of dazzling or scintillating lights, usually in elaborately coloured patterns), depression or a radical change of mood without reason.

A migraine headache can be aborted by quickly indulging in violent exercise, snuff-induced sneezing, or administration of ergotamine (unless the subject is pregnant). Many women have found their own means of averting the attack by employing some personal shock therapy.

Glaucoma 23a and **23b:** often glaucoma will steal up insidiously on an unsuspecting subject, but often it will herald its coming by such premonitory signals as:

Seeing rainbows around lights – a distinct sign of glaucoma that should bring the subject to the ophthalmologist immediately. The earlier he gets medical care *the more* of his eyesight will be saved.

Brow aches and misty vision can also be early symptoms.

Temporal arteritis 33: possible early signs are pain while chewing, pain in the teeth and ear and back of the head.

Deafness in infants and children 48 and **49:** a surprising number of children are born with some hearing loss, a condition that is often undetected not only by teachers but by parents as well.

Infant before the age of six months: normally, babies startle easily – if a baby does not cry or look frightened or respond in any way upon hearing a sudden loud sound, his hearing should be checked.

Infant after nine months: all 'good' babies who lie quietly in their cots should be treated with some suspicion. A baby who sleeps through all kinds of noises may have some hearing loss. Without being seen, make a sound that is louder than normal noises, not enough to frighten him but just enough to attract his attention. At this age he is capable of identifying sound direction and will turn in the direction of the sound unless he has hearing loss. Watch his speech development, if it is slower than it should be he may have a hearing problem. If your child also seems sluggish and inattentive, don't feel that he is mentally retarded. Children learn by imitation; he cannot imitate or understand a sound he cannot hear.

Babies who have had measles, mumps, scarlet fever, diphtheria, chicken pox, or whooping cough should be checked for hearing loss.

A deaf child or a partially deaf child can be helped immeasurably if the parents are aware of his condition. He can be sent to a special school and often have his deafness cured with proper early medical attention.

Pulmonary tuberculosis 112: occasionally TB creeps up with no significant symptoms and occasionally it appears masked in the guise of a comparatively milder disease, such as influenza, but when the flu-like ailment lasts too long (beyond four or five days) and the fever remains after a week, TB becomes a possibility.

Other factors that should arouse suspicion include a child's failure to gain weight, a patient's loss of weight and increasing rather than diminishing fatigue, pleurisy and mild chest pains, an ache when breathing, rapid, shallow breathing; consistent low-grade temperature (37·8° to 38·3°C, 100° to 101°F), some loss of vital capacity, and a red line on the gums.

If the x-rays are negative but the tuberculin test is positive, the patient should immediately be put on isoniazid and other anti-tuberculosis drugs even if he does not have a cough.

Heart disease 123, 124, 125, 126: many of the following symptoms of heart disease can also be indicative of minor ailments; if a number of them occur simultaneously, however, it would be wise to have a thorough physical examination.

Shortness of breath: if walking up a short incline produces breathlessness, an unfamiliar symptom, this is cause enough to consult a doctor.

Fatigue: fatigue that seems to be increasing, although coming on slowly over weeks and months, needs investigation.

First effort of the day: if the first activity causes some pain around the chest or even some discomfort and has been happening frequently, this is a significant symptom.

Irregular or rapid pulse: an irregular or rapid pulse that occurs without provocation generally requires medical attention.

Yellow marks or lumps on the skin: most frequently found around the eyelids, these deposits are cholesterol patches stored under the skin by the body because it cannot metabolize the fat properly. The cholesterol may also be stored on the interior of the arteries. On the skin it's called xanthoma, on the arterial walls it's called atherosclerosis.

Swelling (oedema) of the ankles or legs: may come and go.

Slight giddiness: if it occurs occasionally over a period of time, this symptom is worth a visit to the doctor.

Sweating: heavy sweating that is not normally characteristic may be just a phase or it may herald some cardiovascular disorder.

Nosebleed: if colds and sinus problems have been ruled out, an unusual nosebleed can indicate weakened blood vessels from arterio-atherosclerosis or high blood pressure. Occasionally, however, nosebleeds occur for no reason at all.

Cyanosis (blue patches on the skin): most often this symptom is indicative of cardiac trouble, although frostbite, chilblains, and some respiratory disorders can also cause cyanosis.

Middle-aged and sedentary: a sedentary person in this age bracket is a target for a heart attack.

Muscular persons who have been overweight since age twenty-five: statistics show that such a person is far more prone to heart disease.

A family tendency to diabetes or high blood pressure: this is a greater risk category. An annual check-up is in order.

The cholesterol belt: a palate with an especial fondness for eggs, milk, butter, cheese, chocolate, coconuts, heavy meats, and sweets.

Smoking: a prime factor in heart disease.

Menopause: women past the menopause are no longer safe from heart attacks; they have the same probabilities as men.

Long-sustained obesity: this will eventually overtax the heart.

Kidney problems: kidney diseases increase susceptibility to heart disease.

Diabetes: diabetics have a far higher rate of heart attacks than non-diabetics.

Pulse does not slow up upon lying down: normally the pulse rate is faster when a person is standing than when he is lying down; if there is no difference, it may indicate heart disorder.

Post-exertion heart rate: a minute after exertion either sustained or of short duration, the heartbeat should show a significant drop. If it drops only a few points, it may indicate some loss of heart accommodation.

Stroke 139: stroke susceptible people are those who have the beginnings of high blood pressure, show signs of diseased blood vessels, have a high cholesterol level, have a family history of diabetes, or who are obese or heavy smokers.

If symptoms of approaching stroke are recognized and medical care is immediately instituted, the stroke can be either prevented or held in check for many years. A stroke is not inevitable.

The following symptoms are all characterized by their briefness. Lasting for several minutes or more often for only a minute with no aftereffects, the patient is lulled into believing the symptoms are not significant, and, consequently, he dismisses and ultimately forgets them. They are, however, early warning signals – harbingers of disaster if the warning is not acted upon.

Hearing loss may be partial or complete for moments or a few minutes.

Nausea, most particularly if it comes and goes quickly.

A numbness or prickling on the face, arms, legs, and side, especially if only on one side.

Falling without known cause either while conscious or blacking out for a few moments. Return to consciousness is full and complete.

A temporary difficulty in swallowing that is unrelated to any cause.

A momentary difficulty in speaking, such as stammering or a thickness in the throat or tongue.

A headache throbbing in consonance with the heartbeat, of very brief duration and without reason.

Amnesia lasting only a few seconds.

Double vision, a temporary aberration, returning quickly to normal sight.

A difficulty in understanding the written and the spoken word, lasting only a few minutes.

A temporary loss of voluntary muscle control, lasting from seconds to a minute or two.

An inability to feel pain or temperature, usually on one side of the face or the body, that disappears quickly.

A brief loss of muscular coordination in the leg, arm, or one side of the body.

A brief paralysis or weakness, usually moderate, of both legs or both arms.

Dizziness – a feeling that everything is spinning, lasting a few seconds.

An inability to recognize persons or things that passes quickly.

Early treatment can prevent a stroke.

Regional enteritis 168 (Crohn's disease, ileitis): although the full-blown disease occurs in middle age, the early indications of regional enteritis appear between the ages of twenty and thirty when it can be controlled or even cured. Later, even control is extremely difficult.

A view held by most psychiatrists is that regional enteritis strikes at emotional, highly geared people who are tense, angry, or resentful and are unable to do something external about their real or assumed indignations and so internalize them. The early symptoms are anaemia, malnutrition, transient migratory (changing) arthritis, abscesses and fistulas around the anus, and weight loss.

Appendicitis 178: a simple early sign of appendicitis is the inability or decreased ability of the patient to hold up his right leg. The earliest direct sign is a vague discomfort in the mid-abdomen that slowly concentrates in the lower right quadrant. A combination of these two indications should alert the patient.

Sprue 180: sprue has a long premonitory period before the full onset of the disease, the single symptom then being very foul-smelling, frothy stools which should prompt the subject to take some action. Early treatment can often effect a complete cure before sprue can actually make its appearance.

Uraemia 207: kidney diseases that gradually lead towards uraemia often develop symptoms months and even years before uraemia becomes apparent. A routine blood test of a healthy appearing subject might show a small increase in blood urea nitrogen (BUN); when coupled with such other not very significant symptoms as excessive urination, lassitude, and general fatigue, a rise in BUN should alert both the patient and the doctor to the possibility of oncoming uraemia, a dangerous disease.

Prolapsed uterus 224: the early signs before the uterus has dropped are a dragging sensation in the lower abdomen, backache while standing or on exertion, and frequency of urination, symptoms that should send the patient to the doctor. Early treatment and medical care can often prevent surgery, which is almost always a hysterectomy.

Toxaemia of pregnancy 246 (preeclampsia): although early warnings of this disease are often vague and not well-defined, it is most wise to take serious note of them, because the ultimate development, eclampsia, is a grave, violent disorder that causes much suffering and is too frequently fatal.

The early symptoms are a loss of appetite, persistent and unexplained weakness, headaches, and, most significantly, an uneasy sick feeling that cannot be shaken off. A combination of these symptoms may turn out to be innocuous, but if it is preeclampsia, the hypochondria will have been justified.

Prostatitis 249: before prostatitis becomes fully developed, some early warning symptoms are in evidence: low-grade fever, some fatigue, a greater frequency of urination (often when asleep), and an inability to completely empty the bladder. These symptoms, especially in a man over fifty, should prompt the subject to see his doctor, who, more than likely, can stave off the full-fledged attack.

Juvenile rheumatoid arthritis 260: often heralded by the unexplained appearance of a high fever, a transient rash, but most frequently by some form of iritis, juvenile rheumatoid arthritis can often be prevented by early medical care.

Iritis can precede by weeks, months,

even years the onset of symptoms of the joints.

Herpes simplex 304: (cold sores, fever blisters): a viral skin eruption around the corners of the mouth that can recur again and again, the approach of herpes simplex blisters is often signalled by a tingling, itching, and other symptoms that are often quite individual. Recognized early, the outbreak can be staved off by applying very hot water or collodion.

Heat exhaustion 313b: heat exhaustion usually gives ample warning before collapse occurs. Working, exercising, or lying in a hot sun can bring on this disorder or worse. The early signals are dizziness, vertigo, a sudden weakness, nausea, a dimming or blurring of vision, and often mild muscular cramps. To avert heat exhaustion, a person should lie down in a cool place with his head lower than his body, sip water *slowly* for half an hour, and take a salt tablet.

Diabetes 332: persons susceptible to diabetes include those born of diabetic parents, overweight women over forty, women who have borne babies over 4kg, 9lb, women who have had repeated miscarriages, and persons with thyroid conditions. An early sign of diabetes is cramp in the calves of the legs. Susceptible people would be well advised to take medical advice to determine whether they are on the road to diabetes. Early diagnosis can minimize the disease enormously.

Diabetic coma: a diabetic coma never comes on suddenly; it is usually preceded by increased urination and thirst, nausea, drowsiness, giddiness, air hunger, a flushed but cold face, a sweetish breath and a subnormal temperature.

Gout 334: after two or more attacks of gout quite often a patient will recognize the advance warning, such as a tingling in the joints, of subsequent attacks. An immediate intake of colchicine can often abort the painful siege completely or at least minimize its intensity. Another sign of an impending attack of gout is depression, which is more easily noticeable by a wife or business associate who can see it coming and advise the gout sufferer.

Hyperthyroidism 340 (Graves' disease): a feeling of weariness and exhaustion for no apparent reason, nervousness, restlessness, and irritability forewarn of hyperthyroidism. A swelling of the neck confirms the diagnosis.

The ailment in this early form is now poised, waiting for some triggering mechanism, such as fright, grief, a shock, or prolonged strain, to set it off. An early medical consultation should include full revelation of every possible symptom. Additional early warning symptoms are patches of white unpigmented skin and enlarged breasts in the male.

Scarlet fever 359: early treatment can minimize this disease.

Chicken pox 372: two weeks before the eruption of chicken pox, the child usually has a peculiar diarrhoea of very soft stools.

Cancer: note the following early warning signals:

Any change in bowel or bladder habits.

Any sore that does not heal.

Any unusual bleeding or discharge from any place.

Any lump, tumour, thickening in the breast or elsewhere.

Indigestion or difficulty in swallowing.

Obvious change in a wart or mole.

Prolonged hoarseness or nagging cough.

Lung cancer 411: the early symptoms are deceptively moderate – slight chest pain, mild cough, some wheezing, some shortness of breath. If all these conditions exist, a doctor should be consulted.

Cancer of the retina 414: a whitish appearance of the pupil is the earliest noted symptom, usually seen by the parent of a child.

Hodgkin's disease 416: months before the lymph node enlargement, which is the definitive sign of this disease, there is an early warning symptom of severe and persistent pruritis (general itching).

Breast cancer 420: a lump in the breast (although eighty per cent of them are not cancer), a retraction of a nipple that has not occurred before, an indentation in the breast, and bleeding or discharge from a nipple are cause for immediate medical examination.

Cancer of the oesophagus 429: the early warning symptoms, which are usually ignored, include difficulty in swallowing and a vague feeling of pressure beneath the breastbone.

Stomach cancer 430: The mild early warning signals – heartburn, distension of the abdomen, a vague heaviness in the upper abdomen, and a rapid satiation at meals – are usually attributed to other disorders.

Cancer of the colon and rectum 434: the early symptoms may be a chronic history of ulcerative colitis, a persistent change in bowel habits, particularly a narrowing of the stools, rectal bleeding, and constipation followed by diarrhoea.

TABLES, TESTS, AND GUIDES

Table 1: Salt in our diet
Foods to avoid in salt-free diets:
All tinned foods except those marked salt-free
All margarines except those marked salt-free
All relishes and prepared dressings
All prepared meats, such as sausages, frankfurters, corned beef, and bacon
All tomato sauces including ketchup
All smoked foods
All pickled foods
Such vegetables as beets, celery, kale, and spinach
Baked goods: cakes, sweet or dry biscuits, pastries, and white bread
All prepared flours, prepared deserts, and almost all prepared cereals
All prepared foods that have more than one ingredient, such as bouillon cubes, malted milk, soups, mustard, potato crisps, and a vast multitude of others
Beer and soda
Such proteins as kidneys, caviar, olives, and all seafood
Cheese and all butter not identified as salt-free
In general, more foods contain salt than anyone would suspect. It is always essential to read the label (no matter how fine the print) on all packaged or prepared foods. In addition, salt can be innocently ingested, as in sedatives, laxatives, and even drinking water.

A salt-free diet should never be undertaken without medical advice. A diet totally free of sodium can be harmful; only a doctor knows each individual's needs.

The salt content is listed in milligrams per 100 grams, 3½ ounces of food. Here is a partial list from the *Composition of Foods* edited by B. K. Watt and A. L. Merrill issued by the US Department of Agriculture.

Grapes	0·4	Baby food (vegetable and chicken)	307
Sweet corn	0·7	Gelatin (dessert powder)	318
Apples	1	Soup (chicken)	382
Apricots	1	Pancakes	425
Bananas	1	Baby food (oatmeal)	437
Blueberries	1	Doughnuts	401
Grapefruit	1	Bread	400 to 600
Asparagus	2	Salad dressing	500 to 1,300
Wheat	3	Peanut butter	607
Potatoes	4	Chocolate	615
Peanuts	5	Pizza	702
Lettuce	9	Tuna (canned in oil)	800
Onions	10	Bran flakes	925
Jams, preserves	12	Margarine	987
Broccoli	15	Crabmeat (canned)	1,000
Cashew nuts	15	Cornflakes	1,005
Mushrooms	15	Bacon (cooked)	1,021
Beans	19	Waffles (prepared mix)	1,029
Cream (light)	43	Frankfurters	1,100
Carp	50	Cheese, American	1,136
Chicken	50	Biscuit (prepared mix)	1,300
Milk	50	Pickles (dill)	1,428
Beets	60	Pretzels	1,680
Pork	70	Corned beef (cooked)	1,740
Bluefish	74	Popcorn	1,940
Herring (fresh)	74	Caviar	2,200
Lamb	75	Olives	2,400
Eggs	122	Bacon, Canadian (cooked)	2,555
Asparagus (canned)	236	Olives (Greek)	3,288
Beans (canned)	236	Beef (chipped, dried)	4,300
Cake	from 200 to 400	Herring (salt)	6,231
Peas (canned)	236	Soy sauce	7,325
Pie (apple)	301	Cod (salted)	8,100
		Bouillon cubes	24,000

Excess salt has been proven to raise blood pressure in many human beings. Salt also causes fluid retention in the body. Five grams a day is all that an individual needs. The average man eats 20 grams per day, decreasing his life-span and affecting his general health.

Table 2: Low cholesterol diet

Almost all fish

Chicken and fowl of all kinds

Cottage cheese

Skim milk (not the 99 per cent fat-free kind; regular milk is 97 per cent fat free. True skim milk contains a fraction of one percent of fat)

Egg white (the yolk has the highest cholesterol content of any food)

Yogurt (the best is made from skim milk)

Very lean meats
Cereals
Fruit
Vegetables
Special note:
Yogurt: although made from whole milk and therefore high in cholesterol, yogurt is paradoxically one of the best anticholesterol foods known. According to recent investigations there seems to be a substance in yogurt which lowers cholesterol in the body.*

Mushrooms: this food is not only anticholesterol but also antiviral. Recent investigations have indicated that it can prevent or reduce polio and flu in animals.† The Japanese have isolated a chemical from mushrooms called 'eritadenine' which lowers cholesterol in the blood.

Table 3: Foods high in cholesterol

Egg yolk
Almost all organ meats (especially brain)
Animal fat
Regular meat with normal fats
Hydrogenated vegetable oils
Shortening (lard in particular)
Bacon
Seafood
Shellfish
All dairy products except skim milk and products made of skim milk
Chocolate
Cocoa
All baking mixes
All baked goods
Coffee whiteners
Palm kernel oil (in many packaged products)
Coconut oil

Table 4: Saturated fats

A saturated fat is any fat that hardens at room temperature, such as butter, lard, and bacon fat. Polyunsaturated fats are, for the most part, liquid at room temperature.

Any fat that has been hydrogenized, a term used in margarine, has been saturated. Partially hydrogenated means, of course, partially saturated. The margarine manufacturers have neglected to state how much is 'partial', so there's no way of judging the amount.

With the exception of coconut oil, all vegetable or nut oils are low in saturated fats and high in polyunsatured fats. The same is true of fish oils. Whale blubber, for example, has three times as much polyunsaturated oil as saturated, which may account for the low incidence of heart disease among the Eskimos.

Goat and buffalo milk have the highest amount of saturated fat, twice as much as unsaturated. Cow's milk has two-fifths more saturated fats than unsaturated, while human milk has equal amounts of each.

Saturated fat (which includes cholesterol) has been implicated in the development of arterio-atherosclerosis.

* Dr George V. Mann of the National Heart and Lung Institute, USA.
† According to Dr Kenneth W. Cochran, professor of epidemiology, University of Michigan School of Public Health, USA.

Table 5: Exercise tests to determine cardiovascular fitness

(New physical fitness heart tests)

Test A: Step up and down from a 20cm, 8in high stool or box 48 times a minute (24 round trips) for three consecutive minutes. Then sit down and after waiting one minute, take your pulse.

The following determinations indicate your fitness:

| Condition | Pulse rate | |
	Men	Women
Excellent	67	75
About average	79	85
Average	90	95
Poor	160	110

Test B: A simpler but less accurate test is to take your basal pulse rate (your pulse as soon as you open your eyes after a night's sleep before getting out of bed). If your pulse is in the forties (per minute), you are of athletic calibre, able to participate in any competitive sport. If it's in the fifties, you are extremely fit, capable of any vigorous sport, such as running, mountain climbing, skiing, and the like. If your pulse is in the sixties, it's about normal.

Cardiovascular exercises: calisthenics are not the best. Climbing, jogging, and swimming are far, far better. For men who have been sedentary for long years, vigorous exercises must be approached with caution and only upon the advice of a doctor.

The best benefits from cardiovascular exercises are derived when the effort makes you sweat. The heart rate should rise into the 120s (not over 145 if you're middle-aged). Jogging a mile every day in ten minutes is ideal.

Negative signs indicating unfitness after exercise are faintness, some dizziness, unusual shortness of breath, and pallor. A doctor should be consulted on how to get in shape, gradually.

After a normal jog of a mile there should be no feeling of exhaustion. Within ten minutes the heart and breathing should be back to normal. Check your heart rate and breathing rate before the run and afterwards. Ordinarily a ten- or eleven-minute jog of a mile should bring on some feeling of exhilaration and well-being. Often a healthy person will feel more energetic after the run than before.

Table 6: Oral hygiene

1. Checkups: regular visits to your dentist or dental hygienist to scale down the tartar that forms between the teeth and the gums as a result of the calculus in the saliva, and twice yearly examination for possible new cavities or lesions in the mouth, tongue, and gums are advised.

2. Sugar: avoid sweets as much as possible. It is better to eat a larger quantity of sugary foods once a day than smaller quantities several times a day. If you do eat sweets, rinse immediately. It is important to get the sugar off your teeth in a matter of minutes. The bacteria working on your teeth on a film of sugar reach their maximum effectiveness within a quarter

of an hour. Try to avoid sucking sweets; lollipops and the like for children are reprehensible. For those who need sweets, substitute figs, dates, raisins, or any other fruit.

3. Rinsing: it is a good idea to rinse not only after eating sweets, but also after eating foods high in acidity. such as orange juice, which eat away the enamel.

4. Between the teeth: use unwaxed dental floss to get at the food particles the toothbrush cannot reach. Use it as often as you can. Soft wedge-shaped toothpicks and the water pic are also recommended for intradental cleansing.

5. Fluorine: if the water supply in your community has not been fluorinated,

ask your dentist for a fluorine mouth rinse or toothpaste or tablets that can be taken internally.

6. Toothbrushing: the preoccupation with brushing the teeth has superseded its value. This belaboured form of oral hygiene is not as effective as was once thought. No amount of brushing can stave off decay or gum diseases. Many cultures where no brushing is practiced have a lower incidence of caries than those who do. Brushing, nevertheless, can be useful if it is done in moderation, for heavy brushing can and does rub away the thin enamel.

Ask your dentist or chemist for 'disclosing tablets', which when chewed, stain the plaques (gummy, transparent, very sticky films of sugar and bacteria that cannot be seen until stained by the harmless colouring of the disclosing tablet). Brush the stained plaques with a soft natural bristle (not hard nylon).

7. White teeth: teeth are rarely pure white; they have a yellowish cast to them despite the toothpaste advertisements. You cannot brush them

until they turn white, you can only brush off the enamel to expose the even yellower dentin underneath. There is no dentrifice that can whiten teeth. If they are discoloured, your dentist can remove the stains.

8. Mouthwash: plain or salt water used twice a day will help keep your mouth clean. You need no chemist's preparation unless you want to smell of wintergreen or oil of cloves or whatever. Commercial mouthwashes, no matter how pleasant-tasting or unpleasant (some manufacturers deliberately make them unpleasant in order to give the buyer the feeling that this mouthwash is strong and powerful), do nothing really about sterilizing your mouth or nullifying bad breath; they only mask the odour – and the masking of the breath only lasts a few minutes.

9. Chewing: as often as possible, chew on hard, firm food, which will not only invigorate the gums but will also cleanse the teeth and strengthen them. (No, this does not include toffee, caramels, or hard nougats.)

Table 7: A test for hearing loss
An ear specialist can test for hearing loss with an audiometer, which can be increased decibel by decibel. A 20-decibel loss means you have difficulty hearing in a theatre. A 30-decibel loss means you cannot hear well in a living room and you are in need of a hearing aid. A 50-decibel loss indicates you cannot hear well even on the telephone.

Self-test: answer yes or no to the following questions:

Do you hear better on the telephone than in normal room conversation?

Do you often misunderstand what is being said on television?

Do you frequently find it necessary to

cock your ear with your hand to hear better?

Do you often give up listening to someone because he is difficult to hear? (This has only been happening lately.)

Do you misunderstand what people are saying?

When you place a ticking watch at the ear opening and then on the bone behind the ear, do you hear better on the bone?

If any of the above questions are answered yes, you are suffering from some hearing loss and should consult a doctor.

Table 8: Postural drainage
Postural drainage is a method by which secretions from the bronchi and the lungs are drained by placing the head lower than the chest. The position will induce or aggravate coughing with the desired result of bringing up phlegm.

About five minutes twice a day, morning and evening, is the indicated procedure.

The classic position of leaning over the bed from the abdomen down is not advised, because of the danger of falling

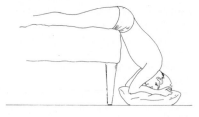 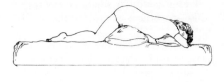

(*Drawings by Julian A. Miller*)

and of exposure to the dust on the floor, which may cause an allergic reaction in dust-sensitive patients:

The best method involves placing a strong heavy cushion under the groin of the patient. He leans over it, his face on a cloth, his chest supported by smaller pillows. In this way he is relaxed and comfortable:

Table 9: Modified yoga breathing

Exercise A: Stand erect, hands at the sides, in front of a mirror, with windows wide open.

Inhale slowly through the nostrils, filling your lungs with air from the abdomen first, then the lower chest, and finally the upper chest to near full capacity. While inhaling, raise your hands slowly overhead so that when inhalation is complete your hands are directly overhead, touching. In this form of inhalation the lower part of the lungs are equally involved (normally they are neglected). Hold your breath, with your hands remaining up, for a few seconds. Exhale slowly as your arms are owly brought back to the sides. Repeat the exercise four times.

Exercise B: Repeat the inhalation as in A, but exhale rapidly, completely through the mouth, as you drop your hands just as quickly to your sides. Repeat the exercise four times.

Exercise C: Repeat the inhalation as in A, but exhale slowly and *forcibly* through a narrow opening in the mouth puckered as if for whistling, as if blowing up a resistant balloon. Repeat the exercise two to four times.

Exercises A, B, and C should be done as one set, three times daily.

Table 10: Tests for lung efficiency

Expiration test: A watch with a second hand is needed.

Take a deep breath; then, with mouth wide open, blow out as fast and as hard as possible. Normal time required is three to four seconds (slightly less time for a young person, slightly more for an older person). Six seconds or longer indicates some obstruction of the lungs which could mean chronic bronchitis, emphysema, and other pulmonary ailments.

Chest expansion: Measure the chest with a tape measure after normal exhalation – for males run the tape measure across the nipples; for females, just under the breasts. Measure again at the fullest point of expansion and at the peak of inhalation. Expansion should be a minimum of 3 to 5 centimetres, 1½ to 2 inches. If it is less, the lungs have lost elasticity and should be checked by a doctor.

Snider match test: Light a book match and hold it six inches from your mouth. Take a very deep breath; then, keeping your mouth wide open, blow out the light. If there is a deficiency in pulmonary function it will be difficult or impossible to do this. Failure indicates that your vital capacity has been seriously decreased.

Table 11: How to avoid constipation

Eat regularly.

Move your bowels at the same time every day by deliberately developing the habit. The best time is a half hour or so after breakfast.

Spend at least ten minutes at stool. Never strain; be relaxed, read a newspaper, magazine, or such.

Get plenty of physical exercise.

Drink a half glass of hot water a half hour before breakfast every day. Drink a total of eight glasses of fluids daily, two of which should be fruit juice.

Laxatives are absolutely inadvisable. Eat fruit, rough vegetables, bran, high bulk foods, whole grain breads, and whole grain cereals.

If all these efforts do not work, take a bulk-producing agent (any psyllium product; Metamucil is well known). Plantago seed is equally effective and much cheaper (nonprescription). You might also try a stool softening agent, such as dioctyl sodium sulphosuccinate.

If you are still having difficulty, an ounce of mineral oil taken with some fruit juice before retiring may help. However, this practice must never become a habit, since mineral oil interferes with the absorption of all fat-soluble vitamins, such as A and K.

When a reasonable bowel regime has been finally established, slowly withdraw the above agents over a period of weeks.

Retraining will take from ten days to a month.

Table 12: How to avoid swallowing air (aerophagia)

1. Sighing: people sigh at work or during stress periods, often without being aware they are doing so. Each sigh means a swallow of air. If you can't avoid stress, try to become aware of sighing so that you can stop yourself.

2. Eating: never bolt your food or eat while you are upset – you are swallowing air. Exhale after chewing or just before swallowing.

3. Drinking: do not wash down your food. Drink liquids at the end of a meal. Do not sip or gulp liquids; drink slowly from a glass or cup and keep your upper lip submerged by tilting the glass.

4. Food and drink: avoid all carbonated drinks from soda pop to champagne; avoid all foods that have air whipped into them (malted milk, milk shakes, whipped butter, anything whipped, very porous cakes). If you are suffering from aerophagia, keep away from such notorious vegetables as beans, cabbage, and brussels sprouts. Don't drink very hot beverages – unconsciously you will draw in air to cool them.

5. Tobacco: smoking increases the saliva flow, excess saliva increases swallowing, excess swallowing increases air intake.

6. Swallowing: many aerophagists swallow air in order to bring up gas (more air), but more air is swallowed than is brought up; consequently, each attempt to get relief by swallowing air actually worsens the condition.

7. Bowel movements: don't delay a bowel movement; heed every urge. Delay means that the normal gas in the colon will collect and cause bloating.

Table 13: Standard table of desirable weights for men and women

Age: 25 or over. Shoes: 5cm (2in) for women, 2·5cm (1in) for men. Clothes: indoor.
Nude weight: deduct 2 to 3kg (5 to 7lb) for men; 1 to 2kg (2 to 4lb) for women.

Women

cm	small frame	average	large frame
147 (4'10")	42kg (92lb)	46kg (101lb)	54kg (119lb)
150 (4'11")	43kg (94lb)	47kg (104lb)	55kg (122lb)
152 (5')	44kg (96lb)	49kg (107lb)	57kg (125lb)
155 (5'1")	45kg (99lb)	50kg (110lb)	58kg (128lb)
157 (5'2")	46kg (102)	51kg (113lb)	59kg (131lb)
160 (5'3")	48kg (105lb)	53kg (116lb)	61kg (134lb)
163 (5'4")	49kg (108lb)	54kg (119lb)	63kg (138lb)
165 (5'5")	50kg (111lb)	56kg (123lb)	65kg (142lb)
168 (5'6")	52kg (114lb)	58kg (127lb)	66kg (146lb)
170 (5'7")	54kg (118lb)	59kg (132lb)	68kg (150lb)
173 (5'8")	55kg (122lb)	60kg (136lb)	70kg (154lb)
175 (5'9")	57kg (126lb)	62kg (140lb)	72kg (158lb)
178 (5'10")	59kg (130lb)	63kg (144lb)	74kg (163lb)
180 (5'11")	61kg (134lb)	65kg (148lb)	76kg (168lb)
183 (6')	63kg (138lb)	67kg (152lb)	79kg (173lb)
185 (6'1")	64kg (142lb)	68kg (156lb)	81kg (178lb)

Men

cm	small frame	average	large frame
157 (5'2")	51kg (112lb)	56kg (124lb)	64kg (141lb)
160 (5'3")	52kg (115lb)	58kg (127lb)	65kg (144lb)
163 (5'4")	54kg (118lb)	59kg (130lb)	67kg (148lb)
165 (5'5")	55kg (121lb)	60kg (133lb)	69kg (152lb)
168 (5'6")	56kg (124lb)	62kg (137lb)	71kg (156lb)
170 (5'7")	58kg (128lb)	64kg (141lb)	73kg (161lb)
173 (5'8")	60kg (132lb)	65kg (145lb)	75kg (166lb)
175 (5'9")	62kg (136lb)	67kg (149lb)	77kg (170lb)
178 (5'10")	64kg (140lb)	69kg (153lb)	79kg (174lb)
180 (5'11")	65kg (144lb)	71kg (158lb)	81kg (179lb)
183 (6')	67kg (148lb)	74kg (162lb)	84kg (184lb)
185 (6'1")	69kg (152lb)	75kg (166lb)	86kg (189lb)
188 (6'2")	71kg (156lb)	78kg (171lb)	88kg (194lb)
191 (6'3")	73kg (160lb)	80kg (176lb)	90kg (199lb)
193 (6'4")	74kg (164lb)	82kg (181lb)	93kg (204lb)
196 (6'5")	76kg (168lb)	85kg (186lb)	95kg (209lb)

Table 14: The daily morning stretch

Stretching is invaluable for all ages, but it is particularly essential for the sedentary and for the middle-aged.

Yoga stretching should begin in the morning before getting out of bed. As soon as your eyes open, while you are still contemplating facing the day, begin your first exercise.

1. Extend one leg downwards so that it becomes longer than the other (you must feel it in the calves, ankles, and toes). Do the same with the other leg. Alternate legs, four or five times on each.

2. Now stretch one arm outward until it feels longer than the other; stretch it as far as it will go, until you feel the tension at the shoulders, wrist, and fingers. Next stretch the arm upwards. Follow the same procedure with the other arm. Alternate arms four or five times.

3. Stretch your neck, moving it from side to side as far as it will go; then arch your back to its utmost. Relax. Do this exercise until you feel you've had enough.

4. Get out of bed. Before running to the bathroom or jumping into your clothes, stretch – stretch any part of the body you feel so inclined. Do not hurry. Your body, now relaxed, might just possibly help relax your mind as well.

Table 15: How to lift a heavy weight

Keep your feet apart (about 30 centimetres, 1 foot) and stand near the object. Bend at the knees, pick up the object, and rise slowly, using your legs to do so, never your back, until your knees are straight.

Hernia develops from using your back muscles rather than your legs.

Table 16: Tests and additional signs of pregnancy

Montgomery's glands: usually unnoticeable, Montgomery's glands, small prominences on the areolas (the dark-ringed circles around the nipples), enlarge during pregnancy.

Jorissenne's sign: pregnancy is indicated when the pulse does not accelerate upon changing from a horizontal to an upright position.

Jacquemier's sign: after the fourth week of pregnancy a violet-coloured spot will appear on the mucous membrane of the vagina just below the urethral orifice.

Table 17: The Semans technique for impotence and frigidity

The following techniques designed to improve sexual performance were developed by Dr James Semans of Duke University, USA.

Impotence: a therapy suitable for both impotence and premature ejaculation, the basic idea is love-making without sexual intercourse. The period of time spent in this procedure may take days, weeks, and even months. The form of love-making is not prescribed but is left completely to the parties concerned. Each session takes place in the nude; the man is stimulated and aroused to the point of near-orgasm. At this critical moment, the woman seizes his penis firmly between the shaft and the head, thumb on the underside and two fingers on the upper part, holding it for three to six seconds. For some reason, as yet unknown, this action will head off an orgasm and often return the penis to flaccidity. During the course of each session the point of near-orgasm should be reached several times. At the end of the session, if necessary, ejaculation should be allowed.

Later, closer intimacies are tried with closer contact between the genitalia but never actual penetration. The woman must always be able to manually control and prohibit ejaculation.

No attempt should be made to have intercourse until both parties agree that he is ready. When this stage is finally achieved, insertion of the penis into the vagina should be accomplished as calmly as possible. Upon entry, he should remain quiet and unmoving for a considerable length of time. When he feels he has gained some control, slow and guarded movements may begin.

Of course there will be accidents and failures, but following this procedure has proven effective in clinics and at home, and many have been helped.

The basic idea behind this sytem is that a man's fear of failure – of either not being able to become erect or, if he does so, of ejaculating prematurely – is eliminated. He cannot have anxiety about failure since there is nothing he has to achieve, or anyone to satisfy but himself – the sex act being forbidden. Thus he can relax and just enjoy making love. Eventually he will also learn to relax when he performs the act. Frigidity: as in male therapy, sex play is substituted for the sex act. There is no time limit, no schedule – the play is continued as long as it takes the woman to reach and maintain some level of sexual satisfaction (not necessarily an orgasm). Again, no sexual intercourse is engaged in during this period of acclimatization, even if it takes weeks or months.

The time spent in bed during this sex play is considerably longer than if a natural course was being followed, concluding with the male orgasm, which always terminates the act. Here there are no conclusions, just relaxation and pleasure – no tensions, no compulsions, no anxieties. The woman need only please herself. In this sex play she can no longer be just the spectator of her partner's drive for completion; she is the sole reason and occasion for the event. Thus she can not be neutral and will find it difficult to be unresponsive.

However, some consideration should be observed for the male partner at the end of each session, to avoid his being left frustrated.

Many of the causes that may have induced frigidity in the woman, such as fear, a feeling of incompetence, ignorance of her own body, ignorance of clitoral function, self-repression, past sexual traumas (rape, near-rape, unhappy male encounters), can be overcome by this form of sexual therapy.

Table 18: Lotions for sunburn and suntan

As good as any commercial preparation, and considerably less expensive and more effective, all of the following can be prepared by a pharmacist without a medical prescription.

Protection against sunburn:
aminobenzoic acid N.F.   6 grains
titanium dioxide U.S.P.   3 grains
hydrophilic ointment (quantity sufficient to make 60 grains) or
red petrolatum jelly

Soothing ointment after burn:
zinc oxide (enough to make it into a paste)
calamine lotion
glycerin (about 20 per cent)
rose water

Suntan lotion:
mineral oil   45 per cent
sesame oil   45 per cent
wintergreen oil   10 per cent
any perfume for scent, if so desired

Table 19: Wood ticks: how to remove them

Wood ticks are found everywhere in brush and wooded areas throughout the summer season. Brown or speckled brown, they are very flat with an extremely hard protective covering and are about 3 millimetres, ⅛ of an inch in size.

Ticks attach themselves to clothing or the fur of animals and later make their way to the skin where they burrow in by a painless bite, the most common sites being hairy places, such as the pubic region, under the arms, and especially on the scalp. Within a day or so, after feeding on blood and tissue fluids, they will grow to half an inch (over 1 centimetre).

It should be noted, however, that not all ticks are carriers of infection, just as all mosquitoes are not disease carriers.

Ticks should *never* be touched by bare fingers or *crushed* on the skin, which only contaminates the skin with the body fluid of the tick. Removal can best be accomplished by putting a drop of kerosine, turpentine, or gasoline on its body. If these substances are not available, grease or oil of any kind can be used (this interferes with its respiration). After application, the tick should be pulled off gently with tweezers. Trying to remove a tick frantically or too energetically may leave the head or mouth parts embedded in the skin, which then will require the aid of a doctor. Afterwards the area should be washed with soap and water and disinfected if possible.

Table 20: How to check for breast cancer

Once a month, preferably within a week after your menstrual period, check yourself for lumps in the breasts. This simple self-examination takes only a few minutes and can save your life. Breast cancer is curable if caught in time.

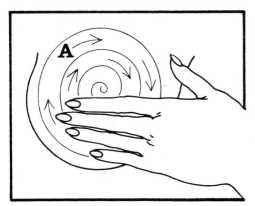

A procedure by means of which a woman can check herself for breast cancer is outlined in this series of illustrations.

In the shower or bath, while your skin is still wet and slippery, touch every part of each breast, starting at A in the drawing reproduced here and following the arrows. Keep the fingers flat and feel gently for a lump or thickening.

If you find a spot that feels thick, lumpy, or unusual, see your doctor.

Most of the time these aberrations are benign, but only a doctor can tell.

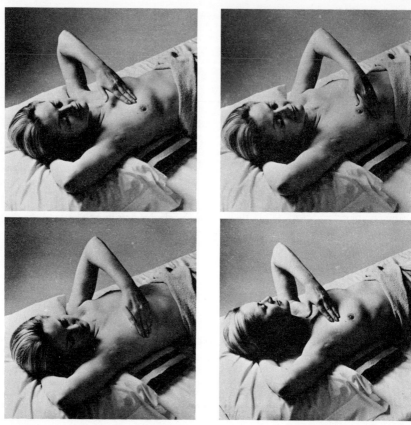

Now do a more thorough check lying down. Put one hand behind your head. With the other hand, fingers flattened, gently and lightly press your breast. Then reverse and check the other breast.

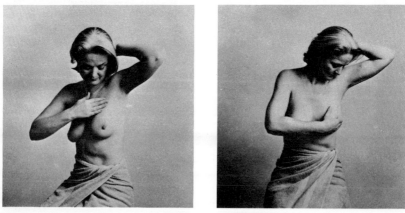

Now repeat the same procedure, this time sitting up but with your hands still behind your head. Then reverse and check the other breast. Finally, the procedure should be repeated one more time, this time while standing. If you do find a lump, the chances are eight to ten that it is benign; but you should see your doctor at once. (*American Cancer Society*)

Table 21: Aspirin

Aspirin is a marvellous drug, but it does have side effects, some of which can be serious, especially to the susceptible. The following aspirin facts should be noted:

Taking more than two aspirin at one time will not increase its effectiveness.

People who have asthma or who are allergic are more sensitive to aspirin. About one out of five will respond badly to it.

Aspirin is dangerous for those who are taking anticoagulating drugs, because aspirin itself is something of an anticoagulant and frequently will cause bleeding in the stomach.

Aspirin is dangerous for those who suffer from or are prone to ulcers.

Aspirin is dangerous for pregnant women; it can injure the foetus.

Aspirin is dangerous for those who are under antidiabetic medication or antigout therapy.

Aspirin can cause heartburn, nausea, dizziness, ringing in the ears, deafness, stupor, and even death.

Aspirin can get too old to use. If the bottle has a vinegary smell or if the pills look uneven or furry, throw them away.

Taking forty aspirins in one day can kill.

The cheapest aspirin and the most expensive are identical in action, purity, and effectiveness. In addition, despite the expensive advertising, there is no difference between buffered, compounded, or coated. Alka-Seltzer and its many equivalents are valuable because the aspirin is already dissolved in water. (The quickest way for aspirin to work is to take it in warm water.) Alka-Seltzer, however, also contains a considerable amount of sodium, which is contra-indicated for those who are suffering from high blood pressure or other heart ailments or who are obese.

Aspirin is a very good all round medication. Don't use it unless you absolutely must. Under no circumstances should you overuse it. It's a powerful drug – respect it.

Table 22: Emergency lifesaving technique: heart-lung resuscitation

(Artificial respiration and external cardiac compression)

Seconds count. While waiting for the doctor or ambulance, the heart attack victim can be kept alive by quick action. Anyone can perform this first aid, but it needs coolness and determination.

Usually the victim has had an arrest of not only his heartbeat but also his breathing. Resuscitation is best managed by two people, one to administer artificial respiration and the other to apply external cardiac compression.

The patient should be placed on his back on a hard surface, such as the floor (a bed or couch will not do). Point his chin upwards. Make sure his mouth and throat are cleared of all obstructions. Pinch his nose shut so that no air will escape when you blow into his mouth at a rate of no less than twelve breaths a minute (once every five seconds; for a child, once every three seconds). (Seconds can be determined by counting one thousand, two thousand, three thousand, four thousand, five thousand, which gives you five seconds.)

The patient's chest will expand moderately with each breath; if it doesn't there is some obstruction, which should be quickly investigated. Take your mouth away after each breath to allow the air to be exhaled. Artificial respiration should be kept up rhythmically until the patient is breathing or until help arrives.

The other rescuer will at the same time (coordination is not necessary) apply cardiac compression. He places one palm on the lower end of the breastbone (the notch at the end of the breastbone is too far down) the other hand on top of the first hand and at right angles to it. The rescuer now puts his full weight on his hands, keeping both arms stiff, in

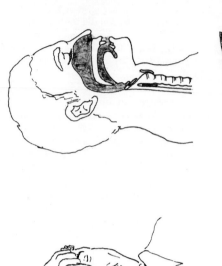

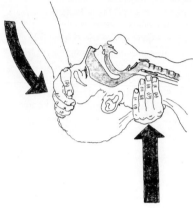

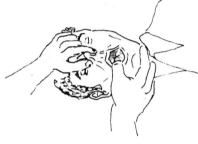

Cardio-pulmonary resuscitation. Before mouth-to-mouth resuscitation can be initiated, the victim's airway must be opened; here, the airway is shown first closed, and then opened by shifting the victim's head into the second position illustrated. Finally, the victim's nose is pinched shut and his jaw pulled forward and mouth-to-mouth can begin. (*Julian A. Miller*)

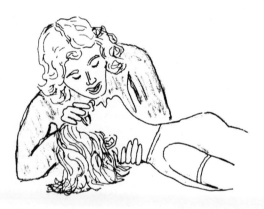

a steady rhythm of sixty to seventy times a minute (less than once a second will have little value). For children, the rhythm should be twice a second. The breastbone will move down about 4 to 5cm, 1½ to 2in. If there is no response after several minutes, try a sharp blow on the breastbone – it might just do the trick. At any rate, continue cardiac compression until professional help arrives.

If one person is obliged to do both jobs, it is, admittedly, difficult, but not impossible. Bear in mind that breathing

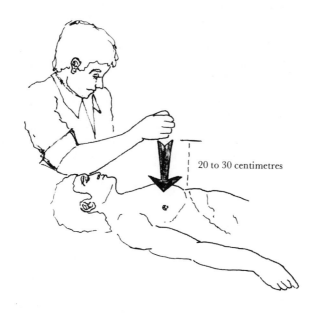

20 to 30 centimetres

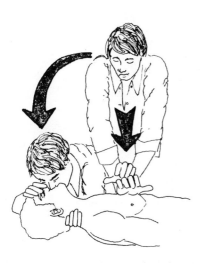

Before external cardiac massage can be initiated, it is necessary to administer a precordial thump. The rescuer can then begin applying cardiac compression while his partner administers mouth-to-mouth resuscitation. Coordination between their movements is not necessary. External cardiac massage for an infant is shown in the last illustration. (*Julian A. Miller*)

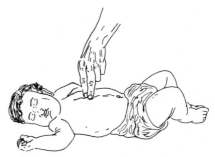

comes first. Artificial respiration is applied first, for five breaths, then cardiac compression. Later establish a pattern of one breath after five heart thrusts. Heart compression must never be delayed for longer than five seconds.

Do not be squeamish or discouraged. Keep at it even *after* you feel it is hopeless. There have been any number of cases in which a victim revived after more than an hour of resuscitation efforts.

543

Table 23: What to do in the event of a nosebleed

Get the patient to sit in a chair with his head erect; throwing the head back accomplishes nothing except to divert the blood into the throat. Strange as it may sound, vigorously blowing the nose may stop the haemorrhage or at least reduce it to a trickle – a nose filled with clotted blood must be cleared or bleeding will not stop.

After expelling all such matter, a pledget of dry cotton should be inserted into the affected nostril and fingertip pressure applied to the exterior of the nose, directed towards the cotton wool plug for a period of five or six minutes. Ice packs on the back of the neck are of no value.

If blood continues to flow into the back of the throat despite the above measures, the bleeding point is probably located posteriorly. In this uncommon event, the services of a doctor should be obtained without delay.

Table 24: Calorie chart

All the foods listed below are in the quantity of 100 grams (3½ ounces).

Fruit	calories
Cantaloupe	25
Grapefruit	30
Orange	33
Strawberries	37
Peach	46
Pineapple	52
Apple	60
Pear	60
Blueberries	61
Peaches (tinned)	68
Grapes	70
Pineapple (tinned)	80
Bananas	90
Dried figs	270
Dates	285

Dairy	calories
Skimmed milk	36
Milk	70
Cottage cheese	95
Eggs (2)	150
Single cream	204
Double cream	325
Cream cheese	370
Swiss cheese	370
Cheddar cheese	400
Butter	720
Margarine	720

Starches	calories
Spaghetti	150
Whole-wheat bread	240
Rye bread	250
White bread	275
Biscuits	342
Rice	360
Cornflakes	372
Doughnuts	425

Vegetables	calories
Mushrooms	11
Cucumber	12
Lettuce	15
Courgette	16
Tomato	20
Spinach	20
Aubergine	24
Green pepper	25
String beans	25
Cabbage	25
Carrots	30
Broccoli	30
Onions	32
Peas	70
Corn	85
Broad beans	95
Potato, baked, mashed	100
Avocado	245
Chick-peas (garbanzos)	290
Tinned pork and beans	290
Lentils	290
Potatoes (French-fried)	300
Potato chips	540

Beverages	calories
Coffee	0
Tea	0
*Ginger ale	35
*Coca Cola	46
*Apple juice	50
*Beer	50
*Cocoa	90

* Less than half a cup

†Gin, vodka	135
†Scotch whisky	140
†Blended whisky	145
†Rum	150

Meats, poultry, fish *calories*

Fish (cod, haddock)	70
Clams	81
Lobster	88
Halibut	126
Beef liver	140
Herring	190
Sardines	215
Corned beef	216
Bologna	225
Tuna (tinned)	250
Frankfurters	250
Lamb	260
Turkey	265
Chicken	285

Salmon (tinned)	290–325
Beef	325
Oysters	350
Hamburger meat (mince)	360
Pork (ham)	400
Bacon	610

Desserts *calories*

Gelatin (no sugar)	65
Ice cream	205
Pies	250
Jams	275
Pretzels	360
Chocolate (with milk, nuts)	530

Miscellaneous *calories*

Sugar	285
Peanuts, roasted or shelled	560
Peanut butter	576
Mayonnaise	696
Lard	900

† A measure and a quarter

A BRIEFING FOR GOOD HEALTH AND LONG LIFE

Good health does not mean the absence of disease – although many would settle for that – it means,, rather, ebullience, fitness, and vigour. The average Westerner reaches bodily old age long before chronological old age. We are proud of ourselves, of the skills and techniques that have made life so much easier and more comfortable. Unfortunately, making life easier is not consonant with making it healthier; generally, an easier life is a shorter life.

Consider the average man under thirty. His body is more middle-aged than young. Put him to the test, the test for buoyant youth, which is what he should be at that age. Can he run 200 metres? Can he run up two flights of stairs without stopping or without being unduly winded? Can he swim a short city block? The fact is he cannot. Only a small percentage of men have managed to guard and preserve their youth and health by keeping themselves fit.

The body is constantly at war, from birth to old age, against the environment, against bacteria, viruses, and microorganisms of every kind. In order to fight these constant battles the body must be in good physical condition. A lack of fitness makes one vulnerable to every kind of disease, all of which are waiting in the wings, waiting for the opportunity.

Our culture seems to be dedicated to indolence. We drive to work, take lifts up to the office, sit at a desk, sit at lunch, drive back home, sit at dinner, and then sit at a movie or TV for several hours and then to bed. We are spectators instead of participators. It is no different for the business woman, although the housewife fares better. She is far more active, cleaning the home, washing clothes, shopping, carrying, lifting, keeping up with her children and their needs. She is in far better shape than her sedentary husband and statistics prove it.

The notion that the easy life will preserve us is utterly false. Man is not a machine – unlike the automobile, he does not last longer with disuse. In man, the more he doesn't use his body, the *less time it will last.* A horse trainer knows that his horse must run and exercise every day. All animals, including man, need to be exercised. Man is a physical animal – his legs are more than half of his body; he was made to walk, run, climb, carry, and, yes, even to fight when necessary with his hands, feet, and heart. Man needs daily vigorous constant physical activity to keep him toned up and healthy.

Our civilization has contributed to many marvellous advancements and has reduced pain and misery, but we must not let civilization overwhelm us. The mystique of living requires each of us to be vessels of energy – the more energetic we are, the more energy we have.

Air pollution: now endemic all over the world, air pollution has certainly contributed to the sudden rise in lung cancer, emphysema, bronchitis, and other respiratory diseases – how much, no one can say but we do know that it is prodigious. More than forty substances have been identified in the atmosphere of our cities, from damaging to downright toxic (hydrocarbons, nitrogen oxides, nitrogen dioxides, smoke, heavy dust, sulphur oxides, carbon monoxide, and many others).

Rural communities are hardly immune – some areas are hit hard, particularly where mining, smelting, and cement factories are situated. Lead, zinc, antimony, every kind of metal poisoning, and scores of other toxic substances that are spewed into the air contribute to deadly air pollution.

All of us, everywhere, country or city, are breathing in asbestos fibres (from the linings of car brakes), a newly discovered danger that can cause progressive lung disease.

What is the answer? How do we avoid this hazard that hangs over us? Persons who have delicate lungs or are frail in health or are elderly should remove themselves from smog areas if possible. If not, then periodic trips away from polluted regions is essential. The alternative is a whole spectrum of diseases, many of which will shorten life considerably.

Water pollution: pollution of our water – lakes, rivers, and streams – has become a risk.

Our oceans, upon which life on land is intimately related, is now also in danger. Such pollutants as mercury, lead, toxic pesticides, radioactive wastes from radioactive ores, and unwanted toxic substance are being dumped into the oceans. There is not much each individual can do to avoid this hazard except fight to preserve our waters and to keep our ever-expanding industries from overwhelming us.

Noise pollution: a new hazard and a serious one to our health, consistently loud noises can reduce body efficiency, severely extend stress, cause ulcers, raise blood pressure, induce headaches, cause accidents, raise cholesterol levels, and, of course, produce deafness. Listening to rock music for hours is no small contributor to an irreparable loss of hearing, in addition to causing a multitude of other body disorders. Loud consistent noise should be recognized as a health hazard; it can cause sickness.

To fight this health hazard, everyone should make an effort to keep loud sounds out of the home by carpeting, heavy curtains, and various other soundproofing means. Noise is, generally, something each of us can do something about.

Doctoring – too much and too little: too much doctoring can only be matched in harmfulness by too little. The person who has a hoarse voice for weeks or the person who finds blood in his urine and neglects to see a doctor is, of course, committing a serious crime against himself. But too much doctoring is just as bad.

Drugs and medication: wherever possible, all drugs, all medication should be avoided, including aspirin. All drugs are harmful, generally a calculated risk in which the curative value of the drug exceeds the danger of its use. If the disease is comparatively minor and the symptoms are minor, it is better to try to get by without medication. Many diseases cured by drugs may leave side effects that may remain for a long time and can affect health.

The discovery of antibiotics represents the most magnificent advance in curing many diseases, but too little might not kill all the bacteria and thus leave a resistant strain in the body. In addition, antibiotics can cause severe allergic reactions and occasionally result in serious complications. They should never be self-administered.

Radiation: no one doubts the immense value and importance of x-ray in detecting disease, in identifying broken bones, and in the treatment of cancer, but it can, nevertheless, be dangerous. Both American and Russian authorities have warned that the sharp rise of leukaemia in recent years is due to years of exposure to x-ray. Most mothers of leukaemic children have had more x-rays (before conception and during pregnancy) than mothers of normal children. Radiologists suffer from leukaemia eight times more frequently than other doctors.

It is true we are exposed to radiation from cosmic rays, from the sun, and from radioactive minerals in the earth, but they are generally minimal, with the exception of the sun's ultraviolet radiation, which can induce cancer of the skin.

From 450 to 600 Rs (an R is a roentgen, a measure of x-ray; also called a rem – a roentgen equivalent in man) is fatal to half the people exposed; they will die of radiation sickness. The other half may go on to succumb later to leu-kaemia or other diseases. The effect of cumulative radiation is not yet fully understood. Some authorities (for ex-ample, Dr Shields Warren of Harvard Medical School) believe it is truly cumu-lative, that each x-ray exposure keeps adding up until after a number of years a dangerous level is reached, and five to twenty years later leukaemia will strike.

Some authorities believe that x-ray is like any injury or burn and will heal without any aftereffects, while others feel that the healing is never fully complete. Indeed, no one knows for sure how radi-ation really affects us.

Other long-range dangers, besides leu-kaemia, anaemia, and a susceptibility to infection, are sterility, malfunctioning of the embryo in pregnant women, and injury to the sperm.

Chest x-rays are no longer employed to detect TB; in any event, today practically every hospital has new x-ray equipment that is a hundred times less lethal but just as efficient as the earlier machines. Even so, x-rays are kept to a minimum.

Radioactive strontium 90 is second on the list of radiation dangers. It is found in human food wherever calcium is found (milk, for example) and now affects everyone in the world. It is stored in the bone for life. Strontium 90 has appeared as a result of all the nuclear bomb testing that has been carried out by many coun-tries throughout the world and is a grow-ing hazard. Strontium is very similar to calcium, and where calcium is not fully available, plants will absorb strontium instead. Within another decade many authorities predict a considerable rise in leukaemia directly traceable in good part to strontium 90.

Nutrition, vitamins, and obesity: it is not always true that we are what we eat, but what we eat can make a great deal of difference in our bodies and even our minds.

Meat is not essential; fowl and fish are far better, containing much less saturated fats (see *Table 4*) and much less choles-

terol. What is often lacking in the diet is fluorine, iron, vitamin A, and calcium. Fluorine, essential for teeth and bones, should be obtained in tablet form if it is not available as fluoridated water.

Vitamin A is plentiful in all fresh coloured vegetables, green, yellow, or red. No supplement is needed in the form of pills. Iron, vital for energy and oxygen, is found in raisins, molasses, and dried peas; two ounces a day of raisins will do nicely. Calcium, an essential mineral of the bones and for the clotting of blood, is found in skim milk, fish, nuts, fruits, whole grain cereals, and in the soft edible bones of canned salmon. Whole milk is not essential for adults; generally it is not well tolerated by large portions of the populations, despite popular belief in its nutritional value. Whole milk is a perfect food for suckling infants but not for adults. The fat in whole milk is harmful; skim milk, however, is not only tolerable but an excellent source of calcium.

The height, weight, and intelligence of children is often dependent upon the mother; if she is malnourished or under-nourished during pregnancy it can affect the child for the rest of his life.

An all-vegetarian diet is excellent, pro-viding that milk and eggs are included. Otherwise, the children of such parents will suffer from a lack of calcium and iodine (available in seafood and most fish).

In moderation, coffee, tea, minerals, and cocoa are not harmful, although, like coffee and tea, cocoa also contains caffeine.

Organic food is essentially better, but whether it is that much better, in terms of the trouble in procuring it, not to mention the doubling or tripling of the cost, should be considered. It is always far better to eat food that has not been treated with chemical fertilizer or pesti-cides, but, sad to say, more organic food is sold than grown.

Vitamins are essential for human life, but all the vitamins one needs are easily available in the food that is normally eaten. Vitamin pills are really quite un-necessary unless specifically advised for a specific condition. The maintenance of the vitamin value of foods, however, needs some consideration. The key word is 'less' – less storage time, less cooking time (vitamin C can be destroyed by heat), and less water in cooking.

All the claims of vitamin E exponents have not been shown to be facts; it is not an aphrodisiac; there is no evidence that it improves potency, nor does it cure sterility and impotence. Frankly no one really knows what it does, but since it is in such abundance everywhere – in all wheat and cereal germ, eggs, leafy vegetables, nuts – it is hard to believe that anyone in a developed country would ever be deficient in this nutrient.

The controversial vitamin C, however, is another matter. Dr Linus Pauling has steadfastly maintained that large doses of vitamin C can stop or stave off a cold. This cannot be dismissed out of hand, and the theory has been subjected to numerous investigations. It has been found to be effective for many people – with some it can cause a miraculous cure, with others it has no effect. It is surely worth a try. The indicated dosage during a cold is from 1 to 4 grams (4,000mg). Vitamin C needs daily replenishment since it cannot be stored or manufactured in the body.

Food notes: Sugar has received a very bad press in recent years as a cause for practically every disease (much of this could easily be true). Honey is a substitute, but it is a sugar as well, a little different and perhaps better. When buying honey make sure the label on the bottle or jar identifies the flower from which the honey was derived. If it does not name the flower, the likelihood is that it comes from a commercial hive that has been feeding its bees sugar water.

Real obesity, however, is hazardous to health and longevity; it will raise blood pressure, worsen diabetes and heart disease, and cut down life expectancy. This is not hard to understand, considering that the body has ten to twenty more pounds to carry around, more miles of blood vessels to overwork the heart, and more strain on the glands and other organs.

Fad diets are almost always dangerous. Some may succeed in reducing weight, but they can also be very harmful.

The right approach to weight reduction is to eat all foods but a little less of them. Two slices of bread at breakfast every morning can be cut down to one; two spoonfuls of sugar in a cup of coffee reduced to one and a half. In the course of six months or a year, the weight loss will be considerable.

The real cause of obesity can be under-exercising rather than overeating. Jogging or swimming or a stiff walk every day might burn up only 50 grams a day, but in six months that could mean a loss of 10 kilograms.

Obesity usually begins with the parents. Overstuffing the child, encouraging sedentariness, or not encouraging activity might be the first and most significant cause of this disease (see *Obesity* **347**).

Additives: of additives now in our food, many have never been tested. Each of us consumes about 2·5kg, 5lb of additives yearly.

Colour additives are mostly derived from coal tar (consistently implicated as a carcinogenic agent). Monosodium glutamate, a common additive, destroys the cells of the nervous system. Nitrates or nitrites, which are added to practically all processed meats, including frankfurters and smoked fish, can be changed in the stomach upon meeting other not uncommon substances into a cancer-producing constituent. BHT, a widely used preservative, remains in the body tissue for years. When the body loses weight this additive is dumped into the body proper with as yet unknown effects. The administration of antibiotics to fowl and cattle to keep the bacteria count down, and thus allow the animal to gain weight, ultimately means that some farmer is prescribing antibiotics for the public.

Stilboestrol is given to poultry and cattle to fatten them. Besides being a potent female sex hormone, stilboestrol also destroys vitamin B in the body. Nor is it known how many men like the idea of being fed female sex hormones without their consent.

Smoking: one sure way to shorten life, smoking can cause or increase the chances of:

developing lung cancer (nine times higher than in non-smokers);

suffering a heart attack (twice as high among those who smoke a pack or more a day);

developing emphysema (usually a direct result of smoking);

worsening of a gastrointestinal disorder (ulcers either heal more slowly or become chronic);

reducing birth weight (maternal heavy smoking can affect the foetus);

increasing circulatory ailments (smoking is a serious risk for those suffering from heart or circulatory disorders; it will raise blood pressure, narrow the blood vessels of the legs, fingers, and toes, and is a direct cause of intermittent claudication [pain on walking from narrowed blood vessels] and gangrene of the leg).

New investigations are constantly indicating that smoking is a factor in a large number of diseases.

How to stop smoking

1 Why are you smoking? List the reasons. Be cold-blooded about it. Write it all down on paper.

2 If one of the reasons is that it gives you handling satisfaction by keeping your hands busy, use a fake cigarette.

3 If one of the reasons is that it's possibly a habit and admittedly you often put a cigarette in your mouth without thinking, keep a card inside the cellophane of the pack and tick off every cigarette you smoke. You won't stop smoking, but you will assuredly cut down on the number.

4 If one of the reasons is that you are afraid of gaining weight if you stop, don't worry about that. After you've stopped smoking you can tackle the weight problem. Once you have licked smoking, you will far more easily lick a few extra pounds.

5 If one of the reasons is that you need a cigarette in moments of stress or

tension, try physical exertion, like jogging or swimming – any very active sport will reduce mental tension far better than smoking.

6 If one of the reasons is that you believe you're addicted, bear in mind that not every cigarette you put in your mouth is a craved one. Many of them are in anticipation of a craving, so that a number of them can be eliminated. First try smoking only those cigarettes you feel you must absolutely have. You will discover that your smoking will be cut in half. Secondly, try to give it up completely after a week or so of curtailed smoking. If you fail, you will need professional assistance. Many have been helped by hypnosis or by psychiatric consultation, and many have kicked the habit through group therapy with other addicted smokers.

Those who are serious about giving up smoking usually find some way to accomplish their goal.

Heart: all aspects of heart and health are discussed in *Part 2, Chapter 8*, and in *Early warning signals, Part 3, Heart disease* **123, 124, 125, 126**.

Eye health: all children should have their eyes tested no later than at school entry, regardless of whether they have symptoms or not.

Acute symptoms that must be investigated are: an intolerance of bright lights, persistent blinking, blurring, and spots before the eyes.

Non-acute symptoms that should also be investigated are: an aversion to reading, unusual fatigue after normal eye use, an unusual number of errors in writing, difficulties in concentrating, and headaches, particularly those that radiate to and from an eye.

Good eye health rules

When reading, writing, or doing other close work, the source of light should be steady, nonglaring, and easy to read by. The light should come from behind.

All spectacles must be shatterproof or made of plastic.

Light that shines directly into the eyes should be avoided.

Frosted bulbs or shaded lamps are always better.

The entire room should be lighted, not just the working area.

Indirect lighting is preferred to direct.

When doing extensive reading or writing, the eyes should be rested for a minute or so from time to time by closing them or looking at faraway objects.

Sunglasses at night or in darkened places are not advisable. Even in daylight sunglasses should only be worn in glare conditions, unless otherwise instructed by a doctor (see *Dark glasses syndrome* **18**).

Ear health: persons susceptible to ear infections should try to keep their ears dry.

Poking around in the ear with a toothpick, or matchstick is a good way to puncture the eardrum and infect the middle ear. The drum is not very far inside the canal and can easily be injured.

No earache should be allowed to continue for longer than a day without consultation with a doctor.

Continuous loud noises should be avoided, for a partial hearing loss can result which may become permanent.

Wax should always be removed from the ear – germs like it, an ideal breeding place.

Streptomycin, quinine, and heavy drinking can permanently affect hearing.

Such diseases as tonsillitis, mumps, measles, all streptococcal infections, the flu, pneumonia, meningitis, and syphilis can cause hearing impairment and ear disorders.

Swimming in doubtful pools or polluted waters can be risky.

The nose should be blown properly. One wrong blow can cause an inner-ear infection, which may last for months. When blowing the nose, one nostril should be kept open as well as the mouth.

Fatigue and stress: one of the prime causes of fatigue, besides disease, is stress. Any form of nervous tension can sap one's energy. It has been estimated that seventy-five per cent of all fatigue is psychological. Anxiety, depression, maladjustment, conflict, and boredom can induce great fatigue. Overwork, although often used as a complaint, is rarely the cause.

No matter how deeply fatigued a person may feel, if he is suddenly confronted with a dangerous or threatening situation, his fatigue will suddenly vanish like a magician's handkerchief. If a person is bored, the promise of excitement will do the same.

There are, however, a few diseases that can cause exhaustion: insufficient insulin in diabetes, any heart disorder that impairs circulation, a low thyroid hormone output, and obesity (a result of carrying around excess weight).

Fatigue cannot be cured by pep pills, extra vitamins, tonics, yeast tablets, liver extracts, or mineral capsules. If the reason is not organic, vigorous exercise will, in almost all cases, dispel fatigue. Exercise will keep the adrenal glands in high gear and improve circulation by bringing more oxygen into the body.

Indolence is another significant cause. When wild animals are domesticated their enforced (caged) idleness causes their adrenal glands to shrink. The same happens to man when he lives in voluntary physical indolence.

Stress has been blamed for every ill of man, and while some of this may be true, basically we are all well-equipped with the glands and hormones necessary to handle stress, to withstand the hazards of life. Stress is part of living. The caveman battling to bring down a mammoth for food for his tribe or family was under just as much stress as modern man labouring to keep his head above water at his job.

Basically how we handle stress means a great deal in terms of health and longevity. An animal that gets into a dangerous spot, a cat, perhaps, suddenly confronted by a huge, hostile dog, screams, claws, spits, and fights, but when she has managed to survive the encounter, the stress does not linger on. Within a few minutes she is her old self, as if the incident had never happened.

Not so with many of us. A bad incident is often relived and agonized over for days and weeks.

Stress can cause or worsen certain disorders – headache, chronic fatigue, and moderate stomach upsets are tolerable, but others, high blood pressure, ulcers, and asthma, are killers.

If one cannot handle stress properly, some self-evaluation is in order. An urgent talk with wife, husband, friend, relative, or a psychiatrist is indicated.

Relaxation: a divine gift, relaxation allows us to rest, recoup, and recover, to let go of all the pressures, so that the next round of pressures can be attacked with renewed vigour. It is vital for good health. Some people, even though they lie down or sit in an easy chair, never relax; they are still running, battling only in a sitting or lying position.

There are two excellent ways of relaxing; one is by vigorous physical activity and the other is a superb Oriental method.

Engaging in a vigorous sport or activity that requires total concentration can bring about full relaxation. Skiing, horseback riding, tennis, jogging, and swimming are excellent. It is almost impossible to worry about a business deal when negotiating a steep downhill run, returning an opponent's serve, or enduring the small agony of pushing one's body to unusual limit, as in running. Reading a book, watching football, or listening to music is nowhere near as effective.

The Oriental system requires lying face down on a bed, couch, or floor with the arms and legs slightly outstretched; from the head down each part of the body is relaxed separately and in turn. Starting with the eyes, each eyeball is relaxed one at a time. Relaxing means letting go, like untensing a muscle. Concentration is then focused onto the neck, relaxing every muscle; then the shoulders, deliberating on each one, one at a time, loosening up all the tightness. Next the right arm, first the upper arm, then forearm, the wrists, and hands. The same procedure is followed with the left arm. Afterwards the chest, the abdomen, the hips, the groin,

thighs, knees, legs, ankles, feet. The entire body can be relaxed in this fashion in ten minutes.

After the entire body has been mentally massaged in this way, total repose should be continued for fifteen minutes or longer. A half hour of this form of relaxing can be as effective as a night's sleep.

Sex: sexual frustration is a prime cause of mental problems and physical disorders; it can lead to all the stress ailments and a few more besides. Everyone must make some accommodation to this driving force, adjusting one's sexual needs to reality, which means devoting enough time and energy to this pursuit.

A good marriage is perhaps the best answer, but if this is not immediately available, each one must find his own private answer. Most of us cannot live well or in good health without some basic sexual satisfaction. Good health in mind and body is not possible without proper sexual fulfilment.

Good health and travel: everyone should carry a Medical Card in his wallet, which indicates his personal pertinent medical history; for example, it might indicate an allergy to penicillin or some other substance, or that he is a diabetic or an epileptic. In case of an accident or unconsciousness, a Medical Card can be a lifesaver.

When travelling in tropical countries carry insect repellent and never wade in any natural body of water. In doubtful countries, drinking the local water can be hazardous; it is best to confine oneself to wine, beer, and carbonated drinks. The same holds true for ice (although bacteria and other micro-organisms cannot survive boiling, they do survive freezing). Only vegetables and fruit that can be peeled should be eaten raw. Pork and rare beef should be avoided.

Plenty of rest is strongly advised when crossing one or more time zones. Jet lag can be alleviated by drinking a glass of water (or other liquids) for every hour aloft, for the body becomes dehydrated on long trips.

A medical travelling kit is useful. It

should contain paregoric for diarrhoea, medication for motion sickness and respiratory infections, sleeping pills, insect repellents, antacids, aspirin, water purification tablets, a Red Cross first-aid book, and a supply of antibiotics. In addition, some doctors advise carrying 50gm, two ounces of Chlorox – one drop in 1 litre, 1 quart of water will kill all the pathogens within ten minutes.

Exercise and fitness: bulging muscles do not indicate fitness; rather, fitness is indicated by cardiovascular health, stamina, endurance, and good physical tone. Lifting weights only develops muscles, nothing much more. Calisthenics are better, but the regimen is rarely continued long enough to do any good. To achieve real fitness, treat yourself to jogging, swimming, cycling, brisk walking, and other sustained exercises.

When walking for exercise the pace must be brisk and continued for a minimum of an hour daily. Walking leisurely is no exercise at all.

At least two hours should elapse after a meal before jogging. When jogging the arms and shoulders should occasionally be shaken to prevent them from tightening up, and frequent deep breaths will help both in relaxation and in oxygen intake. The entire body in all its separate parts should be as loose as possible. Each step should land on the heel, roll onto the ball of the foot, and then take off in one continuous motion. If this method is uncomfortable, try landing on the whole foot (the weight slightly more on the ball of the foot) with as little jolting of the body as possible. Running only on the balls of the feet will cause tension and soreness in the leg and foot muscles.

A daily jogging regimen (at least a mile or two daily) will eventually lower the pulse rate at rest by ten points or more. This lowered pulse rate can save 10,000 extra heartbeats a day (as if the heart has rested two to three hours daily).

The human body is far more likely to rust out than wear out; the more it is used the better it will function. If it is not kept well exercised it will begin to falter, not only in musculature but in the glands, heart, lungs, and all the vital organs. Whenever possible, one should walk rather than drive, climb stairs rather than take the lift, move frequently instead of remaining seated for long periods of time. Walk to work, at least part of the way if the whole distance is too far.

A brisk hour-walk every day will not only deliver major health benefits in terms of fitness but will also burn up 5kg, eleven pounds a year. It will also increase the oxygen level, decrease nervous tension, and expand capillaries, as well as reduce body fat.

Fitness is not possible without proper, daily, vigorous, meaningful exercise. Whatever the exercise, it must not be an unpleasant chore; forcing the body out of indolence may be acutely uncomfortable, but the daily challenge and victory over culturally acquired body passivity should be rewarding and even exhilarating (see *Tables 5, 9,* and *14*).

Long life: Sweden has the longest life expectancy, 72 years for the male. Most of the African nations are at the bottom, with 32 years for Upper Volta, and Gabon on the very bottom with a life expectancy of 25 years!

Women on the average live four to seven years longer than men.

The following rules and guidelines can extend life for ten years or longer.
1 Marriage: strange, and perhaps unbelievable to many of us, married people are longer-lived than single persons. They spend less time in hospitals, are generally happier, healthier, and more successful than their unblissful single counterparts.
2 Sex: sexual activities should never be given up at any age. The truth is that the more one continues his sexual life the more one is capable of practising it. Continuation of sex is related to longer life.
3 Understanding the physical self: each of us should know his limitation in regard to food, drink, activity, allergies, and responses to pressure and live within his limitations. The body should

be taxed for maximum health but never overtaxed.

4 Retirement: a human being, like his heart, must keep on working or expire. Although retirement is often compulsory at a certain age, idleness can be deadly. The statistics are overwhelmingly poor for those who stop being active. One must find a new enterprise, perhaps less strenuous, and keep on working.

5 Pessimism: continued chronic pessimism is always a losing game with the outcome considerably hastened. Pessimism can cut down the life-span as sure as any fatal disease. One of the great secrets of long-lived people is their joy in living, which can often keep them alive beyond their normal lifespan.

6 Cholesterol and saturated fats: enough has been said about them elsewhere in this book. Most of us know the harm these substances can do to the heart and circulation (see *Tables 2, 3, and 4*).

7 Nutrition: knowing the value of different foods can add years to life. Nutrition-aware people do themselves and their families a great service by buying only wholesome, nourishing foods as opposed to packaged high-additive foods, by reading the labels, by avoiding foods that are known to be harmful or those that don't 'look right', by reading the dates on bread, milk, and fresh juices. A nutritionally conscious person walks into a supermarket as if into a hostile land.

8 Salt: salt is a hidden item in all processed foods and in a large number of dairy products (butter, cheese, and margarine). It is also present in practically all processed breakfast cereals and processed food normally considered sweet. Salt in excess will cut down the lifespan. As indicated many times, read the labels.

9 Women over forty-five: a cervical smear every year is advisable; all such women should examine their breasts carefully once a month (see *Table 20*). For those who have a family history of breast cancer, a mammography once every year or every six months is suggested.

10 Obesity: obesity and long life are contradictory. Rapid diets, fad diets, and trick diets can be even more harmful (see *Obesity* **347**).

11 Alcohol: in small amounts alcohol may be beneficial, but excess drinking can shorten life.

12 Drugs and medication: a basic rule for good health and a long life is to keep away from all drugs and medication as much as possible. This includes aspirin (see *Table 21*), antihistamines, tranquillizers, and sleeping pills, unless ordered by a doctor.

13 Relaxation: the tensions of life must never be allowed to build up. The practice of daily relaxation is basic to a long life (see *Relaxation* above).

14 Tension: prolonged tension is destructive; it can lead to many diseases that can shorten life (see *Fatigue and stress* above).

15 Exercise: a minimum of twenty minutes (more is better) should be spent at some vigorous sport or activity – jogging, swimming, mountain climbing, tennis, cycling, skiing, or very brisk walking (5 to 6 kilometres an hour) – not once a week or at weekends but daily.

16 Vacation: if a vacation cannot be taken whenever needed, a heavy work pattern should be broken up with holiday weekends.

17 Fresh air: inhabitants of smog-ridden areas must get out of it from time to time to give their lungs a chance to recover. The unrelieved breathing of polluted air will cut down on the durability of the lungs. A long life is not possible without healthy lungs.

18 Symptoms: all vague and uneasy symptoms should eventually be discussed with a doctor.

There are signs, however, that may indicate a dangerous condition. If any one of the following symptoms exist, medical consultation is imperative, even if only to rule out a serious disease:

The appearance of blood anywhere, in

the urine, in the stools, in vomit, or in a cough.

The appearance of a tumour or a lump anywhere or an unusual swelling of the lymph nodes.

An unusual shortness of breath, pain in the chest, paralysis of any part of the body, an unexplained loss of weight, and heavy night sweats.

A cloudy or bloodshot eyeball, sunken eyeballs, a loss of vision, blurring or narrowing of the visual field, dilated pupils, seeing halos around lights or seeing a shower of sparks.

Abnormal or discoloured fingernails, white leg with a prominent vein, black skin, yellow deposits under the skin, dead-white numb skin, cyanosis anywhere, and clubbing of fingers.

Persistent hoarseness, consistent anaemia, sustained fever, dizziness, fainting, personality changes, and headaches if one has never had them before.

19 X-ray: one should always ask: Is this x-ray absolutely essential? Radiation can cut down the life span. ·

20 Accidents: if one follows all the above guidelines and is basically careless in driving a car or crossing the street or not putting on a safety belt, he'll be just as dead as if he had totally ignored the rules. Being the healthiest person in the cemetery is not a valuable accomplishment.

The human body remains to this day an awesome mystery, and though daily we learn more and more about it, the profound secrets of the body are yet to be discovered. It is like a light in the darkness; the larger the illuminated area, the larger the area of surrounding darkness. The human body defies our logic; it functions with a wisdom that perplexes us. Some people will die of a bee sting, others will survive the bite of a cobra.

The body wants to live and will survive incredible blows, but it cannot fight well without the mind's full cooperation. In the absence of accidents, the philosophical thought that no one dies without giving his consent is generally true. One can give his consent by carelessness, recklessness, indifference.

A long life need not be characterized by managing to survive many ailments. Many of these ailments can be bypassed. Good health, admittedly, is harder to come by when reaching middle age and beyond; it does require greater efforts to attain it, but the few who devote themselves to this end unquestionably live longer.

Eventually we are all caught by that dark hunter, but those of us who are constantly active and constantly moving around are more difficult targets and less easily caught.

Glossary of medical terms

The words in this glossary are medical terms used in this book. Many medical words not listed below are fully explained in the text.

abscess A collection of pus formed by the disintegration of surrounding tissues

acetone A sweet, fruity substance (ketone) found in normal urine and in larger quantities in the urine of diabetics

achlorydia Absence of hydrochloric acid secretion in the stomach

acid-base balance The mechanism by which acids and alkalies are kept in equilibrium; disturbance of this balance results in acidosis or alkalosis

acidosis Decreased alkalinity of the blood

acoustic Pertaining to sound or hearing

acupuncture An ancient Chinese system of medicine in which needles are inserted into the body at three-hundred-odd points for therapy and anaesthesia. As yet no suitable explanation has been found for its frequent effectiveness

adenoids A tonsil-like growth in the back of the nasal passage in the throat

adhesion Tissues growing together abnormally after an inflammation, injury, or surgery

aerosol A spray for sterilizing the air or an atomized solution for inhalation

albumin A protein found in the whites of eggs, in plants, and in animals; when found in the urine, it usually indicates a number of diseases

alkalosis Excessive alkalinity of the blood or tissue fluids

allergen Any foreign substance towards which the body becomes hypersensitive

allergist A doctor who specializes in the treatment of allergies

alveoli A tiny cluster of minute air sacs that make up most of the lung tissues

amphetamine Any of a group of drugs that is a powerful stimulant and appetite inhibitor

amylase An enzyme from the pancreas that converts starches into sugar; also found in saliva

anaerobic (1) When referring to exercise, energy that is not provided by inspired oxygen. (2) Without oxygen (*anaerobic bacteria* are able to live without oxygen)

analgesic A drug that reduces pain

anaphylaxis A shock reaction to an allergic substance, such as animal serum, bee sting, and so on

androgen A hormonal substance that produces male characteristics (testosterone)

anaesthesia Loss of the sensation of pain, usually induced by the administration of a drug in order to perform painful procedures

aneurysm A weak, bulging section of an artery, often in the aorta, which can rupture

angina A sensation of choking or extreme pressure (*angina pectoris*, pain and pressure in the chest)

animal serum Serum obtained from an animal rendered immune against a disease-causing microorganism, which is then injected into a patient with that disease

anoxia Lack of oxygen in the body

aorta Largest artery in the body, receiving all the blood from the heart before circulating throughout the body

anterior chamber The aqueous chamber of the eye between the cornea and the iris and lens

antibiotic Any of a group of drugs that kills or inhibits the growth of bacteria or rickettsia

antibodies A substance produced by the body and circulated in the blood for defence against disease-causing microorganisms and antigens that have gained entry into the body

anticoagulant A substance that slows the clotting of the blood

antiemetic A drug or substance that prevents vomiting

antigen A foreign substance in the body (bacteria, toxins of bacteria, foreign blood cells, and so on) that induces the formation of antibodies

antihelmintic (anthelmintic) A drug that is destructive to worms

antihistamine Any of a variety of drugs that opposes the effects of histamine in the body; used in allergic conditions, such as hay fever, serum sickness, and for alleviation of cold symptoms

antipyretic Any medication that reduces fever

antirheumatic Any medication that combats rheumatism

antispasmodic Any substance that prevents spasms

antitoxin A substance capable of counteracting or neutralizing toxins or poisons that gain entrance into the body

Apgar score A system for scoring an infant's condition a minute after birth, including heart rate, respiration, muscle tone, colour, and response to stimuli

aphasia Loss or impairment of the ability to use words or speech

apicectomy Surgical removal of the apex of a tooth root

appetite, hunger Appetite is an acquired desire for food; hunger is the need for food

areola A pigmented ring around a central point, such as the area around a nipple

arrhythmia Irregular heartbeat

arteriole A very minute artery that leads into the capillaries

arteriosclerosis A thickening and hardening of the arteries of the body

articular Pertaining to a joint

ascites An abnormal accumulation of fluid in the abdominal cavity

aspiration The removal of fluids or gases from the body by suction; inhalation of foreign material into the lungs

asymptomatic Without symptoms

atherosclerosis A generalized condition of the arteries with plaques of fatty material (cholesterol and other saturated fats) and calcium on the inside of the arterial wall (arterio-atherosclerosis is a combined word referring to the hardness and inelasticity of the arteries resulting from the formation of hardened fatty plaques)

atrophy A shrinking, wasting away, or reduction of a tissue, muscle, or organ

audiology The science of hearing

aura A premonitory sensation that precedes an epileptic seizure or migraine headache

Australia antigen An antigen discovered in some patients with viral hepatitis; also known as hepatitis-associated antigen

autoimmune disease Several diseases of unknown origin in which the body is strangely unable to distinguish between foreign invaders and its own tissues, so that it produces antibodies against itself, often causing serious harm

autonomic Spontaneous, self-controlling

autonomic nervous system That part of the nervous sytem that functions without conscious control, innervating the blood vessels, heart, glands, liver, and so on

bacteraemia An infection in which bacteria have entered the bloodstream

bactericide Any medication that kills bacteria

basal metabolism A measurement of the amount of energy the body uses at rest by determining the amount of oxygen intake

benign Not recurrent nor malignant

bifocal lens Two lenses cemented together, the upper one for distance, the lower one for close vision

bile A bitter alkaline secretion from the liver that aids in digestion and is stored in the gallbladder

bile duct A tube carrying bile from the liver and gallbladder to the small intestine

biliary Pertaining to bile

biliary colic Pain caused by gallstones

biopsy The surgical removal of minute bits of tissue for microscopic study

bitemporal Both temples

bovine Pertaining to cattle

bronchodilator Any substance that will dilate the bronchi

B_{12} A vitamin extracted from the liver that is essential for the formation of red blood cells; a specific medication for pernicious anaemia

bubo A painful swelling of the lymph gland in the groin and under the arm

buccal Pertaining to the cheek

bursa A sac-like cavity filled with a sticky fluid that is used as a lubrication over the bony prominences of the body to prevent friction

calcification A hardening of tissues resulting from deposits of calcium

calculus A stony mass in the bladder, kidney, or gallbladder, *dental calculus* is tartar that accumulates on the teeth

capillary A very tiny blood vessel

cardiovascular Pertaining to the heart and blood vessels

cardioverter An electrical device to shock the heart into action

carditis Inflammation of the heart

carotene A yellow pigment found in vegetables, fruits, and eggs, which converts to vitam A

carotid Arteries of the neck

cartilage The gristle attached to the bone to provide better articulation of the joints

catheter Any of a variety of tubes for insertion into the body to remove fluids

cerebrovascular Pertaining to blood vessels of the brain

cervix, cervical Pertaining to the neck; also to the neck of an organ, such as the cervix of the uterus

chancre A hard, primary syphilitic ulcer

chemotherapy Treatment with chemicals and drugs

Cheyne-Stokes respiration A form of breathing that occurs in some patients with heart, kidney, or vascular disease. At first breathing is slow and shallow; it then increases in depth and rapidity until it reaches a maximum, upon which it begins to decrease until it stops for ten to twenty seconds. The entire process is then repeated

chiropractor One who practises manipulative treatment in the belief that all diseases are caused by pressure on the spinal nerves and can be corrected by spinal adjustments

cholesteatoma A tumour of the middle ear

cholesterol A fatty wax-like substance essential to the human body, which is found in the brain, blood, and bile and is manufactured by the liver. A redundance of this substance through the intake of animal fats, egg yolk, and milk products can be dangerous to the circulatory system by being deposited on the inner linings of the arteries and narrowing them

choline One of the B-complex group of vitamins, important in the metabolism of fats

chordee The painful downward curvature of the penis in erection, either congenital or resulting from gonorrhoea

chorea (St Vitus's dance) A disease of the nervous system seen most often in rheumatic fever that is manifested by irregular, jerky, rapid movements of the face, legs, and arms

choriocarcinoma An extremely rare but extremely malignant cancer, usually of the uterus and testes; also known as *chorioepithelioma*

chorioepithelioma see *choriocarcinoma*

cirrhosis of the liver A hardening, thickening, and degeneration of the liver cells, causing the growth of fibrous tissue and the ultimate destruction of the liver

clitoris A small body of highly sensitive erectile tissue situated above the vagina, corresponding to the male penis

clubbing (of the fingers) Fingertips become broad and bulbous due to a heart or lung disease

colic An intermittent, spasmodic pain, usually abdominal; in *biliary colic*, paroxysms of pain from gallstones

collateral circulation Auxiliary blood vessels that expand and take over when an artery is blocked so that the necessary blood can be supplied to the deprived area (usually around the heart)

collodion A viscous liquid preparation smelling of ether and highly flammable, used chiefly for cementing dressings and sealing wounds. When applied dries to a strong transparent film

colostomy A surgical procedure that provides an artificial anus in the colon

comedo A blackhead

concussion A brain injury from a blow on the head or a violent jarring

congenital Existing at birth

conjunctiva Membrane that covers the front of the eyeball and the eyelid

contracture A permanent contraction of a muscle from a spasm or paralysis

cortisone A hormone from the adrenal glands, also made synthetically, with important medical uses

coryza The common cold

cosmetic factor Serving to preserve or create a good appearance or beauty

crisis The turning point or critical period of a disease; a sharp paroxysm of pain in the course of a disease

cyanosis Blueness of the skin caused by insufficient oxygen in the blood

cyst A sac containing fluid or a semisolid substance

cystoscope An instrument for interior examination of the bladder and ureter. It is introduced through the urethra into the bladder

defibrillation Stoppage of the fibrillation of the heart and the restoration of natural rhythm by the use of drugs or an electrical instrument

dehydration The loss of more water than is taken into the body, a serious aspect of disease

dementia A deterioration of the brain with resultant impairment of intellect, willpower, and memory; behaviour may be confused and irrational

diaphragm The muscle that separates the chest from the abdomen. *Vaginal diaphragm:* a ringed rubber cup that blocks entrance to the cervix of the uterus for contraceptive purposes

diastole The interval between heartbeats, indicating the condition of the arteries at rest; the lower of the two figures in recording blood pressure (120/80)

diathermy A treatment to produce heat in the body tissues by passing high frequency electric currents through them

digitalis An important medication, derived from the foxglove plant, used in the treatment of heart ailments

dilatation Expansion of a vessel, organ, or the pupil of an eye

dilatation and curettage (D & C) A surgical procedure in which the cervix of the uterus is dilated and the uterus is scraped with a curette.

disc, disk A pad of cartilage between the veterbrae of the spine

disclosing tablet A chewable tablet that stains and exposes plaques on the teeth

diuresis An increase in urination that is accompanied by a reduction in oedema of the tissues; a *diuretic* is a medication that brings this about

diverticulum A blind pouch (like a tiny balloon) opening from a hollow organ, usually from the oesophagus or the colon

Down's syndrome Mongolism, a congenital defect marked by retardation, a sloping forehead, flat bridge of the nose, and an Oriental appearance

dropsy An old term for oedema, the collection of fluid in the body

duodenum The first part of the small intestine that is connected to the stomach

dyslexia Disorders of reading, writing or learning

dyspepsia Acid indigestion

dyspnoea Shortness of breath

eclampsia A very serious toxic disorder of late pregnancy marked by severe convulsions and coma

electrocardiograph An electrical instrument that records variations and changes in heart action, used in determining heart disorders

electrolyte Dissolved salts and alkalies normally found in the blood and tissue fluids

embolism The obstruction of a blood vessel by an *embolus*, which is a blood clot

encephalogram An x-ray photograph of the brain

endocrine Glands whose secretions are absorbed directly into the bloodstream, occasionally referred to as ductless glands

enzyme An organic substance that causes other compounds to split into simpler compounds; a catalyst

epididymis The small cordlike mass on the back of each testicle in which the sperm are stored

epigastric Pertaining to the region over the pit of the stomach

erythematous Marked by redness of the skin

eustachian tube A rather narrow canal from the middle ear to the back of the throat for the maintenance of proper air pressure within the ear

exophthalmic Pertaining to protruding eyeballs

exotoxin A toxin (poison) excreted by bacteria

extrasystole A premature heartbeat

exudate A substance that is excreted or oozed

faecal Pertaining to the faeces

fallopian tubes The tube that connects each ovary to the uterus, through which an egg from the ovary passes to the uterus

fibrillation A tremor or twitching of a heart muscle rather than a beat

fibrinogen A clotting agent in the blood manufactured by the liver

fibroid A degeneration in which tissue resembles fibre

fissure A slit, break, or crack

fistula An abnormal channel leading from a hollow organ to a free surface

flatus Intestinal gas passed through the rectum

foetus The unborn child beyond the third month of pregnancy; prior to the third month it is called an embryo

folic acid One of the B complex vitamins, important in blood formation and essential in the treatment of certain forms of anaemia. Found in green leafy vegetables, yeast, liver, and mushrooms

fontanelle The soft spot on the top of an infant's head where the skull bones have not yet joined

forceps Surgical pliers for grasping and holding body parts; obstetrical forceps fit around an infant's head, and are designed to assist in birth

fulminate Sudden onset, explosive, rapidly worsening

galloping rhythm Heart sounds resembling

the gallop of a horse that are indicative of heart trouble

gamma globulin A protein substance normally occurring in the blood that stimulates and participates in the production of protective antibodies

gangrene The localized death of tissue resulting from the blood supply being cut off

gastrectomy The surgical removal of a part or all of the stomach

gastric lavage The washing out of the stomach

gene Part of a chromosome, a basic unit that determines hereditary traits

gingivitis Inflammation of the gums

glans The head of the penis or head of the clitoris

glucose A sugar (dextrose) produced in the body from starchy foods, a main source of energy

glucose tolerance test A test for early diabetes

gluten Vegetable albumin found in wheat and other grain

glycogen A substance manufactured from dextrose by the liver, which also stores it and reconverts it back to glucose (blood sugar) when needed

glycosuria Sugar in the urine

goitrogen A substance found in certain foods (notably the cabbage family) that in excessive amounts induces goitre

gonad A sex gland, either an ovary or a testicle

gram (gm) A unit of weight of the metric system (about 30gm equal an ounce)

granulation The formation of small, rounded granules of flesh that usually occurs in early stages of healing ('proud flesh' is excessive growth of this tissue)

gross motor play Involving large movements, such as running, wrestling, and so on

gumboil A swelling of the gum from an abscess at the root of a tooth

gumma A firm mass of tissue, as a tumour, occurring almost anywhere in the body as a result of late syphilis

gynaecology The branch of medicine dealing with diseases of women

haematology The branch of medicine dealing with the blood and its diseases

haemodialysis The cleansing of the blood of waste material by passing it through a special membrane, usually as applied to an artificial kidney machine

haemolysis The destruction of red blood cells

hernia The protrusion of an organ or part of an organ through a weak spot in the muscles that contain it; a rupture. Most common area is the groin (*inguinal hernia*) in which men are most susceptible; *hiatus hernia* occurs in the oesophagus

Hippocratic face The facial appearance of those dying from a long illness: dark brown or leaden skin, hollow eyes, loose, relaxed lips, drawn, pinched face, contracted ear lobes turned outward

hormone A substance secreted by an endocrine gland that affects activities of the body or various organs

hyperkinesis An excessive amount of mobility

hyperlipaemia An excessive amount of fat in the blood

hypertension High blood pressure

hyperthermia An unusually high temperature; the treatment of disease by raising the temperature

hyperthyroidism Overactivity of the thyroid glands

hypertrophy An abnormal enlargement of an organ or tissues

hypodermic Inserted under the skin

hypoglycaemia Abnormally low blood sugar

hypothyroidism Underactivity of the thyroid gland

iatrogenic Any disorder or disease induced by medical care, usually injudicious treatment or overtreatment on the part of a doctor

idiopathic Of unknown cause, not resulting from any known disease, often peculiar to the patient

ileostomy A surgical procedure to create an artificial opening into the ileum (lower portion of the small intestine)

impacted tooth A tooth so placed in the jawbone that eruption is impossible

impotence Inability of the male to achieve erection for the sexual act. In the great majority of cases, it is of psychosomatic origin. Impotence does not mean sterility

incontinence Inability to contain or control urination or defecation

infarct An area of tissue destruction resulting from obstructed circulation, as in heart attack

inositol A part of the vitamin B complex, believed to inhibit tumour growth

insulin A hormone produced by the pancreas and essential for sugar metabolism

intention tremor Involuntary trembling

occasioned or triggered when voluntary movement is attempted

intercurrent infection Occurring while another disease is in progress

intra-abdominal Within the abdomen

intussusception The telescoping in on itself of a portion of the intestines; if not corrected, it may cause strangulation of that section of the bowel

iris The coloured part of the eye, between the lens and cornea with the pupil in the centre

jaundice A yellow tint to the skin, whites of the eyes, and mucous membrane

jugular A vein on each side of the neck

keratosis A hard, grey, horny growth on the skin, such as a wart or callous

labia majora The hairy folds of skin (lips) on either side of the vulva

labia minora The folds of mucous membrane within the labia majora

labyrinth Intricate communicating passageways, particularly of the internal ear

lavage The washing out of a cavity, eg, the stomach

lesion Any localized diseased change of an area on the skin or an organ, such as a rash, boil, blister, abscess, sore, and so on

leukorrhoea A white viscous vaginal discharge

libido Conscious or unconscious sexual desire and drive

lobar Pertaining to a lobe, a defined section of an organ with boundaries

lordosis Exaggeration of the normal forward curve of the spine, with the abdomen thrust forward, the shoulders back; late pregnancy is a temporary lordosis

lymph The clear (sometimes yellowish) watery fluid found in lymph vessels and around body cells

lymph nodes (glands) Oval-shaped nodules along lymph vessels, which filter out germs and foreign bodies

malabsorption The defective absorption of food

malaise A feeling of general body discomfort

malignant Life-threatening, usually refers to cancer

malocclusion Poor alignment of teeth so that the upper and lower teeth do not mesh properly.

malpractice Negligent or callous medical treatment by a doctor or a nurse

mcg (microgram) One thousandth of a milligram

meatus An opening or passageway, such as the external opening of the urethra

melanoma A highly malignant tumour of the skin, usually from a mole

membrane A thin layer of tissue that lines a tube, covers an organ, or separates one part from another

menarche The first menstrual period, somewhere between tenth and seventeenth year

meningococcus The bacterium that causes cerebral meningitis

mestasis Secondary growth

metabolism The aggregate of all the chemical processes constantly taking place in the body, including those that use energy to convert nutrients into protoplasm and those that release energy in breaking down protoplasm

mg (milligram) A thousandth of a gram

microorganism A bacterium or protozoan not visible to the naked eye

migratory arthritis Changing in concentration from one joint to another

mitral valve The valve at the left side of the heart that takes in oxygenated blood to the main pumping chamber, the left ventricle

mucoid Similar to mucus

mucous membrane (mucosa) The membranous moist lining of the nose, mouth, gastrointestinal tract, and vagina

mucus A watery secretion from the mucous membrane, usually thin but in the presence of infections can be heavy, thick, and sticky

nasopharynx The back of the throat above the soft palate

necrosis Death of a localized section of tissue

needle suction See *aspiration*

neurosurgery Surgery of the nervous system

nitroglycerin An explosive liquid, of great medical use in angina pectoris, asthma, and stroke

nocturia Excessive night urination

nodule A small hard lump, a small node

nystagmus An involuntary rhythmic jerky movement of the eyes when they are turned sharply to the right or left, characteristic of many nervous disorders

obstetrics The branch of medicine that deals with pregnancy and childbirth

obstruction A blockage of any passage of the body that interferes with normal function

occiput The back part of the head

occlusion An obstruction; also closure of the upper and lower teeth

oculist An *ophthalmologist*, a doctor who specializes in the care of the eyes

oedema A collection of fluid in the tissues

oestrogen Female hormone; can also be produced synthetically

ophthalmic Pertaining to the eyes

opiate A narcotic containing some form of opium; also, any drug with similar properties

optician A technican who grinds lenses and fits glasses

optometrist A person trained and licensed to examine the eyes and prescribe glasses

orthodontist A dentist who specializes in the prevention and correction of crooked, irregular, and maloccluded teeth

orthopaedist A doctor who specializes in the correction of deformities and diseases of the bones, joints, muscles, and spine

osteopathy A system of treating disease by the massage and manipulation of the bones

ovulation The maturing of an egg cell and its release from the ovary, occurring once every twenty-eight days in a mature woman

oxygenation The saturation of a substance with oxygen

pacemaker A special node in the right auricle of the heart that triggers the heart and sets the pace. *Electronic pacemaker:* a mechanical device implanted inside the chest wall to substitute for the damaged or diseased natural pacemaker

palliative A medication or treatment for the relief of pain but usually without curative value

palpate To examine or identify by feeling with the hand

pancarditis Inflammation involving all the structures of the heart

papilla A small nipple-shaped elevation

papilloma A benign tumour of the skin or mucous membrane

parenteral An injection of a substance or medication into the body in any way other than by swallowing

particulate Made up of separate particles

past-pointing The inability to accurately place a finger on a selected point, such as nose, elbow, or other places

pathogen Any substance or organism that can cause disease

peptic Concerning digestion or concerning pepsin, a protein-digesting enzyme found in the stomach

perceptive deafness Deafness in which the nerve is damaged as opposed to conduction deafness in which the sound is blocked from reaching the nerve

perforation A hole, usually made by an ulcer

pericardium The tough membranous sac that encloses the heart

perineum The region between the anus and the genitals

periodontal Located around the tooth

periphery The outer edge

peristalsis The wave of muscular contraction that pushes food along the oesophagus into the intestinal tract

peritoneum The membrane that lines the abdominal wall

pernicious Destructive, harmful, life-threatening

pessary A device placed in the vagina to either support the uterus or prevent conception

phimosis The constriction of the end of the penis by a tight inelastic foreskin, making erection impossible or extremely painful

phlebitis Inflammation of a vein, which may lead to the formation of a clot

phlegm Mucus, sputum

photophobia An intolerance for light, especially bright lights

phrenic (1) Pertaining to the diaphragm. (2) Concerning the mind

physiotherapy Treatment with physical and mechanical means

pinpoint bleeding Tiny blood vessels bleeding into the skin and mucous membrane, causing purplish spots

PKU (phenylketonuria) A congenital metabolic defect that leads to mental degeneration and early death if left untreated

plaque Patch or film of unnatural formation such as that found in atherosclerosis on inside of the arteries

platelets Tiny, colourless corpuscles, about a quarter of the size of a red blood cell, that are essential in blood clotting

pneumococcus An oval-shaped bacterium enclosed in a protective capsule, of which there are more than seventy-five types, responsible for pneumonia, meningitis, otitis media, and dozens of other serious diseases

podiatrist One who treats foot ailments, a chiropodist

polyp A benign tumour on a stalk

postpartum Occurring after childbirth

preeclampsia A toxic condition of late pregnancy characterized by high blood pressure, fluid retention, and kidney malfunction, which may lead to eclampsia

premature ejaculation A psychogenic disorder in which a man ejaculates before his penis has entered the vagina

proctitis Inflammation of the membranes of the rectum

proctoscope A tubular instrument with a light source that permits a view of the interior of the rectum

productive cough A cough in which mucus or sputum is expectorated

progesterone The female hormone that prepares the uterus for reception and development of a fertilized egg

projectile vomiting Vomiting of such force as to hurl the material a foot or two from the body, usually without nausea

prolapse The falling down of an organ from its usual place

prophylaxis Preventive treatment

prothrombin A substance in the blood that forms thrombin, essential for clotting

protozoa The lowest division of the animal kingdom, including such one-celled animals as the amoeba and paramecium, some of which can cause disease

pruritis Severe itching

psychogenic Of mental origin

psychoneurosis Mild to moderately severe mental disturbance characterized by exaggerated defences against unresolved emotional conflicts

psychosomatic disorders Diseases traced to emotional factors

psychotherapy Treatment of disease, especially nervous disorders, by mental rather than physical means (eg, hypnosis, analysis, and so on)

psychotic episode A period of insane behaviour

pudendum (pl. *pudenda*) The external female sex organs, usually the vulva

pulmonary Pertaining to the lungs

pulp The interior of a tooth, composed of soft tissue containing nerves and blood vessels

purulent Containing pus, suppurating

pyloric sphincter The narrow muscular opening between the stomach and the duodenum that opens and closes to allow food to pass through

R Abbreviation for roentgen, a unit of radiation

RA Abbreviation for rheumatic arthritis

rad Acronym for *r*adiation *a*bsorbed *d*ose; *radiation* in medical terms is treatment with a radioactive substance, including x-ray

rales Abnormal sounds from the lungs or bronchi

regurgitation Throwing up of undigested food, usually of infants, actually a spitting up of food not as severe as vomiting. Also, the

backward flow of blood through a leaky heart valve

rel Acronym for *r*adiation *e*xposure *l*imit, the recommended limit of accumulated exposure of an individual to radiation to prevent excess

rem Acronym for *r*oentgen *e*quivalent in *m*an

remission An abatement of symptoms without medical treatment

remittent Alternately abating and returning

resect To cut out part of an organ or tissue

resorb To absorb again

respirator An 'iron lung', a mechanical breathing device for those whose breathing muscles are paralysed

retardation Delayed mental or physical response, mental deficiency

retinopathy Any noninflammatory disorder of the retina

Rh factor A hereditary factor in the blood that can cause complications if the mother is Rh negative and the foetus is Rh positive

sac A pouch or bag-like covering of an organ or a cyst

St Vitus's dance (chorea) A nervous disease with involuntary jerky motions

salivation Excessive secretion of saliva

Salmonella A genus of bacteria that causes food poisoning

scatology The scientific study and analyses of faeces

scoliosis Sideways curvature of the spine

sebaceous glands Tiny glands located on the outer layer of skin that secrete an oily substance known as sebum

self-limited disease A disease that without treatment runs a definite course within a limited time

semen The fluid produced by the prostate gland that contains the sperm and is expelled through the urethra at orgasm

seminal vesicles Sacs lying behind the bladder which are attached to the prostate and that, among other things, act as storage organs for the sperm and exude a thick, viscous fluid which forms part of the semen

sepsis A generalized poisoning (toxicity) of the body from bacterial infection

septicaemia Blood poisoning from infectious organisms

serum The clear liquid of the blood after the blood has coagulated, which contains antibodies; a vaccine from animals rendered immune against a disease-causing organism and injected into a patient with the same disease

sinus A hollow enclosed space, in particular

one of several air-filled cavities in the head connected with the nose; an opening

sippy diet A special bland milk diet for patients with peptic ulcers

sitz bath A tub of water that covers only the hips and buttocks, used to relieve pain anywhere in the pelvic area

slough A mass of dead tissue cast off from living tissue

smut A fungus disease of plants; the dusty black powder from this disease

soft palate The roof of the mouth near the throat

spasm The sudden, severe, involuntary contraction of a muscle, preventing function and causing pain

spasticity Tension of muscles causing stiff and awkward movements

sphincter A circular 'purse-string' muscle that surrounds and controls the opening and closing of an orifice in valve-like fashion, such as the anal sphinctre

sphygmomanometer The common instrument that measures blood pressure

spider angioma (spider nevus, vascular spider) A branched growth, resembling a spider, of dilated capillaries of the skin

spinal cord A long cord-like structure of nerves beginning in the brain and extending inside the vertebral column to the pelvic area

spinal tap The withdrawal of cerebrospinal fluid from the spinal cavity by needle for use in diagnosis of disease

spirochete A bacterium, shaped like a screw, that can be harmless or can cause syphilis and other virulent diseases

spontaneous Occurring without external cause; *spontaneous fracture* – a fragile bone that breaks with little or no external cause

spore An inactive form of a microorganism that is resistant to destruction but is capable of becoming reactivated

sputum The sticky, viscous secretion that forms within the bronchi and is expelled by coughing or hawking

stapes The tiny stirrup-shaped bone of the middle ear

staphylococcus (staph) Spherical bacteria, which grow in clusters, they are the cause of a large variety of diseases and are most resistant to antibiotics

sternum The breastbone

steroid Any of a variety of hormones, natural or synthetic, similar to and as effective as cortisone

strangulation Constriction of a part of the body, usually the bowels or the throat

strangury Painful and interrupted

urination from spasmodic muscular contraction of the urethra and bladder

streptococcus Bacteria that grow in chains and cause a wide variety of diseases

stricture A narrowing or tightening of a duct or passageway from an inflammation, injury, or obstruction

subacute Intermediate between chronic and acute

suppurate To form pus

syndrome A number of symptoms that characteristically occur together

systemic Pertaining to the whole body rather than a part

systole The contraction of the heart, representing the greatest force exerted by the heart and the highest degree of resistance from the arterial walls; the higher of the two figures in recording blood pressure (120/80)

tachycardia Very rapid heartbeat

Tay-Sachs disease A degenerative disorder of the brain in infants with fatal consequences

tenesmus Painful straining to empty the bladder or the bowels without success

testosterone Male sex hormone

thorax The chest

thrombosis The formation of a blood clot that blocks a blood vessel

tinnitus A ringing or other noises in the head

tonometer An instrument for measuring pressure or tension within the eye, used for determining glaucoma

topical Local, pertaining to a definite area

tourniquet Any band applied around a limb to constrict blood flow and control bleeding

toxaemia Blood poisoning due to the poisonous products of bacteria emanating from a local site causing fever, diarrhoea, vomiting, disorders of the heartbeat and respiration and finally shock

toxin A poison produced by germs

trachea The windpipe

tracheotomy (tracheostomy) Cutting an artificial hole in the windpipe below the level of the larynx to prevent asphyxiation resulting from an obstruction in the throat

trauma An injury or wound

triglycerides Fatty compounds manufactured by the liver that are important in the body's metabolism; intake of large amounts of this substance has been implicated in heart disease

truss A device to hold a hernia in place

tubercle A small nodule or prominence, especially a mass of cells produced by the tubercle bacilli characteristic of tuberculosis

ulcerogenic Causing ulcers
unproductive Of a cough that does not bring up sputum
unsymptomatic Without symptoms
urea frost White flaky deposits of urea appearing on the skin of patients with advanced uraemia
ureter The tube through which urine moves from the kidney to the bladder
urethra The tube through which urine moves from the bladder to the exterior of the body
uvea The iris and choroid of the eye

vaginitis An inflammation of the vagina, with discharge and discomfort
varix (pl. *varices*) Varicose
vas deferens The narrow vessel through which sperm pass from the testes to the seminal vesicles
vasoconstrictor A drug that constricts or narrows the blood vessels
vasodilator A drug or substance that dilates the blood vessels

vector A carrier of a disease, especially an insect or animal
venereal disease Any disease that is contracted through sexual intercourse
venous Pertaining to the veins
ventricle Either of the two lower chambers of the heart from which blood is pumped to the arteries; a small cavity
vermiform Shaped like a worm
viraemia The presence of viruses in the blood
vital capacity The maximum amount of air that can be sucked into the lungs in a forced respiration

wheals Hives, temporary swellings of the skin, appearing like large mosquito bites, usually due to allergy
white leg Phlebitis of the femoral vein with whiteness and swelling of the leg
wisdom tooth The last molar tooth on each side of the upper and lower jaw

Index of symptoms

fainting 63
  preceded by dizziness 63
false membrane:
  in mouth 99
  in throat 115
fatigue 36–7
  with anaemic symptoms 37
  with fever 38
  with headache 38
  plus rapid heartbeat 129
  with shortness of breath 120–
  121
  and weight loss 55
  see also Lethargy; Weakness
feet:
  arch, painful 187
  calluses 173
  corns 173
  cracked skin 173
  enlarged 187
  flatfeet 187
  sole, painful 187–8
  swollen 49, 188
  ulcers and infection 188
feminization (male) 166
fever 38–9
  and difficulty in swallowing
  114
  erratic 39
  high 39
    with delirium 59
    and headache 39–40
    and profuse sweating 48
    and shortness of breath 40
    sustained 40
  with inflammation of joints
  191
  low-grade, with inflammation
  of joints 191–2
  with pain in abdomen and
  vomiting 138
  recurrent attacks 45–6
  and severe headache 73
  and shortness of breath 122
  and sore throat 116
fingers:
  clubbed 188–9
  disorders of fingernails 189
  enlarged 190
  frostbite 186
  loss or deformity of 189
fits, *see* Convulsions
flatulence 144–5
flushing 70–71
  (female) 160
foods, distaste for certain 144
fractures, spontaneous 185
freckles 174
freezing of the extremities 186
frigidity 162
frostbite 186

gas, *see* Belching; Flatulence
genitals:
  blisters on 155
  enlarged 155
  itching of 155
  loss of pubic hair 156
  smallness of 156

sores on 156
tumours of 156
ulcers of 156
unpleasant odour 157
see also Penis; Vagina
giddiness, *see* Dizziness
groin:
  enlarged lymph nodes in 155
  lump or mass in pelvis
  (female) 162
  lump in pubic region (male)
  166
growth, retarded 36
gums:
  bleeding 107
    and bad breath 97
    as part of general bleeding
    107–8
  bleeding socket 108
  boils on. 108–9
  gangrenous 108
  painful 108
  pockets in 108
  receding 108
  swollen(inflamed) 108
  ulcers on 108–9
  tumours on 108–9

hair:
  baldness 170
  dandruff 170
  excess 170
  falling 170–71
  lifeless 171
halitosis 96
hands:
  enlarged 190
  palsied 190
  puffy 49, 190
head:
  bulges in 72
  enlarged 77
  prominent blood vessels 77
  softening of bones in 77
  twisting to the side 77
headaches 72–3
  and chills and fever 32–3
  and convulsions 58
  and dizziness 60–61
  and fatigue 38
  and high fever 73
  in infants and children 73–4
  and mental ability
    impairment 66
  moderate or dull 74
  and muscular cramps (aches
    or spasms) 196
  radiating 74
  severe:
    and dizziness 60–61
    and fever 73
    and intermittent 75
    and vomiting 76–7
  and sweating 47
  throbbing 75–6
  variable 76
  and vomiting 148
hearing loss 90

heartbeat:
  extra 126
  irregular, premature or
    skipped beat 126–7
  palpitation 127
  and shortness of breath 123
  rapid 127–8
    extreme 128
    plus fatigue or weakness 129
    plus jaundice 129
    with pain in chest or
      abdomen 129
    and shortness of breath 123
  slow 130
heartburn 145
height:
  excessive 185
  loss 185
hiccups 40–41
hip:
  dislocation of 190
  pain in 190
hoarseness 117–8
  and difficulty in swallowing
  115
hot flushes 160
hunger 41
hyperactivity 63

impotence 167–8
indigestion 145–6
insomnia 63–4
intercourse, painful (female)
  162
irritability 64
itching 174–5
  rash 175
    with blisters 175–6
    intense, with 175
    red spots over entire body
    175
    without 175

jaundice 176
  anaemia with 30
  mild 176
    and vomiting 176
  plus pain in abdomen and
    vomiting 138
  plus rapid heartbeat 129
  severe 176–7
    and vomiting 177
    and weight loss 55
jaw:
  pain in 109
  protruding 109
  stiff 109
joints:
  bad weather ache in 190
  deformity of 190
  inflammation:
    with fever 191
    with low-grade fever 191–2
    without fever 192
  lumps around 192
judgement, impaired 66

kidney, *see* Urinary tract

Index of diseases

spinal curvature 407, 486
spine:
  curvature of 407, 486
  osteoporosis of 405
spotted fever (meningitis) 210–211
sprains:
  ankle 410–11
  wrist 410
sprue:
  adult nontropical 343–4
  childhood nontropical 344
squamous cell carcinoma 502–503
squint (strabismus) 220–1
staphylococcal pneumonia 276–8
staphylococcal gastroenteritis 328
stenosis (obstruction in the peptic ulcer) 325
sterility:
  in men 397–8
  in women 381–2
stiff neck 407
sting, hypersensitivty to (anaphylactic shock) 416–17
stomach:
  cancer of 515
  food poisoning 327
  haemorrhage due to peptic ulcer 325
  mucous lining of:
    inflammation of (gastritis, gastroenteritis) 321–2
    sore on (peptic ulcer) 322–5
  opening to small intestine, narrowing of (obstruction in peptic ulcer) 325
  perforation due to peptic ulcer 325–6
  surgical removal of, syndrome following 326–7
stomatitis:
  aphthous 253–4
  gangrenous 255
  herpetic 253
  traumatica 255
strabismus (cross-eye, walleye, squint) 220–21
strawberry marks 430
streptococcal throat (pharyngitis) 250–51
stroke (cerebrovascular accident) 309–11
sty 229
sudden infant death (SID) 489
sunburn 429–30
sunstroke 429
swimmer's ear (external otitis) 237
syphilis:
  congenital 369
  early (primary and secondary) 366–8
  hidden in pregnancy 387
  late (tertiary) 368–9
systemic diseases that affect the eye 230–31

systemic lupus erythematosus 432

tachycardia 303
tapeworm 483
teeth, *see* Tooth
temporal arteritis 227
temporal lobe seizures (epilepsy) 206
temporomandibular joint disorder 266–7
tennis elbow (bursitis) 403–4
tertiary syphilis 368–9
testicle(s) 395–6
  cancer of 512–13
  cysts in scrotum around 396
  epididymus, inflammation of, (epididymitis) 396
  inflammation of (orchitis) 396
  undescended 395–6
tetanus (lockjaw) 466–7
thiamine deficiency 458
threadworms 482
three-day measles 473
throat:
  adenoiditis 249
  cancer of 518–19
  diphtheria 464–5
  quinsy 249–50
  simple sore and strep (pharyngitis) 250–51
  tonsillitis 249
  vocal cords, benign growths on 251
thrombophlebitis 311–12
thrush (moniliasis):
  of mouth 253
  of vagina 378
thyroid gland:
  cancer of 507–8
  enlargement of (goitre) 451
  overproduction of hormone by (hypothyroidism) 450–1
  underproduction of hormone by (hypothyroidism) 449–450
thyrotoxicosis 450–51
tic douloureux (neuralgia) 208
tics 213–14
tissue, connective, disorders of:
  lupus erythematosus (discoid and systemic) 432
  scleroderma 432–3
tobacco, eye disorders resulting from 227–8
toenail, ingrown 412
tongue, disorders of:
  black hairy tongue 257
  cancer of 517–18
  geographic tongue 257
  glossodynia 257
  ranula 257–8
  scrotal tongue 257
  tonguetie 256–7
tonsillitis 249
tooth:
  abrasion 262
  abscess 261–2

broken or chipped 264
cavity 260–61
contact between, poor (malocclusion) 262–3
decay 260–61
eruption 264–5
evulsed (knocked-out) 264
extraction complications 263–4
grinding of teeth (bruxism) 265
impaction (wisdom tooth) 264
implantation 264
knocked-out 264
missing 264
pulp, infection of (pulpitis) 261
replantation 264
wisdom, impaction of 264–5
torticollis, spasmodic 407
toxic hepatitis 350–5
toxic nodular goitre 450–51
toxoplasmosis 481
trachoma 221–2
traumatic stomatitis 255
traveller's diarrhoea 470–71
trench mouth 252–3
trichinosis (trichiniasis) 481–2
trichomoniasis (*Trichomonas vaginalis*) 371–2
trick knee 410
trigeminal neuralgia 208
tubal pregnancy 289
tuberculosis (TB) 279–82
  of the joints and bones 404
tumour(s):
  of the brain 212–13
  of the breast, benign 381
  fibroid uterine 379–80
  of the mouth 256
  ovarian 380
  See also Cancer
Turista, La (traveller's diarrhoea) 470–71
twitching 213–14
typhoid fever 468–9
typhus 483–4

ulcerative colitis 335–7
ulcerative gingivitis (trench mouth) 252–3
ulcer of the oesophagus 317–18
undescended testicle 395–6
uraemia:
  acute 364–5
  chronic 364–5
urethritis, nonspecific 371
urticaria (hives) 414–15
uterine sarcoma 511
uterus:
  cancer of 511
  fibroid tumours in 379–80
  inflammation in 378
  prolapsed 379
uveal disease (choroiditis) 225

vaginal inflammation (leucorrhoea, vaginitis,